A

CONSUMERS

DICTIONARY OF

COSMETIC INGREDIENTS

A

CONSUMER'S

DICTIONARY

OF COSMETIC

INGREDIENTS

SEVENTH EDITION

Complete Information About the Harmful and Desirable
Ingredients Found in Cosmetics and Cosmeceuticals

RUTH WINTER, M.S.

THREE RIVERS PRESS
NEW YORK

THREE RIVERS PRESS and the Tugboat design are registered trademarks of
Random House, Inc.

Previous editions of this work were published in
1972, 1976, 1984, 1994, 1999, and 2005.

Library of Congress Cataloging-in-Publication Data
Winter, Ruth, 1930–
A consumer's dictionary of cosmetic ingredients / by Ruth Winter.—7th ed.
Includes bibliographical references.
1. Cosmetics—Dictionaries. I. Title.
TP983.A55.W57   1999
668'.55'03—dc21   98-44781

ISBN 978-0-307-45111-8

Printed in the United States of America

7 9 10 8

Seventh Edition

To my husband, Arthur Winter, M.D.;
my daughter, Robin Winter-Sperry, M.D.;
my son-in-law, Jonathan Sperry;
my sons, Craig and Grant; and my grandchildren,
Samantha, Hunter, and Katelynd

CONTENTS

INTRODUCTION

Why You Need This Book

Are you afraid of aging?

Does a wrinkle on your face cause you to panic and make you fear you are becoming unattractive and unemployable?

Do you believe a fragrance can make you irresistible?

Are you willing to spend your hard-earned money to buy expensive cosmetics that promise you a cure for whatever flaw you think you may have?

If you answer yes to these questions, you have become a pawn of the manipulative cosmetic industry. These geniuses of marketing have convinced you and most of society of the following:

- Aging and wrinkles are to be greatly feared.
- Natural body odors are mortifying.
- Cosmetics can cure anything.

I really do admire the cleverness of cosmetic producers and sellers—even if they don't like me because I reveal to you what is really in their products. But I believe they are still fabulous sociologists, psychologists, and marketers. They know before anyone else what we want or should want, and they immediately build upon those desires to sell us what we may or may not need. From the department store counter to the drugstore to the Internet, they have given us literally thousands of choices of cosmetics. As you will read in this dictionary, some of the potions and powders are excellent and fulfill their promises, many of the compounds do nothing and are actually fraudulent, and some may be damaging to our health because they contain toxins or cancer-causing agents.

You may be asking yourself at this point: "Well, doesn't the FDA protect us?" The answer is NO!

Cosmetics have always been a low priority at the U.S. Food and Drug Administration (FDA), but now its regulatory powers have been weakened to the point where they are almost nonexistent.

WHY ARE COSMETIC REGULATIONS SO LIMITED?

The agency's regulations were determined more than seventy years ago when it was wrongly assumed that the skin is an impermeable barrier that prevents chemicals from penetrating into the body. Scientists now know that this is not true, yet most consumers and cosmetic companies are concerned only with allergic reactions and skin irritations. But what of systemic absorption, toxicity, and chronic effects? What degree of absorption is there when a cosmetic is left on the face (as a makeup base might be for twelve hours) or spread over the entire body (like suntan lotions)? What is the impact when these products are used for many years?

No one knows. Cosmetic companies do know that an increasingly popular way to deliver drugs is "transdermally."

All we know is that cosmetics can affect us outwardly and inwardly, so the question becomes, What safeguards does the FDA have today?

THE FDA'S COSMETIC SAFETY REGULATIONS

The following quote is directly from the current *FDA Handbook:*[1]

> *Although the FD&C Act does not require that cosmetic manufacturers or marketers test their products for safety, the FDA strongly urges cosmetic manufacturers to conduct whatever toxicological or other tests are appropriate to substantiate the safety of their cosmetics. If the safety of a cosmetic is not adequately substantiated, the product may be considered misbranded and may be subject to regulatory action unless the label bears the following statement: "Warning—The safety of this product has not been determined."*[2]

WHY IS THE FDA SO POWERLESS?

The Report of the Subcommittee on Science and Technology on the FDA Science and Mission at Risk presented answers.[3] The committee said its major findings were as follows:

- The FDA cannot fulfill its mission because its scientific base has eroded and its scientific organizational structure is weak.

- The FDA cannot fulfill its mission because its scientific workforce does not have sufficient capacity and capability.

- The FDA cannot fulfill its mission because its information technology (IT) infrastructure is inadequate.

---

[1] Grimes & Reese, *FDA Handbook,* Guide and Reference Material, 2008, Idaho Falls, ID.
[2] Ibid.
[3] *FDA Science and Mission at Risk: Report of the Subcommittee on Science and Technology,* prepared for the FDA Science Board, November 2007, Washington, DC.

Inspections have declined while the work assigned to the FDA has skyrocketed. In 2008, the United States imported more than $2 trillion worth of products sent to the United States by an estimated 825 major importers, through more than 300 ports of entry. The FDA projects a total of 18.2 million import lines a year, 9 percent of which is cosmetic products. The FDA is also responsible for overseeing more than ninety thousand U.S. facilities where food, drugs, and other products are manufactured, processed, or stored. Twenty-one cents of every dollar spent by consumers goes toward products the FDA is supposed to regulate. The Office of Regulatory Affairs (ORA) is the lead office for all FDA field activities. The largest portion of ORA's work involves postmarket inspections of foods, human drugs, biologics, animal drugs and feeds, and medical-device manufacturers (nothing is designated specifically for cosmetics). The FDA has about 3,472 full-time employees associated with field activities with a requested budget at $542,534,000. They are sometimes helped by state health inspectors.[4]

Why is the FDA so beleaguered and underfunded? No matter how skilled and well intentioned the staff may be, they are being smashed under an impossible workload. Unless consumers like you and savvy organizations such as those listed on pages 559–64 lobby effectively for changes, nothing will happen.

In the meantime, I have written both *A Consumer's Dictionary of Cosmetic Ingredients* and *A Consumer's Dictionary of Food Additives* to give you the information you need to make wiser choices in the almost unregulated marketplace. For example, anyone can go into the cosmetics business without notifying the FDA. If you don't believe it, the following is directly from the *FDA Handbook:*[5]

Voluntary Registration

Although the FD&C Act does not require cosmetic firms to register manufacturing establishments or formulations with the FDA or make available safety data or other information before a product is marketed in the United States, manufacturers or distributors of cosmetics may submit this information to the agency voluntarily. Voluntary registration and assignment of a registration number by the agency does not denote approval of a firm or product by the FDA. Any use of a registration number in labeling must be accompanied by a conspicuous disclaimer phrase as prescribed by regulation.

Cosmetic companies that wish to participate in the voluntary registration forward data to the FDA. Only an estimated 35 to 40 percent of the companies are honorable enough to inform the FDA of the ingredients they are using. But since the last edition of *A Consumer's Dictionary of Cosmetic Ingredients,* there is a new game being played. A significant number of the companies are "registering" their names with the FDA and then saying in their ads "Registered with the FDA" in an attempt to have us believe their product has been approved by the agency.

The truth is the FDA admits it cannot require companies to do safety testing of their cosmetic products before marketing. Neither cosmetic products nor cosmetic

---

[4] FDA Activities—Office of Regulatory Affairs, 2009.
[5] Grimes and Reese, FDA's *Cosmetics Handbook,* http://www.mlmlaw.com/library/Guides/fda/coshdbok.htm.

ingredients are reviewed or approved by the FDA before they are sold to you. Recalls taken by the cosmetic industry to call back products that present a hazard, or that are somehow defective, are voluntary. The FDA is not permitted to require recalls of cosmetics but does monitor companies that conduct a product recall.

The FDA can only take action against a company if complaints are made by consumers or health providers and the complaints are registered. For this edition, I found out the FDA no longer has a database of reports of adverse effects from cosmetics. When I asked why, a very frustrated FDA staff member said, "Because our staff and our money have been cut!"

Although there are no full-time field agents assigned to cosmetics, investigators in district offices may be assigned "as the need arises." The FDA is supposed to collect cosmetic product samples as part of its rate plant and import inspections.

The FDA reports that it has 1.75 professional staff persons per year to process submitted cosmetic forms and maintain computer files at a cost of $97,465 per year. (Don't you wonder what a .75 professional looks like?) Since cosmetic companies are always worried about the competition stealing their formulas, the FDA assures the registrants that their information is locked in a safe and guarded by 1.75 professionals—presumably except when a guardian has to eat lunch or go to the restroom. Then the door is locked.[6]

While consumer and industry assistance has been significantly reduced or eliminated, the FDA has increased its Internet presence, and its website offers statements such as: "The FDA does not function as a private testing laboratory"; "The FDA is prohibited from recommending private laboratories to consumers for sample analysis"; and "Consumers may consult their local phone directory for testing laboratories."

If the FDA does wish to remove a cosmetic from the market, it must first prove in a court of law that the product is injurious to users, improperly labeled, or otherwise violates the law. Such court cases in the past have cost the budget-strapped agency millions and the companies with their powerful lawyers and political clout almost always win.

Again, this is directly from the *FDA Handbook:*

With the exception of color additives and a few prohibited ingredients, a cosmetic manufacturer may, on his own responsibility, use essentially any raw material as a cosmetic ingredient and market the product without approval. The law requires that color additives used in food, drugs and cosmetics must be tested for safety and approved by the FDA for their intended uses. A cosmetic containing an unlisted color additive; i.e., a color additive which has not been approved by the FDA for its intended use, is considered adulterated and subject to regulatory action. The color additives approved for use in cosmetics are listed [see them in this dictionary]. The use of the following ingredients is either restricted or prohibited in cosmetics: bithionol, mercury compounds, vinyl chloride, halogenated salicylanilides, zirconium complexes in aerosol cosmetics, chloroform, methylene chloride, chlorofluorocarbon

---

[6] FDA Supporting Statement for Cosmetic Product Voluntary Reporting Program, OMB No. 0910–0030; 2004.

*propellants, and hexachlorophene [see all in the dictionary]. The agency also
considers as adulterated cosmetics nail products containing methyl methacrylate monomer or those containing more than 5% formaldehyde. Although not
prohibited by law or regulation, in addition, the manufacturers of cosmetic
fragrance products have voluntarily agreed to not use or to limit maximum
use levels of certain selected ingredients which have been found to cause
depigmentation, irritation, neurotoxicity, or phototoxicity or allergic reactions.* (See all the restricted or prohibited chemicals in this dictionary.)[7]

Is there anyone at the FDA who deals with a consumer's physical problems
caused by cosmetics or ingredients not explicitly prohibited by the FDA?

There are regulatory enforcers and criminal investigators under CFSAN, the
FDA's Center for Food Safety and Applied Nutrition. The personnel are responsible for a wide variety of products, including foods, seafood, wine beverages less
than 7 percent alcohol (including wine coolers), bottled water, food additives, infant
formulas, dietary supplements, and cosmetics. Each of these products is used dif-
ferently and regulated under a different part of the FDA Act and thus has slightly
different investigational requirements. Do you think it is important that the FDA
conducts appropriate investigations and follow-up on adverse events attributed to
cosmetic products?[8]

How many expert regulators are there on CFSAN's staff to enforce the above?
Five, at this writing. How many do they have on staff for all the products potentially
involved in criminal activity? Three![9]

This does not mean no one is watching the cosmetic stew. The trade organization Personal Care Products Council (PCPC; formerly the Cosmetic, Toiletries and
Fragrance Association) is doing an admirable job and has established its own safety
assessment system, the Cosmetic Ingredient Review (CIR). It has a six-member
Steering Committee chaired by the president and CEO of the council (from the
industry); a dermatologist representing the American Academy of Dermatology; a
toxicologist representing the Society of Toxicology; a consumer representative from
the Consumer Federation of America, and the council's executive vice president for
assessing the safety data. Since its establishment in 1976 CIR panels have reviewed
1,298 ingredients as of August 2006. (You can read about them in the dictionary.)
Of that number,

- 781 ingredients were found safe as used.
- 408 ingredients were determined safe with qualifications.
- 119 ingredients could not be evaluated because of insufficient data.
- 9 ingredients were cited unsafe.

The basic purpose of the review is to gather information from the scientific literature and from company files on the safety of cosmetic ingredients. It alerts the

---

[7] *FDA Handbook,* op. cit.
[8] Inspection References, *Investigations Operations Manual,* 2008, updated February 2, 2008.
[9] Ibid.

FDA and makes that information publicly available without any private review or comment. Thus far, members have questioned the safety of ingredients—such as 6-methyl coumarin and musk ambrette (*see both*)—and these substances have been voluntarily removed by PCPC member companies. However, proponents of increased cosmetic regulation argue that participation in this voluntary compliance system is low. In addition, critics contend the CIR is an industry-funded expert panel established to conduct safety assessments of cosmetic products, yet has only reviewed 11 percent of cosmetic ingredients since 1976.[10]

In 2007, the trade organization the Cosmetic Toiletries and Fragrance Association's (CTFA) board of directors changed its name, as mentioned, to the Personal Care Products Council (PCPC) because "the change represented a new, broader and more contemporary name to better represent the association's growing and diverse membership." In addition, the board chose a new motto for the association: *Committed to safety, quality and innovation.* The PCPC states that its members produce the majority of the cosmetics on the market. We should be grateful that there are scientists testing ingredients for us. The cosmetic companies, however, are politically astute. Such self-testing and efforts at self-regulation fend off potential outside regulation by government agencies. And the cosmetic manufacturers contribute heavily to political campaigns, including the presidential race. It is in their own interest, of course, to avoid using an ingredient that might be found at some later date to be potentially harmful. Adverse publicity can instantly kill a product into which millions of dollars have been invested.

THE STATE OF STATE COSMETIC REGULATIONS

Due largely to consumer pressure, some states have been formulating stricter regulations concerning cosmetics.

MAKING UP INTERNATIONALLY

Since the commerce in cosmetics is global today, there has been an effort to "harmonize" labeling and regulations. In 2011, the global makeup market is forecast to have a value of $32.1 billion, an increase of 27.8 percent since 2006.[11]

The European Union (EU) has worked toward agreement on ingredient terms to ease marketing across the borders in countries representing nine different languages. The U.S. Office of Cosmetics and Colors (OCAC) has considered these harmonizing requests on a case-by-case basis, in line with its legal responsibilities under the Fair Packaging and Labeling Act (FPLA) to promulgate regulations "necessary to prevent the deception of consumers or to facilitate value comparisons."

Labeling can be confusing because the EU likes to use fancier names and botanic monikers for certain cosmetic ingredients. For instance, what we call *water* is called *aqua* by the EU and what we label as *mineral oil,* they call *paraffinum liquidum. Butyrospermum parkii* is the EU's name for our *shea butter. Lentinus edodes* is the EU's name for *shiitake mushroom.* The EU also designates colors by number such as *CI60730* for the hair coloring we call *violet 2,* while the Japanese called it

---

[10] Environmental Working Group Cosmetics Petition, infra note 234.
[11] Datamonitor's Make-up: Global Industry Guide, Decision News Media (SAS), December 10, 2008.

murasaki 401. As much as possible, such names have been cross-referenced in the dictionary for you, since many of the cosmetics you buy may be made overseas.

You will also read in the dictionary how some ingredients are banned in the Asian market and the European Union but allowed in the United States. The European Union, Japan, Canada, and the United States do not agree on the safety of some colors, for example. The FDA says that this is a complicated issue, due to factors such as the requirements that only colors approved for use in the United States by the FDA are allowed to be added to cosmetics and that, for some of these "approved" colors, only those specifically tested and certified in FDA-approved laboratories may be used in cosmetics for the U.S. market. On the other hand, Britain, at this writing, is banning some colors used in the United States because they have been linked to hyperactivity in children. The Japanese coloring Acid Yellow 40, for example, which the Japanese label Ki402, is not approved for use in either the United States or the European Union.

REACH

During the great effort at harmonization and cooperation among the countries, one European regulation has stirred up the most anxiety. It is called REACH, which stands for Registration, Evaluation & Authorization of Chemicals. It is a controversial, comprehensive European law that is supposed to make sure proposed and already-available chemicals are safe. To ensure a high level of protection, this law requires data to be submitted on human and environmental safety. It applies to all chemicals made in the EU, or imported into the EU, including certain natural substances and those substances used in cosmetic products. It is intended to address any public concern about the use of chemicals. Probably the most difficult "harmonization" among countries concerns REACH's efforts to ban cosmetic testing on animals.

TESTING COSMETICS ON ANIMALS

The practice of testing cosmetics on animals started in 1933 when an American woman used a Lash Lure mascara to darken her lashes. Her eyes first burned, then she went blind and died. Following this incident, in 1938 the U.S. Food and Drug Association passed an act to protect the public from unsafe, risky cosmetic products.

Today, EU experts say that it is a common view among the general public that in order to define the safety of finished cosmetics products it should be sufficient to test them directly on human volunteers. The EU maintains this type of evaluation is adequate to reveal any acute toxic effects of a product. It is absolutely insufficient, however, for identifying those effects, such as systemic toxicity, carcinogenicity, and teratogenicity for which the only test methods currently scientifically acceptable are those developed in animals. Alternative methods, experts say, to evaluate long-term toxic effects of ingredients on humans may take more than twenty years for the damage to become evident.[12]

The most controversial and widely used animal test is the Draize eye irritancy test, which involves putting drops of the substance in question into the eyes of albino

---

[12] Directive 2003/15/EC of the European Parliament and of the Council, February 27, 2003, Amending Council Directive 76/768 EEC on the approximation of the laws of the member states relating to cosmetic products.

rabbits. Investigators then note if any redness, swelling, cloudiness of the iris, or corneal opacity occurs. In addition, they measure the eye's ability to repair any damage. Draize is difficult to replace with a single alternative test because it measures three different areas of the eye. Replacing Draize will probably take a combination of alternative tests, but the combination has not yet been developed.

Many companies, because of the sentiment against using animals for testing, now label their cosmetics *cruelty free,* which implies that products have not been tested on animals. How do many companies back up their claims today that their products are "cruelty free"? A cosmetics manufacturer told me that some are now paying humans to test cosmetics rather than using four-legged animals. A private labeler who supplies products to many name-brand companies told me his firm *does* tests on animals, but the large companies that buy his products say that they *don't.* However, if a company uses older cosmetic ingredients that have long ago been tested on animals, they can still say their "new" cosmetic versions have not been tested on animals.

Incidentally, cosmetic manufacturers took the word *animal* out of their ingredient labels but not out of the ingredients. Hydrolyzed animal protein, for example, is now called hydrolyzed collagen. Desamido collagen is used in "anti-aging creams" and also has had the word *animal* removed from its label, even though it is made with animal proteins. Dozens of cosmetic ingredients are derived from animals. You will be able to identify them with this dictionary.

Animal welfare groups say thirty-eight thousand animals die needlessly in the EU every year in tests for new products. In 1991, the EU put forward a clause that prohibited marketing of cosmetic products containing ingredients or combinations of ingredients tested on animals. The EU proposed a ban on the testing of cosmetics on animals in 1993 and gave a deadline of 2009 for "cruelty-free" cosmetics. The law did go into effect in 2009, but under the exemptions, when products need to be checked for their toxicity or their effect on fertility, animal testing will be allowed to continue until 2013. The ban also outlawed the sale in the EU of cosmetics that have been tested on animals in other parts of the world. The proposed EU law does not ban existing products that have been tested on animals in the past. The ban is aimed at forcing cosmetic makers to switch to alternatives to animal testing, such as test-tube methods—if those are shown to be effective. Britain, Germany, Austria, Belgium, and the Netherlands have already banned cosmetic tests on animals, but unlike the EU law, such bans do nothing to stop products tested on animals being imported from abroad. Most of Europe's cosmetic testing is carried out in France and Italy.

Progress on Substitute Tests

Some countries, notably the United States and Japan, legally require safety tests to be conducted on animals. Although it is unlikely that animal testing will be fully phased out, the EU is working hard to develop alternatives. Implementing this legislation requires a strategy to find alternative tests, so that human health can be protected.

In November 2005, for the first time, the European Commission and a number of companies and trade federations active in various industrial sectors launched a joint initiative called the "European Partnership for Alternative Approaches to

Animal Testing" (EPAA) whose purpose is to promote the development of new "3R" methods: refine, reduce, replace. The European Centre for the Validation of Alternative Methods (ECVAM) is the site where research is done to develop the new and, it is hoped, equally effective test to replace animals in industries. ECVAM—which has a staff of sixty—collaborates on cosmetics with the European Cosmetic Toiletry and Perfumery Association (COLIPA). In April 2007, the first tests in laboratories were introduced. These new methods, the European Partnership hopes, will lead toward the end of using rabbits in skin and eye irritancy tests. A cell culture that mimics human skin is also being employed to help evaluate the potential skin irritancy of chemicals. Two other methods identify severe eye irritants using animal tissues from slaughterhouses, which would otherwise be discarded.

The European Commission has launched a new website, Tracking System for Alternative Test Methods Review Validation and Approval (TSAR). It is designed to track the development of new alternative test methods that should replace, reduce, and refine current animal testing. You can track it yourself if you have access to a computer: http://tsar.jrc.ec.europa.eu/.[13]

SOME CHANGES MADE

This is the seventh edition of *A Consumer's Dictionary of Cosmetic Ingredients*. Since the sixth there have been a lot of changes, some of them very good and some of them unsettling. Here is a sampling:

- The FDA, the World Health Organization, the EU, the PCPC, and the ASEAN have all put their regulations and some—but certainly not all—of their ingredients on the Web (see pages 559–64).

- The FDA is now allowing cosmetic companies to *self-affirm* whether their products are generally recognized as safe (GRAS). (*See* GRAS in the dictionary.) In the past, the GRAS designation gave some comfort because the FDA had either studied the ingredient or through "grandfathering" had found it to be safe after long-term use. Why shouldn't a company self-proclaim its chemical compound as "safe"? It is good for sales but not necessarily for us.

- Many cosmetic ingredients are now made in China, where the Chinese government has little oversight. Unsanitary conditions and unregulated sources of raw material are all too common, but the government says it is working on correcting inadequacies. For example, China's Ministry of Health issued an emergency notice, asking that certain illegal cosmetic ingredients be recalled by their manufacturers. The ingredients were dexamethasone, chloramphenicol, metronidazole or hydrocortisone acetate, which are all banned raw materials in their cosmetics (see all in dictionary).[14] China in 2006 issued proposed regulations banning more than twelve hundred substances in cosmetics. Zhang Heyong, the director of the China Quality Association for Pharmaceuticals, said "weak government supervision and lack of compulsory

---

[13] http://ec.europa.eu/health/ph_risk/risk_en.htm.
[14] China Sourcing Forum by Editorial Staff, "Ministry of Health Recalls Ten Chinese Cosmetics," November 27, 2007.

testing of ingredients lead to safety worries. The regulations, which reflect similar requirements in the European Union, have been strengthened after angry consumers demanded cosmetics be made safe."[15]

- Imported cosmetic products from all over the world flood into U.S. ports but remain almost entirely uninspected. The U.S. Interagency Working Group on Import Safety reported to the president that federal agencies cannot and should not attempt to physically inspect every product entering the United States: "Doing so would not only bring international trade to a standstill, but would also distract limited resources from those imported goods that pose the greatest risk. Instead, we have to be smarter about what we do. While we acknowledge it is not possible to eliminate all risk with imported and domestic products, being smarter requires us to find new ways to protect American consumers and continually improve the safety of our imports. We recommend working with the importing community to develop approaches that consider risks over the life cycle of an imported product, and that focus actions and resources to minimize the likelihood of unsafe products reaching U.S. consumers."[16]

IS IT A COSMETIC, A DRUG, OR A FOOD?

There are many innovations in cosmetics both here in the United States and abroad. You will read about them throughout this book. However, innovations can bring problems. One of the growing conundrums since the last edition is whether a product designed to improve our appearance is a drug, a cosmetic, a food, or a combination of the three. Even the Center for Food Safety and Applied Nutrition and the Federal Drug Administration are confused about a product's legal status, and the agencies' staffs state that this confusion will impede investigational use of complaint system information. Of course, it's worth noting that at this writing, such a complaint system no longer exists.[17]

A newly named category—*nutricosmetics*—involves eating and drinking your skin care to improve your looks from the inside and out. It is becoming increasingly popular, and includes food-based cosmetics such as vitamin C collagen and vitamin-fortified skin care yogurt with avocado.

In the last edition of this book, the so named *nutraceuticals* were just starting to become publicized. They are compounds of natural, bioactive chemicals that have nutrients and immune-building or medicinal properties.

Feeding your skin by applying a nutraceutical or a nutricosmetic not only improves your health, it also provides wealth for the cosmetic companies. One company is selling Inside-Out, a vitamin-infused lipstick with a gel-based outer core to deliver long-lasting pigment coverage and an inner core to deliver the nutrients.[18]

---

[15] "China to Ban 1,200 Substances from Cosmetics Production," December 19, 2006; www .peopledaily.com.cn.
[16] *Protecting Americans Every Step of the Way: A Strategic Framework for Continual Improvement in Import Safety: A Report to the President,* Interagency Working Group on Import Safety, September 10, 2007.
[17] "Is It a Cosmetic, a Drug or Both? (Or Is It Soap?)" at http://www.cfsan.fda.gov/~dms/cos-218.html.
[18] Sara Mason, "Makeup Meets Skin Care," *Skin Inc.,* posted December 5, 2007.

Following is some information that will help you penetrate the subtle crossovers. It is directly from the *FDA Cosmetics Handbook:*

> *The FD&C Act defines cosmetics as articles intended to be applied to the human body for cleansing, beautifying, promoting attractiveness, or altering the appearance without affecting the body's structure or functions. Included in this definition are products such as skin creams, lotions, perfumes, lipsticks, fingernail polishes, eye and facial make-up preparations, shampoos, permanent waves, hair colors, toothpastes, deodorants, and any material intended for use as a component of a cosmetic product. Soap products consisting primarily of an alkali salt of fatty acid and making no label claim other than cleansing of the human body are not considered cosmetics under the law.*[19]

THE COSMETICS-DRUG CONNECTION

Products that are cosmetics but are also intended to treat or prevent disease, or otherwise affect the structure or functions of the human body, are also considered drugs and must comply with both the drug and cosmetic provisions of the law. Examples of products that are drugs as well as cosmetics are anticavity toothpastes (e.g., "fluoride" toothpastes), hormone creams, suntanning preparations intended to protect against sunburn, antiperspirants that are also deodorants, and antidandruff shampoos.

Most currently marketed cosmetics that are also drugs are over-the-counter drugs. Several are new drugs for which safety and effectiveness had to be proved to the agency before they could be marketed. A new drug is a drug that is not generally recognized by experts as safe and effective under the conditions of intended use or that has become so recognized but has not been used to a material extent or for a material time under such conditions.

The regulatory requirements for drugs are more extensive than the requirements applicable to cosmetics. For example, the FD&C Act requires that drug manufacturers register every year with the FDA and update their lists of all manufactured drugs twice annually. Additionally, drugs must be manufactured in accordance with current good manufacturing practice regulations as codified as Adulterated or Misbranded Cosmetics.

The PCPC, however, has been vigorously pursuing efforts to convince the FDA's Center for Drug Evaluation and Research to adopt "reasonable regulatory standards for products considered as both cosmetics and drugs."

A category particularly troublesome to the United States and the European Union concerns sunscreens and suntan products. The two cannot agree whether the goods are cosmetics or drugs: the FDA believes some of them are drugs, and the EU believes they are all cosmetics.

FUN IN THE SUN WITH A COSMETIC OR DRUG

We humans can't stay indoors all the time, and we do enjoy going out on a bright sunny day. Dermatologists have warned for years, however, that exposure to solar

---

[19] *FDA Cosmetics Handbook,* op. cit.

rays can induce skin cancer—including the life-threatening melanoma—and speed the aging of skin.

What's the difference between UVA and UVB? The "burning" sun rays are ultraviolet B (UVB) that peak during midday. The "aging rays" are believed to be the ultraviolet A (UVA) because they penetrate deeper into the skin and cause cumulative damage. UVA radiation does not cause the painful sunburn that is a result of exposure to UVB radiation; therefore, it is hard to detect. UVA was once thought to be "safe," but now researchers report both UVA and UVB can increase the risk of skin cancer.

Suntan products generally are sunscreening preparations that permit penetration of ultraviolet radiation to allow for best tanning results. When used as directed, consumers may remain in the sun for a predetermined time period without risking a sunburn. The sunburn protection is provided by sunscreen active ingredients, such as cinoxate and homosalate (*see both* in the dictionary). Sunscreens of variable potency protect against the adverse effects of ultraviolet (UV) radiation. They are considered over-the-counter (OTC) drugs by the FDA and cosmetics by the EU. Both agencies consider *suntanning* products cosmetics, products that just help you become tan without the sun, whereas *sunscreens*—sunblocks, sunscreen gels, creams, and liquids (also known as suntan lotions)—are lotions, sprays, or other topical products. They help protect the skin from the sun's potential cancer-causing radiation. Besides checking the ingredient label, you can look for the Skin Cancer Foundation's Seal of Recommendation on the label or in the packaging. The seal is awarded to sun protection products that have an SPF of 15 or greater, validated by testing on twenty people, does not produce phototoxicity or contact irritation, and has substantiated claims for water resistance. Following the FDA guidelines, a "water-resistant" product must maintain its SPF after forty minutes of water immersion, and a "very-water-resistant" product after eighty minutes (www.skincancer.org).

The FDA tried to prevent companies from using a sun protection factor (SPF) above 30 in sunscreens. SPF is a rating scale indicating how much time you can expose your skin to the sun before you will burn when using a particular sunscreen. The FDA did not think above 15 was effective and that furthermore it might encourage consumers to stay in the sun longer. The PCPC successfully lobbied against the restriction in 2002.

The current FDA regulations curb to some degree *sunscreen* label warnings, discarding the liberal old "prevents cancer of the skin" in favor of versions of "Sun Alert: the sun causes skin damage. Regular use of sunscreens over the years may reduce the chance of skin damage, some types of skin cancer, and other harmful effects due to the sun." The FDA has been influenced by epidemiologists, who maintain that it is not very healthy for light-complexioned people to expose themselves to long-term UV radiation, even when protected by "effective" sunscreens.

Some newer *suntan* products of interest are capsules intended for ingestion and containing mostly beta-carotene and canthaxanthin (*see both*). These color additives enter the bloodstream and are partially deposited in skin tissue, giving the skin a tanlike color. Neither color additive is approved for this particular use, and products containing them are considered by the FDA to be adulterated. Some reports of adverse reactions associated with tanning pills have mentioned stomach cramps, hepatitis, nausea, diarrhea, and deposition of the color in the retina of the eye.

It has become common practice to add sunscreening ingredients of variable potency to cosmetics to protect against the adverse effects of UV radiation exposure. In a study done at Case Western Reserve University, in Cleveland, Ohio, it was shown that cosmetic preparations containing sunscreening ingredients are indeed protective against the sun's rays and should therefore be encouraged.[20]

Dr. John Bailey, the former director of the FDA Office of Cosmetics and now an executive with PCPC, pointed out that there is a difference between "photoaging" from the sun and chronological aging: "Cosmetics can't do anything about the latter."

Cosmetic companies believe they can—or at least say they can.

COSMECEUTICALS—A COSMETIC DRUG FOR WRINKLES?

The modern age of the cosmeceutical began with the approval of Johnson & Johnson's Retin-A as a topical anti-acne drug in 1973. A serendipitous observation was made that the product not only got rid of pimples, it reduced the appearance of wrinkles. Johnson & Johnson subsequently sought approval for a related vitamin A product, Renova. After much controversy, it was recommended for approval in April 1992 by an FDA advisory panel for the treatment of fine wrinkling, mottled hyperpigmentation (liver spots), and roughness associated with sun damage.

Medical reports that a vitamin A derivative could reverse some sun damage and fade wrinkles fueled a whirlwind of interest in the cosmetic field. Some companies rushed to market vitamin A products. One of them, Cosmetic Laboratory Sales, took a full-page ad in the tabloid the *Star,* September 28, 1993, promoting "free retinol Vitamin A crème when you purchase Alpha/H, Alpha Hydroxy Creme, Medical Science's New Age Reversal Formula." The ad went on to say that "Direct from leading medical journals, plus fashion magazines like *Vogue* and *Cosmopolitan,* comes the 'bombshell announcement' of a wondrous discovery that can help you grow away lines and signs of age in a brand-new, smooth-as-silk complexion and make you look 10 to 15—why even a whole generation—younger."

The number of commercial products containing the acids exploded, jumping from around five in 1990 to two hundred by 1994.

By 1997, highly respected companies were in the mix. Neutrogena, for example, introduced its Healthy Skin Antiwrinkle Cream with retinol. It contains a combination of moisturizers and vitamin B_5, which is claimed to "increase moisture levels and skin firmness" and "even out skin tone." It was a big seller.

Because alpha-hydroxy acids (AHAs) are somewhat irritating and may cause increased sensitivity to the sun, the trend, at this writing, is toward beta-hydroxy acids. These contain salicylic acid, long used in acne medicines. Both the alpha and the beta acids are exfoliants that cause the shedding of superficial skin cells. In the youth market, such products are sold to get rid of oily, blackhead-dotted top layers of skin. As one cosmetic manufacturer told me, however, you can grind up apricot pits and rub them on your face and get the same effect.

---

[20] C. A. Elmets, A. Vargas, and C. Oresajo, "Photoprotective Effects of Sunscreen in Cosmetics on Sunburn and Langerhans Cell Photodamage," *Photodermatology, Photoimmunology and Photomedicine* 3 (June 9, 1992): 113–20.

Remember, FDA regulations say that if a substance changes structure, it is a drug and must undergo rigorous scientific and expensive bureaucratic evaluations. If it is a cosmetic, you can just put it on the market. If you look and listen to the promotion of many cosmeceuticals, you would think they change structure, and now some of them do, but the cosmetic companies want them to be considered cosmetics. The cosmetic producers say their AHA exfoliants do not change the structure of the skin, just peel off the dead layers, and therefore the products are cosmetics.

Zoe Draelos, M.D., professor of dermatology at Wake Forest University, disagrees. She said at a meeting of cosmetic dermatology in 1998 that "These acids can alter the stratum corneum [*see* the dictionary] 20 to 30 layers deep, particularly in formulations with a pH of 3 or lower. . . . Even cosmetic products with AHA concentration at or below 10 percent and at a pH of at least 3.5 are penetrating the skin further than necessary. When patients feel stinging or burning, they think, 'Good, the product is working,' when in fact the pain they feel relates to the fact that the acid has penetrated the dermis and is interacting with the dermal nerve endings." That technically makes AHAs a topical application.

The FDA's National Center for Toxicological Research (NCTR) is currently investigating the effects of long-term exposure to AHAs to determine whether the AHA (glycolic acid) may increase the potential for cancer when skin is exposed to the sun. Researchers found that topical application of glycolic acid at concentrations as low as 4 percent and for as short a duration as four days can alter the skin's response to UV radiation.

DISCRIMINATE AGAINST THE HYPE

The *FDA Handbook* states:

A cosmetic is misbranded if its labeling is false or misleading, if it does not bear the required labeling information, or if the container is made or filled in a deceptive manner.

Nevertheless, cosmeticians don't call a wrinkle a wrinkle: it's a "dermatologic corrugation." But no matter what it is called, wrinkles, liver spots, dry skin, and gray hair are all potential goldmines for cosmetic companies. Today's arsenal of chemicals have some ingredients that may actually work. The trick is to know which may be based on scientific evidence and which are just fantasies. This book can help you decide between benefit and blather.

Some argue that while Congress intended to safeguard the health and economic interests of consumers with the federal Food, Drug, and Cosmetic Act, it also meant to protect a manufacturer's right to market a product free of excessive government regulation. And in an industry that sells personal image, especially images of beauty and sex appeal, not allowing any inflated claims would certainly hurt the marketing. Most cosmetics, of course, contain ingredients that are promoted with exaggerated claims of beauty, of long-lasting effects to create an image. It's up to the consumer to believe it or not. Dr John Bailey, former director of the FDA's Office of Cosmetics and now executive vice president for science at the Personal Care Products Council, says you really have only the manufacturers' representations to rely on for these products. Price doesn't necessarily correlate to product performance, but if a woman buys an expensive, elegant formulation that may or may not work, if it makes her feel real good, then she's gotten her money's worth.[21]

Cosmetic labels that claim a product is "dermatologist tested," "sensitivity tested," "allergy tested," or "nonirritating" carry no guarantee that you won't have a reaction, and what you have in a bottle is not necessarily what you have on the skin in a few minutes. Alcohol and/or water may evaporate and you may be left with a very different compound than what is listed on the bottle.

In the United Kingdom, advertised claims are subject to close scrutiny by watchdog organizations, broadcast advertisements must be precleared by Clearcast, and both broadcast and print advertisements are scrutinized by the Advertising Standards Authority (ASA). These organizations require robust scientific evidence to substantiate claims being made. The ASA is the independent body set up by the advertising industry to police the rules laid down in the advertising codes. The ASA is committed to protecting consumers and creating a level playing field for advertisers. To find out more, visit www.asa.org.uk.

The United Kingdom's ASA went after Estée Lauder, the giant cosmetic company, in 2009 for claiming in an advertisement that by using the Tri-Aktiline Instant Deep Wrinkle Filler consumers would "Start to see your wrinkles disappear INSTANTLY." Another claim in the advertisement purported: "After 4 weeks of continued use: 83% reported improvement in the appearance of lines. After 8 weeks of continued use: clinical studies measured a 45% visible reduction in wrinkle depth and length."[22]

Estée Lauder said the claim "68% of subjects reported a visible filling of wrinkles" was based on the results of the consumer evaluation study on fifty women. They said 68 percent of subjects (thirty-four women) responded to the question "How would you rate the effectiveness of 'the product' for . . . immediately filling-in fine lines/wrinkles" by reporting that Tri-Aktiline was extremely, very, or somewhat effective. However, they did not submit the method or results of the evaluation study in full.

They said the claim "After 4 weeks of continued use: 83% (41 women) reported improvement in the appearance of lines" was supported by the consumer evaluation study. They said participants responded to the question "How would you describe the degree of improvement in the appearance of your fine lines and wrinkles after 4 weeks of use?" and 82 percent reported a slight, moderate, or dramatic improvement. They acknowledged that the ad had claimed "83% reported improvement in the appearance of lines" but argued that that was an error unlikely to render the claim misleading. Estée Lauder said they also carried out a clinical test on twenty-three women to assess the effectiveness of Tri-Aktiline in reducing the appearance of lines and wrinkles after four and eight weeks of use. They said this supported the claim that consumers would see a significant improvement in their lines and wrinkles after four weeks as 83 percent of the subjects in the clinical study had a significant improvement in their wrinkles after four weeks, based on objective measurements. They believed that the percentage of people demonstrating an

---

[21] Bailey, op. cit.
[22] ASA Adjudications: Estée Lauder Cosmetics Ltd t/a Good Skin Labs, 73 Grosvenor Road, London W1K 3BQ, January 7, 2009.

improvement in wrinkle reduction mirrored the results of the consumer study and therefore proved the claims were true and consistent with consumer expectations. They said the data from the clinical study showed that after eight weeks of product use, Tri-Aktiline reduced the appearance of lines and wrinkles by an average of 45 percent.

In a beauty salon, I recently saw an ad for L'Oréal's New Visible Lift. It said "Our first make-up with an age serum inside. Visibly reduce lines by 31%." I had to wait until I returned home so I could use a magnifying glass to read an almost illegible line at the bottom of the page that said: "Results based on a 4-week clinical study." How many subjects? Who did the study? Was it just asking a few women what they thought of their wrinkles after four weeks? Who knows? Not us.

Another antiwrinkle cosmetic that is still under the radar at this writing claims to do the same as BOTOX, the expensive injectable agent that temporarily diminishes or eliminates lines and wrinkles on the face by relaxing underlying facial muscles. It is derived from *botulinum toxin* type A, a bacterium-produced neuromuscular toxin that can be deadly in a pure state. It is used in a highly diluted form. The FDA has approved botulinum toxin treatment for alleviating eye-muscle disorders and smoothing frown lines. This treatment is often used in conjunction with facial plastic surgery procedures such as a face-lift or eyelid lift to maximize its cosmetic benefit. The results usually last between three to six months, though results will vary based on the patient and the area injected. A company is now marketing Botox Cosmetic, which it says does not require injections. Faitox-25 wrinkle creams cost $55 for 1 ounce to $200 per .5 oz for its eye wrinkle cream. They claim to do the following:

- Boost new collagen production
- Even out skin tone and restore clarity
- Reduce expression lines and deep furrows
- Firm, tone, and increase skin's elasticity

Manufacturers claim that the product is collagen that actually supports the structure of our skin, making it firm and resilient. Faitox-25 Botox wrinkle cream with Argireline and Matrixyl 3000, the company says, is the first Botox alternative wrinkle cream that combines three scientifically advanced ingredients that rival the results of the injectable Botox. The company says that "Argireline, at 25%, is a wrinkle relaxing peptide, a brand name for Acetyl Hexapeptide-3. Argireline mimics the actions of Botox by relaxing muscle contractions that create wrinkles. Faitox-25 Botox alternative wrinkle cream contains the highest concentration of Argireline available today." The product's website has no address or phone number, but through its URL (http://www.synovialabs.com/) I did find a company: Jabalabs.com at 14080 Nacogdoches, Suite 64, San Antonio, TX 78247; toll free 888-508-4510. The website is support@jabalaabs.com and the company sells Faitox-25, but you have to order five bottles at a time. Jabalabs does carry the statement that cosmetic companies are supposed to carry if they have not come under the FDA umbrella:

"The statements made within this website have not been evaluated by the Food and Drug Administration. These statements and the products of this company are not intended to diagnose, treat, cure, or prevent any disease."

The fact is that if cosmetic chemists could put "youth in a bottle," they would deserve the Nobel Prize or at least the Ponce de Leon Fountain of Youth Award. Yet, in a society that fears growing old, you can be subjected to such claims. Even in the global recession, at this writing, another company, La Prairie, is still selling its Skin Caviar Luxe Cream, an anti-aging longevity serum, which "Re-firms, Re-plumps and Re-ignites skin's luminosity" for the customer who has "multiple aging concerns, including loss of luminosity and firmness." Price? $375 for one fluid ounce. You can obtain the same cream in a jeweled jar for $2,000. The numbered jar includes 1.7 ounces and comes with a certificate of authenticity. This is a prime example of the container costing more than the cosmetic inside. The website is http://shoplaprairie.com/store/viewPrd.asp?.

Cosmetic companies also do not want the price of their ingredients publicized. If you read labels, you'll see that water and alcohol are two of the most commonly used ingredients. One French perfumer was asked, for example, how much the ingredients in a perfume selling for $230 per ounce in a department store really cost. His answer: "Four to six dollars."

Another reason the prices may not be publicized is because it is illegal to price-fix. Some of the major department stores like Macy's, Nordstrom's, and Bloomingdale's were accused of price-fixing, and although they claimed no wrongdoing, they agreed in a class action settlement in February 2004 to give away $175 million in cosmetics and perfumes. The cosmetics were given out from January 20 to 27, 2009, to consumers who bought products from the stores listed in the suit between May 1994 and July 2003. The free products included mascara, moisturizers, and fragrances sold by L'Oréal, Estée Lauder, and Chanel, who were among the list of manufacturers from which consumers could claim products. After January 27, the giveaway ended and wasn't scheduled to be repeated.

ORGANIC OR NATURAL—WHAT'S THE DIFFERENCE?

"Natural" can mean anything to anybody. "There are no standards for what 'natural' means," says Dr. Bailey of the PCPC. "They could wave a tube [of plant extract] over the bottle and declare it natural. Who's to say what they're actually using?" "Natural," according to the FDA, implies that ingredients are extracted directly from plants or animal products as opposed to being produced synthetically. There is no basis in fact or scientific legitimacy, the FDA says, to the notion that products containing natural ingredients are good for the skin.[23]

"Natural" doesn't mean pure or clean or perfect either. According to the cosmetic trade journal *Drug and Cosmetic Industry,* all plants [including those used in cosmetics] can be heavily contaminated with bacteria, and pesticides and chemical fertilizers used to improve crop yields." Still, more and more "botanicals" are being added to cosmetics, including anti-aging products and other "treatment" and beautifying ingredients. Botanicals compose the largest category of cosmeceutical addi-

[23] Bailey, op. cit.

tives found in the marketplace today. Their use is unregulated and often unsupported by science, and their purported therapeutic properties remain largely unexplored.

Some botanicals that may benefit the skin include: green tea extract, ferulic acid, and grape seed extract. Natural, organic, and environmentally friendly products have carved out a stable and profitable niche in the cosmetic sector, but competition is intensifying as new brands contend with established players. The market opportunity is clear, but delivering on promises of natural and organic products in a highly critical marketplace isn't always easy, especially without clear definitions and regulations. As traditional differences between natural food and beauty dissolve, the natural movement is establishing its place in the cosmetic industry.

Deciding what is really "organic" is a constant problem. Cosmetic companies won their fight to ensure that the USDA maintains a certification program for organic personal care products. The authority decided to reverse its decision to drop the certification system following a concerted campaign by industry members and lobby groups. Since the cosmetic companies do not have to register their ingredients with the FDA or USDA, they can decide, if they want to, that their product is organic.[24] As consumers increasingly want to buy "green products" that do not harm themselves or the atmosphere, the cosmetic companies are more than ready to provide for the growing demand. According to *Organic Monitor,* the international market for natural and organic cosmetics is expected to generate billions in sales, with Europe and the United States accounting for the most customers. However, the terms "natural" and "hypoallergenic" are not necessarily interchangeable, as anyone who has ever had poison ivy knows. While cosmetic companies often try to exploit this confusion of terms, this dictionary will help you understand which "natural" drugs are actually hypoallergenic.

HYPOALLERGENIC

In 1975, the FDA tried to publish regulations defining hypoallergenic cosmetics as cosmetics with a lower potential for causing an allergic reaction. These regulations were defeated by two cosmetic companies, Almay and Clinique, who claimed consumers already understood that hypoallergenic products were no panacea against allergic reactions. The courts eventually held for the companies.

Hypoallergenic implies that products making this claim are less likely to cause allergic reaction. There are no prescribed scientific studies required to substantiate this claim, the FDA says. Likewise, the terms "dermatologist tested," "sensitivity tested," "allergy tested," or "nonirritating" carry no guarantee that products won't cause skin reactions.

Hypo means "less than," and hypoallergenic means only that the manufacturer feels that the product is less likely than others to cause an allergic reaction. Although some manufacturers do clinical testing, others may simply omit perfumes or other common problem-causing ingredients.

Dr. Bailey says that, with limited funds and personnel, the FDA Office of Cosmetics and Colors must concentrate more on risk than on claims. Although preservatives partly protect against infection, they can irritate the eye and skin in some sensitive persons. Additionally, some people may be allergic to fragrances or

---

[24] Simon Pitman, "Cosmetics Companies Win Battle Over Organics Certification," *CosmeticsDesign,* August 2005.

other ingredients in a cosmetic, such as rosin (also called colophony), nickel, and lanolin. They may develop tearing, itching, and redness of the eyes, or swelling and flaking of the eyelids. Allergic persons may need to try different "hypoallergenic products" until they find one that is safe for them. For instance, pencil eyeliner and powder eye shadow may cause less irritation than liquid liner and liquid shadow.

FRAGRANCE—THE SWEET AND SOUR SMELL OF SUCCESS

The greatest artists in the cosmetic business are the "noses"—those remarkably scent-sensitive people who create fragrances, sometimes with as many as two hundred or more ingredients. These mix masters can combine chemicals and make you think you smell freshly baked bread, a new car, or Chanel perfume. One of the reasons we do not have specific ingredients for "fragrances" or "flavors" is that these noses don't want to give their secret formulas away. Even federal labeling regulations recognize this and require that only the words *perfume* or *fragrance* be added to the label.

Pleasant aromas are derived from a spectacular number of substances, including plant materials and synthetic chemicals. Perfumers can even improve on nature. Certain natural flower scents, for instance, cannot be extracted, yet the experts, using various chemicals, can reproduce the same aroma we smell in the actual blossom. Because of the complexity of perfume formulas, it is difficult but possible for competitors to break them down and reproduce them.

Since fragrances are intended to vaporize, and they do contain plant and floral derivatives as well as many other chemicals, they frequently cause allergic reactions. A less-frequent side effect of perfume is a skin pigmentation called berloque dermatitis. With new awareness that chemicals can be delivered to the body not only through ingestion and absorption through the skin but also by inhalation of scent, federal and industrial scientists are concerned that some of the volatile ingredients in cosmetics may have an adverse systemic effect. In fact, the fixative AETT was voluntarily removed from cosmetics after it was shown to be a nerve toxin in animals. At this writing, there is additional concern about another fixative, musk ambrette, being a nerve toxin. ASEAN has banned it in cosmetics (*see* page 39).

The big problem with fragrances is that some people are hypersensitive to them. The advertisers who place perfume samples in magazines have to enclose them because so many people are allergic. Even those who spray passing customers in department stores get into trouble if they spray someone allergic with a fragrance. Furthermore, as you will read in the dictionary section, of all cosmetics, fragrances have the most ingredients, as well as the most potentially harmful ingredients. Fragrance producers use many chemicals that are toxic as well as allergenic. A woman in 2009 won a suit against her employer because a co-worker would not stop wearing a perfume that caused the woman's lung problem to worsen.

The Flavor Experts Manufacturing Association (FEMA) is aware of the problems that may arise from their industry's products. The association conducts frequent workshops to foster self-regulation. At one in 2000, Dr. Barbara Hall of Sureconsult said the fragrance industry understood that effective self-regulation is necessary to avoid health concerns and ensure the confidence of customers. Furthermore, Hall claimed that, unlike governmental authorities, self-regulatory bodies such as the International Fragrance Association (IFRA) are able to keep up with the speed of new scientific developments.

She added that dermatologists and the industry must cooperate more closely to identify the formulation of fragrances that cause allergies in patients. They should be able to perform mix tests and advise patients to avoid certain fragrances altogether rather than carry out more expensive patch tests.

As of now, fragrance manufacturers are often left without feedback on which ingredients are likely to have provoked allergic reactions. Hall said IFRA runs an information scheme for dermatologists should they need fragrance ingredient information. Cooperation initiatives such as this were called for from both sides to create a healthy flow of information.

RACE, CULTURE, AND COSMETICS

Women of color—African American, Hispanic, Middle Eastern, and Asian—have different cosmetic color needs than Caucasian women. The cosmetic companies, as well as dermatologists, are currently investigating the differences in skin sensitivity and grooming techniques between different ethnicities. Sensitive skin is a complex problem with genetic, individual, environmental, occupational, and ethnic implications, and the development of cosmetics and toiletries designed especially for different ethnic skin and hair types is under way.

The number one concern of black women, according to the experts, is uneven skin tone, primarily hyperpigmentation, which are dark spots or dark areas on the skin. Other concerns include blemishes, splotchiness, excessive oiliness, dry patches, and ashiness; the quest is on to find products that are gentle but effective enough to treat these concerns but that will not trigger any additional damage. Dry skin can be a particular problem for African Americans. It's uncomfortable, and it's also easily noticed because of its grayish, "ashy" appearance. Using moisturizers can help, although people with acne may find these products worsen that condition. Ashiness can also affect the scalp. Industry sources report that black women spend approximately three times more on hair care products and styling than other women. Pomades that make the hair more manageable can decrease scalp dryness. But if pomade spreads to the forehead during sweating, it can block pores, leading to a condition called acne cosmetica.

Although African Americans have been the focus of ethnic marketing in the past, Latinos are now the fastest-growing ethnic group, and cosmetic companies are marketing to many different ethnicities.

This edition of *A Consumer's Dictionary of Cosmetic Ingredients* includes unique products traditionally used by Asians, Middle Easterners, and Africans, as well as lists some of the potential side effects, such as high lead levels from kohl and ochronosis from the overuse of bleaching creams.

Ethnic minorities, now one-third of the U.S. population, are expected to become the majority by 2042. Ethnic consumers generally buy and use more makeup and are more playful with color. "When compared to the general population, ethnic women have a high percentage rate of makeup usage, beauty spending and the number of beauty brands purchased," says Delia Grant, Avon's senior manager for U.S. marketing, color.[25]

---

[25] Sara Mason, "Ethnic Cosmetics Fit New Beauty Paradigm." Posted December 12, 2008, from www.GCImagazine.com.

Cosmetic companies are eager to gain sales in cosmetics in the opportune, relatively untapped Muslim market, but cosmetic products have to satisfy Muslim values. Although they note that in theory wearing cosmetics is *hamam,* for the bath, a significant proportion of Muslim women do wear cosmetics and those who do may well prefer a *halal* (permitted) version. Labeling *halal certified* usually means that the cosmetic contains no animal ingredients and has not been tested on animals. That means Muslim and Orthodox Jewish women will have to read this dictionary carefully because many cosmetic products today are derived from animals, including most gels.

Colgate-Palmolive has a number of toothpaste products that are certified halal and the Australian firm Almaas produces halal color cosmetics such as mascaras and eye shadows.

In addition, The Body Shop, although not certified halal, is an example of a successful retailer in the Middle East having taken a strong stance against animal testing and using a number of natural ingredients in its products.

We know that cosmetic companies are aimed at appealing to a multiethnic market, but what other underserved categories do they have in their sights? Men, of course.

FOR MEN ONLY

For more than a decade, the beauty industry has considered men as a potential growth area, but the sector had been somewhat disappointing. The most successful companies making for-men-only products acknowledge that men are fundamentally wash-shave-and-walk-out-the-door types, but these companies are still trying to persuade men to take the next steps: moisturize and protect. In the old days, men were forced to use women's products if they wanted moisturizers and concealers, but now men have these cosmetics made especially for them. One company, Aramis's Lab Series for Men, introduced Trifecta Triple Effect Formula, which the company says reduces excess shine, shrinks pores, and smoothes the skin.[26] Trifecta is said to use "a gentle, non-acid technology to rid the skin of dry, flaky cells and provide hydration." Its ingredients include antioxidants: green tea, tocopheryl acetate, and algae. Other ingredients are caffeine, polymers, sclareolide, sodium hyaluronate, palmitoyl pentapeptide, and acetyl glucosamine.

Mintel Beauty Innovation, which keeps track of cosmetic categories and sales, has seen a dramatic increase in the number of new personal care products launched for men. In 2008, Mintel tracked more than 500 new men's personal care products in the United States, a substantial increase from the 375 launched in 2007. Globally, Mintel recorded more than 3,600 new men's personal care product launches in 2008.[27]

Mintel Beauty Innovation sees rapid growth in four areas of advanced male grooming:[28]

1. Lip-, eye- and hand-specific: Premium and mass-market brands alike now offer products for men that promise to enhance certain areas of the body.

---

[26] Briony Davies, "Men's Grooming: Worth the Hype?" Posted December 10, 2007, from the December 2007 issue of *GCI Magazine.*
[27] "Mintel Reports Growth in Men's Care," posted December 16, 2008.
[28] Find this article at http://www.gcimagazine.com/marketstrends/consumers/men/36235724.html.

Clarins Men Lip Guard and Jack Black Industrial Strength Hand Healer emphasize functionality, not preening, to appeal to ordinary men. Still, other products such as L'Oréal Men Expert eye cream and the 4VOO Shape and Shine Nail Set target men seeking a flawless appearance.

2. Makeup and self-tanning: Makeup for men is still a superpremium, niche market in the United States, but Mintel Beauty Innovation has seen many new brands emerge recently. Jean Paul Gaultier Monsieur and Clinique Skin Supplies for Men remain key players. Many personal care brands, including L'Oréal, also feature self-tanning products for men.

3. Anti-aging and exfoliating ingredients: Men's grooming lines increasingly boast semiscientific claims based on anti-aging or exfoliating ingredients. Biotherm Homme's High Recharge Non-Stop Moisturizing Anti-Fatigue Concentrate uses the anti-aging ingredient ginseng, but others have included coenzyme Q10 or creatine for anti-aging benefits. Exfoliation has become a focus as well with products like Unilever's Axe Skin Contact Smoothing Shower Scrub featuring cactus milk to exfoliate and smooth the skin.

4. Organic, natural, and ethical: Mintel sees organic and natural products driving growth in many sectors; men's personal care is no exception. John Allan's facial moisturizer features natural ingredients, while Aveda Men uses organic ingredients in its hair care. The Body Shop has long promoted ethical causes and opposed animal testing.

Recent innovations, including men's makeup, have put men's cosmetics on track. Euromonitor International, which keeps track of the global men's grooming sector, maintains it is sizable, at a value of $21.7 billion, although it accounts for only 8 percent of value sales in the cosmetics and toiletries market as a whole and is smaller than price-pressured commodity sectors (e.g., oral hygiene and bath and shower products). In terms of dynamism, the sector grew 5 percent in fixed exchange rate terms in 2006—approximately on par with the entire cosmetics and toiletries market.

Euromonitor says that maturation in the traditional men's grooming areas of shaving products and deodorants, which accounted for 79 percent of total sector sales in 2006, is holding back growth. Even burgeoning demand from the emerging markets and the niche appeal of newer men's grooming subsectors—such as moisturizers, exfoliators, and hair-styling products—is proving insufficient to halt the slowdown.

One of the newer cosmetic pitches for men's products is aimed at their penises. I am not kidding. First the cosmetic magicians convinced women that vaginas needed perfumes and creams, and now they are working their sales pitch toward men.[29]

MensMax, the manufacturer of the penis moisturizer RestoreMax, has published the results of research suggesting that more and more men are ranking penis skin care as important. In a survey of a hundred American men, the company claimed

---

[29] http://www.mensmax.com. "RestoreMax™ Penis Skin Care Treatment," posted 2009.

that 23 percent considered penis skin care an important part of their daily routine compared with 16 percent in similar research the previous year. The promotion says that it will help men deal with the "Daily bombardment of stresses."

The company said a variety of complaints associated with the stresses and strains of modern life lay behind the trend. Chemicals found in latex condoms, lubricants, and spermicidal creams were all reported to have the potential to produce reactive and irritating effects. Other environmental factors, such as the confinement and excess heat generated from tight pants, were mentioned as causes of dryness. MensMax goes on to say that sexual intercourse can leave the penis feeling sore, irritated, chafed, and raw. However, the most frequently stated issue was age. Male skin tends to become drier with age so that older men often suffer from reduced sensitivity, elasticity, and texture. MensMax.com concluded its research saying the penis is subject to a "gauntlet of torture" every day and that to restore it to health men should rub RestoreMax onto the shaft of their penis twice a day and always after sex.

MensMax is not the only company to be specializing in intimate personal care products. At the HBA Global Expo in 2009 in New York, a conference session entitled "Personal Care: The New Intimacy" was dedicated to the rise of the intimate in the industry.

Companies have figured out that men want speed of application and makeup that is not obvious. One company is offering Brow & Eyelash Gel to groom eyebrows into place, promoting the product as a "must" for men with shapeless and unruly brows, like *60 Minutes*'s Andy Rooney. The promotion notes that the "flake-free formula also helps define eyes by imparting a subtle luster to eyelashes" and "may also be used to help tame sideburns and mustaches."

Clinique, at this writing, has introduced Clinique Skin Supplies for Men Moisture Surge Extra Oil-Free gel. The ads say: "This super-hydrating gel is suited for men's skin after a day in the sun or a long plane flight. It contains ingredients such as aloe, trehalose, palmitoyl tripentapeptide-3 and glycerin." The gel, Clinique proclaims, "helps retain moisture in the skin and buffers daily environmental aggressors."

The cosmetic marketers have also recognized that millions of men in middle age have to seek a new job or career because of economic downturns and layoffs, downsizing, or burnout. Such men are ripe for products that may make them appear younger and more attractive. This trend will foster the purchase of grooming aids, hair colors, and new wardrobes.

THE CHILDREN'S MARKET
Babies and Young Children

While cosmetic companies are increasing marketing to the aging, men, and people of color, they are also aiming at another group—babies and young children.

There are perfumes for children and lipsticks for mothers who want to smell like children. The Nordstrom department store chain sells lip balm for babies with an Internet ad that says: "Kiehl's Baby Lip Balm . . . This gentle, emollient lip balm has been formulated for infants and children as a safe way to provide soothing relief and moisturization to the lip area for $7.50 a stick. Mild enough to be used on nose and cheeks." The store adds: "Pediatrician tested. Sensitivity tested to minimize allergy risk. Not tested on animals." The business also sells Kiehl's Baby Nurturing Cream for Face & Body: "This gentle formulation is a unique blend of natural ingredients to moisturize and soothe baby's delicate skin. Massage cream with shea butter, apricot kernel oil and purified honey nurtures skin, leaving it smooth and soft. Gentle enough for use on baby's face to help moisturize and even out dry patches." And also stated: "Pediatrician tested. Sensitivity tested for daily use and tested to minimize allergy risk. Not tested on animals." You can buy a 6.8-ounce tube for $18.50.

The children's market is estimated at $3 billion to $5 billion and growing 5 to 8 percent a year. One reason: children now make up one-fifth of the U.S. population, and a growing number of companies are catering to their needs. An analysis of Information Resources Inc. (IRI) sales data from 2002 shows that in the largest segment, oral hygiene, 4.2 percent of all the products sold were designed especially for children. For soap and bath products, kid-specific products accounted for 2.6 percent of sales. For shampoo and conditioner, 3.4 percent of sales were of children's products. Sales of children's sun care products are hot, accounting for 11.6 percent of all sales, perhaps fueled by parents' concerns over potential long-term sun damage to their kids.[30]

But there is trouble in the crib. A French health charity launched a high-profile campaign against the "toxic cocktail" of baby cosmetic products distributed in their country's maternity wards. Le Comité pour le Développement Durable en Santé (C2DS) hit the headlines in September 2008 in the French national press to alert the public to the presence of parabens, EDTA, BHA, and bisphenol A (*see all* in dictionary) in baby cosmetics.[31]

The organization gathered doctors, chemists, and cancer specialists to raise the alarm over the potential danger of these products on newborn babies whose skin is particularly permeable. Professor Dominique Belpomme, who is president of the cancer research charity ARTAC, told the press that the accumulative cocktail effect of the baby products was unknown. She said the current situation is absolutely unacceptable from the point of view of public health. Many of the chemicals flagged by the C2DS are commonly accused of presenting health dangers in cosmetics.

Health Canada recently banned the chemical bisphenol A (BPA) from baby bottles and recommended it for inclusion in the government's list of toxic substances.

No such move has been made in Europe, where the European Food Safety Authority reviewed the scientific data on BPA in July 2008, and reaffirmed its safety at the existing limits.

There is still trouble in the United States, though, with baby contact chemicals. Research published in the medical journal *Pediatrics* found that as the use of baby care products rose, so did the concentration of phthalates (*see* in dictionary), which are used in many fragrances. Infants and toddlers exposed to baby lotions, shampoos, and powders carry high concentrations of hormone-altering chemicals in their bodies that might have reproductive effects, according to a new scientific study of babies born in Los Angeles and two other U.S. cities. The lead scientist in the study,

---

[30] U.S. Mintel International Group Ltd., "Children's Personal Care Products," August 1, 2003.
[31] Guy Montague-Jones, "Health Association Raises Alarm Over Baby Cosmetics," Cosmetics Design-Europe.com, September 19, 2008.

Dr. Sheela Sathyanarayana of the University of Washington's Department of Pediatrics, said the findings suggested that many baby care products contain a variety of phthalates that enter children's bodies through their skin. In the study, doctors tested the urine of 163 children between the ages of 2 months and 28 months born in Los Angeles, Minneapolis, and Columbia, Missouri, between 2000 and 2005. All had detectable amounts of at least one type of phthalate, and more than 80 percent had seven or more types.[32]

Manufacturers do not list phthalates as ingredients on labels, so it is unknown which products contain them. The researchers at the University of Washington and the University of Rochester stressed that the potential effects on babies were uncertain. The study is the first, however, to report that skin transfer may be a main route of exposure for babies.

"Phthalate exposure is widespread and variable in infants. We found that mothers' reported use of infant lotion, infant powder and shampoo was significantly associated with . . . urinary concentrations," the scientists wrote in the new study.

In the study, babies exposed to baby lotion, shampoo, and powder had more than four times the level of phthalates in their urine than babies whose parents had not used the products. The highest levels were reported in babies under eight months old, and those exposed to lotions. More than half the mothers in the new study reported using baby shampoos on their infants within twenty-four hours of the urine tests; about one-third had used lotion and 14 percent used powder within the same time period. No link was found to baby wipes or to diaper creams.

The highest concentrations in the babies were for a phthalate known as MEP, which comes from DEP, the compound used in fragrances. One baby had an extremely high level of MEP—4.4 parts per million.

There was criticism of Dr. Sathyanarayana put out on the Public Relations Newswire by the Center for Individual Freedom (CFIF) that she did not reveal her conflict of interest since she is active in efforts to ban phthalates.

Previous animal and human research suggests that early exposure to some phthalates could reduce testosterone and alter reproductive organs, particularly in males. The three phthalate compounds found in the highest concentrations in babies in the study were linked to reduced testosterone in a 2006 study of newborns in Denmark.[33] Some scientists theorize such changes in hormones could lead to fertility problems and male reproductive disorders.

Phthalates, in addition to helping cosmetics retain fragrance and color, are used as plasticizers in some vinyl. A 2008 California law banned six types in children's toys and feeding products. But no federal or state law in the United States prohibits their use in personal care products or cosmetics.

Representatives of the fragrance and cosmetics industries said they were surprised by the University of Washington study findings and questioned their validity. They said only one phthalate compound is used in baby products, and it is found in such low levels that they doubt it could explain high concentrations found in the babies.

---

[32] Dr. Sheela Sathyanarayana, "Baby Care Products: Possible Sources of Infant Phthalate Exposure," *Pediatrics* 121, no. 2 (February 2008): e260–e268 (doi:10.1542/peds.2006-3766).
[33] Marla Cone, "Study Finds High Levels of Chemicals in Infants Using Baby Cosmetics," *Los Angeles Times,* February 4, 2008, http://www.latimes.com/news/custom/scimedemail/la-me-babies4feb04,0,6725249.story.

In their report, the scientists advised parents who want to reduce their baby's exposure to stop using lotions and powders unless their doctors recommend them for medical reasons. They also suggested limiting use of shampoos and other products. Many adult lotions and other personal care products also contain phthalates.

Europe has banned some phthalates in baby toys and cosmetics, but not the DEP found in fragrances.

Trade associations, here and abroad, defend baby products. Responding to the French C2DS campaign, the Fédération des Entreprises de la Beauté (FEBEA) sought to reassure consumers that baby cosmetics are safe.

The manufacturers are not only appealing to parents, they are targeting youngsters directly. Manufacturers have signed licensing agreements to market everything from Barbie sunblock to Spider-Man power toothbrushes to Harry Potter hand soap. Kids aged four to twelve spend $40 billion annually and influence $500 billion more in family purchases, according to James McNeal, author of *The Kids Market: Myths and Realities* (Paramount Books). Because children can be quite vocal in urging their parents to purchase a particular product, many adults would rather indulge their children's desires for a certain flavor of toothpaste than for a box of candy or toy.[34]

The French trade association said all cosmetics are thoroughly tested and that under the EU Cosmetics Directive, products aimed at children under three must undergo a specific evaluation process. In the EU, certain ingredients that are permitted for use in ordinary cosmetics are banned or restricted in products for young children and babies.

TWEENS AND TEENS

The young and the restless are just as great a market as their baby brothers and sisters. By age thirteen, 71.6 percent of children use blusher, 84.9 percent use lip gloss, and 94.1 percent use hair conditioner. Teens represent a large consumer group, comprising more than 40 million consumers and spending $155 billion a year, according to the Geppetto Group in New York. Of that total, $8 billion a year is spent on girls' health and beauty aids.[35]

Johnson & Johnson released a moisturizing skin care range designed for teens who do not suffer from problem skin in an attempt to cash in on the increasingly affluent young consumer group. The range will be part of the Clean and Clear brand, which is already well known for products designed for oily and problem skin; however, this will be the first time the brand is targeting teenagers with normal to dry skin.

Teens with dry skin, according to the company, have been ignored. The range Clean and Clear Soft includes a night cream formulated to replace lost moisture overnight, a product that hitherto has been more associated with the anti-aging market rather than products for young consumers. In addition, the range includes a day moisturizer that contains SPF 15 in order to protect the skin from UV rays. Similarly, moisturizers containing sun protection factor are often associated with products designed for older skin; however, the move mirrors widespread concern about the laissez-faire attitude adopted by some teenagers regarding sun protection.

---

[34] U.S. Mintel International Group Ltd., "Children's Personal Care Usage Trends Data Monitor," December 2008, page 68, http://www.researchandmarket.com/reportinfo.asp?report_id=683445.
[35] Melanie Marchie, "Girl Power: Teens Hit the Cosmetics Scene," *Household & Personal Products Industry*, September 1, 2001.

The range also includes a treatment product, the Soft Steam In-Shower Facial, designed to hydrate the skin when applied for a minute in the shower.

The Procter & Gamble Company is manufacturing a line of personal care products exclusively for "'tween and teenage boys." The items available to these "minor men" will include antiperspirant/deodorants and personal cleansers. As a mother of two boys, I would encourage that effort.[36]

Leading players in the teen sector will benefit from increased brand recognition, which may translate into brand loyalty later in life.[37]

INGREDIENT CREATIVITY

As I pointed out in the beginning, cosmetic companies are not only great marketers, they are creative. Here are just a few of the innovative products available at this writing:

- Revlon provides a lip-changing experience with Renewist Lipcolor, delivering SPF 15 along with its patent-pending ProCollagen Moisture Core.

- From the spa sector, Jane Iredale launched Sugar&Butter, a lip duo that combines a natural exfoliator featuring beeswax and organic brown sugar with a tinted lip plumper of cool mint and ginger. The active ingredient is palmitoyl oligopeptide, the natural tripeptide (*see* in dictionary) "which stimulates collagen synthesis and helps diminish lines."

- Purify Me Body Mask, a deep cleanser and intensive moisturizer for body skin (not just the face anymore). The Body Shop's Spa Wisdom bath and body range includes a hydrating gel called On a High Hydrating Puree. Origins has launched Spice Odyssey Foaming Body Rub, whose formulation is based on the Moroccan spice mixture for cooking, *ras el hanout,* meaning "best of the best," featuring seven herbs and spices, twenty essential oils, and four exfoliants.

- Body butters are being added to many body care brand portfolios. Examples include Honey Olive Neroli massage body butter within the Boots Mediterranean range, Opal London's Water Lily & Almond Spa body butter, and Tisserand Aromatherapy Organic Lavender & Bergamot Body Butter.

- Oils are another upcoming format, already popular in Germany and quickly catching on as a versatile and less greasy alternative to body creams, butters, and balms. The Body Shop's Monoi Miracle Oil is a light, nongreasy coconut oil scented with gardenia flowers for use as a moisturizer on the body or even as a prewash on the hair. Bio-Oil, from the South African skin care company Union-Swiss, is claimed by the company to be one of the fastest-growing skin care products worldwide. The unique ingredient in Bio-Oil is PurCellin Oil, a rapidly absorbed "dry oil" that can be used to reduce the appearance of scars, stretch marks, and uneven skin tone and is recommended for dehydrated or aging skin.

---

[36] Diana Dodson, "Global Fragrance Market Booms," http://www.gcimagazine.com/market$trends/segments/finefragrance/15520492.html, posted February 11, 2008, from the February 2008 issue of *GCI* magazine.
[37] Katie Bird, "Teen Market Further Targeted by Johnson & Johnson," http://cosmeticsdesign.com, April 2, 2008.

- Energizing Formulations in Skin Care to pep up your face. French skin care brand Daniel Jourance Océ Vie radiance revitalizing face cream contains the marine active ingredient thermophiline, an ingredient that helps protect and revitalize skin, and Rock samphire, a "sensory ingredient" known for its stimulating properties. It also claims that its texture and fragrance with essential oils "infuses the skin with a wave of freshness and well-being." Energizer is an energizing face cream that contains botanical ingredients, amino acids, and vitamin B, said to promote the production and storage of energy in the cells.

- Another French brand, Mademoiselle Bigondi, has launched a range of moisturizers that can be customized to your needs and moods.

- Détoxifiant is a detoxifying cream with ivy and sunflower and rice extracts and is said to protect the skin against urban aggression, leaving a protective veil on the skin. Eclat du Teint is a radiance care cream that contains fermented black tea extracts, which the producer claims gives a peachlike complexion to gray and dull skin. Light-reflecting microprisms help to illuminate the complexion, leaving it brighter and clearer.

I could go on and on with the product promotions that sometimes make P. T. Barnum, the ebullient circus promoter, seem like an introvert. Although the majority of cosmetics are perfectly safe and sometimes effective, there are some that may or may not be harmful. The scientists either haven't investigated them or can't make up their minds. Take nanotechnology, for example.

NANOTECHNOLOGY

What is nanotechnology and why is it important to cosmetic manufacturers despite the warnings of scientists, government agencies, and consumers? Nanotechnology is the ability to measure, see, manipulate, and manufacture things usually between 1 and 100 nanometers. A nanometer is one-billionth of a meter; a human hair is roughly 100,000 nanometers wide. The applications of nanotechnology range from practical to fantastic to potentially dangerous. Although the nanotechnology industry is just starting out, it is already booming. It is projected to capture 14 percent of the $2.6 trillion global manufacturing market, says the UN Environment Program (UNEP). In contrast, it made up less than 0.1 percent just three years ago.[38]

Some critics of nanotechnology say that nanoparticles could easily be inhaled, absorbed through the skin, or built up in the environment. Others have likened the materials to asbestos, which is now known to cause lung cancer and other diseases. When nanoparticles in cosmetics penetrate the skin and move around the body, what happens to them? No one knows because at this writing, they are untraceable.

A recent report based on research from U.S. scientists, for example, shows that nanoparticles used in certain sun cream formulations can affect the brain cells of mice by upsetting the chemical balance and potentially causing neurological damage. The study, carried out by Bellina Veronesi of the U.S. Environmental Protection Agency and published on the website Nature.com, looked at the effects of nano-sized Titania,

---

[38] Nanopublic: UNEP Report on Nano and the Environment, February 5, 2007.

now commonly used in sun cream formulations and often labeled titanium oxide, on cultures of microglia mice cells.[39] Although Veronesi stressed that the research does not necessarily imply that the Titania grains are harmful to the human body and other experts have aired caution over the interpretation of the findings, it does add to a growing body of research that suggests potential risks might exist when certain compounds are reduced to nano size.

PCPC, the U.S. cosmetic trade group, released a paper on the application of nanotechnology in personal care products. "The nanoparticles used in sunscreens provide important sun protection benefits, helping reduce the risk of skin cancer," said John Bailey, executive vice president of science at PCPC. "These sunscreen ingredients have been used safely for many years and have been evaluated and approved by the FDA and independent scientists. They are transparent and aesthetically pleasing, and therefore encourage greater consumer use."[40]

The PCPC says that the FDA concluded in 1996 that smaller, micronized particles of titanium dioxide are not new substances and that there is no evidence demonstrating that these micronized particles are unsafe.

Dr. Andrew Maynard, science adviser to the Project on Emerging Nanotechnologies, is an internationally recognized expert on airborne particles. According to Maynard, aerosol sprays can produce breathable particles a few micrometers in size that can remain airborne for long periods of time and can reach the sensitive deep lung if inhaled. Once deposited, there is the possibility of chemicals or nanoparticles (if present) in the droplets causing damage.

David Rejeski, the director of the Project on Emerging Nanotechnologies at the Woodrow Wilson International Center, says: "We are about to be inundated with hundreds, if not thousands, of new products but governments are not ready. Industry and trade groups are not prepared. A research strategy for addressing possible human health or environmental risks is not in place, and the public is not informed."

In his testimony before the U.S. House of Representatives Committee on Science, Rejeski put forward a number of practical recommendations to address these challenges. They include carefully planned and adequately resourced research into possible environmental, health, and safety risks; an integrated oversight regime that is transparent, efficient, and predictable; a one-stop shop for businesses, especially small and medium-sized companies, to help with nanotechnology commercialization; and greater public engagement.[41]

A report from the United Nations (UN) has called for tighter regulation on nanotechnology, which is already being used to develop drugs, cosmetics, and other commercial products. In its annual report of the global environment, the UNEP said that "swift action" was needed by policymakers to properly evaluate nanotechnology. The UNEP report stated that priority must be given in assessing the potential risks of nanomaterials already being mass-produced.[42]

---

[39] David Biello, "Do Nanoparticles and Sunscreen Mix?" *Scientific American,* posted August 20, 2007.
[40] "Cosmetic Industry Releases Scientific White Paper on Use of Nanoparticles in Personal Care Products," posted October 10, 2006, http://redorbit.com/news/health/687483/cosmetic_industry_releases_scientific whitepaperonuseofnanoparticles/index.html.
[41] david.rejeski@wilsoncenter.org, Director, Project on Emerging Nanotechnologies Expertise Technology policy/assessment.
[42] *"Tighter Controls" for Nanotechnology: A Report from the United Nations (UN),* February 7, 2007, Annual Global Ministerial Environment Forum.

BUGGY COSMETICS

Every time you open a bottle of foundation or case of eye shadow, microorganisms in the air have an opportunity to rush in, but adequately preserved products can kill off enough germs to keep the product safe. European rules state that makeup's "best before" date is thirty months from manufacture, but only products that last less than six months have to be stamped with an expiry date. Makeup artists recommend you have a clear-out before then anyway, and toss your mascara in particular after three or four months. Powder blusher lasts two years and cream blusher eighteen months. Eye shadow should be replaced after a year, while lipsticks and glosses can be kept for two years, as can lip and eye pencils, as long as you keep them sharpened.

Occasionally, however, a product will be seriously contaminated. According to FDA data, most cases of contamination are due to manufacturers using poorly designed, ineffective preservative systems and not testing the stability of the preservatives during the product's customary shelf life under normal use conditions.

Expiration dates are, for practical purposes, a rule of thumb, and a product may expire long before that date if it has not been stored and properly handled. On the other hand, products stored under ideal conditions may be acceptable long after the expiration date has been reached. Generally, cosmetics are formulated and tested for a shelf life of one to three years under normal storage conditions.

Contaminated makeup is the result of either inadequate preservation or product misuse. But contamination doesn't necessarily translate into serious injury for the user. Cosmetics are not expected to be totally free of microorganisms when first used or to remain free during consumer use.

Since ancient history women have worn cosmetics to enhance the appearance of their eyes. Most people who wear eye makeup never have a problem related to makeup use. Some women can, however, develop an allergic reaction, infection, or injury of the eye or eyelids. These problems can range from minor annoyance, such as tearing of the eyes, to visual loss or even blindness. Who has problems with eye makeup? Contact lens wearers and people with allergies or sensitive skin are more likely to experience problems while using eye cosmetics. However, anyone who wears eye makeup should be aware of basic safety tips to help prevent injury or infection. (See safety tips below.)

The most serious problem related to eye makeup involves injury to the cornea (the clear front surface of the eye), often during application of the cosmetic. A mascara or eyeliner wand or a fingernail can scratch the cornea (corneal abrasion). Occasionally a corneal abrasion can become infected, leading to a potentially blinding corneal ulcer. Corneal injuries are usually painful and always require prompt medical attention.

All eye cosmetics contain preservatives that retard the growth of bacteria in the makeup. If you moisten your eye cosmetics with saliva or even tap water or lend them to others, you are taking a chance and possibly seriously contaminating your product.

There's something else that is definitely taboo when using makeup—sharing! Sharing cosmetics means sharing germs, and the risk, though small, isn't worth it.

But what about the testers commonly found at cosmetic counters? They are even more likely to become contaminated than the same products in an individual's home. Many stores now use little pieces of sponge or cotton-tipped swabs. But leave it to the techies to solve an old problem. IBM and EZFace, Inc., have introduced the Virtual Mirror Kiosk, a virtual reality tool that will allow consumers to "try on" cosmetics at the beauty counter. With the tool, customers are able to snap a digital self-portrait using the kiosk's camera, scan the bar code of the product they've chosen, and virtually apply it to their hair, face, eyes, or lips for approval.[43] The robot cosmetician will also suggest products that work with your skin tones and features.

CONVINCING US WE STINK AND ARE CONTAGIOUS

Do you smell? Are you covered with germs? For years, cosmetic companies have been trying to convince us we must mask all natural odors. Women, particularly, were told they needed products to disguise their "feminine odor." Now the promoters are after both men and women with "body washes." They are in the process of brainwashing us about the need to have special cleansing products and that germs are hiding everywhere. Antibacterials have been added to soaps, deodorants, and toothpastes and have become somewhat controversial. Some scientists believe that because we use so many germ killers in our products, we may not build natural immunity to germs or we may become victims of germs that have mutated. (*See* Triclosan, the germicide in many antibacterial soaps, in this dictionary.)

An estimated 79 percent of liquid soaps and 29 percent of bar soaps now contain triclosan—an antibiotic designed to kill a wide variety of germs. However, it seems this trend for cleanliness could actually be too effective and lead to bacterial resistance. This in turn can contribute to the incidence of MRSA, methicillin-resistant *Staphylococcus aureus,* a type of bacteria that has become resistant to many antibiotics and quickly killed a beautiful model in 2009. She was one of an increasing number of victims of the often deadly infection.

Scientists have been warning that antibacterials in soap and cosmetic products are increasing the resistance of bacteria, which have the potential to persist for up to forty years.

NAILING NAIL PROBLEMS

Nail problems compose about 10 percent of the conditions dermatologists treat. Changes in nails, such as discoloration or thickening, can signal health problems, including liver and kidney disease, heart and lung conditions, anemia, and diabetes. Common nail problems include white spots after an injury to the nails, vertical lines under the nails caused by nail injury or certain drugs and diseases, and bacterial infections, most often due to injury. Fungal infections cause about half of all nail disorders. Women who have nail wraps or artificial nails are particularly susceptible to a fungal infection, onychomycosis. Before an artificial nail is applied, the surface of the nail is usually abraded with an emery board. This procedure damages the nail surface and creates a possible source of fungal infection. Additionally, an emery board used on a fungus-infected nail can introduce the fungal infection to an uninfected nail on the same person or to the next emery board user. Fungal infections can also occur when water becomes trapped under acrylic nail tips or wraps.

---

[43] Sara Mason, "2 in 1: Makeup Meets Skin Care," posted November 8, 2007, from the November 2007 issue of *GCI* magazine.

ARE THERE TOXINS IN YOUR COSMETICS?

You will find information on toxins when you look through the pages of this book. Are toxins harmful to your body? We are told that a minute amount of a poison such as furans and arsenic compounds (*see* in dictionary) won't hurt us. How about multiple toxins that we eat, drink, breathe, and put on our skins? No one really knows, although you will see opinions of scientists in the listings. It is difficult to determine if there are toxins in your body unless you become really sick or show chronic symptoms. Toxins may kill quickly. It is almost impossible to tell if other potential deadly ingredients, such as cancer-causing agents, are in your cosmetics because they may take twenty years or more to do their deadly deed. (*See* Toxicokinetics.)

ARE THERE CARCINOGENS IN YOUR COSMETICS?

There are certainly well-known carcinogens in some cosmetics despite the supposed protection of the Delaney Amendment. The amendment was part of the 1958 law requested by the Food and Drug Administration. The law stated that food and chemical manufacturers had to test additives before they were put on the market and the results had to be submitted to the FDA. The Delaney Amendment specifically states that no additive may be permitted in any amount if tests show that it produces cancer when fed to humans or animals or by other appropriate tests. Ever since it was enacted the food and chemical industries have tried to get it repealed. Efforts have been made to substitute a negligible-risk standard to processed food. Up until 1996, the EPA observed different safety standards for raw and processed foods. For the latter, it used the zero-risk standard established by the Delaney Amendment. That standard, however, proved to be impractical and even counterproductive, according to the EPA and manufacturers. It prohibited foods from carrying minute traces of carcinogenic compounds, while exempting many toxic chemicals that were registered before the amendment was enacted. As a result, regulators were forced to allow the use of toxic chemicals while barring safer alternatives. Congress repealed the Delaney Amendment in the Food Quality Protection Act of 1996 for pesticides, substituting the negligible-risk standard that had long been used to set tolerances for raw foods. This standard allows residues of potentially carcinogenic pesticides as long as there is a "reasonable certainty of no harm" to consumers. In practice, regulators will approve a pesticide application only if it will cause no more than one additional cancer case per million people who consume it over a lifetime. Congress has held hearings to examine the pros and cons of liberalizing the Delaney Amendment. At this writing, debates on the issue were in progress. Some coal tar colors, nitrites, and nitrates that are considered cancer-causing additives are permitted in foods. All the cancer-causing agents allowed in food are also in cosmetics, and additional ones are also in the mix.

The most difficult issue in the identification of ingredients and contaminants in cosmetics concerns cancer-causing ingredients. Senator Edward Kennedy drew attention to findings made by the investigative branch of Congress, the General Accounting Office, during a 1997 congressional debate on how to strengthen the FDA. The GAO has identified more than 125 cosmetic ingredients suspected of causing cancer, as well as others that may cause birth defects. Testing for mutagenicity—breaks in the genetic material of bacteria—can screen many chemicals inexpensively and rapidly. Almost all chemicals known to be carcinogenic in humans have been shown to be mutagens in these systems. However, not all mutagens are necessarily carcinogenic. Thus, animal studies, which cost approximately $300,000 to thoroughly test an ingredient, are needed. All ingredients that cause cancer in humans cause cancer in rats and mice, with the exception of trivalent arsenic. Whether all chemicals that cause cancer in animals cause cancer in humans is a matter of debate, but many scientists in the cancer field believe they do.

Two contaminants found in cosmetics have been shown to cause cancer. One is *n*-nitrosodiethanolamine (NDELA), which penetrates easily through the skin when in a fatty base. This contaminant appears to be produced by the interaction of two otherwise safe ingredients—for example, the amines (surfactants, emulsifiers, and detergents) and nitrites or nitroso compounds such as in the preservative 2-bromo-2-nitropane-1,3-diol (BNPD). The other carcinogen is 1,4-dioxane, a contaminant of raw materials. It is believed that about one-third of the emulsion-based cosmetics containing polyoxyethylene derivatives have it in amounts ranging from 1 percent to over 25 percent.[44]

Like in the mines, where canaries warned miners of danger before they could smell the gas, beauticians, barbers, manicurists, and others who work with cosmetics are our canaries. They have a high rate of certain cancers not as common in the general public. For example, hairdressers are at greater risk of developing bladder cancer because of the chemicals present in the hair dyes they use daily, claims research published in *The Lancet Oncology*.

The conclusion was reached by a panel of scientists at the International Agency for Research on Cancer (IARC) in Lyon, who were brought together in 2008 to review the evidence on the cancer link that has built up over the past fifteen years, according to press reports.

In their report published in *The Lancet Oncology,* Dr. Robert Baan said: "A small but consistent risk of bladder cancer was reported in male hairdressers and barbers."[45]

Although the panel was agreed that regular occupational exposure to hair dye increased cancer risk, they found data on personal use inconclusive. The evidence was judged to be insufficient to make a definitive conclusion on the carcinogenicity of hair dye when exposure is limited to personal use.

Concerns about Specific Chemicals

The scientists also reviewed the data related to the cancer-causing potential of aromatic amines and organic dyes and added the following chemicals to IARC's list of probable and definite carcinogens.

- Ortho-Toluidine, carcinogenic
- 4-Chloro-ortho-toluidine, probably carcinogenic
- 4,4'-Methylenebis, carcinogenic
- Benzidine-based dyes, carcinogenic

---

[44] FDA's *Cosmetics Handbook,* U.S. H.H.S., Washington, D.C., October 15, 1992, pp. 9, 11–12.
[45] Robert Baan, Kurt Straif, Yann Grosse, Béatrice Secretan, Fatiha El Ghissassi, Vincent Cogliano, "Carcinogenicity of Carbon Black, Titanium Dioxide, and Talc," on behalf of the WHO International Agency for Research on Cancer Monograph Working Group, *The Lancet Oncology* 7, no. 4, pp. 295–96, April 2006.

The report was published as Volume 99 of the monographs of the IARC, which is an arm of the World Health Organization (WHO).

The publication of the findings adds to the mounting body of studies, including a recent report by a UK consumer magazine that found that several highly allergenic and potentially carcinogenic chemicals are still widely used in hair dyes without being properly labeled.

A check for this seventh edition in 2009 showed that the National Toxicology Program (NTP) found the testing site had planned to study talc but has now withdrawn it from the lineup. Maybe they are there somewhere, but there were no cosmetics tested or scheduled to be tested for toxicity.

It has been reported that prolonged inhalation of talc can cause lung problems because it is similar in chemical composition to asbestos, a known lung irritant and cancer-causing ingredient in its powdered state. There is no known acute toxicity, but there is a question about talc being a cancer-causing additive upon ingestion. It is suspected that the high incidence of stomach cancer among the Japanese is due to the fact that the Japanese prefer that their rice be treated with talc. Another common cosmetic ingredient—talcum powder—has also been cited several times as a possible carcinogen. Talcum powder is produced from talc, a magnesium trisilicate mineral, which in its natural form may contain asbestos, a known human carcinogen.

Because of this association with asbestos, all home-use talcum products marketed after about 1973—baby powders, body powders, facial powders—have been required by law to be asbestos-free. Asbestos can cause lung cancer and mesotheliomas (cancers affecting the lining surfaces of the pleural and peritoneal cavities). It has been suggested that talcum powder may be carcinogenic to the covering layer of the ovaries through the migration of talcum powder particles (applied to the genital area, sanitary napkins, diaphragms, or condoms) through the vagina, uterus, and fallopian tubes to the ovary. Several epidemiologic studies have examined the relationship between talcum powder and cancer of the ovary. Findings are mixed, with some studies reporting a slightly increased risk and some reporting no association. A case-control study published in 1997 of 313 women with ovarian cancer and 422 without this disease found that the women with cancer were more likely to have applied talcum powder to their external genital area or to have used genital deodorant sprays. Women using these products had a 50 to 90 percent higher risk of developing ovarian cancer.[46]

The FDA issued a statement that the agency had become aware of a new National Toxicology Program (NTP) study showing an association between the topical application of diethanolamine (DEA) (*see* in dictionary) and certain DEA-related ingredients and cancer in laboratory animals. For the DEA-related ingredients, the NTP study suggests that the carcinogenic response is linked to possible residual levels of DEA. Although DEA itself is used in very few cosmetics, DEA-related ingredients such as oleamide DEA, lauramide DEA, and cocamide DEA are widely used in a variety of cosmetic products. These ingredients function as emulsifiers or foaming ingredients and are generally used at levels of 1 to 5 percent. The FDA statement says the agency takes these findings very seriously and is in the process of carefully eval-

[46] D.W. Cramer et al., "Genital Talc Exposure and Risk of Ovarian Cancer," *International Journal of Cancer* 81 (1999): 351–56.

uating the studies and test data to determine the risk, if any, to consumers. The FDA says that if its evaluation of the NTP data indicates a health hazard exists, it will advise the industry and the public and will consider its legal options under the authority of the Food, Drug and Cosmetic Act. In other words, we will all probably have a few more wrinkles before any "action" is taken.

Ingredients in a wide variety of cosmetics and personal care products can mimic the effects of the hormone estrogen. Scientists are concerned that even at low levels, these environmental estrogens may work together with the body's own estrogen to increase the risk of breast cancer. Although risk factors are known to include the loss of function of the susceptibility genes BRCA1/BRCA2 and lifetime exposure to estrogen, the main causative agents in breast cancer remain unaccounted for, according to a British researcher, P. D. Darbre of the University of Reading, who published a paper in the *Journal of Applied Toxicology* in 2003. The British researcher noted that underarm cosmetics might be a cause of breast cancer, because these cosmetics contain a variety of chemicals that are applied frequently to an area directly adjacent to the breast. Darbre wrote the strongest supporting evidence comes from unexplained clinical observations showing a disproportionately high incidence of breast cancer in the upper outer quadrant of the breast, just the local area to which these cosmetics are applied. A biological basis for breast carcinogenesis could result from the ability of the various constituent chemicals to bind to DNA and to promote growth of the damaged cells. Like a voice crying in the wilderness, Darbre said: "Multidisciplinary research is now needed to study the effect of long-term use of the constituent chemicals of underarm cosmetics, because if there proves to be any link between these cosmetics and breast cancer then there might be options for the prevention of breast cancer."[47]

There are so many potential cancer-causing agents in cosmetics. It seems foolish, if you know about the proven or suspected chemicals, to use the cosmetics containing them. Cosmetics are not a matter of life and death unless you are very, very vain or work in Hollywood.

THE REAL KEY TO SAFETY IS YOUR OWN KNOWLEDGE

If you are young and your hormones and your oil glands are very active, your skin is supple but may pop out with pimples. As your skin ages, collagen and elastin, the tissues that keep it supple, weaken. Your skin becomes thinner and loses fat, so it looks less plump and smooth. While these changes are taking place, gravity participates by causing your skin to sag and wrinkle.

This book can help everyone, young and old, decide which cosmetics actually help and which will just make matters worse. And what about getting your money's worth? "Just because it costs more doesn't mean it's better!" This has been one of the major themes of all editions of *A Consumer's Dictionary of Cosmetic Ingredients,* but now it is echoing through the colorful, scented halls of the cosmetic, toiletries, and fragrance industry itself. A fierce battle is raging to sell products to a changing population in hard economic times.

---

[47] P. D. Darbre, "Underarm Cosmetics and Breast Cancer," *Journal of Applied Toxicology* 23 (2003): 285–88, Division of Cell and Molecular Biology, School of Animal and Microbial Sciences, University of Reading, P.O. Box 228, Whiteknights, Reading RG6 6AJ, UK; p.d.darbre@reading.ac.uk.

Cosmeticians in stores who choose the right color makeup for you and say "you look beautiful" are fading fast. They are being replaced by mass marketers and samples in magazines and offers on the Internet. Add to that the frenzied lifestyle today and customers don't have time to have makeup applied or flit from counter to counter to choose a product.

The once-very-particular prestige cosmetic companies, as a result, are now out to sell us their products anywhere they can, from cable TV, direct mail, beauty salons, and, yes, even in the territory of the broad marketers—the supermarket and the drugstore and infomercials. Supermarkets now account for about 12 percent of the mass beauty product market.

Naysayers said it wouldn't work if you couldn't smell a perfume or dab a foundation on your wrist, but it has; and often you can find good prices on the Internet—but watch out for the handling and/or mailing charges that sometimes make the item as expensive or more expensive than if you bought it at a local store. Be careful of the offer of free samples because you may, as I was, be unexpectedly signed up for a whole year's supply of an expensive product. You won't have a cosmetician giving you advice and telling you how beautiful you look online but you will save time, a precious commodity in this busy world, and some sites do offer advice.

MIRROR, MIRROR—WHO'S FAIR?

We have become more savvy consumers. We are reading labels and recognizing that often the only difference between an expensive cosmetic and an inexpensive one is the cost of the package and the hype. There is a 500 to 1,000 percent spread between cost and sales price in cosmetics. This margin is needed, according to manufacturers, to meet heavy promotional expenses.

Today's customers seem to be attracted by the promise of scientific benefits, a belief that is being exploited by the current crop of advertisements for beauty products.[48]

"Put this on your skin, and you will be irresistible." If we believe a cream can take away wrinkles or a mascara can make us alluring, what's the harm? So we pay $50 for ten cents' worth of ingredients. Maybe the psychological lift is priceless.

On the other hand, cosmetics may cost us more than we really want to pay. If a cosmetic ingredient may cause an allergic reaction or contribute to the cancer burden, that's quite another matter. If we take a drug with side effects, the risk may be worth it because we may need the drug to regain or maintain our health. Although they may be rewarding psychologically, are cosmetics worth any risk?

LABEL WARNINGS—PAY ATTENTION

Experts in the field of safety often say that consumers do not read, never mind pay attention to, warnings on product labels. Misuse of some cosmetic products can cause problems that range in severity from mild rash to skin burns, or from burning eyes to blindness. Sometimes the label print is too small for those without 20/20 vision.

---

[48] Cosmetics and Toiletries USA, 2003; Klinegroup.com.

CHOOSE YOUR COSMETICS WISELY

Until the time the public demands tighter controls over cosmetics, your greatest protection is your own knowledge. The cosmetic companies are very sensitive to consumer desires, and both the industry and the FDA may respond to reports of untoward effects from a cosmetic. But they can't do so if no one tells them about it.

The purpose of this dictionary is to enable you to look up cosmetic ingredients listed alphabetically. The dictionary includes most of the cosmetic ingredients in common use, a large percentage of which have been kept secret, including many of the so-called trade secret ingredients. If a cosmetic company declares an ingredient a trade secret, it does not have to be listed on the label but the list must end with "and other ingredients."

HOW TO USE THIS BOOK

Although unique in content, this dictionary follows the format of most dictionaries. The following are examples of entries with any explanatory notes that may be necessary:

ABIETIC ACID • Sylvic Acid. Chiefly a texturizer in the making of soaps. A widely available natural acid, water insoluble, prepared from pine rosin, usually yellow and composed of either glassy or crystalline particles. Used also in the manufacture of vinyls, lacquers, and plastics. Little is known about abietic acid toxicity; it is harmless when injected into mice but causes paralysis in frogs and is slightly irritating to human skin and mucous membranes. May cause allergic reactions.

We have learned that abietic acid is also known as sylvic acid, that it is a naturally occurring rosin acid, which as a texturizer maintains consistency in soaps, and we discovered its noncosmetic uses and its known toxicity. Source material for the comments on toxicity is indicated in the notes at the end of the dictionary.

ALLANTOIN • Used in cold creams, hand lotions, hair lotions, after-shave lotions, and other skin-soothing cosmetics because of its ability to help heal wounds and skin ulcers and to stimulate the growth of healthy tissue. Composed of colorless crystals, soluble in hot water, it is prepared synthetically by the oxidation of uric acid (*see*) or by heating uric acid with dichloroacetic acid. It is nontoxic.

Allantoin, we can see, is a synthetic product derived from uric acid. By looking up uric acid, we learn that it derives from urine and is used as a sunburn preventative.

Terminology in this dictionary generally has been kept to a middle road between what is understandable to the technician and to the average interested consumer, while at the same time avoiding oversimplification of data. Once again, if in doubt, look up alphabetically any term listed that seems unfamiliar or whose meaning has been blunted by overuse, such as isolate, extract, demulcent, emollient, or even shampoo. I have also listed the organizations and their abbreviations as well as the frustrating initials used by all sorts of agencies.

The Generally Recognized as Safe (GRAS) List was established in 1958 by Congress. Those substances that were being added to food over a long time, which under conditions of their intended use were generally recognized as safe by qualified scientists, would be exempt from premarket clearance. When a cosmetic ingredient is also a food additive that is listed as GRAS, the designation has been noted, even though no premarket clearance is required for cosmetic ingredients.

With *A Consumer's Dictionary of Cosmetic Ingredients,* you will be able to work with current and future labels to determine the purpose and desirability or toxicity of the ingredients listed. For the first time, you will have the knowledge to choose the best cosmetics for you. By checking on a product's ingredients, as listed on the label, you can eliminate many products and choose those that are harmless, even beneficial, and you save money and reward those manufacturers who deserve your purchases. With the aid of this book, you will be able to know a great deal more about the cosmetics you have been using. See organizations and government agencies concerned with cosmetics in the Appendix.

Abbreviations Frequently Used in This Book

ASEAN	Asian Association of Southeast Asian Nations
ASP	The FDA's full up-to-date toxicology information has been sought.
BANNED	The substance was formerly approved as a cosmetic ingredient but is now banned; there may be some toxicology data available.
CIR	Cosmetic Ingredient Review
E	Approved or used by the European Union
EAF	There is reported use of the substance, but the FDA has not yet been assigned it for toxicology literature search.
ECHA	European Chemicals Agency
EU	European Union
FAO/ WHO	An international group of experts from the World Health Organization and the Food and Agriculture Organization of the United Nations
FDA	Food and Drug Administration
GRAS	Generally Recognized as Safe
JECFA	Joint Expert Committee on Food Additives under FAO/WHO
NEW	There is reported use of the substance, and the FDA has an initial toxicology literature search in progress.
NIL	Although listed as added to food, the FDA has no current reported use of the substance, and therefore, although toxicology information may be available in the Priority-Based Assessment of Food Additives (PAFA) database, it is not being updated.
NUL	The FDA has no reported use of the substance and there is no toxicology information available in PAFA.
OTC	Over-the-counter
SIN	Substitute It Now
UK	United Kingdom
USDA	United States Department of Agriculture

A

ABEYANCE • The term used by the FDA that includes petitions that were filed and were found after detailed review by the Office of Food Additive Safety (OFAS) of certain cosmetic colorings to be deficient. OFAS does not actively work on petitions in abeyance. When all the information required to address the deficiency or deficiencies is provided, a petition can be refiled and assigned a new filing date.

ABIES • *A. alba, A. balsamea, A. pectinata, A. sibirica.* Essential oils derived from a variety of pine trees. They are used as natural flavoring ingredients and to scent bath products. Ingestion of large amounts can cause intestinal hemorrhages.

ABIES ALBA LEAF WAX • A wax obtained from the needles of *Abies alba* (*see above*). It is used as a skin-conditioning ingredient and as a skin protectant.

ABIES PECTINATA OIL • The volatile oil from *Abies alba* (*see*) used as a fragrance ingredient.

ABIETIC ACID • Abietinol. Abietol. Sylvic acid. Chiefly a texturizer in the making of soaps. A widely available natural acid, water insoluble, prepared from pine rosin, usually yellow and composed of either glassy or crystalline particles. Used also in the manufacture of vinyls, lacquers, and plastics. Little is known about abietic acid toxicity; it is harmless when injected into mice but causes paralysis in frogs and is slightly irritating to human skin and mucous membranes. May cause allergic reactions.

ABIETYL ALCOHOL • Increases thickness. *See* Abietic Acid.

ABITOL • Dihydroabietyl Alcohol. Used in cosmetics, plastics, and adhesives. *See* Abietic Acid.

ABRADE • Scrape or erode a covering, such as skin.

ABRASIVE • Natural or synthetic cosmetic ingredients intended to rub away or scrape the surface layer of cells or tissue from the skin.

ABSOLUTE • The term refers to a plant-extracted material that has been concentrated but that remains essentially unchanged in its original taste and odor. For example, *see* Jasmine Absolute. Often called "natural perfume materials" because they are not subjected to heat and water as are distilled products. *See* Distilled.

ABSORBENT • An ingredient or cosmetic that has the capacity to absorb.

ABSORPTION BASES • Compounds used to improve the water-absorbing capacity and stability of creams, lotions, and hairdressings. Lanolin-type absorption bases are mixtures of lanolin alcohols, mineral oil, and petrolatum (*see all*). Also used as bases are cholesterol and beeswax (*see both*).

AC • Abbreviation for anticaking agent.

ACACIA • Gum Arabic. Catechu. Acacia is the odorless, colorless, tasteless dried exudate from the stem of the acacia tree, grown in Africa, the Near East, India, and the southern United States. Its most distinguishing quality among the natural gums is its ability to dissolve rapidly in water. The use of acacia dates back four thousand years, when the Egyptians employed it in paints. Medically, it is used as a demulcent to soothe irritations, particularly of the mucous membranes. It can cause allergic reactions such as skin rash and asthmatic attacks. Oral toxicity is low, but the FDA issued a notice in 1992 that catechu tincture had not been shown to be safe and effective as claimed in OTC digestive aid products. *See also* Vegetable Gums and Catechu Black.

ACACIA DEALBATA LEAF WAX • *Acacia dealbata.* Mimosa, Silver Wattle. Obtained from the leaves of a prickly Egyptian shrub. It is used as a skin-conditioning ingredient, emollient, and skin protectant. Used in moisturizers, cleaning products, blushers, eye shadow, and foundations. It is considered a poisonous house plant.

ACACIA FARNESIAN EXTRACT • Acacia Extract. Flowers and stems of *Acacia farnesiana*. It is used as an astringent.

ACACIA FARNESIANA GUM • AEC Gum Arabic. *Acacia senegal* Gum. Widely used all over the world, it acts as an adhesive in mascara, bath soaps, and detergents as well as in body and hand preparations, except for shaving creams. It is also used in hair colorings.

ACAI • Brazilian plum-colored berry that contains antioxidants, amino acids, essential omegas, fibers, and protein and is being promoted as an anti-aging product. The acai berry comes from a group of palms located in Central and South America and is known to be among the most nutritious foods found in the Amazon. Acai can be found in many skin care cosmetics and hair care products.

ACANTHOPANAX SENTICOSUS • Extract of Eleuthero Ginseng. Siberian Ginseng. A plant material derived from *Acanthopanax senticosus*. A skin-conditioning ingredient related to siloxanes and ginseng (*see both*).

ACEFYLLINE METHYLSILANOL MANNURONATE • Used as a skin-conditioning ingredient. Prepared from theophylline, an alkaloid (*see*) with caffeine found in tea leaves. Theophylline, however, is usually prepared synthetically.

ACENOCOUMAROL • Previously known as nicoumalone in the United Kingdom. An anticoagulant medicine used to prevent blood clots. May cause rash, diarrhea, allergy, hair loss (alopecia), damage to the liver, nausea and vomiting, bruising, increased tendency to bleed, and inflammation of the pancreas (pancreatitis). Prohibited in cosmetics in the UK except when used in a fragrance.

ACER • *A. pseudoplantanus, A. saccharinum*. Mountain Maple. It acts similarly to tannin (*see*).

ACEROLA • *Malpighia glabra*. Derived from the ripe fruit of the West Indian or Barbados cherry, grown in Central America and the West Indies. A rich source of vitamin C. Increasingly used as an antioxidant in skin care products that target redness and inflammation.

ACESULFAME K • Sunette. Sweet One. Non-nutritive sweetener two hundred times sweeter than sugar. Animals that were fed acesulfame developed tumors more often than animals not given it.

ACETAL • A volatile liquid derived from acetaldehyde (*see*) and alcohol and used as a solvent in synthetic perfumes such as jasmine. Also used in fruit flavorings (it has a nut-like aftertaste) and as a hypnotic in medicine. It is a central nervous system depressant, similar in action to paraldehyde but more toxic. Paraldehyde is a hypnotic and sedative whose side effects are respiratory depression, cardiovascular collapse, and possible high blood pressure reactions. No known skin toxicity.

ACETALDEHYDE • Ethanal. An intermediate (*see*) and solvent in the manufacture of perfumes. A flammable, colorless liquid with a characteristic odor, occurring naturally in apples, broccoli, cheese, coffee, grapefruit, and other vegetables and fruits. Used as a fragrance ingredient in cosmetics. Also used in the manufacture of synthetic rubber and in the silvering of mirrors. It is irritating to the mucous membranes, and ingestion of large doses may cause death by respiratory paralysis. Inhalation, usually limited by intense irritation of the lungs, can also be toxic. May cause skin irritation.

ACETAMIDE MEA • N-Acetyl Acid Amide. N-Acetyl Ethanolamine. Used as a solvent, plasticizer, and stabilizer (*see all*). Used in hair conditioners and skin creams and as a foam booster and thickener. It is also used in shampoos, tonics, dressings, and other hair products. Crystals absorb water. Odorless when pure but can have a mousy scent. A mild skin irritant with low toxicity. Has caused liver cancer when given orally to rats in doses of 5,000 milligrams per kilogram of body weight. The CIR Expert Panel (*see*) found that it is safe at concentrations not to exceed 7.5 percent. The Panel found, however, that it may form nitrosamines (*see*). The Joint Expert Committee on Food Additives (JECFA) noted in 2006 the available toxicity data for this substance indicated that it was clearly carcinogenic in both mice and rats, and although the mechanism of tumor formation is unknown, the possibility of gene toxicity cannot be discounted. The JECFA considered it inappropriate for such a compound to be used as a flavoring agent or for any other food additive purpose and agreed that acetamide would not be evaluated according to the Procedure for the Safety Evaluation of Flavoring Agents. A mild skin irritant with low toxicity. FDA reports it in use but has, as of this writing, not yet done a thorough toxicology search. EAF

ACETAMIDOETHOXYBUTYL TRIMONIUM CHLORIDE • Used in hair conditioners, skin-conditioning ingredients, and other miscellaneous products. *See* Quaternary Ammonium Compounds.

ACETAMINOPHEN • A coal tar derivative, it is widely used as a pain reliever and fever reducer. It is used as an antioxidant and stabilizer in cosmetics.

ACETAMINOPROPYL TRIMONIUM CHLORIDE • Antistatic ingredient used in conditioners, bath soaps, detergents, and shampoos. *See* Quaternary Ammonium Compounds.

ACETAMINOSALOL • Derived from ammonia and salicylic acid (*see both*), it absorbs ultraviolet light.

ACETANILID • Acetanilide. A solvent used in nail polishes and in liquid powders to give an opaque matte finish. It is also used in fragrances. Usually made from aniline and acetic acid (*see both*). It is of historic interest because it was the first coal tar analgesic and antifever ingredient introduced into medicine. It is a precursor of penicillin and is used as an antiseptic. It is sometimes still used in medicines but is frowned upon by the American Medical Association since there are other related products with less toxicity. It can cause a depletion of oxygen in the blood upon ingestion and eczema when applied to the skin. It caused tumors when given orally to rats in doses of 3,500 milligrams per kilogram of body weight.

ACETARSOL • Acetarsone. Used in mouthwashes, toothpaste, and vaginal suppositories. Thick white crystals with a slight acid taste. Soluble in water. The lethal dose in mice is only 4 milligrams per kilogram of body weight. May cause sensitization.

ACETATE • Salt of acetic acid (*see*) used in perfumery and as a flavoring used in liquor, nut, coffee, vanilla, honey, pineapple, and cheese flavorings for beverages, ice cream, sherbets, cakes, cookies, pastries, and candy.

ACETIC ACID • Ethanoic Acid. Glacial Acetic Acid. Solvent for gums, resins, and volatile oils. Styptic (stops bleeding) and a rubefacient (*see*). Also used as a fragrance ingredient and pH adjuster. A clear colorless liquid with a pungent odor, it is used in freckle-bleaching lotions, hand lotions, and hair dyes. It occurs naturally in apples, cheese, cocoa, coffee, grapes, skim milk, oranges, peaches, pineapples, strawberries, and a variety of other fruits and plants. Vinegar is about 4 to 6 percent acetic acid, and essence of vinegar is about 14 percent. In its glacial form (without much water) it is highly corrosive, and its vapors are capable of producing lung obstruction. Less than 5 percent acetic acid in solution is mildly irritating to the skin. GRAS for packaging only, not for direct ingredient in product. It caused cancer in rats and mice when given orally or by injection. Banned in cosmetics by ASEAN (*see*).

ACETIC ANHYDRIDE • Acetyl Oxide. Acetic Oxide. Colorless liquid with a strong odor, it is derived from oxidation of acetaldehyde (*see*). It is used as a dehydrating and acetylating ingredient (*see both* Dehyrated and Acetylated) and in the production of dyes, perfumes, plastics, food starch, and aspirin. It is a strong irritant and may cause skin bumps and eye damage.

ACETOIN • Acetyl Methyl Carbinol. A flavoring ingredient and aroma carrier used in perfumery, it occurs naturally in broccoli, grapes, pears, cultured dairy products, cooked beef, and cooked chicken. As a product of fermentation and of cream ripened for churning, it is a colorless, or pale yellow, liquid or a white powder. It has a buttery odor and must be stored in a light-resistant container. Mildly toxic by injection under the skin. A moderate skin irritant. When heated to decomposition, it emits acrid smoke and fumes. GRAS. ASP

ACETOLAMIDE • *n*-Acetyl Ethanolamine. Used in hair-waving solutions and in emulsifiers. *See* Ethanolamines.

ACETONE • A colorless, ethereal liquid derived by oxidation or fermentation and used as a denaturant (*see*) and as a solvent in nail polish removers and nail finishes. It is obtained by fermentation and is frequently used as a solvent for airplane glue, fats, oils, and waxes. It can cause peeling and splitting of the nails, skin rashes on the fingers and elsewhere, and nail brittleness. Inhalation may irritate the lungs, and in large amounts it is narcotic, causing symptoms of drunkenness similar to ethanol (*see*). In 1992, the FDA proposed a ban on acetone in astringent (*see*) products because it had not been shown to be safe and effective as claimed.

ACETONITRILE • Methylacyanide. Colorless liquid with a pleasant odor. Used as a solvent in extraction processes and for separation of fatty acids from vegetable oils. Also used in nail glue remover and fragrances. Toxic by skin absorption and inhalation. On the Canadian Hotlist (*see*). Banned in cosmetics by ASEAN and the UK except in fragrances. It is number 184 on the CERCLA (*see*) Priority List of Hazardous Substances. *See also* Artificial Nail Remover.

3-(a-ACETONYLBENZYL)-4-HYDROXYCOUMARMIN AND ITS SALTS • Banned in the United Kingdom except in fragrances. *See* Acetone, Benzene, and Coumarin.

ACETOPHENETIDIN • *See* Phenacetin.

1-ACETOXY-2-METHYLNAPHTHALENE • A hair coloring. *See* Naphthalene.

ACETUM • *See* Vinegar.

ACETYL ACETONE • *See* Pentane.

ACETYL ARGININE • *See* Arginine and Vinegar.

ACETYL BENZOYL PEROXIDE • Benzo-benzone. White crystals that decompose slowly. It is an active germicide and disinfectant and is used for bleaching flour. It is toxic by ingestion and a strong irritant to the skin and mucous membranes. Benzoyl peroxide is on the Canadian Hotlist (*see*). Also banned by the EU in cosmetics.

ACETYL CYSTEINE • Used in skin products as an antioxidant and conditioner. In medicines, it is used to relieve mucous congestion of the nose, sinuses, and airways. Because it alters the action of mucus in the stomach, acetylcysteine has been found to cause digestive problems, especially in people with peptic ulcers.

ACETYL DIPEPTIDE-1 CETYL ESTER • Amino acids combined with esters (*see both*), it is used in hair and skin conditioners.

N-ACETYL DISHYDROSPHINGOSINE • An alcohol combined with an amide (*see both*), it is used in skin and hair conditioners.

ACETYL ETHYL TETRAMETHYL TETRALIN (AETT) • While not banned, the FDA frowns upon its use because it has been found to cause serious neurotoxic disorders and discoloration of internal organs. UK has banned it in cosmetics except for fragrances.

ACETYL GLUCOSAMINE • Used as a skin-conditioning ingredient in cosmetics, glucosamine is found in chitin (*see*), cell membranes, and protein and sugar complexes in the blood. It has become popular as an anti-osteoarthritis medication.

ACETYL GLUTAMIC ACID • Used in skin conditioners. *See* Glutamic Acid and Acetylated.

ACETYL GLUTAMINE • Used in skin conditioners. *See* Glutamic Acid and Acetylated.

ACETYL GLYCERYL RICINOLEATE • Used in skin conditioners. *See* Castor Oil.

ACETYL HEXAMETHYL INDAN • A fragrance ingredient. Derived from coal tar, it may be irritating to the skin and eyes.

ACETYL HEXAMETHYL TETRALIN • Used in perfumes, it is closely related to acetyl ethyl tetramethyl tetralin, which was voluntarily removed from perfumes when it was reported that it caused nerve damage in animals. The "hexyl" component was inserted to make the fragrances less volatile and less allergenic.

ACETYL HEXAPEPTIDE-1 • Derived from proteins, it is used in skin conditioners. It is a "tanning" ingredient.

ACETYL HEXAPEPTIDE-3 • Argireline. It is an artificially created peptide (a chain of six amino acids) developed by a Spanish company, and it works by limiting the nerve signals that tell your facial muscles to move (so the effect is something like Botox). It is claimed to relax muscle contractions within minutes of application. It does not paralyze muscles like Botox but reduces muscle contractions. In testing, acetyl hexapeptide-3 reduced wrinkle depth by reportedly 27 percent after thirty days of daily use, the company says. Long-term use of this active ingredient is supposed to produce a benefit similar to Botox and lines can become more shallow and less pronounced in time. Little scientific research has been done to prove this works, which doesn't mean that it may be without value.

ACETYL HISTIDINE • Derived from protein, it is an amino acid used in emollients and other skin creams as a humectant (*see*).

ACETYL MANDELIC ACID • A pH (*see*) adjuster. *See Mandelic Acid.*

ACETYL METHIONINE • Methenamine, used to process fat in cosmetics. An acetylated (*see*) amino acid (*see*) used in skin conditioners.

ACETYL PENTAPEPTIDE-1 • Derived from proteins, it is used in skin conditioners.

ACETYL PROPIONYL • Yellow liquid. Soluble in water. Used as a butterscotch or chocolate-type flavoring. *See* Propionic Acid.

ACETYL TETRAPEPTIDE-2 • Derived from proteins, it is used in skin conditioners.

ACETYL TRIBUTYL CITRATE • A fragrance ingredient and plasticizer used in nail polish products and eyebrow pencils, eyeliners, mascara, and mudpacks.

ACETYL TRIETHYL CITRATE • A clear, oily, essentially odorless liquid used as a solvent. *See* Citric Acid.

ACETYL TRIETHYLHEXYL CITRATE • A plasticizer and emollient.

ACETYL TRIPEPTIDE-1 • Derived from proteins, it is used in skin conditioners.

ACETYL TRIOCTYL CITRATE PECTIN • Citrus Pectin. A jelly-forming powder obtained from citrus peel and used as a texturizer and thickening ingredient to form gels with sugars and acids. Light in color.

ACETYL TYROSINE • Used in suntan gels, creams, and liquids. Widely distributed amino acid (*see*), termed nonessential because it does not seem to be necessary for growth. It is used as a dietary supplement. It is a building block of protein and is used in cosmetics to help creams penetrate the skin. The FDA has asked for further study of this additive that is GRAS. *See* Acetylated.

ACETYL VALERYL • *See* Valeric Acid and Acetic Acid.

ACETYLATED • Any organic compound that has been heated with acetic anhydride or acetyl chloride to remove its water. Acetylated lanolins are used in hand creams and lotions, for instance. Acetic anhydride produces irritation and necrosis of tissues in the vapor state and carries a warning against contact with skin and eyes.

ACETYLATED CASTOR OIL • Skin conditioner. *See* Castor Oil and Acetate.

ACETYLATED CETYL HYDROXYPROLINATE • Used in skin conditioners, it is derived from ammonia and amino acids (*see both*).

ACETYLATED GLYCOL STEARATE • Used as an emulsifying ingredient, stabilizer, and skin conditioner. *See* Acetylated and Glycols.

ACETYLATED HYDROGENATED COTTONSEED GLYCERIDE • Used as a skin conditioner and emollient. *See* Cottonseed Oil.

ACETYLATED HYDROGENATED LANOLIN • Skin conditioner. *See* Lanolin and Hydrogenation.

ACETYLATED HYDROGENATED LARD GLYCERIDE • Skin conditioner ingredient. *See* Lard.

ACETYLATED HYDROGENATED TALLOW GLYCERIDES • Skin conditioner ingredient. *See* Tallow and Hydrogenation.

ACETYLATED HYDROGENATED VEGETABLE GLYCERIDE • *See* Vegetable Oils.

ACETYLATED LANOLIN • An emulsifier and emollient. Repels water better than plain lanolin and does not form emulsions. It is used as a water-resistant film when applied to the skin and reduces water loss through the skin. It is used as an emollient and gives that "velvety feel" to baby products and to skin, hair, and bath preparations such as creams, lotions, powders, and sprays. It is used in lipsticks, creams, shaving preparations, cleansing products such as cold creams, liquids, and pads, and eye makeup as well as hair conditioners. It is also in suntan gels and mud packs. The CIR Expert Panel (*see*) found it safe in the early 1980s but is considering new information to determine if the final safety assessment should be reaffirmed, amended, or have an addendum. *See* Lanolin.

ACETYLATED LANOLIN ALCOHOL • Hair and skin conditioner. Used in eye shadows, skin moisturizers, talcum, suntan gels, hair grooming aids, colognes, and toilet water as well as bath soaps and baby powders. The CIR Expert Panel (*see*) found it safe. *See* Acetylated Lanolin.

ACETYLATED LANOLIN RICINOLEATE • A lanolin derivative, it is a skin conditioner. *See* Lanolin and Castor Oil.

ACETYLATED LARD GLYCERIDE • An emollient and skin conditioner. *See* Lard and Glycerol.

ACETYLATED PALM-KERNEL GLYCERIDES • *See* Acetylated and Palm Kernel Oil.

ACETYLATED SUCROSE DISTEARATE • Ingredient in skin conditioners. *See* Sucrose.

ACETYLATED TALLOW • *See* Acetylated and Tallow.

ACETYLCHOLINE AND ITS SALTS • Used as a catalyst in cosmetics. A chemical neurotransmitter that is released by nerve cells and stimulates either other nerve cells or muscles and organs throughout the body. This neurotransmitter is believed to be involved in memory function. Acetylcholine also dilates the blood vessels and helps to move food through the intestines. In a chloride solution for the eye, it causes contraction of the iris, resulting in contraction of the pupil. Used after eye surgery. No adverse reactions reported for a 1 percent solution. On the Canadian Hotlist (*see*). ASEAN has banned it and its salts in cosmetics. The United Kingdom has banned it except for use in fragrances.

ACETYLENE CHLORIDE • Used in the manufacture of cosmetics. *See* Vinyl Chloride.

ACETYLENE DIUREA/FORMALDEHYDE/TOSYLAMIDE CROSSPOLY-MER • A film former. *See* Formaldehyde.

ACETYLISOEUGENOL • Isoeugenol acetate. White crystals with a spicy, clovelike odor, it is used in perfumery, especially for carnation-type odors and for flavoring.

ACETYLMETHIONYL METHYLSILANOL ELASTINATE • A protein derivative, it is an ester of methionine and elastin (*see*). Used in hair and skin conditioners.

ACETYLPHYTOSPHINGOSINE • Derived from proteins, it is used in hair and skin conditioners.

ACETYLMETHYLCARBINOL • *See* Acetoin.

ACETYL-P-AMINOPHENOL • *See* Phenyl Acetaldehyde.

ACETYLSALICYLIC ACID • *See* Aspirin.

ACHILLEA MILLEFOLIUM • An extract of yarrow (*see*), it is widely used in hair dressings and other hair grooming aids, shampoos, skin care products, face masks, and cleansing lotions, liquids, and pads.

ACHYRANTHES FAURIEI • Hinatainokozuchi. Japanese weed that belongs to the cockscomb family, contains a steroidlike substance. This species possesses sharp spines at the bases of the utricles and is thus a possible source of mechanical injury. Phototoxicity following ingestion has also been reported. *See* Amaranthus Caudatus.

ACHYROCLINE SATUREOIDES • Macela, marcela, birabira, marcela-damata, hembra marcela, Juan blanco, macela-do-campo, marcela hembra, camomila-nacional, marcelita, mirabira, viravira, wirawira, yatey-caa, yerba de chivo. A medium-size aromatic annual herb that produces small white flowers with yellow centers and serrated green leaves. It is indigenous to much of tropical South and Central America and is found throughout Brazil. It is widely used in folk medicine. Used for its anti-inflammatory and analgesic actions in skin products.

ACID • An acid is a substance capable of turning blue litmus paper red and of forming hydrogen ions when dissolved in water. An acid aqueous solution is one that has a pH (*see*) of less than 7. Water has a pH of 7. Citric acid, widely used in cosmetics, has a 2.3 to 3.5 pH in solutions.

ACID AMMONIUM SULFATE • *See* Quaternary Ammonium Compounds.

ACID BLACK 1 • A diazo dye (*see*).

ACID BLACK 52 • A monoazo color (*see*).

ACID BLACK 131 • Nigrosine. It is a greenish blue-black. Acid colors are made by adding acids such as adipic (*see*) and tartaric to obtain various shades. Toxicity depends upon ingredients used. *See Colors and Acid Dyes.*

ACID BLUE 1 • A triphenylmethane group (*see*) color.

ACID BLUE 3 • A triphenylmethane group (*see*) color.

ACID BLUE 9 • A triphenylmethane group (*see*) color.

ACID BLUE 9 ALUMINUM LAKE • *See* Triphenylmethane Group and Lakes, Color.

ACID BLUE 9 AMMONIUM SALT • A color classed chemically as a triphenylmethane group (*see*) color. The CTFA-adopted name for certified (*see*) batches of this color is FD & C Blue No. 1 (*see*).

ACID BLUE 62 • Classed chemically as an anthraquinone (*see*) color.

ACID BLUE 74 • An indigoid color.

ACID BLUE 74 ALUMINUM LAKE • *See* Indigo and Lakes, Color.

ACID BROWN 13 • A coal tar hair coloring. Classed as a nitro coloring.

ACID DYES • The ability of these dyes to color and to remain fast during washing and exposure to light varies greatly. The ones that give the best water and light fastness are the compounds that are combined with metals. They are widely used in inexpensive dyes for plastics, varnishes, and some pigments.

ACID FUCHSIN • *See* Azo Dyes.

ACID GREEN 1 • A nitro (*see*) color.

ACID GREEN 25 • Classed chemically as an anthraquinone (*see*) color, the name can be applied only to batches of uncertified colors. The CTFA-adopted name for certified (*see*) batches of this dye is D & C Green No. 5 (*see*).

ACID GREEN 50 • A triphenylmethane color. *See* Triphenylmethane Group and Acid Dyes.

ACID ORANGE 3 • A nitro (*see*) color. A hair dye ingredient, it is mutagenic. Oral cancer-causing studies in rats and mice did yield clear evidence of carcinogenic activity in female (but not in male) rats and in female mice. The results of a skin cancer study in mice exposed to hair dye formulations containing 0.2 percent Acid Orange 3 were negative. The CIR Expert Panel concluded that irritation and sensitization data on Acid Orange 3 are absent. Since the label requirements set by the FDA, however, advise patch-testing instruction, individuals who might have an irritation/sensitization reaction would be able to avoid significant exposure. On the basis of the animal and clinical data, the CIR Expert Panel concluded that Acid Orange 3 "is safe for use in hair dye formulations at concentrations less than 0.2 percent." *See also* Acid Dyes.

ACID ORANGE 6 • A monoazo color (*see*). *See also* Acid Dyes.

ACID ORANGE 7 • A color classed as a monoazo (*see*). The name can be used only when applied to uncertified batches of this dye.

ACID ORANGE 24 • A diazo dye (*see*), the name can be applied only to uncertified batches of this color. The CTFA adopted name for certified batches is D & C Brown No. 1 (*see*).

ACID RED 14 • A monoazo color (*see*).

ACID RED 18 • A coal tar hair coloring, it is classed as a monoazo color (*see*).

ACID RED 18 ALUMINUM LAKE • *See* Acid Red 18 and Lakes, Color.

ACID RED 27 • A monoazo color (*see*). The name can be used only when applied to batches of color that have not been certified (*see*). Use of this color certified as FD & C Red No. 2 is prohibited in cosmetic products in the United States. Its use as a cosmetic colorant may also be restricted in other countries.

ACID RED 33 • A monoazo color (*see*), the name can be applied only to uncertified batches. The CTFA-adopted name for certified (*see*) batches is D & C Red No. 33 (*see*).

ACID RED 35 • A monoazo color (*see*), it is the disodium salt of napthalenedisulfonic acid. It is very soluble. Determined by NIOSH to be a positive animal carcinogen.

ACID RED 51 • A xanthene color (*see*), the name can be applied only to uncertified batches of color. The CTFA-adopted name for certified (*see*) batches is FD & C Red No. 3 (*see*). This name can be used only when applied to batches of colors that have not been certified. Use of this color certified as FD & C Red No. 3 is prohibited in the United States. Its use as a cosmetic colorant may also be restricted in other countries.

ACID RED 52 • A xanthene color (*see*).

ACID RED 73 • A diazo dye (*see*).

ACID RED 87 • A xanthene color (*see*), it is the sodium salt of Solvent Red 43 (*see*). The name can be used only when applied to uncertified batches of this dye. The CTFA-adopted name for certified (*see*) batches is D & C Red No. 22 (*see*).

ACID RED 92 • A xanthene color (*see*), it is the sodium salt of Solvent Red 48 (*see*). The name can be applied only to uncertified batches of this dye. The CTFA-adopted name for certified (*see*) batches of color is FD & C Red No. 28 (*see*).

ACID RED 95 • A xanthene color (*see*), it is the sodium salt of Solvent Red 73 (*see*). The name can be applied only to uncertified batches of this dye. The CTFA-adopted name for certified (*see*) batches is D & C Orange No. 11 (*see*).

ACID RED 184 • A coal tar hair coloring classed as a monoazo color (*see*).

ACID RED 195 • A coal tar hair coloring classed as a monoazo color (*see*).

ACID VIOLET 9 • A coal tar dye used in hair coloring, it is classed as a xanthene color (*see*).

ACID VIOLET 43 • An anthraquinone (*see*) color, the name can be applied only to uncertified batches of this dye. The CTFA-adopted name for the certified (*see*) batches of this color is Ext. D & C Violet No. 2 (*see*).

ACID YELLOW 1 • A nitro color, the name can be applied only to uncertified batches of this dye. The CTFA-adopted name for the certified (*see*) batches of this color is Ext. D & C Yellow No. 7 (*see*).

ACID YELLOW 3 • A mixture of the disodium salts of the mono- and disulfonic acids of indanedione, a class of indirect-acting anticoagulants. The name can be applied only to uncertified batches of this dye. The CTFA-adopted name for the certified (*see*) batches of this color is D & C Yellow No. 10 (*see*).

ACID YELLOW 23 • A pyrazole (*see*) color, the name can be applied only to uncertified batches of this dye. The CTFA-adopted name for the certified (*see*) batches of this color is FD & C Yellow No. 5 (*see*).

ACID YELLOW 23 ALUMINUM LAKE • A coal tar color used in hair dye. *See* Acid Yellow 23 and Lakes, Color.

ACID YELLOW 73 • Classified as a coal tar dye, the name can be applied only to uncertified batches of this dye. The CTFA-adopted name for the certified (*see*) batches of this color is D & C Yellow No. 7 (*see*).

ACID YELLOW 73 SODIUM SALT • A fluoran color, the name can be applied only to uncertified batches of this dye.

ACID YELLOW 104 ALUMINUM LAKE • An insoluble salt of Sunset Yellow. The name may be used only when applied to batches of uncertified colorants. The CTFA name for certified (*see*) batches is FD & C Yellow No. 6 (*see*).

ACIDOPHILUS • *Lactobacillus acidophilus*. A type of bacteria that ferments milk and is used to treat intestinal disorders. It changes the intestinal flora. Yogurt containing live cultures of these bacteria reportedly decreases by a third the number of vaginal yeast infections in women. Acidophilus is used in emollients in cosmetics; it is also widely used to prevent and to relieve diarrhea, especially when taking antibiotics. *See also* Yogurt.

ACIDOPHILUS/GRAPE FERMENT • Obtained by the fermentation of grapes by acidophilus (*see*). Used in anti-aging skin creams. *See* Acidophilus and Grape Extract.

ACINTOL • *See* Tall Oil.

ACNE • Skin pores become plugged with an oily substance, sebum, and other materials such as pigment, dead cells, and bacteria. If the plug (comedo) remains just beneath the surface, it appears as a very small, round, whitish bump, a "whitehead." If it reaches the skin surface, it looks like a black dot, a "blackhead." In some cases, the plugged pore may burst, thereby releasing its oily contents into the surrounding tissue and causing inflammation. This results in the formation of pimples, pus-filled lesions, or even cysts, cavities containing a sticky fluid. When a makeup product claims that it does not cause comedos, it means it has not been found to plug pores and cause acne.

ACONITINE • Principal alkaloid of *Aconitum napellus* (*see*) and its salts. Banned by the ASEAN (*see*) in cosmetics. The UK bans it in cosmetics other than as a fragrance. *See* Aconitum Napellus Leaves and Roots.

ACONITUM NAPELLUS LEAVES AND ROOTS AND GALENICAL PREPARATIONS • Aconite is found in various regions, from hilltops to forests. It grows best in moist and dimly lit areas. The word *Aconite* is derived from Acona city, which is part of Eraclea country (Britinia, in Asia Minor). It is believed that the plant originated in Acona. "Aconite" also comes from the Greek word *acona*, which means rock, because the plant grows at the foot of mountains. *Aconitum reclinatum* Gray (white flowers) and *Aconitum uncinatum* (blue flowers) are found in the mountains of Georgia and northward to Ohio and New York, in shadowy woods, on slopes, and along creeks. When applied to the skin, it causes a tingling sensation followed by numbness. Aconite liniments were once used extensively to treat neuralgia, sciatica, and rheumatism. Aconite is a component of a number of multi-ingredient preparations. *Aconitum* species are used as anti-inflammatory agents in traditional Chinese medicine. The lethal dose for adults is about 5 milligrams, and it reputedly has been used as a murder weapon. Banned by the EU and ASEAN (*see*) in cosmetics.

ACOPHYLLUM NODOSUM • Brown algae. Used in skin conditioners. *See* Algae.

ACORNS • Akarn. The name means "fruit of the forest trees," and it is the nut of the oak. Acorns are used in teas and in food as a nutrient and to soothe skin. They contain tannins, flavonoids, sugar, starch, albumen, and fats. They were used by American Indians to treat diarrhea and as a food staple.

ACORUS CALAMUS • Sweet Flag. Sweet Sedge. Derived from the herb *Acorus calamus*. The rhizome contains essential oil, mucilage, glycosides, amino acid, and tannins. The oil is obtained by steam distillation of the stem or root and is used as a flavoring ingredient and in perfumery. Calamus root is an ancient Indian and Chinese herbal medicine used to treat acid stomach, irregular heart rhythm, low blood pressure, coughs, and lack of mental focus. Native Americans would chew the root to enable them to run long distances with increased stamina. Externally, it was used to induce a state of tranquility. Banned as a food additive by the FDA.

ACRYL GLUTAMATE • A surfactant. *See* Glutamate.

ACRYLAMIDE • Colorless, odorless crystals soluble in water and derived from acrylonitrile and sulfuric acid. It is used in the manufacture of dyes and adhesives, and in permanent-press fabrics, nail enamels, and face masks. It is toxic by skin absorption.

ACRYLAMIDE COPOLYMER • A film former and thickener. *See* Acrylamide.

ACRYLAMIDE/SODIUM ACRYLATE • A polymer of acrylamide and sodium acrylate monomers. *See* Acrylamide and Acrylates.

ACRYLAMIDES/DMAPA • Film-former on hair and skin. May cause allergic skin reaction. Used in hair products and moisturizers.

ACRYLATES/METHOXY PEG METHACRYLATE COPOLYMER • A film former used in hair fixatives. *See* Acrylamide and Acrylates.

ACRYLAMIDOPROPYLTRIMONIUM CHLORIDE/ACRYLAMIDE CO-POLYMER • An antistatic ingredient and film used in hair products. *See* Acrylamide.

ACRYLATES • Salts or esters of acrylic acid used as thickening ingredients and as constituents of nail polishes. Strong irritants. *See* Acrylic Monomer.

ACRYLATES/ACETOACETOXYETHYL METHACRYLATE COPOLYMER • A film former and hair fixative. Also used to thicken liquids. *See* Acrylates.

ACRYLATES/ACRYLAMIDE COPOLYMER • Provides a continuous film for nail enamels or to control film formation in hairsprays. *See* Acrylates.

ACRYLATES/C10–30 ALKYL ACRYLATE CROSSPOLYMER • Synthetic polymers (*see*) used in sunless tanning products. *See* Alkyl and Acrylates.

ACRYLATES/AMMONIUM METHACRYLATE COPOLYMER • *See* Acrylates and Ammonium.

ACRYLATES COPOLYMER • Synthetic polymers (*see*) made up of acrylic acid, methacrylic acid or one of their esters (*see*). Used as a binder, film former, hair fixative, and suspending ingredient. Widely used in cosmetics in such products as nail polish, blushers, base coats and undercoats, mascara, eye shadows, powders, makeup preparations, deodorants, cleansing products, and hairsprays. *See* Acrylates.

ACRYLATES/DIACETONEACRYLAMIDE COPOLYMER • A film former. *See* Acrylates Copolymer.

ACRYLATES/OCTYLACRYLAMIDE COPOLYMER • A film former. *See* Acrylates Copolymer.

ACRYLATES/STEARETH-50 ACRYLATE COPOLYMER • A thickening ingredient. *See* Acrylates Copolymer.

ACRYLIC MONOMER • A tough rubbery material first used in fake nails in the cosmetic industry. It was once used to fill teeth. Fake nails usually consist of acrylates, a catalyst such as peroxide, and a plasticizer (*see all*). To be effective, the compound must be stiff at room temperature. If inhaled, the acrylates can cause allergic reactions in humans. Lethal to rats when inhaled. Can penetrate rubber gloves. May contain hydroquinone, benzoyl peroxide, and tertiary amines (*see all*). Benzyol peroxide is on the Canadian Hotlist (*see*).

ACRYLIC RESINS • Polymers (*see*) of acrylics. Used in waxy oils, base coats, protective coatings, and waterproofing. If inhaled, acrylates (*see*) can cause allergic reactions in humans.

ACRYLINOLEIC ACID • *See* Cyclocarboxypropyloleic Acid.

ACRYLONITRILE COPOLYMERS • Used in packaging materials. When heated to decomposition it emits acrid smoke and irritating fumes. It is 274 on the CERCLA (*see*) Priority List of Hazardous Substances. The ECHA (*see*) says it should be SIN (substitute it now).

ACRYLONITRILE POLYMER WITH STYRENE • Used in coatings and films in packaging materials. No restrictions, but cyanide and its compounds are on the Community Right-to-Know List (*see*). The ECHA (*see*) advises SIN (substitute it now). *See also* Styrene.

ACTINIC DAMAGE • Skin damage caused by the sun.

ACTINIC KERATOSES • AK. Roughness and thickening of the skin caused by overexposure to the sun's ultraviolet rays. Actinic keratoses, also called solar keratoses, age spots, or liver spots, are scaly lesions that are often brown in color. The lesions usually begin to appear in middle age and may increase in number as individuals grow older. Although sometimes referred to as precancerous lesions, the actual incidence of squamous cell carcinoma in preexisting actinic keratoses is about 1 in 1,000 annually per individual.

The primary concern of patients seeking treatment for actinic keratoses is more often cosmetic than medical.

ACTINIDIA CHINENSIS • Derived from *Actinidia chinensis,* the kiwi plant. *See* Kiwi Extract.

ADANSONIA DIGITATA • Derived from *Adansonia digitata,* cream of tartar tree. The oil is used in skin conditioners. The powder is used as a thickening ingredient.

ADDITIVE • Substances added to cosmetics to improve, preserve, or make the user appear more attractive.

ADENINE • Vitamin B_4. Derived from tea or yeast. Used in skin conditioners.

ADENOSINE • White crystalline powder with mild saline or bitter taste. It is isolated by the hydrolysis of yeast nucleic acid.

ADENOSINE PHOSPHATE • *See* Adenosine Triphosphate.

ADENOSINE TRIPHOSPHATE • Adenylic Acid. An organic compound that is derived from adenosine (*see*). A fundamental unit of nucleic acid, it serves as a source of energy for biochemical transformation in plants, photosynthesis, and also for many chemical reactions in the body, especially those associated with muscular activity. Used in skin conditioners.

ADEPS BOVIS • Fat from cows. Name cannot be used on American labels but is used in European cosmetic labels. United States lists the ingredient as tallow.

ADEPS SUILLUS • Fat from swine. Name cannot be used on American labels but is used on European labels. United States lists the ingredient as lard.

ADI • Abbreviation for Acceptable Daily Intake.

ADIANTUM CAPILLUS-VENERIS • Derived from *Adiantum capillus-veneris*. *See* Maidenhair Fern Extract.

ADIPIC ACID • Hexanedoic Acid. Colorless, needlelike formations, fairly insoluble in water; found in beets. A buffering and neutralizing ingredient impervious to humidity. Used in hair color rinses, nylon manufacture, and plasticizers. Lethal to rats in large oral doses. No known human toxicity.

ADIPIC ACID DIHYDRAZIDE • The CIR Expert Panel (*see*) concludes the available data are insufficient to support the safety of this ingredient as used in cosmetic products. *See* Adipic Acid and Hydrazine. Hydrazine is banned in cosmetics by the EU.

ADIPIC ACID/EPOXYPROPYL DIETHYLENETRIAMINE COPOLYMER • A "bodying" ingredient and film former that combines chemically with the amino acid cysteine to give "body" to hair. Shampooing removes it.

ADIPIC ACID/NEOPENTYL GLYCOL/TRIMELLITIC ANHYDRIDE COPOLYMER • A film former. *See* Adipic Acid.

ADONIS VERNALIS AND ITS PREPARATIONS • False Hellebore. Bird's Eye. Found in the lime-rich soil of eastern and southern Europe and in Asia, it contains resins and plant hormones. It has been used as a tonic for the heart. It is used in cosmetics in some anti-aging creams. On the Canadian Hotlist (*see*). Banned in cosmetics by the EU and ASEAN (*see*). Allowed in fragrances by the UK.

ADRENAL GLAND • About the size of a grape, your two adrenal glands lie on top of each of your kidneys. Each adrenal gland has two parts. The first part is the medulla, which produces epinephrine and norepinephrine, two hormones that play a part in controlling your heart rate and blood pressure. Signals from your brain stimulate production of these hormones. The second part is the adrenal cortex, which produces three groups of steroid hormones. The hormones in one group control the levels of various chemicals in your body. For example, they prevent the loss of too much sodium and water into the urine. Aldosterone is the most important hormone in this group. The hormones in the second group have a number of functions. One is to help convert carbohydrates or starches into energy-providing glycogen in your liver. Hydrocortisone is the main hormone in this group. The third group consists of the male hormones androgen and the female hormones estrogen and progesterone. Anti-androgens with steroid structure banned from cosmetics by ASEAN (*see*).

ADSORBATE • A powdered flavor made by coating liquid flavoring on the surface of a powder such as cornstarch, salt, or maltodextrin (*see*).

ADSORPTION • The attachment of a substance such as a liquid or gas to the surface of a solid.

AEGOPODIUM PODAGRARIA • Derived from *Aegopodium podagraria*. *See* Saint John's Wort.

AEROSOL • Small particles of material suspended in gas.

AEROSOL SHAVING CREAMS • *See* Shaving Creams.

AEROSOLS • Many cosmetic sprays, particularly hair care products and fragrances, are sold in aerosol containers. The first aerosol patent was actually issued in 1899 but was not used until 1940, when insecticides were first packaged in self-dispensing gas-pressurized containers. Freon, the most commonly used group among aerosol gases, is a lung irritant and central nervous system depressant and in high concentrations can cause coma. More than a hundred people, mostly young Americans, have died from sniffing aerosol gases for "kicks." These gases can cause severe irregular heartbeat. In addition to Freon, hair sprays contain PVP (polyvinylpyrrolidone, *see*) or shellac. PVP is believed to be cancer-causing. In addition, thesaurosis, a condition in which there are foreign bodies in the lungs, has been found in persons subjected to repeated inhalation of hairsprays. The aerosol container can become a lethal weapon, acting as a flamethrower if near a fire and a shrapnel bomb if heated. It has been known to explode when placed too near a radiator or heater. Also, aerosol gases turn into toxic gases: fluorine, chlorine, hydrogen fluoride, and chloride, or even phosgene, a military poison gas. Aerosol hair dyes and "hot" shave creams were made possible by compartmentalization of the container. However, in the case of the hot shave cream, there was unreliable mixing of the chemicals and skin rashes resulted. In powder products, the inhalation of powder or the silicones can damage the lungs. In 1972, the Society of Cosmetic Chemists reported that powder aerosols evidence a high particle retention in the lungs and profound pulmonary effects. Tests showed large powder particles in twenty-three separate areas of the lungs. In addition, Freon, the propellant, cannot be considered inert, that is, lacking in chemical activity or in an expected biologic or pharmacologic effect. Many products have been placed in hand pump containers because of the concern about aerosols.

AESCULUS HIPPOCASTANUM • *See* Horse Chestnut.

AFTER-BATH LOTIONS • *See* Cologne.

AFTER-SHAVE LOTIONS • *See* Shaving Lotions.

AGAR • Japanese Isinglass. Used as an emulsifier and emollient in cosmetics and as a substitute for gelatin in foods. Extracted from various seaweeds found in the Pacific and Indian oceans and the Sea of Japan. It is also used as a bulk laxative. It is an occasional allergen.

AGAROSE • Extract of the seaweed *Graceilaria* and used in skin conditioners as a humectant and thickener.

AGAVE LECHUGUILLA • American Aloe. Native to the warm part of the United States and known by its heavy, stiff leaf and tall panicle or spike of candelabralike flowers. The leaves are used for juice, employed in cosmetics as an adhesive, and used in medicines as a diuretic. The fermented juice is popular in Mexico for its distilled spirit (mescal). Some species are cultivated for their fibers, which are used in thread and rope. No known skin toxicity.

AGE SPOTS • *See* Skin Bleach.

AGRIMONY EXTRACT • An extract of *Agrimonia eupatoria,* an herb found in north temperate regions. It has yellow flowers and bristly fruit. It contains tannins, flavonoids, nicotinic acids, vitamins B and K, iron, and essential oils. Mentioned in medical literature as early as 63 B.C., it has been used in American folk medicine as an astringent (*see*) and an analgesic, as well as to stop bleeding and to treat inflammations. It is also used in ointments and boluses to shrink hemorrhoids, as a tonic, and to treat abscesses in gout.

AGROPYRON REPENS • *See* Couch Grass Root Extract.

AGOUTI • A protein on melanocyte receptors that triggers melanin (*see*) production. It is being developed for skin lightener products.

AHA • Abbreviation for alpha-hydroxy acids (*see*).

AHNFELTIA CONCINNA • Derived from *Ahnfeltia concinna*. From an algae, it is used in skin conditioners.

AILANTHUS ALTISSIMA • Derived from *Ailanthus altissima,* a small family of East Indian and Chinese trees, also called tree of heaven. Used in skin conditioners.

AKA • Followed by a number this signifies the Japanese name for a coloring. Some are not approved for use in the United States but most are.

ALANINE • Colorless crystals derived from protein. Believed to be a nonessential amino acid. It is used in microbiological research and as a dietary supplement in the L and DL forms. The FDA has asked for supplementary information. It is now GRAS for addition to food. It caused cancer of the skin in mice and tumors when injected into their abdomens.

ALANROOT OIL • *Inula helenium.* Benzyl cyanide. Elacampade. Scabwort. Prohibited by UK and FDA when used as a fragrance ingredient. Harmful to the skin. Allergenic.

ALBUMEN • A group of simple proteins composed of nitrogen, carbon, hydrogen, oxygen, and sulfur that are soluble in water. Albumen is usually derived from egg white and employed as an emulsifier in foods and cosmetics. May cause a reaction to those allergic to eggs.

ALBUMIN • *See* Albumen.

ALCLOXA • Aluminum Chlorhydroxy Allantoinate. *See* Allantoin.

ALCOHOL • Ethyl Alcohol. Ethanol. Alcohol as a solvent is widely used in the cosmetic field. Many cosmetics consist largely of alcohol: after-shave lotion, bubble bath, cologne, cold cream, deodorant, freckle lotion, face packs, hair lacquer, hair tonic, liquid face powder, mouthwash, nail polish remover, perfume, preshaving lotion, shampoo, shaving cream, skin lotion, spray deodorant, suntan lotion and oil, and toilet water. Alcohol is manufactured by the fermentation of starch, sugar, and other carbohydrates. It is clear, colorless, and flammable, with a somewhat pleasant odor and a burning taste. Medicinally used externally as an antiseptic and internally as a stimulant and hypnotic. Absolute alcohol is ethyl alcohol to which a substance has been added to make it unfit for drinking. Rubbing alcohol contains not less than 68.5 percent and not more than 71.5 percent by volume of absolute alcohol and the remainder of denaturants, such as perfume oils. Since it is a fat solvent, alcohol can dry the hair and skin when used in excess. Toxic in large doses.

ALCOHOL DENAT • This identifies an approved formula of denaturants in accordance with the European Union's labeling. American manufacturers can use the traditional SD Alcohol (*see*) label or change to this.

ALCOHOL FREE • In the past this has meant that certain cosmetic products do not contain ethyl alcohol (or grain alcohol). Cosmetic products, however, may contain other alcohols, such as cetyl, stearyl, and cetearyl alcohol, or lanolin (*see all*), which are known as fatty alcohols.

ALDEHYDE, ALIPHATIC • A class of organic chemical compounds intermediate between acids and alcohols. Aldehyde contains less oxygen than acids and less hydrogen than alcohols. Formaldehyde (*see*), a preservative, is an example of an aldehyde widely used in cosmetics. Benzaldehyde and cinnamic aldehydes are used to scent perfumes. Most are irritating to the skin and gastrointestinal tract.

ALDIOXA • Aluminum Dihydroxy Allantoinate. Astringent, antiperspirant prepared with the skin-healing salts of aluminum chlorhydroxy allantoinate (*see*). Used as an astringent, keratolytic, tissue stimulant, and buffer in cosmetics. Nonsensitizing and non-irritating. The CIR Expert Panel (*see*) says that there is not enough information about this additive to judge its safety in cosmetics.

ALDOL • Made from acetaldehyde, which occurs naturally in apples, broccoli, cheese, coffee, grapefruit, and other vegetables and fruits. It is a colorless, thick liquid used in the manufacture of rubber and in perfumes. It has also been used as a sedative and hypnotic in medicine. May cause contact dermatitis.

ALEURITIC ACID • A yellowish solid obtained from shellac (*see*). It is used in perfumes.

ALEURITES MOLUCCANA • Kukui. Fatty acids derived from *Aleurites moluccana* are used in skin conditioners. *See* Kukui Nut Oil.

ALFALFA EXTRACT • Lucerne. Extract of *Medicago sativa*. A natural cola, liquor, and maple flavoring ingredient for beverages and cordials. Alfalfa is widely cultivated for forage and is a commercial source of chlorophyll. It is used in cosmetics as a source of proteins and vitamins.

ALGAE • From seaweed and pond scum. Algae is claimed to prevent wrinkles and to moisturize the skin, but the American Medical Association denies any validity for algae's therapeutic benefits. However, seaweed products are widely used in cosmetics for many purposes. *See* Alginates.

ALGIN • The sodium salt of alginic acid (*see*).

ALGINATES • All derivatives of alginic acid are designated "algin" (ammonium, calcium, potassium, and sodium). These gelatinous substances are obtained from certain seaweeds and used as emulsifiers in hand lotions and creams and as thickening ingredients in shampoos, wave sets, and lotions. They are also used as barrier ingredients (*see*) in hand creams and lotions, in the manufacture of celluloid, as an emulsifier in mineral oil, and in mucilage. Sodium alginate from brown seaweed is used as a thickener in dentifrices, but the FDA is testing the sodium form (largely used in ice cream) for short-term mutagenic birth-deforming, reproductive, and subacute effects. Alginates are also used as stabilizers and water retainers in many foods.

ALGINIC ACID • A stabilizer in cosmetics, it is obtained as a highly gelatinous precipitate. The sodium carbonate (*see*) extracts of brown dried seaweeds are treated with acid to achieve a gelatin. Resembles albumen or gelatin (*see both*). Alginic acid is slowly soluble in water, forming a very thick liquid.

ALIPHATIC ALDEHYDE • *See* Aldehyde.

ALIZARIN • Turkey Red. Occurs in the root of the madder plant and was known and used in ancient Egypt, Persia, and India. Today it is produced synthetically from anthracene, a coal tar. It yields different colors, depending upon the metals mixed with it. Colors used in cosmetics are turkey red, blue, orange, red, rose, black, violet, lilac, yellow, and dark brown. It is also used to dye wool. Can cause contact dermatitis.

ALKALI • The term originally covered the caustic and mild forms of potash and soda. Now a substance is regarded as an alkali if it gives hydroxyl ions in solution. An alkaline aqueous solution is one with a pH (*see*) greater than 7. Sodium bicarbonate is an example of an alkali that is used to neutralize excess acidity in cosmetics.

ALKALI SULFIDES • Alkaline Earth Sulfides. Depilatories. The EU calculates 2 percent as sulfur pH to 12.7. Label must list "Avoid contact with eyes."

ALKALOID • A vegetable substance with an organic nitrogen base capable of combining with acids to form crystalline salts. Alkaloids exert a strong biological response in humans, even in small amounts. Chemical alkaloids end in *-ine*, such as betaine from beets, caffeine from coffee beans, and cocaine from the leaves of the coca plant.

ALKANES • Hydrocarbons (*see*) that can be either gaseous, liquid, or solid. They occur naturally in petroleum and natural gas, and include methane, propane, and butane. Also called paraffin. The group of alkanes as a whole is called the alkane series or the methane or paraffin series. Its first six members are methane, ethane, propane, butane, pentane, and hexane. EU considers them a high priority for the study of potential adverse effects to the environment, and some may be cancer-causing agents.

ALKANET ROOT • *Alkanna tinctoria.* A red coloring obtained from extraction of the herblike tree root grown in Asia Minor and the Mediterranean. Its name is from the Spanish *alcana,* from the Arabic *al-hena,* for henna, *Lawsonia inermis.* Used as a copper or blue coloring (when combined with metals) for hair oils and other cosmetics. May be mixed with synthetic dyes for color tints. Formerly used as an astringent.

ALKANNIN • A red powder and the principal ingredient of alkanet root (*see*). Used as an astringent in cosmetics and to color cosmetics and food.

ALKANOMIDES • Fatty acid alcohols used chiefly as detergent additives. Also as low foam and rust protection and is ecologically friendly.

ALKANOLAMINES • Compounds used in cold creams and eyeliners as a solvent and to adjust pH (*see*) and composed of alcohols from alkene (a saturated fatty hydrocarbon) and amines (from ammonia). These compounds are viscous, colorless liquids that form soaps from fatty acids (*see*). Triethanolamine (*see*) is an example.

ALKOHL • A form of kohl (*see*) used in Saudi Arabia.

ALKYL • Meaning "from alcohol," usually derived from alkane. Any one of a series of saturated hydrocarbons such as methane. The introduction of one or more alkyls into a compound makes the product more soluble. The mixture is usually employed with surfactants (*see*), which have a tendency to float when not alkylated.

ALKYL ARYLPOLYETHYLENE GLYCOL ETHER • A dispersant for preshave lotions, but basically a wetting ingredient. It rarely sensitizes or irritates human skin.

ALKYL BENZENE SULFONATE • A detergent used in bubble bath and shampoo. Prolonged feeding to animals showed no evidence of toxicity, but such ingredients are known to be defatting and therefore drying to the skin.

ALKYL SODIUM SULFATES • Used in shampoos because they have cleaning power and wash out of the hair easier than soap. A basic alkyl sulfate shampoo formula: sodium lauryl sulfate, 15 percent; behenic acid, 3.5 percent (*see both*); water, 81.5 percent. These sulfates were developed by the Germans when vegetable fats and oils were scarce. A large number have been made. They are prepared from primary alcohols by treatment with chlorosulfuric or sulfuric acid. The alcohols are usually prepared from fatty acids (*see*). For example, lauric acid makes a soap effective in hard water. If it is reduced to lauryl alcohol and sulfated, it makes sodium lauryl sulfate, a widely used detergent. The alcohol sulfates are low in acute and chronic toxicity, but they may cause skin irritation.

ALKYL SULFATES • Surfactants (*see*) used in foods, drugs, and cosmetics. The Germans during World War II developed these compounds when vegetable fats and oils were scarce. A large number of alkyl sulfates have been prepared from primary alcohols by treatment with sulfuric acid; the alcohols are usually prepared from fatty acids (*see*). Alkyl sulfates are low in acute and chronic toxicity but may cause skin irritation. The final report to the FDA of the Select Committee on GRAS Substances stated in 1980 that there is no evidence in the available information that it is a hazard to the public when used as it is now and it should continue its GRAS status with limitations on amounts that can be added to food.

ALKYLAMIDO BETAINE COCOAMIDOPROPYL BETAINE • *See* Coconut Oil and Surfactants.

ALKYNE ALCOHOLS, THEIR ESTERS, ETHERS, AND SALTS • The following perfume ingredients have been banned or restricted in cosmetics by EU and ASEAN (*see*) because they may cause skin irritation: allyl cinnamate, allyl cyclohexaneacetate, allyl cyclohexanepropionate, allyl heptanoate, allyl hexanoate, allyl isovalerate, allyl octanoate, allyl phenoxyacetate, allyl phenylacetate, and allyl 3,5,5-trimethylhexanoate.

ALLANTOIN • Used in cold creams, hand lotions, hair lotions, after-shave lotions, and other skin-soothing cosmetics because of its ability to help heal wounds and skin ulcers and to stimulate the growth of healthy tissue. Colorless crystals, soluble in hot water, it is prepared synthetically by the oxidation of uric acid (*see*) or by heating uric acid with dichloroacetic acid.

ALLANTOIN ACETYL METHIONINE • *See* Allantoin.

ALLANTOIN ASCORBATE • Allantoin (*see*) with ascorbic acid (*see*) salt.

ALLANTOIN BIOTIN • Allantoin (*see*) with B-complex vitamins.

ALLANTOIN CALCIUM PANTOTHENATE • A combination of the salt of the B-complex vitamin and the healing ingredient allantoin (*see*). Used to soothe the skin in emollients.

ALLANTOIN GALACTURONIC ACID • Allantoin (*see*) and galacturonic acid, which is derived from pectin (*see*). Used for skin soothing, conditioning, and protection.

ALLANTOIN GLYCYRRHETINIC ACID • Used as a skin-protecting and -soothing agent. The CIR Expert Panel (*see*) has listed this as top priority for review. *See* Allantoin and the derivative of licorice root, Glycyrrhetinic Acid.

ALLANTOIN POLYGALACTURONIC ACID • *See* Allantoin and Galacturonic Acid.

ALLANTOINATE • A salt of allantoin (*see*).

ALLERGEN • A substance that provokes an allergic reaction in the susceptible but does not normally affect other people. Plant pollens, fungi spores, and animal danders are some of the common allergens.

ALLERGIC CONTACT DERMATITIS • ACD. Skin rash caused by direct contact with a substance to which the skin is sensitive. Symptoms include a red rash, swelling, and intense itching. Blisters may develop and break open, forming a crust. In severe cases, the rash and blisters may spread all over the body. A variety of substances can cause the condition. The most common is poison ivy. Others include industrial chemicals, metals, cosmetics, deodorants, mouthwashes, dyes, certain types of textiles, and medicines, as well as local treatments with ointments and local application of antibiotics. ACD may develop at any age. Its precise prevalence is unknown but is thought to affect a significant percentage of the population. The disease may be acute or chronic. It is less common than skin rashes caused by irritants but more serious because relapses commonly occur and may force a person to change jobs. Symptoms may appear seven to ten days after the first exposure to an allergen. More often, the allergic reaction doesn't develop for many years and may require many repeated low-level exposures. Once the sensitivity does develop, however, contact with the triggering allergen will produce symptoms within twenty-four to forty-eight hours. An attack builds in severity from one to seven days. Even without treatment, healing often occurs in one or two weeks, although it may take a month or longer. The rash does not spread on one's body, nor can it be spread to another person. The extension of the rash is caused by renewed contact with whatever triggered the initial outbreak. Some substances, such as film developers, rubber chemicals, and beryllium, can cause symptoms other than the classic red rash and blisters. In some cases, ACD may look like hives. Detailed questioning about the work and leisure activities and the pattern of the rash often reveals its source.

ALLERGIC REACTION • An adverse immune response following repeated contact with otherwise harmless substances such as pollens, molds, foods, cosmetics, and drugs.

ALLERGY • An altered immune response to a specific substance, such as ragweed or pollen, on reexposure to it.

ALLIUM CEPA OR SATIVUM • *See* Garlic Extract.

ALLYL ALCOHOL • Perfume ingredient. It is classified as a toxic and irritant substance. The EU says "Use only when the level of free allyl alcohol in the ester is less than 0.1%." And it further said that the restriction is based on the delayed irritant potential of allyl alcohol.

ALLYL ALPHA-IONONE • Synthetic scent. Reputedly the most floral and most violetlike of all the ionones (*see*). Used in detergents, alcoholic lotions, fabric softeners, antiperspirants, foam baths, bleaches, deodorant sticks, shampoos, detergents, and soap.

ALLYL CAPROATE • *See* Caprylic Acid.

ALLYL ISOTHIOCYANATE • *See* Mustard Oil. Banned by the EU and ASEAN (*see*) in cosmetics.

ALLYL HEPTANOATE • *See* Heptanoic Acid.

4-ALLYL-2-METHOXYPHENOL • *See* Eugenol.

ALLYL PELARGONATE • Liquid, fruity odor, used in flavors and perfumes.

ALMOND • *Prunus amygdalus.* The oil is obtained from a small tree grown in France, Spain, and Italy. Almond oil has been reported by researchers to lower cholesterol. It is used as a flavoring ingredient in the United States. It is distilled to remove dihydrocyanic acid (prussic acid), which is very toxic. Almond meal is used to create soothing skin preparations. Almond paste was a favorite early European cleanser. Almonds also contain amygdalin, which serves as the basis of laetrile, a controversial anticancer drug that the FDA will not permit to be sold on the market.

ALMOND MEAL • A powder obtained by pulverizing blanched almonds and used in various cosmetics and perfumes. It is used in skin abrasives. *See* Bitter Almond Oil for toxicity.

ALMOND MILK • A creamy mixture of blanched almonds, acacia (*see*), sugar, and water blended to a smooth paste and sieved. Used as a demulcent, especially in organic cosmetics. *See* Bitter Almond Oil.

ALMOND OIL • Used in brilliantines and spice flavorings. *See* Bitter Almond Oil.

ALMOND PASTE • A favorite early European cleanser. Made from the dried ripe seeds of the sweet almond. *See* Bitter Almond Oil for toxicity.

ALMONDAMIDE DEA • Fatty acids from almond (*see*).

ALMONDAMIDOPROPALKONIUM • Fatty acids derived from almond oil (*see*). Used as an antistatic ingredient and hair-conditioning ingredient.

ALNUS FIRMIFOLIA • Derived from *Alnus firmifolia,* a member of the alder family found in the Andes and north temperate zones. Has a woody, conelike fruit.

ALOE VERA • *Aloe perryi, A. barbadensis.* First-aid plant. A compound expressed from the leaf of the aloe, which is a South African lilylike plant. There are more than 300 species. Only a few have been used medicinally. Aloe is employed for its supposed softening benefits in skin creams. It contains 99.5 percent water, aloins, polysaccharides including glucosans, anthraquinones, glyco proteins, sterols, saponins, albumen, essential oil, silica, phosphate of lime, a trace of iron, and organic acids. Used medicinally for more than 3,000 years, it is referred to in the Bible. Ancient Egyptian women and today's women use it for softening benefits in skin creams. In the West, aloe gel, which is derived from the thin-walled mucilaginous cells of the plant, is considered an effective healing ingredient for the treatment of burns and injuries. A diluted liquid is taken daily for its enzyme-promoting activity. It is used to regulate menstruation. It is also used to counteract wrinkles and to regulate female hormones. Used in bitters, vermouth, and spice flavorings for beverages and alcoholic drinks. Cross-reacts with benzoin and Balsam Peru in those who are allergic to these compounds. In 1992, the FDA proposed a ban on aloes in oral menstrual drug products because it has not been shown to be safe and effective for its stated claims. There is no scientific evidence that aloe vera has any benefits in cosmetics according to the American Medical Association.

ALOE VERA GEL • *See* Aloe Vera.

ALOIN • A mixture of active principles obtained from aloe (*see*). Yellow crystals with a bitter taste. Cosmetics manufacturers eliminate it from their finished aloe vera gel because of adverse effects on the skin. Banned by the FDA in 1992 as an ingredient in laxatives.

ALPHA-ARBUTIN • White Mask. Skin whitener. Derived from bearberry (*see*), alpha-arbutin has long been praised as a natural skin brightener and has been used for several years throughout Asia. Formulations made with alpha-arbutin, a more stable and effective brightening ingredient than beta-arbutin, are offered in the form of a soft paper sheet presaturated with alpha-arbutin solution, along with moisturizing glycerin, serine, and botanical brighteners.

ALPHA BISABOLOL • A synthetic bisabolol.

ALPHA-GLUCAN OLIGOSACCHARIDE • A carbohydrate used in skin and hair conditioners.

ALPHA-HYDROXY ACIDS • AHA cosmetics are believed to have derived from the "chemical peels" that dermatologists and plastic surgeons have used for years. The peels, typically trichloroacetic acid, phenol, resorcinol, and salicylic acid, help remove undesirable signs of skin aging, such as discoloration, roughness, and wrinkling. The chemicals cause the skin to lose its outer layer, or peel off, revealing a fresher-looking layer of skin. Known as chemical exfoliation, the procedure is done in doctors' offices so that doctors can control the process and prevent deep skin burns from the highly acidic solutions. Cosmetics manufacturers began to market similar but milder versions of these chemical peels containing AHAs for salon and at-home use around 1989. They quickly caught on, and by 1992, mass marketing had begun. Typically, AHA products sold to consumers have an AHA concentration of 10 percent or less. The concentration of AHA products used by trained cosmetologists may run between 20 and 30 percent, while those used by doctors can range from 50 to 70 percent.

The following are the AHAs used in cosmetic products: glycolic acid, lactic acid, malic acid, citric acid, glycolic acid plus ammonium glycolate, alpha-hydroxyethanoic acid plus ammonium alpha-hydroxyethanoate, alpha-hydroxyoctanoic acid, alpha-hydroxycaprylic acid, hydroxycaprylic acid, mixed fruit acid, triple fruit acid, tri-alpha hydroxyfruit acids, sugarcane extract, alpha hydroxy and botanical complex, L-alpha hydroxy acid, glycomer in cross-linked fatty acids alpha nutrium. Though sold to consumers mainly in face and body creams and lotions, AHAs also can be found to a lesser degree in other cosmetics, such as shampoos and cuticle softeners. Available everywhere, from discount pharmacies to fine department stores, the products typically range in price from a few dollars to as much as $60 a bottle.

The FDA has a particular concern about AHAs because, unlike traditional cosmetics, AHAs seem capable of penetrating the skin barrier. In reviewing the limited data on AHAs, the FDA concluded in a 1996 report that certain formulations of AHA products can affect the skin in a manner similar to that of chemical peels—that is, increasing cell turnover rate and decreasing the thickness of the outer skin. The effect depends on the product's pH level (a measure of its acidity), the AHA concentration, and the AHA vehicle cream, as well as how the product is used (e.g., frequency of use and where on the skin it is applied). Sun sensitivity, an additional concern, arose as the FDA prepared its 1996 report on AHA safety. Some people who had reported adverse reactions cited increased sun sensitivity. In addition, one industry-sponsored study found that participants whose skin was exposed to 4 percent glycolic acid twice daily for twelve weeks developed minimal skin redness with

13 percent less ultraviolet (UV) radiation exposure than normal. Three participants developed minimal redness with 50 percent less UV exposure than normal. Another study that looked at the effects of glycolic acid on production of sunburn cells (markers for UV-induced skin damage) found that people who received the AHA product in the presence of UV radiation experienced twice the cell damage in areas where the AHA had been applied than those who were treated with the non-AHA product. The FDA's concern is that people who are sensitive to sunlight may be particularly susceptible to UV rays, which can damage the skin and, over a long period, can cause skin cancer.

In 1997, the CIR Expert Panel—the cosmetic industry's self-regulatory body for reviewing and addressing safety of cosmetic ingredients—concluded that the AHA's glycolic acid and lactic acid and their related chemical compounds are safe for use in products intended for consumer use when the AHA concentration is 10 percent or less, the final product has a pH of 3.5 or greater (lower numbers indicate greater acidity), the final product is formulated in such a way that it protects the skin from increased sun sensitivity, or its package directions tell consumers to use sunscreen products. For AHA products used by trained cosmetologists, the CIR Expert Panel concluded that formulations of glycolic acid and lactic acid at concentrations of 30 percent or less and a pH of 3.0 or greater intended for only "brief" use at one time followed by thorough rinsing and daily use of sun protection are safe. The panel's conclusions actually serve as guidelines for cosmetics manufacturers, Dr. Bailey of the PCPC says. "This means that each manufacturer of an AHA product should conduct appropriate testing on their products to measure whether or not the product increases the sensitivity of the user to UV radiation and, if so, should add sun protection to their product and warn consumers to take extra steps to protect themselves at all times."

Meanwhile, the FDA continues to study AHA safety. Scientists at the National Toxicology Program and the FDA studied hairless mice for one year under simulated solar light to determine the relationship between AHAs and increased risk for skin cancer. The mice did develop skin cancer from the simulated sun, but AHAs did not have an effect on the process—and in fact, salicylic acid *delayed* the appearance of skin tumors. The FDA and dermatologists will advise consumers who use AHA products to follow these precautions:

- Always protect your skin before going out during the day. Use a sunscreen product with an SPF (sun protection factor) of at least 15. Wear a hat with a brim of at least 4 inches (about 10 centimeters). Cover up with lightweight, loose-fitting, long-sleeved shirts and pants.

- Buy products with adequate label information: for example, a list of ingredients to see which AHA or other chemical acids are in the product; the name and address of the manufacturer or distributor, which can serve as the contact if a problem or question arises; and a statement about the product's AHA concentration and pH level. The first two pieces of information are mandatory; the third is optional. Consumers can call or write the manufacturer, however, to get information about a product's AHA concentration and pH level.

- Buy only products that comply with the CIR Expert Panel's 1997 recommendations—that is, products with an AHA concentration of 10 percent or less and a pH of 3.5 or greater.

- Do a skin-sensitivity test on a patch of skin if you are a first-time user of any AHA product or are using a different brand or a product with a different concentration or pH than you are used to.

- Follow the instructions on the label.
- Do not exceed recommended applications. You won't get "younger" any faster.
- Stop using the product immediately if you experience adverse reactions. Signs of adverse reactions include stinging, redness, itching, burning, pain, and bleeding or change in sun sensitivity. Even mild irritation is a sign that the product is causing damage. Despite what the manufacturer may indicate on the product label, dermatologists say cosmetics shouldn't sting or cause irritation.

The FDA issued a guidance in 2005 suggesting that AHA labels state the following: "Sunburn Alert: This product contains an alpha hydroxy acid (AHA) that may increase your skin's sensitivity to the sun and particularly the possibility of sunburn. Use a sunscreen and limit sun exposure while using this product and for a week afterwards." *See also* Salicylic Acid and Exfoliation.

ALPHA-LIPOIC ACID • Lipoic Acid. Thioctic Acid. Derived mainly from dietary sources such as spinach, liver, and brewer's yeast, although the body does manufacture small supplies of its own. Used as an antioxidant in skin creams to "fight age damage." Discovered in 1951, it was first thought to be a vitamin. Because it dissolves in both water and fat, this so-called universal antioxidant reportedly is more effective than most antioxidants in combating free radicals (*see*) and is able to scavenge more wayward free-radical cells than most antioxidants, which tend to dissolve in either fat or water but not both. Alpha-lipoic acid can reach tissues composed mainly of fat, such as the nervous system, as well as those made mainly of water, such as the heart. It is being studied as a treatment for diabetes.

ALPHA OLEFIN SULFONATE • *See* Sulfonated Oils.

ALPHA TERPINEOL • *See* Terpineol.

ALPHA TOCOPHEROL • *See* Tocopherols and Vitamin E.

ALTHEA ROOT • *Hibiscus moscheutos.* Marshmallow Root. A natural substance from a plant grown in Europe, Asia, and the United States. The roots, flowers, and leaves are used externally as a poultice. The dried root is used in strawberry, cherry, and root beer flavorings for beverages. The boiled root is used in ointment to soothe skin and mucous membranes.

ALTHEA ROSEA POWDER • The dried, crushed flowers of *Althea rosea. See* Marshmallow Root.

ALUM • Potash Alum. Aluminum Ammonium. Potassium Sulfate. A colorless, odorless, crystalline, water-soluble solid used in astringent lotions, after-shave lotions, and as a styptic (stops bleeding). Also used to prevent aluminum chloride (*see*) from causing skin irritation in antiperspirants. In concentrated solutions, alum has produced gum damage and fatal intestinal hemorrhages. It has a low toxicity in experimental animals, but ingestion of 30 grams (an ounce) has killed an adult human. It is also known to cause kidney damage. The Food and Drug Administration issued a notice in 1992 that potassium alum and ammonium alum have not been shown to be safe and effective for stated claims in OTC products, including astringent drug products. No specific harmful effects reported in cosmetics.

ALUMINA • A natural or synthetic oxide of aluminum occurring in nature as bauxite and corundum. The aluminum hydroxide (*see*) formed is washed, dried, and used as an extender for cosmetic colors in which opacity is not desired. High concentrations of alumina may be irritating to the respiratory tract, and lung problems have been reported in alumina workers. No known skin toxicity.

ALUMINUM ACETATE • Burow's Solution. A mixture including acetic acid and boric acid, with astringent and antiseptic properties, used in astringent lotions, antiperspirants, deodorants, and protective creams. It is also used as a fur dye, in fabric finishes, in waterproofing, and as a disinfectant by embalmers. Ingestion of large doses can cause nausea and vomiting, diarrhea, and bleeding. Prolonged and continuous exposure can produce severe sloughing of the skin. It also causes skin rashes in some persons.

ALUMINUM BEHENATE • The aluminum (*see*) salt of behenic acid (*see*).

ALUMINUM BENZOATE • *See* Aluminum Salts and Benzoic Acid.

ALUMINUM BROMOHYDRATE • Aluminum Bromide. White, yellowish, deliquescent crystals derived by passing bromine over heated aluminum. The waterless form is highly corrosive to the skin. It is used in bromation, alkylation, and isomerization. EU bans bromine in cosmetics.

ALUMINUM CAPRYLATE • *See* Aluminum Salts.

ALUMINUM CHLORHYDROXIDE • *See* Aluminum Chlorohydrate.

ALUMINUM CHLORHYDROXY ALLANTOINATE • Used in after-shave lotions and other astringents. Also used as a buffer. Nonsensitizing and nonirritating. *See* Allantoin.

ALUMINUM CHLORIDE • The first antiperspirant salt to be used for commercial antiperspirant products and still the strongest available in effectiveness. It is also antiseptic but can be irritating to sensitive skin, and it does cause allergic reactions in susceptible people. Lethal to mammals upon ingestion of large doses.

ALUMINUM CHLOROHYDRATE • The most frequently used antiperspirant in the United States. Causes occasional infections of the hair follicles. May be irritating to abraded skin and may also cause allergic reactions, but it is considered by cosmetic manufacturers as one of the least irritating of the aluminum salts.

ALUMINUM CHLOROHYDRATE COMPLEX • *See* Aluminum Chlorohydrate.

ALUMINUM CHLOROHYDREX • A derivative of aluminum chlorohydrate (*see*) combined with propylene glycol, making it soluble in alcohol. It is used in deodorants and in antiperspirants. *See* Aluminum Salts.

ALUMINUM CITRATE • The salt of aluminum hydroxide and citric acid. *See* Aluminum Salts.

ALUMINUM DIACETATE • *See* Aluminum Salts.

ALUMINUM DICETYL PHOSPHATE • An aluminum salt used as an emulsion stabilizer. *See* Aluminum Salts.

ALUMINUM DICHLOROHYDRATE • An antiperspirant ingredient. *See* Aluminum Salts.

ALUMINUM DICHLOROHYDREX PEG AND PG • Aluminum dichlorate and propylene glycol in which some of the water molecules have been replaced by the propylene glycol. Used as an astringent. *See* Aluminum Salts and Propylene Glycol.

ALUMINUM DILINOLEATE • The aluminum salt of dilinoleic acid (*see*).

ALUMINUM DIMERATE • The aluminum salt of dimer acid. *See* Aluminum Salts.

ALUMINUM DIMYRISTATE • Used in soaps. *See* Aluminum Salts and Myristic Acid.

ALUMINUM DISTEARATE • A binder that holds loose powders together when compressed into a solid cake form. On the basis of the available information the CIR Expert Panel (*see*) found it safe in the early 1980s but is considering new information to determine if the final safety assessment should be reaffirmed, amended, or have an addendum. *See* Aluminum Stearates.

ALUMINUM FLUORIDE • Less toxic on ingestion than other fluorides, it is used to inhibit fermentation and in toothpaste. Fluorine concentration must not exceed 0.15

percent in a product. The EU label is required to say: "Contains aluminum fluoride." *See* Fluoride.

ALUMINUM FORMATE • Used as an antiperspirant to make other aluminum salts less acid and corrosive to fabrics. *See* Aluminum Salts and Formic Acid.

ALUMINUM GLYCINATE • *See* Aluminum Salts.

ALUMINUM HYDRATE • Gloss White. Usually obtained as a white, bulky, amorphous powder. Practically insoluble in water but soluble in alkaline solution. Used as an adsorbent, emulsifier, and alkali in detergents, antiperspirants, and dentifrices. Used medicinally as a gastric antacid. No longer permitted as a coloring in cosmetics.

ALUMINUM HYDROGENATED TALLOW GLUTAMATE • The aluminum salt of tallow (*see*) used in face powders.

ALUMINUM HYDROXIDE • Mild astringent and alkali used in antiperspirants, dentifrices, and dusting powders. A white, gelatinous mass used as a drying ingredient, catalyst, adsorbent, and coloring ingredient in many cosmetic processes. A leavening ingredient in the production of baked goods, as well as a gastric antacid in medicine. Practically insoluble in water but not in alkaline solutions. Aluminum hydroxide has a low toxicity but may cause constipation if ingested. No known skin toxicity. *See* Aluminum Salts and Deodorants.

ALUMINUM ISOSTEARATES/LAURATES/STEARATES • The aluminum salt of a mixture of isostearic acid, lauric acid, and stearic acid (*see all*). Used as a gelling ingredient.

ALUMINUM ISOSTEARATES/MYRISTATES • Myristate is the aluminum salt of a mixture of isostearic acid and myristic acid (*see both*). Used as a gelling ingredient.

ALUMINUM ISOSTEARATES/PALMITATES • Palmitate is the aluminum salt of palmitic acid (*see*) and isostearic acid (*see*). Used as a gelling ingredient.

ALUMINUM LACTATE • The aluminum salts of lactic acid (*see both*).

ALUMINUM LANOLATE • *See* Aluminum Salts.

ALUMINUM METHIONATE • *See* Aluminum Salts.

ALUMINUM MYRISTATES/PALMITATES • Myristate is the aluminum salt of a mixture of palmitic acid and isostearic acid (*see both*). Used as a gelling ingredient.

ALUMINUM PALMITATE • White granules, insoluble in water, used as a lubricant and waterproofing material. Employed as an antiperspirant. *See* Aluminum Salts and Deodorants.

ALUMINUM PCA • The aluminum salt of pyrrolidone carboxylic acid. It is used in skin conditioners. Pyrrolidone is derived from acetylene and formaldehyde. Carboxylic acid is a fatty acid.

ALUMINUM PHENOLSULFONATE • Aluminum Sulfocarbolate. Pink powder, soluble in water, used in preshave astringent-type lotions and spray deodorants for its antiseptic and detergent properties. It is also used in dusting powder. *See* Aluminum Sulfate for toxicity.

ALUMINUM PHOSPHATE • Aluminum Orthophosphate. White crystals, insoluble in water. Used in ceramics, dental cements, and cosmetics as a gelling ingredient. Corrosive to tissue.

ALUMINUM POWDER • A color additive composed of finely divided particles of aluminum. Used in face powders and hair colorings. Permanently listed by the FDA in 1977 for use as a coloring.

ALUMINUM SALTS • Aluminum Acetate. Aluminum Caprylate. Aluminum Chloride. Aluminum Chlorohydrate. Aluminum Diacetate. Aluminum Distearate. Aluminum Glycinate. Aluminum Hydroxide. Aluminum Lanolate. Aluminum Methionate. Aluminum Phenolsulfonate. Aluminum Silicate. Aluminum Stearate.

Aluminum Sulfate. Aluminum Tristearate. These are both the strong and weak acids of aluminum used in antiperspirants to combat body odors. The smell of sweat is caused by bacterial action on moisture. The salts are believed to prevent perspiration from reaching the skin by impeding the action of sweat and to act as an antibacterial. The strong salts may cause skin irritation and damage fabrics, particularly linens and cottons. Therefore, buffering ingredients are added by cosmetics manufacturers to counteract such adverse effects. The salts are also styptic (*see*).

ALUMINUM SESQUICHLOROHYDRATE • An aluminum salt used in antiperspirants and cleansing ingredients. In the United States, it may be used as an active OTC ingredient.

ALUMINUM SESQUICHLOROHYDREX • Aluminum Sesquichlorohydrex PG and PEG. A complex of aluminum sesquichlorohydrate and polyethylene glycol in which some of the water molecules attached to the metal have been replaced by the polyethylene glycol. In the United States, this compound may be used as an active ingredient in OTC drugs and is then called aluminum sesquichlorohydrex polyethylene glycol complex.

ALUMINUM SILICATE • A white mass, insoluble in water, obtained naturally from clay or synthesized, used as an anticaking and coloring ingredient in powders. Also used as an abrasive, bulking ingredient, and opacifying ingredient. Widely used in cold creams, cleansing lotions, dentifrices, mascara, and many other creams and lotions. Essentially harmless when given orally and when applied to skin. *See* Aluminum Salts.

ALUMINUM STARCH OCTENYLSUCCINATE • Dry Flow. Absorbent, anticaking ingredient and thickener, it is used in face powders, body and hand creams and lotions, powders, and after-shave talcs. It is also used in food powders and sprays, eyeliners, deodorants, fragrances, and suntan and tanning products. *See* Aluminum Phenolsulfonate.

ALUMINUM STEARATES • Hard, plasticlike materials used in waterproofing fabrics, in thickening lubricating oils, and as a chewing-gum base component and a defoamer component used in processing beet sugar and yeast. Aluminum tristearate is a hard plastic material used as a thickener and coloring in cosmetics. It is not an approved colorant in the United States. In the European Union, the name must be used, except for hair dye products. It is primarily used in soaps. On the basis of the available information, the CIR Expert Panel (*see*) found it safe in the early 1980s but is considering new information to determine if the final safety assessment should be reaffirmed, amended, or have an addendum.

ALUMINUM SUCROSE OCTASULFATE • The aluminum salt of sulfuric acid combined with sucrose (sugar). It is used in skin conditioners.

ALUMINUM SULFATE • Cake Alum. Colorless crystals, soluble in water, used as an antiseptic, astringent, and detergent in antiperspirants, deodorants, and skin fresheners; also purifies water. It may cause pimples under the arm when in antiperspirants and/or allergic reactions in some people. The Food and Drug Administration issued a notice in 1992 that aluminum sulfate has not been shown to be safe and effective for stated claims in OTC products.

ALUMINUM TRIFORMATE • The aluminum salt of formic acid used as a pH adjuster. *See* Formic Acid.

ALUMINUM TRIPALMITATE/TRIISOSTEARATE • *See* Aluminum Isostearates/ Palmitates.

ALUMINUM TRIPALMITATE/TRIMYRISTATE • *See* Aluminum Myristates/ Palmitates.

ALUMINUM TRISTEARATE • An opacifying ingredient and skin "conditioner."

Used in mascara, tonics, and other hair-grooming products as well as soaps and mascara. On the basis of the available information, the CIR Expert Panel (*see*) concludes that it is safe as a cosmetic ingredient. *See* Aluminum Stearates.

ALUMINUM UNDECYLENOYL COLLAGEN AMINO ACIDS • The aluminum salt of a collagen amino acid, it is used in hair colorings and skin creams as a conditioning ingredient. *See* Collagen and Amino Acids.

ALUMINUM ZINC OXIDE • An antidandruff ingredient, it is also used as a deodorant and opacifying agent. *See* Zinc Oxide.

ALUMINUM ZIRCONIUM HYDROXIDE COMPLEXES • Used as antiperspirant. Concentration restricted to 20 percent by the EU. It is prohibited in aerosol dispensers.

ALUMINUM ZIRCONIUM OCTACHLOROHYDRATE • An aluminum salt used in antiperspirants, astringents, and deodorants.

ALUMINUM ZIRCONIUM PENTACHLOROHYDRATE • An aluminum salt used in antiperspirants. *See* Aluminum Salts.

ALUMINUM ZIRCONIUM TETRACHLOROHYDRATE AND PEG • An aluminum salt of zirconium (*see both*) used in antiperspirants and deodorants.

ALUMINUM ZIRCONIUM TRICHLOROHYDRATE • *See* Aluminum Salts.

ALUMINUM ZIRCONIUM TRICHLOROHYDREX GLYC • Aluminum zirconium trichlorohydrate in which glycine (*see*) is added to replace some of the water molecules that normally cling to metal. It is used in nonaerosol antiperspirants. *See* Aluminum Salts.

AMALAKI • *Phyllanthus emblica.* An herb used for thousands of years in India to treat coughs and eating disorders and to normalize bowel function. It is also used to treat skin diseases and tumors.

AMARANTH • *See* FD & C Blue No. 2.

AMARANTHUS CAUDATUS • *Amaranthus hybridus.* Love-lies-bleeding. Red Cockscomb. An herb used for digestion, bleeding, diarrhea, menstrual pain, as a douche for vaginal discharge, dysentery, and as a food. It has astringent, nutrient, styptic, and diuretic properties and is high in vitamins A and C.

AMBER OIL, RECTIFIED • A perfume ingredient distilled from amber, a fossil resin of vegetable origin, and purified. The oil is pale yellow to yellowish brown and volatile, with a penetrating odor and an acrid taste.

AMBERGRIS • Concretion from the intestinal tract of the sperm whale found in tropical seas. About 80 percent cholesterol, it is a gray to black, waxy mass and is used for fixing delicate odors in perfumery. It is also used as a flavoring for food and beverages.

AMBRETTOLID • Formed in ambrette seed oil. Used as a flavoring and perfume fixative.

AMERCHOL • A series of surface-active lanolin derivatives. Most are soft solids used as emulsifiers and stabilizers for water and oil systems and emollients in cosmetics.

AMERICAN CENTAURY EXTRACT • Extract of the American centaury plant, *Sabatia angularis.* A member of the Gentian family, it is used by herbalists for jaundice. It is a strong antiseptic for cuts and scratches. Also used as a mouthwash.

AMES TEST • Dr. Bruce Ames, a biochemist at the University of California, developed a simple, inexpensive test using bacteria that reveals whether a chemical is a mutagen. Almost all chemicals that are known carcinogens have also been shown to be mutagenic on the Ames test. Whether the test can identify carcinogens is still controversial.

AMETHYST • A mineral consisting mostly of silicon dioxide, used as an abrasive. *See* Silicones.

AMIDE • Derived from ammonia. Used in cosmetics as thickeners, soil removers, and foam stabilizers. Also used as an anti-irritant to prevent "stinging" of other cosmetic ingredients. Cocoamide DEA is an example.

AMIDINOPROLINE • An amine (*see*) used as a humectant in skin conditioners.

AMIDO • Denoting a compound that contains ammonia.

AMINE ACID SURFACTANTS • Acyl Glutamate. Used as anti-irritants in cosmetics to prevent stinging of some cosmetic ingredients.

AMINE OXIDES • *See* Amine Acid Surfactants.

AMINES • A class of organic compounds derived from ammonia. They are basic in nature—synthetic derivatives of ammonium chloride, a salt that occurs naturally. Quaternary ammonium compounds (*see*) used in detergents are examples.

AMINO ACIDS • The body's building blocks, from which proteins are constructed. Of the twenty-two known amino acids, eight cannot be manufactured in the body in sufficient quantities to sustain healthy growth. These eight are called "essential" because they are necessary to maintain good health. A ninth, histidine, is thought to be necessary for growth only in childhood. Widely used in moisturizers and emollients because they are thought to help penetrate the skin.

AMINO BISPROPYL DIMETHICONE • A conditioning ingredient in hair products. *See* Siloxane.

2-AMINO-1,2-BIS(4-METHOXYPHENYL)ETHANOL AND ITS SALTS • Can cause allergic reactions. Banned in cosmetics by the EU and ASEAN (*see*).

AMINOACRYLATES • Contains an amino acid and an acrylate (*see both*).

***p*-AMINOBENZOIC ACID** • Part of the vitamin B complex and found in brewer's yeast, it is sold under a wide variety of names as a sunscreen lotion to prevent sun damage. Also used as a local anesthetic in sunburn products, and medicinally, to treat arthritis. In susceptible people, it can cause a sensitivity to light. In 1992, the FDA proposed a ban on aminobenzoic acid in internal analgesic products because it had not been shown to be safe and effective as claimed. *See* Para-Aminobenzoic Acid.

2-AMINOBUTANOL • An amine used as a pH adjuster. *See* Amino Acids.

AMINOBUTYRIC ACID • *See* Amino Acids and Butyric Acid.

AMINO CAPROIC ACID • *See* Amino Acids and Caproic Acid. Banned in cosmetics by EU and by ASEAN (*see*).

5-AMINO-4-CHLORO-*o*-CRESOL HCL • A hair coloring. *See o*-Cresol and *p*-Cresol.

2-AMINO-6-CHLORO-4-NITROPHENOL • A coal tar hair coloring. The CIR Expert Panel (*see*) concludes this ingredient is poorly absorbed through the skin, suggesting that any systemic effects were unlikely. The panel says that based on animal tests and clinical data this ingredient is safe for use at concentrations up to 2 percent. The EU Scientific Committee on Consumer Products (SCCP) ruled in 2005 that it is of the opinion that the use of 2-Amino-6-Chloro-4-Nitrophenol itself as a semi-permanent hair dye, or as a non-reactive colorant in oxidative hair dye formulations (after mixing with hydrogen peroxide at a ratio between 1:1 and 1:3) at a maximum concentration of 2.0 percent in the finished cosmetic product, does not pose a risk to the health of the consumer. Studies on genotoxicity/mutagenicity in finished hair dye formulations should be undertaken following the relevant SCCP opinions and in accordance with its Notes of Guidance. This hair dye, like many other hair dyes, is a skin sensitizer. *See* Resorcinol.

AMINO-*m*-CRESOL • A coal tar hair coloring. *See* Phenols.

4-AMINO-*m*-CRESOL • Hair coloring. In 2005, the EU evaluated studies and ruled that 4-amino-m-cresol itself as an oxidative hair dye at a maximum concentration of 1.5

percent in the finished cosmetic product (after mixing with hydrogen peroxide) does not pose a risk to the health of the consumer, apart from its sensitizing potential. However, studies on genotoxicity/mutagenicity in finished hair dye formulations should be undertaken following the relevant opinions of the Scientific Committee on Consumer Products and in accordance with its Notes of Guidance. *See* Resorcinol.

5-AMINODIMETHICONE • Used as a skin protectant and in hair sprays. *See* Dimethicone.

AMINODIMETHICONE HYDROXYSTERATE • *See* Amodimethicone and Stearates.

AMINO-2,6-DIMETHOXY-3-HYDROXY-PYRIDINE • A coal tar hair coloring. *See* Phenol.

AMINOETHYLACRYLATE PHOSPHATE/ACRYLATES COPOLYMER • Used in hair products as a film former. *See* Acrylates.

AMINOETHYLPHOSPHINIC ACID • A phosphorous compound used as an ingredient in skin-conditioning products.

AMINOETHYLPROPANEDIOL-AMPD-ACRYLAMIDE COPOLYMER • A synthetic polymer (*see*) containing an ester of methacrylic acid and used in hair sprays. *See* Acrylates.

AMINOETHYLANESULFINIC ACID • Hypotaurine. An amine (*see*) ingredient used as an antioxidant.

5-AMINO-4-FLUORO-2-METHYLPHENOL SULFATE • A hair coloring. *See* Phenols.

2-AMINO-4-HYDROXYETHYLAMINOANISOLE • A coal tar hair coloring. The EU gave manufacturers until July 2005 to submit safety information or the substance will be proposed for a ban. *See* Resorcinol. In 2006, based on the information provided, a margin of safety of 65 has been calculated, suggesting that 2-Amino-4-Hydroxyethylamino-Anisole and its sulfate is not safe for use as a hair dye and should be not present in hair dyes or other cosmetic products.

2-AMINO-3-HYDROXYPYRIDINE • A coal tar hair coloring. The EU gave manufacturers until July 2005 to submit safety information or the substance will be proposed for a ban. In 2008, the SCCP concluded that a formulation containing it in oxidative hair dye of 1.0 percent on the head does not pose a risk to the consumer. *See* Resorcinol and Coal Tar.

4-AMINO-2-HYDROXYTOLUENE • Used in the manufacture of hair dyes. The CIR Expert Panel (*see*) concludes this is a safe ingredient in cosmetics. The panel says that based on the weight of epidemiological studies with this ingredient, there is no indication of it causing cancer. The EU gave manufacturers until July 2005 to submit safety information or the substance will be proposed for a ban. The EU has banned it in cosmetics. *See* Toluene.

AMINOMETHYL-*p*-AMINOPHENOL HCL • A coal tar hair coloring. *See* Coal Tar and Phenols.

AMINOMETHYL PROPANEDIOL • Crystals made from nitrogen compounds that are soluble in alcohol and mixable with water. Used as an emulsifying ingredient for cosmetic creams and lotions and in mineral oils.

AMINOMETHYL PROPANOL • AMP. An alcohol made from nitrogen compounds; mixes with water. Soluble in alcohol and used as an emulsifying ingredient for cosmetic creams and lotions, deodorants, shampoos, after-shave lotions, moisturizers, cleansing products, and in hair sprays. Used in medicines that reduce body water. Prolonged skin exposure may cause irritation due to alkalinity, but in most commercial products the alkalinity is neutralized. It is used in cosmetics up to 10 percent. The available test data do not exceed 1 percent. Therefore, the CIR Expert Panel (*see*) says that concentrations not exceeding 1 percent are safe for use in cosmetics.

4-AMINO-2-NITROPHENOL • The SCCP (*see*) in 2008 concluded that, apart from the risks associated with the use of an extreme sensitizer, the use of 4-Amino-3-Nitrophenol as an ingredient in oxidative hair dye formulations with a maximum on-head concentration of 1.5 percent and in non-oxidative hair dye formulations with a maximum on-head concentration of 1.0 percent does not pose a risk to the health of the consumer. 4-Amino-3-Nitrophenol by itself does not have a relevant mutagenic potential. However, studies on genotoxicity/mutagenicity in finished hair dye formulations should be undertaken following the relevant SCCP opinions and in accordance with its use. Banned in cosmetics by ASEAN. *See* Resorcinol and Aminophenol.

AMINOPHENOL • *m*-Aminophenol. *o*-Aminophenol. *p*-Aminophenol. 2-Amino-5-Nitrophenol. 4-Amino-2-Nitrophenol. 2-Amino-6-Chloro-4-Nitrophenol. *p*-Aminophenol HCL. Aromatic, colorless crystals derived from phenols (*see*), used as intermediates (*see*) in orange-red and medium brown hair dyes. Discovered in London in 1854, aminophenols are also used in the manufacture of sulfur and azo dyes (*see*). Can cause a lack of oxygen in the blood but is less toxic than aniline (*see*) in animals. Solutions on the skin have produced restlessness and convulsions in humans as well as skin irritations. May also cause skin rashes and sensitization, and inhalation may cause asthma. These ingredients have been found to be mutagenic in laboratory tests. They are metabolized in a way similar to acetaminophen (Tylenol), which has been found to have a potential effect on the liver. The CIR Expert Panel (*see*) concluded that although the clinical data for the aminophenols are limited and skin tests in guinea pigs produced some sensitivity, the aminophenols are "safe as cosmetic ingredients in the present practices of use and concentrations." ASEAN has banned 2-amino-4-nitrophenol and 2-amino-5-nitrophenol in cosmetics.

***m*-AMINOPHENOL** • A hair colorant. Based on the information provided, the SCCP is of the opinion in 2006 that the use of *m*-Aminophenol itself as an oxidative hair dye substance at a maximum concentration of 1.2 percent in the finished cosmetic product (after mixing with hydrogen peroxide) does not pose a risk to the health of the consumer, apart from its sensitizing potential. *m*-Aminophenol itself has no mutagenic potential *in vivo*. However, studies on genotoxicity/mutagenicity in finished hair dye formulations should be undertaken following the relevant SCCNFP/SCCP guidance. *See* Aminophenol.

***o*-AMINOPHENOL** • A hair colorant. Banned in the EU and Canada. *See* Resorcinol and *m*-Aminophenol.

***p*-AMINOPHENOL** • A hair colorant. Banned in the EU and Canada. *See* *m*-Aminophenol.

***p*-AMINOPHENOL HCL** • A hair colorant. *See* *m*-Aminophenol.

AMINOPHYLLINE • An approved prescription drug used in the treatment of asthma, it is an ingredient used in many thigh creams (*see*). It is a diuretic (water reducer), blood vessel dilator, and heart stimulant. Its use in cosmetics is unwise and worries the FDA. On the Canadian Hotlist (*see*).

AMINOPROPYL ASCORBYL PHOSPHATE • Used as an antioxidant. *See* Ascorbic Acid.

AMINOPROPYL DIHYDROGEN PHOSPHATE • A skin-conditioning ingredient.

AMINOPROPYL DIMETHICONE • A hair-conditioning ingredient. *See* Dimethicone.

AMINOPROPYL LAURYLGLUTAMINE • An antistatic ingredient used in hair conditioners. Also used as a cleansing ingredient.

4-AMINOSALICYLIC ACID AND ITS SALTS. • Tebacin. Para-Aminosalicylic Acid (PAS). Pamisyl. Derived from phenol (*see*). Banned in cosmetics by the EU and ASEAN (*see*).

AMINOTRIAZINE PENTANE CARBOXAMIDE MIPA • Used in skin conditioners. *See* Amines.

AMLA • Indian Gooseberry. It has long been known in its native India for having protective antioxidant qualities and is increasingly being sought as an additive. It is a traditional Ayurvedic (*see*) rejuvenator and detoxifier. The fruits are widely used in India in jams, syrups, jellies, candies, pickled preserves, relishes, and tomato sauce. The fruit is also being used in functional foods and cosmetics to combat free radicals (*see*). The fruit also contains up to 2 percent natural vitamin C.

AMMI MAJUS AND ITS GALENICAL PREPARATIONS • Bishopsweed, Bishop's weed, Bullwort, Greater ammi, Lady's lace, Laceflower. Contains a furocoumarin in all parts of the plant, but it is especially concentrated in the seed. The compound is photoactive, causing primary photosensitization. Banned in cosmetics by the EU and ASEAN (*see*).

AMMONIA • Liquid obtained by blowing steam through incandescent coke. It is used in refrigerants, in the manufacture of permanent wave lotions and hair bleaches, in the manufacture of detergents, and in cleaning preparations. It may cause hair breakage when used in permanent waves and hair bleaches. It is also used in the manufacture of explosives and synthetic fabrics, herbicides, fertilizers, and pesticides and is one of the top five inorganic chemicals produced in the United States. It has been shown to produce cancer of the skin in human doses of 1,000 milligrams per kilogram of body weight. It is extremely toxic when inhaled in concentrated vapors, and is irritating to the eyes and mucous membranes. *See* Ammonium Hydroxide.

AMMONIA WATER • Ammonia gas dissolved in water. Used as an alkali (*see*) in metallic hair dyes, hair straighteners, and protective skin creams. Colorless with a very pungent odor, it is irritating to the eyes and mucous membranes. In strong solution, it can cause burns and blistering.

AMMONIATED MERCURY • Mercuric Chloride Ammoniated. A white, odorless powder with a metallic taste used in ointment form to combat skin infections and to treat eye disorders. All forms of mercury are poisonous. Topical application may lead to skin rash and other allergic manifestations. Prolonged use may cause skin pigmentation and, when applied too vigorously, it can be absorbed and result in systemic poisoning. Absorption or ingestion may lead to kidney damage. Ingestion also causes stomach pains and vomiting. No longer permitted in cosmetics except in small amounts as a preservative.

AMMONIUM ACETATE • The ammonium salt of acetic acid (*see*).

AMMONIUM ACRYLATES COPOLYMER • Binder and film former. *See* Acrylates.

AMMONIUM ACRYLOYLDIMETHYLTAURATE/VINYL FORMAMIDE COPOLYMER • Emulsion stabilizer and thickening ingredient.

AMMONIUM ALGINATE • *See* Alginates.

AMMONIUM C12–15 ALKYL SULFATE • *See* Quaternary Ammonium Compounds.

AMMONIUM ALUM • Used in astringents and mouthwashes. *See* Alum.

AMMONIUM BENZOATE • White crystals or powder used as a preservative. *See* Benzoic Acid.

AMMONIUM BETA-SISTOSTERYL SULFATE • A hair- and skin-conditioning ingredient. *See* Sterol.

AMMONIUM BICARBONATE • Used as a buffer in thioglycolate cold permanent wave lotions. Occurs in the urine of alligators. Usually prepared by passing carbon dioxide gas through concentrated ammonia water. Shiny, hard, colorless or white crystals; faint odor of ammonia. Used in baking powder formulas for cooling baths. Used medicinally as an expectorant and to break up intestinal gas. Also used in compost heaps to accelerate decomposition. *See* Ammonium Carbonate for toxicity.

AMMONIUM BISULFITE • Colorless, water-absorbing powder that is used as a catalyst in hair-waving formulations.

AMMONIUM CAPRYLETH SULFATE • Used in cleansing products. *See* Capric Acid.

AMMONIUM CARBAMATE • A pH adjuster. *See* pH and Ammonium.

AMMONIUM CARBONATE • A white, solid alkali derived partly from ammonium bicarbonate (*see*) and used as a neutralizer and buffer in permanent wave solutions and creams. It decomposes when exposed to air. Also used in baking powders, for defatting woolens, in fire extinguishers, and as an expectorant. Ammonium carbonate can cause skin rashes on the scalp, forehead, or hands.

AMMONIUM CASEINATE • A hair-conditioning ingredient and skin conditioner. *See* Casein.

AMMONIUM CHLORIDE • Ammonium salt that occurs naturally. Colorless, odorless crystals or white powder, saline in taste, and incompatible with alkalis. Used as an acidifier in permanent wave solutions, in eye lotions, and as a cooling and stimulating skin wash. Also used in bubble baths, hair bleaches, and shampoos. Industrially employed in freezing mixtures, batteries, dyes, safety explosives, and in medicine as a urinary acidifier and diuretic. Keeps snow from melting on ski slopes. If ingested, it can cause nausea, vomiting, and acidosis. As with any ammonia compound, concentrated solutions can be irritating to the skin.

AMMONIUM CITRATE • *See* Citric Acid.

AMMONIUM COCOMONOGLYCERIDES • *See* Coconut Oil and Sulfated Oil.

AMMONIUM COCOYL ISETHIONATE • A cleansing ingredient. *See* Coconut Oil.

AMMONIUM COCO-SULFATE • Used as an emulsifying ingredient and a cleanser. *See* Coconut Oil.

AMMONIUM CUMENE SULFONATE • Benzenesulfonic Acid. Methylated Ammonium Salt. Derived from coal tar or petroleum, it is used as a solvent. *See* Coal Tar.

AMMONIUM DICHROMATE • Orange needles used in dyeing red colors and in synthetic perfumes. Irritating to the eyes and skin, and a suspected carcinogen.

AMMONIUM DINONYL SULFOSUCCINATE • *See* Surfactants.

AMMONIUM DODECYLBENZENESULFONATE • Ammonium Lauryl Benzene Sulfonate. *See* Quaternary Ammonium Compounds and Surfactants.

AMMONIUM FLUORIDE • Used in oral care products and as an antiseptic. Corrosive to tissue. The EU calculates at 0.15 percent when mixed with fluorine compounds. Fluorine concentration must not exceed 0.50 percent. The EU label says "Contains ammonium fluoride." *See* Fluoride.

AMMONIUM FLUOROSILICATE • Strong irritant. Used in oral care products. EU calculates at 0.15 percent when mixed with other fluorine compounds. Fluorine concentration must not exceed 0.15 percent. The EU label says "Contains ammonium fluorosilicate." Also used in glass etching, electroplating, and as a disinfectant in the brewing industry. *See* Fluoride and Silicates.

AMMONIUM GLYCOLATE • A pH (*see*) adjuster widely used in cosmetics such as cold creams, cleansing ingredients, liquids and pads, moisturizing preparations, body and hand preparations (excluding shaving products), and skin care preparations. *See* Glycolic Acid.

AMMONIUM GLYCYRRHIZATE • The ammonium salt of glycyrrhizic acid (*see*). Used in cold creams, lotions, and moisturizers. Also used as a flavoring ingredient. *See* Quaternary Ammonium Compounds.

AMMONIUM HYDROXIDE (OTC) • Ammonia Water. A weak alkali formed when ammonia dissolves in water; exists only in solution. Irritating to the skin and mucous membranes. In 1992, the FDA proposed a ban on ammonium hydroxide in insect bites and sting drug products because it had not been shown to be safe and effective as claimed.

AMMONIUM HYDROLYZED COLLAGEN • Ammonium Hydrolyzed Protein. The ammonium salt of hydrolyzed animal protein. *See* Hydrolyzed Collagen and Surfactants.

AMMONIUM HYDROXIDE • Ammonia Water. A weak alkali formed when ammonia dissolves in water and exists only in solution. A clear, colorless liquid. It is used as a denaturant (*see*) and pH (*see*) adjuster. Used in hair dyes and colors, hair sprays, hair bleaches, mascara, hair conditioners, cold creams and cleansing lotions, shampoos, eyeliners, and shaving creams. It is also used in hair straighteners and as a detergent and for removing stains. It is irritating to the eyes and mucous membranes. It may cause hair breakage.

AMMONIUM IODIDE • An ammonium salt prepared from ammonia and iodine. White, odorless crystals with a sharp saline taste. The crystals become yellow and brown on exposure to air and light. Used in cosmetics as an antiseptic and preservative and in medicine as an expectorant. *See* Iodine for toxicity.

AMMONIUM ISOSTEARATE • The ammonium salts of isostearic acid (*see*). *See also* Surfactants.

AMMONIUM LACTATE • Used as a buffering ingredient, skin conditioner, and humectant. *See* Lactic Acid.

AMMONIUM LAURETH-8 CARBOXYLATE • *See* Lauric Acid and Polyethylene Glycol; *see also* Surfactants.

AMMONIUM LAURETH SULFATE • Ammonium Lauryl Ether Sulfate. A compound that breaks up and holds oils and soil so they can be easily removed from skin or hair. It is used in bubble baths, bath soaps, detergents, cold creams, cleansing lotions, liquids and pads, hair products, and hair rinses. *See* Lauryl Alcohol.

AMMONIUM LAUROYL SARCOSINATE • A hair-conditioning ingredient, surfactant, and cleansing ingredient. *See* Sarcosines.

AMMONIUM LAURYL SULFATE • The ammonium salt of lauryl sulfate derived from the natural coconut alcohols, it is a mild anionic surfactant (*see*) cleanser that is widely used at mild acidic pH values. On the basis of available information, the CIR Expert Panel (*see*) concludes that it is safe as presently used in cosmetic formulations designed for brief use followed by thorough rinsing from the surface of the skin. In products for prolonged contact with skin, concentrations should not exceed 1 percent. *See* Lauryl Alcohol.

AMMONIUM LAURYL SULFOSUCCINATE • *See* Surfactants.

AMMONIUM MONOFLUOROPHOSPHATE • Oral hygiene product EU calculates at 0.15 percent when mixed with other fluorine compounds. Fluorine concentration must not exceed 0.15 percent. The EU label must say: "Contains ammonium mono-fluorophosphate." *See* Fluorine Compounds.

AMMONIUM MONOOLEAMIDO • *See* Ammonia.

AMMONIUM MYRETH SULFATE • *See* Sodium Lauryl Sulfate.

AMMONIUM MYRISTYL SULFATE • The ammonium salt of myristyl sulfate. *See* Myristic Acid.

AMMONIUM NITRATE • Saltpeter. Colorless crystals derived from nitric acid. Used in herbicides and insecticides, as an oxidizer, as a nutrient for antibiotics and yeast, and as a catalyst.

AMMONIUM NONOXYNOL-4-SULFATE • Cleansing material that breaks up and holds oils and soil so that they may be removed easily from the skin or hair surface. Its use in hair colors requires a caution statement and patch test. It is also used in permanent waves, bubble baths, and other hair preparations.

AMMONIUM OLEATE • The ammonium salt of oleic acid (*see*), used as an emulsifying ingredient. It is used in soaps.

AMMONIUM PALM KERNEL SULFATE • A surfactant and cleansing ingredient. *See* Palm Kernel Oil.

AMMONIUM C12–15 PARETH SULFATE • Pareth-25–3 Sulfate. The ammonium salt of a sulfated polyethylene glycol ether and a mixture of C 1215 fatty alcohols (*see*), a cleansing ingredient. *See also* Ammonium Sulfate.

AMMONIUM C9–10 PERFLUOROALKYLSULFONATE • Surfactant (*see*).

AMMONIUM PERSULFATE • Ammonium Salt. Colorless crystals soluble in water, used as an oxidizer and bleach in dyes and skin lighteners. Also as a disinfectant, deodorant, and preservative. It may be irritating to the skin and mucous membranes. In cosmetics, may make hair brittle. Lethal to rats in large oral doses.

AMMONIUM PHENOLSULFONATE • The ammonium salt of phenol sulfonic acid. Used as a preservative and deodorant ingredient. *See* Quaternary Ammonium Compounds.

AMMONIUM PHOSPHATE • Ammonium Salt. An odorless, white or colorless crystalline powder with a cooling taste used in mouthwashes. It is also used in fireproofing textiles, paper, and wood.

AMMONIUM PHOSPHATIDYL RAPESEEDATE • A phosphorous compound, it is used as an emulsifier and stabilizer in emollients.

AMMONIUM POLYACRYLATE • An emulsion stabilizer. *See* Acrylates.

AMMONIUM POLYACRYLAOYLDIMETHYL TAURATE • Synthetic polymer used as a thickener and emulsion stabilizer. *See* Sulfonic Acid.

AMMONIUM PROPIONATE • A preservative. *See* Propionic Acid.

AMMONIUM SALICYLATE • *See* Salicylates.

AMMONIUM SILVER ZINC ALUMINUM SILICATE • A deodorant ingredient. *See* Zinc and Ammonium Nitrate.

AMMONIUM STEARATE • Stearic Acid. Ammonium Salt. A yellowish white powder used as a texturizer in vanishing creams. On the basis of the available information, the CIR Expert Panel (*see*) concludes that it is safe as a cosmetic ingredient.

AMMONIUM STYRENE/ACRYLATE COPOLYMER • Ammonium salt of a polymer of styrene and a monomer of acrylic acid and methacrylic acid used as an opacifier. *See* Acrylates.

AMMONIUM SULFATE • Ammonium Salt. A neutralizer in permanent wave lotions, it is odorless and colorless, either crystals or powder. Industrially used in freezing mixtures, fireproofing fabrics, and tanning. Used medicinally to prolong analgesia. Rats died when fed large doses.

AMMONIUM SULFIDE • A salt derived from sulfur and ammonium, it is used as a neutralizer in permanent wave lotions, as a depilatory, to apply patina to bronze, and in spice flavorings. It has been reported to have caused a death when ingested in a permanent wave solution. Irritating to the skin when used in depilatories.

AMMONIUM SULFITE • Ammonium salt made with sulfuric acid. White, crystalline, soluble in water, almost insoluble in alcohol and acetone. Antiseptic. A preservative in cold permanent waves. *See* Ammonia for toxicity.

AMMONIUM TALLATE • The ammonium salt of tall oil fatty acids. *See* Quaternary Ammonium Compounds.

AMMONIUM TARTRATE • *See* Tartaric Acid.

AMMONIUM THIOCYANATE • Colorless, water-absorbing crystals derived from ammonium cyanide. Used in fertilizers, curing resins, and adhesives. *See* Cyanide.

AMMONIUM THIOGLYCOLATE • The ammonium salt of thioglycolic acid, a liquid with a strong, unpleasant odor that is readily oxidized by air. A hair straightener, antioxidant, and depilatory, it can cause severe burns and blistering of the skin. Large doses injected into the stomachs of mice killed them. The CIR Expert Panel (*see*) concludes this ingredient can be used by individuals at concentrations of up to 14.4 percent if it is used infrequently. It is a cumulative irritant and weak sensitizer.

AMMONIUM THIOLACTATE • The ammonium salt of lactic acid (*see*). Used in permanent waves and in hair straighteners. *See* Thioglycolate.

AMMONIUM VA/ACRYLATES COPOLYMER • *See* Acrylates and Copolymer.

AMMONIUM VINYL ACETATE/ACRYLATES TERPOLYMER • *See* Acrylates.

AMMONIUM XYLENESULFONATE • Ammonium salt of xylene. A lacquer solvent used in nail polishes and in hair preparations. It may be narcotic in high doses. Chronic toxicity or skin effects are not known.

AMNIOTIC FLUID • The fluid surrounding the cow embryo in utero. It is promoted for benefits similar to those of human placenta (*see* Placental Extract) and has limited use in moisturizers, hair lotions, scalp treatments, and shampoos.

AMODIMETHICONE • The silicone polymer. Used in hair products including hair dyes and conditioners, permanent waves, shampoos, hair straighteners, and hair tonics. *See* Amino Acids and Silicones.

AMOMUM AROMATICUM • Derived from *Amomum aromaticum,* an aromatic herb grown in the tropics. It is a member of the Zingiber (ginger) family. It also includes species that bear cardamom and grains of paradise. *See* Ginger Oil.

AMOMUM XANTHIOIDES • A seed extract from a plant, *Amomum,* an Indian spice plant. A genus of aromatic plants. *See* Amomum Aromaticum.

AMORPHOPHALLUS KONJAC • Amorphophallus Konjac Root Powder. Used as an abrasive ingredient. It is from a large plant grown in Japan for its flour. An ingredient expected to increase in use as a gelling additive, thickener, and emulsifier.

AMP • The abbreviation for aminomethyl propanol (*see*).

AMP-ACRYLATES COPOLYMER • A film former. *See* Acrylates.

AMP-ACRYLATES/ALYL METHACRYLATE COPOLYMER • Film former, hair fixative. *See* Acrylates.

AMP-ISOSTEAROYL GELATIN KERATIN AMINO ACIDS/LYSINE HYDROXYPROPYLTRIMONIUM CHLORIDE • Condensed isostearic acid (*see*) with gelatin and the amino acid lysine. Used as an antistatic ingredient in hair and skin products. *See* Quaternary Ammonium Compounds.

AMP ISOSTEAROYL HYDROLYZED COLLAGEN • Collagen (*see*) from animals used in anti-aging products and other emollients.

AMP-ISOSTEAROYL HYDROLYZED ELASTIN • A protein derivative of isosteraic acid and elastin (*see both*). It is used in hair and skin conditioners.

AMP-ISOSTEAROYL HYDROLYZED KERATIN • Protein derived from isosteraic acid and keratin (*see both*). Used in hair conditioners, skin conditioners, and cleansers.

AMP-ISOSTEAROYL HYDROLYZED SOY PROTEIN • Protein derived from soy and isostearic acid (*see both*), used in hair and skin conditioners and cleansers.

AMP-ISOSTEAROYL HYDROLYZED WHEAT PROTEIN • Protein derived from wheat and isostearic acid (*see both*), used in hair and skin conditioners and in cleansers.

AMPD • The abbreviation for aminomethyl propanediol (*see*).

AMPD ACRYLATES/DIACETONEACRYLAMIDE COPOLYMER • Acrylic acid, methacrylic acid, and their simple esters. Used in hair sprays. *See* Acrylates.

AMPD ISOSTEARIC HYDROLYZED PROTEIN • The salt of isostearic hydrolyzed animal protein. Used in hair conditioners, skin conditioners, and cleansing products. *See* Hydrolyzed Protein.

AMPD-ROSIN HYDROLYZED COLLAGEN • The salt of hydrolyzed collagen (*see*). Used in hair and skin conditioners and as a surfactant and cleansing ingredient.

AMPELOPSIS GROSSEDENTATA • Tengcha. A folk medicinal herb used for centuries by the Yao nationality in Hunan Province as a health care beverage. Extracts are used in skin conditioners and emollients. Has antioxidant properties.

AMPHO- • Prefix meaning double or both.

AMPHOTERIC • A material that can display both acid and basic properties. Used primarily in surfactants (*see*), it contains betaines and imidazoles (*see both*).

AMPHOTERIC-2 • A cleansing compound that breaks up and holds oils and soil so that they may be removed easily from the skin or hair surface. *See* Amphoteric.

AMYGDALIN • A glycoside (organic compound) found in bitter almonds, peaches, and apricots. It has been a controversial substance because claims have been made that it can fight cancer in a compound called laetrile. Such claims have been unaccepted by conventional U.S. scientists but the compound is widely available in Mexico.

AMYL ACETATE • Banana Oil. Pear Oil. Obtained from amyl alcohol, with a strong fruity odor. Used in nail finishes and nail polish remover as a solvent, and as an artificial fruit essence in perfume. Also used in food and beverage flavoring and for perfuming shoe polish. Amyl acetate is a skin irritant and causes central nervous system depression when ingested. Exposure of 950 ppm for one hour has caused headache, fatigue, chest pain, and irritation of the mucous membranes. It has been found to stimulate acetylcholine release in the nerve endings and to act as a competitive inhibitor of acetylcholine in isolated nerves. Acetylcholine is a nerve messenger and plays a big part in memory functioning. It is used up to 10 percent in fingernail formulations. The CIR Expert Panel (*see*) concludes this is a safe ingredient in cosmetics.

AMYL ALCOHOL • A solvent used in nail lacquers. It occurs naturally in cocoa and oranges and smells like camphor. Highly toxic and narcotic, ingestion of as little as 30 milligrams has killed humans. Inhalation causes violent coughing.

AMYL BENZOATE • A fragrance ingredient. *See* Benzoic Acid.

AMYL BUTYRATE • Used in some perfume formulas for its apricotlike odor. It occurs naturally in cocoa and is colorless. Also used for synthetic flavorings.

AMYL CINNAMAL • A fragrance ingredient. *See* Cinnamic Acid.

AMYL CINNAMIC ALCOHOL • A solvent used in nail polish removers, waterproofing, and enamelware. *See* Cinnamic Acid.

AMYLCINNAMYL ALCOHOL • A fragrance ingredient. *See* Cinnamic Acid.

AMYL CINNAMIC ALDEHYDE • Liquid with a strong floral odor suggesting jasmine. Used in perfumes and flavorings. *See* Cinnamic Acid.

AMYL DIMETHYL PABA • Used in sunscreens to absorb ultraviolet light from sun's rays to help prevent or lessen sunburn while allowing the skin to tan. *See* Para-Aminobenzoic Acid and Sunscreen Preparations.

AMYL ESTERS • Used in fragrances. *See* Amyl Alcohol and Ester.

AMYL GALLATE • An antioxidant obtained from nutgalls and molds.

AMYL PHENOL • Used in hair-grooming preparations. *See* Phenols.

AMYL PROPIONATE • Colorless liquid with applelike odor used in perfumes, flavors, and lacquers.

AMYL SALICYLATE • Derived from salicylic acid. A pleasant-smelling liquid used in sunscreen lotions and perfumes. *See* Salicylates.

AMYL TRICRESOL • A phenol mercury compound used in mouthwashes. *See* Phenols.

AMYLASE • Used as a texturizer in cosmetics, it is an enzyme prepared from hog pancreases and used in flour to break down starch into smaller molecules. Used medicinally to combat inflammation.

AMYLODEXTRIN • Made from potato and cornstarch, it is an absorbent and thickener.

AMYLOGLUCOSIDASE • Glucose mylase made from the fermentation of *Aspergillus* (*see*) and used in skin conditioners.

AMYLOPECTIN • Amioca. Derived from starch, it is the almost insoluble outer portion of the starch granule. The gel constituent of starch. Forms a paste with water. Used as a texturizer in foods and cosmetics. Obtained from corn. Gives a red color when mixed with iodine and does not gel when mixed with water.

AMYRIS ACETATE • *See* Amyris Oil.

AMYRIS BALSAMIFERA • *Amyris balsamifera*. Bark Oil. Used as a fragrance ingredient.

AMYRIS OIL • *Amyris balsamifera*. The sweet oil distilled from the wood of torchwood and used in perfumery.

ANACARDIUM OCCIDENTALES • Cashew Nut. *Anacardium occidentales*. Small family of tropical American trees that have kidney-shaped fruit. Used in skin conditioners.

ANACYCLUS PYRETHRUM • *Anacyclus pyrethrum*. Mediterranean herb with white or yellow flowers. *See* Pyrethrins.

ANAMIRTA COCCULUS • Fish Berry. A Southeast Asian and Indian climbing plant. Its fruit, *Cocculus indicus,* is the source of picrotoxin, a poisonous alkaloid with stimulant properties. The plant itself has been shown to be effective in treating ringworm. Its crushed seeds are effective against lice and are also traditionally used to stun or kill fish or as a pesticide. The EU banned it in cosmetics.

ANANAS SATIVUS • Pineapple. The common juice from the tropical plant. Contains a protein-digesting and milk-clotting enzyme, bromelin. An anti-inflammatory enzyme, it is used in cosmetic treatment creams. It is also used as a texturizer.

AND OTHER INGREDIENTS • Term used to represent those ingredients that have received trade secret status by the U.S. Food and Drug Administration (FDA).

ANDRO- • Prefix meaning male, as in the male hormone androgen.

ANDROGENS • Male hormones that can stimulate oil glands in addition to other effects on the body. The EU banned anything with androgenic effects in cosmetics.

ANEMARRHENA ASPHODELOIDES • Root extract from *Anemarrhena aspho-*

deloides, a member of the lily family. Used as an anti-inflammatory, demulcent, antipyretic, antibacterial, and nutritive.

ANETHOLE • A flavoring ingredient used in mouthwashes and toothpastes and as a scent for perfumes. Obtained from anise (*see*) oil and other sources. Colorless or faintly yellow liquid with a sweet taste and a characteristic aniselike odor. Chief constituent of anise. Anethole is affected by light and caused irritation of the gums and throat when used in a denture cream. When applied to the skin, anethole may produce hives, scaling, and blisters.

ANETHUM GRAVEOLENS • *See* Dill.

ANGELICA • *Angelica archangelica. A. officinalis.* Masterwort. Archangel. The benefits of this northern European wild herb were said to have been revealed by an angel to a monk during a time of plague. Medicinally, herbalists use it as an astringent, a tonic to improve the circulation and warm the body, and for arthritis pain. The stems, if chewed, reduce flatulence. A beverage of dried leaves with lemon and honey is used as a cure for coughs and colds. Angelica is contraindicated in pregnancy and during menstruation, and in cases of acute gastritis, peptic ulcers, and kidney inflammations. It may also cause photosensitivity.

ANGELICA ROOT AND EXTRACT • *Angelica acutiloba.* Used in inexpensive fragrances, toothpastes, and mouthwashes. Grown in Europe and Asia, the aromatic seeds, leaves, stems, and roots have been used in medicine for flatus (gas), to increase sweating, and reduce body water. Also used as a flavoring in food. When perfume is applied, skin may break out with a rash and swell when exposed to sunlight. The bark is used medicinally as a purgative and emetic. GRAS. EAF

ANGIOEDEMA • Angioneurotic Edema. Acute local swelling, like giant hives, under the skin. The swelling can be very serious if it occurs around the tongue and larynx, causing potential suffocation.

ANGOSTURA BARK • Flavoring ingredient from the bark of trees grown in Venezuela and Brazil. Unpleasant, musty odor and bitter aromatic taste. The light yellow liquid extract is used in bitters, liquor, root beer, and spice flavorings for beverages and liquors (1,700 ppm). Used in cosmetics. Formerly used to lessen fever. GRAS. EAF

ANHYDRIDE • A residue resulting from water being removed from a compound. An oxide—combination of oxygen and an element—that can combine with water to form an acid, or that is derived from an acid by the abstraction of water. Acetic acid (*see*) is an example.

ANHYDROUS • Describes a substance that contains no water.

ANIBA ROSAEODORA • Rosewood. Used in fragrances. *See* Bois de Rose Oil.

ANIGOZANTHOS FLAVIDUS • *See* Kangaroo Paw Flower.

ANILINE • A colorless to brown liquid that darkens with age. Slightly soluble in water, it is one of the most commonly used of the organic bases, the parent substance for many dyes and drugs. It is derived from nitrobenzene or chlorobenzene and is among the top five organic chemicals produced each year in the United States. It is used as a rubber accelerator to speed vulcanization, as an antioxidant to retard aging, and as an intermediate (*see*). It is also used in dyes, photographic chemicals, the manufacture of urethane foams, pharmaceuticals, explosives, petroleum refining, resins, adhesive products, paint removers, herbicides, and fungicides. It is toxic when ingested, inhaled, or absorbed through the skin. It causes allergic reactions. It is a potential human cancer-causing ingredient. It caused cancer in mice when injected under the skin or administered orally. It can also cause contact dermatitis. In a 1991 report of a study of 1,749 workers at the Goodyear Tire & Rubber Company plant in Niagara Falls, New York, it was revealed that workers exposed directly to aniline had 6.5 times the rate of bladder cancer of the average state resident. On the Canadian Hotlist (*see*). Aniline, its salts, and its halogenated and sulphonated derivatives banned in cosmetics by the EU, UK, and ASEAN (*see*).

ANILINE DYES • Coal Tar Dyes. Aniline is a colorless to brown liquid that darkens with age. A synonym for coal tar (*see*) dyes, it refers to a large class of synthetic dyes made from intermediates (*see*) based upon or made from aniline. It is among the top five organic chemicals produced in the United States. Used in the manufacture of hair dyes, medicinals, resins, and perfumes. It is used in carbons, fur dyeing, rubber, photographic inks, colored pencils, and crayons. Most are somewhat toxic and irritating to the eyes, skin, and mucous membranes but are generally much less toxic than aniline itself. These dyes caused tumors in animals whose skins were painted with them. Can cause contact dermatitis. On the Canadian Hotlist (*see*).

ANIMAL COLLAGEN AMINO ACIDS • The word *animal* has been deleted from any name with it, when possible, by the cosmetics manufacturers. *See* Collagen Amino Acids.

ANIMAL ELASTIN AMINO ACIDS • Now called elastin amino acids. *See* Elastin and Amino Acids.

ANIMAL KERATIN AMINO ACIDS • Now called keratin amino acids (*see*).

ANIMAL PARTS • Suspected of being vulnerable to contamination with disease. Adrenal gland, basal ganglia/basal ganglion, sciatic nerve bone marrow, sphingosine phosphatide, brain sphinogomyelin, brain extract, sphingolipid, ceramide B-lactoside, spinal cord, ceramide dihexoside, spleen, cerebellum suprarenal gland, Cerebroside (sulfate), tetraglycosylceramide, cerebrospinal fluid thymus gland (sweetbread), cranial nerves tonsil, collagen (soluble) triglycosylceramide, trisialoganglioside, digalactosylceramide, diglycosylceramides (cytosides), disialoganglioside, dura mater, elastin (source: oxen neck ligaments), eye, galactocerebroside, galactosylcerebroside (sulfate) adrenal gland, rowamyelin, colon (proximal and distal), trinitrophenylaminolauroylglucocerebroside, deer fat trinitrophenylaminolauroylgalactocerebroside, deer antler velvet, ganglioside, glucosylcerebroside, glycerophospholipid, glycosaminoglycan, glycosphingolipid, glycosylceramide, hypothalamus, ileum, intercellular lipids (ICLs), lactocerebroside, lactosylceramide, liposomes, liver, lung, lymph nodes, monoglycosylceramide (cerebroside), monosialoganglioside, N-nervonoyl cerebroside, N-oleoyl cerebroside, N-palmitoyl cerebroside, nasal mucosa, olfactory bulb or gland, pancreas (including pancreatin), phospholipids, pineal gland, pituitary gland, pancreas (including pancreatin), placenta. *See also* ECVAM.

ANIMAL PROTEIN • Name changed to ammonium hydrolyzed collagen (*see*). Prohibited cattle materials means specified risk materials, small intestine of all cattle except as provided in regulations, material from nonambulatory disabled cattle, material from cattle not inspected and passed, or mechanically separated (MS) (Beef). Prohibited cattle materials do not include tallow that contains no more than 0.15 percent insoluble impurities, tallow derivatives, hides and hide-derived products, and milk and milk products. Inspected and passed means that the product has been inspected and passed for human consumption by the appropriate regulatory authority, and at the time it was inspected and passed, it was found to be not adulterated. Mechanically separated (MS) (Beef) means a meat food product that is finely comminuted, resulting from the mechanical separation and removal of most of the bone from attached skeletal muscle of cattle carcasses and parts of carcasses that meet specifications contained in the regulation that prescribes the standard of identity for MS (Species). Nonambulatory disabled cattle means cattle that cannot rise from a recumbent position or that cannot walk, including, but not limited to, those with broken appendages, severed tendons or ligaments, nerve paralysis, fractured vertebral column, or metabolic conditions. Specified risk material means the brain, skull, eyes, trigeminal ganglia, spinal cord, vertebral column (excluding the vertebrae of the tail, the transverse processes of the thoracic and lumbar vertebrae, and the wings of the sacrum), and dorsal root ganglia of cattle thirty months and older and the tonsils and distal ileum of the small intestine of all cattle. No cosmetic shall be manufactured from, processed with, or otherwise contain prohibited cattle materials.

The small intestine is not considered prohibited cattle material if the distal ileum is removed by a procedure that removes at least eighty inches of the uncoiled and trimmed small intestine, as measured from the caeco-colic junction and progressing proximally towards the jejunum, or by a procedure that the establishment can demonstrate is equally effective in ensuring complete removal of the distal ileum. Manufacturers and processors of a cosmetic that is manufactured from, processed with, or otherwise contains material from cattle must establish and maintain records sufficient to demonstrate that the cosmetic is not manufactured from, processed with, or does not otherwise contain prohibited cattle materials. Records must be retained for two years after the date they were created. Records must be retained at the manufacturing or processing establishment or at a reasonably accessible location.

ANIMAL PROTEIN DERIVATIVE • Used in skin conditioners to attract water, thereby helping to maintain the skin's moisture balance. *See* Hydrolyzed Collagen.

ANIMAL SKIN LIPIDS • A mixture of fats derived from animal skin.

ANIMAL TESTING FOR COSMETIC SAFETY • In 1993, the EU first produced a directive that all animal testing would be banned. Animal testing was finally banned in 2009 except in three test areas—reproductive toxicity, repeat-dose toxicity, and toxicokinetics. The sales ban for these tests reaches its deadline in 2013. The FDA neither requires nor bans animal testing. The animals used are mainly albino rabbits for testing cosmetics and mice and rats for most other substances. Cats, dogs, primates, and farm animals account for 1 percent or less of all animal tests, and some cosmetics are tested for skin irritation on human volunteers. The most common test is the Draize test, where the chemicals are placed directly into the eye or onto the skin of an albino rabbit to test for irritation. Tissue cultures used in nonanimal tests often consist of a mass of living cells taken from a mouse and then grown on a culture medium in a glass dish. Many hundreds of dishes of cells can be grown from just a few cells taken from just one living animal. Cosmetics or individual cosmetic ingredients are added to the cells' dish, and any changes in the cells' biochemistry may indicate an adverse reaction caused by the chemical. However, it is difficult to say exactly how that change will translate to irritation or harm in humans. Cosmetic labels may carry phrases like "cruelty free" or "not tested on animals," but this may be misleading. If these phrases are used in the EU, the label is required to state if the testing was carried out on the finished cosmetic or on individual ingredients or combinations of ingredients.

A new skin irritation test from SkinEthic Laboratories has been validated for use by the European Centre for the Validation of Alternative Methods. The Reconstructed Human Epidermis (RHE) test can replace the in vivo Draize rabbit skin test to test the irritation and corrosive potential of cosmetic ingredients and products. With the ban on animal testing coming ever closer, it is important for companies to find reliable alternatives, and according to SkinEthic, the RHE will help reduce animal use in cosmetics testing. The RHE has an overall accuracy of 85 percent according to the company, with a false positive rate of 20 and a false negative rate of 10. With a 42-minute exposure time and a 42-hour incubation time, the model is easy and ready to use, according to SkinEthic. The France-based company also provides the EpiSkin model which was validated by ECVAM (*see*) last year. Like the RHE model, EpiSkin can be used to identify the potential for skin irritation of chemicals and cosmetics, as well as skin corrosion, percutaneous absorption, bacterial adhesion, and pharmacological and toxicological studies. EpiSkin was originally brought to the company's portfolio by L'Oréal, when the cosmetics giant purchased SkinEthic back in 2006. However, the addition of the RHE test to the company's portfolio is not designed to replace or validate EpiSkin, explained SkinEthic's Alain Alonso. Different customer bases explain the concurrent existence of the two tests, he said, and if both continue to be successful, both will be kept on the books. The company is also currently compiling its own data to highlight the robustness of both tests, to further generate consumer trust in its performance in a wide range of situations and chemicals, Alonso added. ECVAM also validated the modified Epiderm Skin Irritation Test (SIT) from U.S.-based MatTek. Increasing the test time of the original SIT test from fifteen to sixty minutes increased the sensitivity of the test and gained it full validation from the European authorities.

No such regulations exist in the United States. The product may say that there has been no animal testing, and the manufacturer may have arranged for the supplier of the ingredients to do the testing for them. Alternatively, companies may simply check the scientific literature to see if tests have been carried out in the past and only use those ingredients that have already been tested. Many ingredients have been around for years. The use in cosmetics of products derived from human tissues or from endangered or protected species, is banned. The main animal products, such as proteins and fats and oils, are used in making soaps and detergents and gels. Musk and civet are obtained from the scent gland of male musk deer, musk ox, and the civet cat. The ambergris from the sperm whale and castoreum from the beaver have also been used in expensive fragrances.

ANIMAL TISSUE EXTRACT • The mixed extract of the skin, testes, and ovaries of the pig, and the thymus, placenta, and udder of the cow. Also called epiderm oil R, it is used in moisturizers and other creams.

ANIONIC SURFACTANTS • A class of synthetic compounds used as emulsifiers in about 75 percent of all hand creams and lotions. An anion is a negatively charged ion that is "surface active." These detergents usually consist of an alkali salt as soap, or ammonium salt of a strong acid. Can be irritating to the skin, depending on alkalinity. Used in shampoos. Whether or not it is irritating to the eyes depends on the compound. Sodium laureth sulfate, for example, is very irritating, whereas triethanolamine (TEA) coco hydrolyzed animal protein is the least irritating. *See* Emulsifiers and Ammonia Water.

ANISALDEHYDE • A fragrance ingredient. *See* Anise.

ANISE • *Illicium verum.* Anise Seed. Dried, ripe fruit of Asia, Europe, and the United States. Used in licorice, anise, pepperoni sausage, spice, and vanilla flavorings for beverages, ice cream, ices, candy, baked goods, condiments, and meats. The oil is used for butter, caramel, licorice, anise, rum, sausage, nut, root beer, sarsaparilla, spice, vanilla, wintergreen, and birch beer flavorings for the same foods as above, excepting condiments but including chewing gum and liquors. Sometimes used to break up intestinal gas. Used in masculine-type perfumes, cleaners, and shampoos. Can cause contact dermatitis.

***p*-ANISIC ACID** • Dermosoft 688. A plant-based natural fungicidal ingredient. Natural-product manufacturers sometimes use essential oils to fight the growth of fungi, but these can cause allergies and vary in their properties depending on their origins. It can be added to formulations with bactericidal ingredients to provide cosmetic products with more complete protection from microbiological deterioration. A flavoring ingredient. Prepared from methoxybenzene. *See* Benzene.

ANISIDINE, *o*-ANISIDINE, *p*-ANISIDINE • Derived from anisole (*see*). Colorless needles. Used in the manufacture of azo dyes (*see*). Can be absorbed through the skin. It is an irritant and sensitizer.

ANISOLE • A synthetic ingredient with a pleasant odor used in licorice, root beer, sarsaparilla, wintergreen, and birch beer flavorings for beverages, ice cream, ices, candy, and baked goods. Also used in perfumery.

ANISYL ACETATE • Colorless liquid with a lilac odor used in perfumery. *See* Anise.

ANISYL FORMATE • Used in perfumery and flavoring. *See* Formic Acid.

ANNATTO • A vegetable dye from a tropical tree. Yellow to pink, it is used in dairy products, baked goods, margarine, and breakfast cereals. Permanently listed as a coloring in 1977.

ANNONA MURICATA EXTRACT • Custard Apple. Used in shampoo to kill lice. *See* Pawpaw Extract.

ANNONA CHERIMALLA • Cultivated in Mexico and in tropical America, it is native to Peru. Contains alkaloids. Used by herbalists for pain in the back.

ANNONA RETICULATA JUICE • Custard Apple. Expressed from the fresh pulp of the custard apple and used in shampoos to kill lice. *See* Pawpaw Extract.

ANTHEMIS NOBILIS • Chamomile. An extract of the *Anthemis nobilis* flower. Widely used in skin conditioners, cleansing products including shampoos and cold creams, face powders, mascara, suntan gels, and in moisturizers. *See* Chamomile.

ANTHOCYANINS • One of the most important and widely distributed groups of water-soluble natural colors, anthocyanins are responsible for the attractive red, purple, and blue colors of many flowers, fruits, and vegetables. Over two hundred individual anthocyanins have been identified, of which twenty have been shown to be naturally present in black grapes, the major source of anthocyanin pigment for food coloration. Used in cosmetics to protect the skin and is being tested to stimulate hair growth. Used in medications to protect capillary blood vessels.

ANTHRACENE OIL • Tar. Yellow crystals with blue fluorescence, it is derived from crude anthracene oil. Used in dyes, calico printing, and in smoke screens. It is a cancer-causing agent and may also cause contact dermatitis, although it has been used to treat eczema and other skin problems. Very toxic to fish. The EU has it for high-priority attention and expects to have a statement on it by October 2009.

ANTHRANILIC ACID • *o*-Aminobenzoic Acid. Yellowish crystals with a sweet taste used in dyes and perfumes. *See* Benzoic Acid.

ANTHRAQUINONE • A coal tar color produced industrially from phthalic anhydride and benzene (*see both*). Light yellow slender prisms, which are insoluble in water. May cause skin irritation and allergic reactions. It is also used as an organic inhibitor to prevent growth of cells and a repellent to protect seeds from being eaten by birds. Caused tumors when given orally to rats in doses of 72 milligrams per kilogram of body weight. It can also cause contact dermatitis.

ANTHRISCUS CEREFOLIUM • Chervil. A Eurasian herb of the Umbelliferae family with short beaked fruit. Celery belongs to this family. It is used as a flavoring ingredient and in perfumery.

ANTHYLLIS VULNERARIA • Kidney Vetch. A legume with yellowish red flowers. A fragrance ingredient. May cause irritation.

ANTIBIOTICS • Six national Swedish agencies have called for a ban on the "unnecessary use" of antibiotics in toiletries, cosmetics, and household cleaners and implements (e.g., kitchen cutting boards). The call came after traces of the antibiotic (or "biocide") triclosan (*see*), which is commonly used in toothpastes, turned up in breast milk. Scientists are concerned that triclosan is very persistent and can accumulate in the environment, where it has been found in fish. They note that it has already been shown to inhibit the human enzyme ENR, which helps the body synthesize fatty acids, and are concerned it could develop further antibiotic-resistant bacteria. Banned in cosmetics by the ASEAN (*see*).

ANTICHOLINERGIC • A substance that blocks the neurotransmitter acetylcholine in the central and the peripheral nervous systems. Acetylcholine plays an important role both in learning and memory and in sending messages from motor nerves to muscles.

ANTICORROSIVE • Added to prevent the corrosion of the packaging or the machinery used to produce a cosmetic. Sodium nitrite and nitromethane (*see both*) are two commonly used but undesirable anticorrosives. The EU regulates anticorrosives in cosmetics.

ANTIFOAMING INGREDIENT • Defoamer. A substance used to reduce foaming due to proteins, gases, or nitrogenous materials that interfere with the manufacture of a product. *See* Silicones.

ANTIGEN • Any substance that provokes an immune response when introduced into the body.

ANTIMICROBIALS • Ingredients added to help reduce the activities of microorganisms on the skin or body. The trade organization Cosmeticsinfo.org says on its website, http://www.cosmeticsinfo.org, "Antimicrobial ingredients are materials that protect against the growth of microorganisms in personal care products, including bacteria, viruses and fungi. Antimicrobial ingredients can also kill organisms that may be present in ingredients that may be used to make products. Antimicrobial personal care products, which are sometimes referred to as antibacterial products, provide an important extra measure of protection for consumers at home and doctors and nurses in hospitals seeking to prevent spread of germs." These products, depending on their formulation and application, kill or inhibit the growth of bacteria that cause skin infections, intestinal illnesses or other commonly transmitted diseases. These include potentially fatal illnesses caused by bacteria such as *Salmonella* and *E. coli*. Such products are regulated by the Food and Drug Administration as over-the-counter (OTC) drugs and have to be shown to be safe and effective for their intended use. There are several different types of OTC drug products that have been established by the FDA. Antimicrobial ingredients play a role in making sure that personal care products are free of microorganisms during storage and after they are opened. Many different types of materials can be used in products, and they are selected based on the specific type of product. A water-based product may use a different type of ingredient (or combination of ingredients) than an oil-based product. The same ingredients that are used to protect cosmetic product integrity may also be used in OTC antimicrobial drug products, although the amount added may be different. For OTC antimicrobial drug products, the amounts allowed are prescribed in the FDA OTC drug monographs for safety and effectiveness (and work as intended).

- Antiperspirants and Deodorants—Antibacterial protection in deodorants enhances personal hygiene by controlling the growth of embarrassing, odor-causing bacteria.

- Soaps—Antibacterial hand and body washes contain an ingredient that kills or controls bacteria that can cause illnesses, odor, or skin infections. Unlike plain soaps, these products leave a very small amount of the antibacterial ingredient on the skin after rinsing to help inhibit the growth of bacteria left behind. Antibacterial soaps and washes are available in bar and liquid form.

- Hand sanitizers—Antibacterial hand sanitizers kill bacteria on hands without soap and water. These products are a good choice when hand washing with soap and water isn't possible.

- Lotions—Antibacterial lotions moisturize rough, dry skin and offer added protection by controlling bacteria. As with antibacterial soaps, a small amount of the antibacterial ingredient in lotions remains on the skin for an extended period of time to help inhibit the growth of bacteria.

• Antibacterial toothpaste and mouthwash—Antibacterial toothpaste and mouthwash products may help prevent plaque and gum diseases such as gingivitis.

The safety of antimicrobial ingredients has been assessed by a number of authoritative bodies. The Cosmetic Ingredient Review Expert Panel (CIREP) has conducted safety assessments of the most frequently used antimicrobial ingredients that are used in personal care products and have found them safe. In addition, the FDA has considered the safety of antimicrobial ingredients as they are used in foods, drugs, cosmetics, and other products regulated by the FDA and has found no reason to dissuade consumers from using these products. In October 2005, the agency expressed concerns, which have also been voiced by some in the scientific community, about the possibility that the products might result in antibiotic resistance. To date, the FDA maintains there is no convincing evidence that products containing antimicrobial ingredients cause increased resistance to antibiotics. Moreover, other jurisdictions, such as the European Union, Japan, and Canada, have assessed the safety of antimicrobial ingredients and found no basis for consumers to stop using products containing these ingredients. *See* Triclosan.

ANTIMONY COMPOUNDS • Antimony Potassium Tartrate. Tartar Emetic. Used in hair dyes. Antimony compounds were recognized as early as 3000 BC. Pastes of antimony powder in fat or in other materials have been used since that date as eye cosmetics in the Middle East and farther afield; in this use, antimony is called kohl. It was used to darken the brows and lashes, or to draw a line around the perimeter of the eye. Obtained from ore mined in China, Mexico, and Bolivia, this silver-white brittle metal can cause contact dermatitis, eye and nose irritation, and ulceration by contact, fumes, or dust. It is used medicinally as an emetic and in the manufacture of bullets and metal bearings and to combat worms. On the Canadian Hotlist (*see*). Banned in cosmetics by the EU, UK, and ASEAN (*see*).

ANTIOXIDANTS • Preservatives that prevent fats from spoiling. Tocopherols and BHA are examples (*see both*).

ANTIPERSPIRANT • Any substance having a mild astringent action that tends to reduce the size of skin pores and thus restrain the passage of moisture on local body areas. The most commonly used antiperspirant compound is aluminum chlorohydrate. Use of zirconium compounds in antiperspirant sprays has been discontinued because of their suspected carcinogens, though they are permissible in creams. Antiperspirants exert a neutralizing action that give them deodorant properties. The FDA classified them as drugs rather than as cosmetics.

ANTISTATIC INGREDIENTS • Plastic polymers accumulate static electricity, which causes dust and other matter to cling. Cosmetics manufacturers add substances such as polyethylene glycols and quaternary ammonium compounds in an effort to counteract static cling.

AO1 • A triphenylmethane color (*see* Acid Blue 9), but the prefix AO1 must be used on Japanese labels.

AO2 • Acid Blue 74, CI 73015. An indigoid color (*see*), this prefix must be used on Japanese products with this color. This ingredient is not approved for use in the United States.

AO201 • CI 73000. Pigment Blue 66. Indigo. The prefix AO201 is required in Japan for this indigoid color.

AO202 • CI 42052. Acid Blue 5. Sodium Salt. AO202 prefix must appear for this blue lake color in Japan.

AO203 • Acid Blue 5, Calcium Salt. AO203 prefix must appear for this blue lake color in Japan.

AO204 • Pigment Blue 64. Indanthrene Blue BC. CI 69825. Approved for use in Japan but not in the United States. The AO204 prefix must appear for this blue lake color in Japan.

AO205 • Blue 4. A trimethan color, the AO25 prefix must be used in Japan.

AO403 • An anthraquinone color, it is not approved for use in the United States or Europe. It must have the AO403 prefix in Japan.

AO404 • Copper. Japan Blue. CI 74160. A phthalocyanine color, it is not approved for use in the United States.

AORTA EXTRACT • Extract of the aorta, the major artery in the body of animals. Used in anti-aging creams.

APIUM GRAVEOLENS • *See* Celery.

APOCYNUM CANNABINUM • Indian Hemp. Canadian dogbane yielding a tough fiber used as cordage by Native Americans; used in folk medicine for pain or inflammation in joints. On the Canadian Hotlist (*see*). Banned in cosmetics by the EU and ASEAN (*see*).

APOMORPHINE AND ITS SALTS • Synthetic morphine. Used for male erectile dysfunction. Banned in cosmetics by the EU and ASEAN (*see*).

APPLE • *Pyrus malus.* Used in organic cosmetics. *See* Apple Stem Cells and Malic Acid.

APPLE BLOSSOM • Used in perfumes and colognes, it is the essence of the flowers from a species of apple tree.

APPLE STEM CELLS • An anti-aging active based on an extremely rare form of apple stem cells has been launched by Mibelle Biochemistry, promising to protect skin stem cells and slow the senescence of hair follicles. Furthermore, the Switzerland-based company has developed a method to cultivate large quantities of the plant cells that allows it to use the benefits of this plant. In vitro and in vivo tests performed by Mibelle have suggested that the ingredient PhytoCellTec Malus Domestica boosts the production of human stem cells, protects human stem cells from stress, and decreases wrinkles. In vitro the extract was applied to human stem cells from umbilical cords and was found to increase the number of the stem cells in culture. Furthermore, the addition of the ingredient to umbilical cord stem cells appeared to protect the cells from environmental stress such as UV light. Another interesting finding was the ability of the ingredient to delay the aging of hair follicles, suggesting a possible use in anti-aging hair preparations. Despite this finding, the company stated that the main focus of the active is skin care for the face.

APRICOT • *Prunus armeniaca.* Fruit and oil. The tart orange-colored fruit. The oil is used in brilliantine, and the crushed fruit is used as a facial mask to soften the skin. For a do-it-yourself facial mask, soak a cup of dried apricots in water until softened, then mix with a small bunch of grapes and 3 tablespoons of skim milk powder. Mix the concoction in a blender, and pat on the neck and face; allow to remain for 15 minutes, followed by a rinse of cool water.

APRICOTAMIDE DEA • A mixture of fatty acids derived from apricot (*see*). Used as a surfactant and thickener.

APRICOT AMIDOPROPYL BETAINE • Fatty acids derived from apricot (*see*).

APRICOT AMIDOPROPYL ETHYLDIMONIUM ETHOSULFATE • A quaternary ammonium compound (*see*) made from apricots and ethosulfate.

APRICOT EXTRACT • *See* Apricot.

APRICOT KERNEL OIL PEG-6 ESTERS • A complex mixture formed from esterification (*see*) of apricot kernel oil. *See* Apricot and PEG.

AQP3 • In a recent publication in the *Journal of Experimental Dermatology,* Alan S.

Verkman, a professor of medicine and physiology at the University of California, questions the safety of a number of anti-aging ingredients that increase the protein aquaporin-3 (AQP3), a member of a family of membrane proteins that play a role in water movement in and out of cells. Having a "cosmeceutical" that "moisturizes" the skin seems like an AQP3 producer would be just the ingredient for expensive anti-aging cosmetics. Dr. Verkman warns, however, there may be an association between the skin production of AQP3 and skin tumor formation. He points out that human squamous cell carcinomas, the second most common form of skin cancer, strongly produce the AQP3 protein. In addition, mice lacking the AQP3 protein failed to form tumors whereas the wild-type mice (mice with the normal AQP3 gene) that underwent the same tumor-inducing conditions formed multiple tumors. Furthermore, in general, the expression of the aquaporin proteins in tumor cells has been found to increase their migration, invasiveness, and metastatic potential, according to the scientist. He notes, however, that there is no data for the effect of AQP3 and the migration of skin cell tumors.

AQUA • The European name for what Americans list on the label as "water."

AQUAPORIN 3 • *See* AQP3.

AQUACACTEEN • An ultrarefined elixir from prickly pear (*Opuntia ficus-indica*) (*see*), this cactus cream is claimed to be high in flavones, vitamins, and antioxidants and minerals as well as having a high content of water-binding compounds. It is claimed to be very soothing to the skin.

ARABIC GUM • *See* Acacia.

ARACHIDETH-20 • A surfactant and emulsifying ingredient. It is a surfactant and cleanser in cosmetic soaps and is used in skin conditioners and moisturizers. *See* Arachidic Acid.

ARACHIDIC ACID • A fatty acid, also called eicosanoic acid, that is widely distributed in peanut-oil fats and related compounds. It is used in lubricants, greases, waxes, and plastics.

ARACHIDONIC ACID • A liquid, unsaturated, fatty acid that occurs in the liver, brain, glands, and fat of animals and humans. The acid is generally isolated from animal liver. A surfactant and emulsifying ingredient, it is used essentially for nutrition and to soothe eczema and rashes in skin creams and lotions. In one study, thus far, it altered the skin's immune response. The CIR Expert Panel (*see*) says it cannot conclude whether this ingredient is safe for use in cosmetic products until such time that the appropriate safety data have been obtained and evaluated.

ARACHIDYL ALCOHOL • A fatty alcohol used as a stabilizer and thickening ingredient. *See* Arachidonic Acid.

ARACHIDYL BEHENATE • A waxy alcohol made from arachidyl alcohol and behenic acid.

ARACHIDYL PROPIONATE • The ester of arachidyl alcohol and *n*-propionic acid used as a wax and as an emollient in lipsticks, skin care products, and body and hand lotions. The CIR Expert Panel (*see*) concludes this is a safe ingredient in the present practices of use and concentration. *See* Arachidic Acid.

ARACHIS HYPOGAEA • *See* Peanut Oil.

ARALIA ELATA • Japanese angelica tree. Upright deciduous tree with large leaves that is hardy, but tends to grow as a suckering shrub in the United Kingdom. The stems are covered in spines. The panicles of white flowers are followed by black fruits. Contains various functional components such as saponins and alkaloids. For a long time in Korean traditional medicine, barks and roots have been used in treating low blood sugar, ulcers, cancer, diabetes, and gastritis. Used in cosmetics as an antioxidant.

ARALIA NUDICAULIS • Wild Sarsaparilla. *See* Sarsaparilla Extract.

ARBITRARY FIXATIVE • An odorous substance that lends a particular note to the perfume throughout all stages of evaporation but does not really influence the evaporation of the perfume materials in the compound. Oakmoss is an example. *See* Fixative and Oakmoss, Absolute.

ARBUTIN • Diuretic and anti-infective derived from the dried leaves of the heath family, genus *Vaccinium,* including blueberries, cranberries, and bearberries, and most pear plants. This may explain why cranberry juice is reputed to ward off and treat urinary tract infections. In cosmetics it is used as an antioxidant and skin conditioner.

ARBUTUS EXTRACT • From the leaves of the evergreen shrub arbutus, found in southern Europe and western North America. It has a white or pink flower.

ARCTIUM, MAJOR and MINOR • Beggar's Buttons. Burdock Root. The roots, seeds, and leaves of this common roadside plant contain an essential oil. The oil contains nearly 45 percent inulin (sugar) and many minerals. Herbalists use it for skin diseases. In modern experiments, burdock root extract has been shown to have antitumor effects. Widely used in cosmetics, in hair products, cold creams, cleansing lotions, night skin care, body and hand lotions, and shampoos, arctium lappa (active ingredient arctiin) extract can, according to a study published in the *Journal of Cosmetics Dermatology,* help protect against chronic tissue inflammation and at the same time stimulate the synthesis of connective tissues such as collagen (*see*).

ARCTOSTAPHYLOS UVA-URSI • Bearberry. Used in skin conditioners, hand preparations, and mud packs.

ARECA CATECHU • Betel Nut. Used in hair conditioners and moisturizers. Also used in suntan gels and shampoos.

ARGAN OIL • *Argania spinosa.* Argan nut oil is pressed from the fruits of the argan tree native to Morocco and known to live up to two hundred years. For centuries, Moroccans have used argan oil in skin care and within their nutritious diet. Argan oil remains one of the rarest oils in the world. A very labor-intensive process, performed primarily by Moroccan women, is required to shell and crush the fruits prior to pressing the oil. Argan oil possesses a remarkable ability to nourish, moisturize, and improve skin elasticity. The oil is high in lipids, including the omega-9 oleic acid and the omega-6 linoleic acid as well as vitamin E. Argan oil can be effective in treating dry skin, eczema, psoriasis, acne, and sunburned skin. It is used for hair care and in formulations for anti-aging products. Its high polyphenol content makes it a strong antioxidant and adds to its stable shelf life. Argan oil possesses anti-inflammatory properties and is a highly beneficial addition to formulations intended to reduce swelling and ease muscular aches and pains.

ARGANIA SPINOSA • Spinosa Oil. *See* Argan Oil.

ARGEMONE MEXICANA OIL • An oil expressed from the leaves of a Mexican poppy. It is used as a skin- and hair-conditioning ingredient.

ARGININE • An essential amino acid (*see*), strongly alkaline. The FDA has asked for further information on the nutrient, which plays an important role in the production of urea (*see*). It has been used for the treatment of liver disease.

ARGIRELINE • A trade name for the peptide acetyl hexapeptide-3 (*see*) that was developed and marketed by Lipotec, which is a Barcelona, Spain, based cosmetics company. Lipotec vigorously defends the patent they hold on Argireline, as it is the company's best-selling product. However, cosmeceutical companies and other producers of skin care products have incorporated Argireline into their antiwrinkle product lines. According to the brief on Argireline available on the Lipotec website, Argireline is marketed specifically as a "cosmetic alternative to Botulinum Toxin A," which is the surgical procedure usually marketed under the trade name Botox. As such, it is an antiwrinkle treatment. Argireline works in the biological pathways of the skin cells by mimicking and destabilizing the receptors essential for muscle contraction. It also acts to inhibit or slow the release of excessive catecholamine (*see*), which is also thought to contribute to wrinkles.

ARGON • An inert gas from the earth's crust. Used as an antioxidant.

ARISTOLOCHIA CLEMATITIS • A woody herb with pungent, aromatic roots. Used in fragrances. It is an established fact that aristolochic acid and its salts, as well as *Aristolochia* subspecies and their preparations, are substances that act as powerful carcinogens. The EU says these substances should therefore be prohibited in cosmetic products.

ARMENIAN BOLE • A soft, claylike red earth. The pigment is found chiefly in Armenia and Tuscany and is used as a coloring material in face powder.

ARMERIA MARITIMA EXTRACT • Derived from an herb that grows along the seacoast in temperate climates.

ARNICA • Wolfsbane. Skin fresheners may contain this herb found in the Northern Hemisphere. The dried flower head has long been used as an astringent and to treat skin disorders, especially in tinctures. It has been used externally to treat bruises and sprains. Ingestion leads to severe intestinal upset, nervous disturbances, irregular heartbeat, and collapse. Ingestion of one ounce has caused severe illness but not death. Active irritant on the skin. Not recommended for use in toilet preparations and should never be used on broken skin.

AROMA • This is the term Europeans use instead of listing individual components of a flavor. In the United States, labels say "flavor."

AROMATHERAPY • The use of scents to relieve everything from stress to a broken heart. Usually promoted by cosmetic manufacturers for bath products and body lotions, it has a long history, and there are some scientific studies now in progress about the use of scent to alter mood.

AROMATIC • In the context of cosmetics, a chemical that has an aroma.

AROMATIC BITTERS • Usually made from the maceration of bitter herbs and used to intensify the aroma of perfume. The herbs selected for aromatic bitters must have a persistent fragrant aroma. Ginger and cinnamon are examples.

ARROWROOT • *Maranta arundinacea.* An ingredient in dusting powders and hair dyes made from the root starch of plants. Arrowroot was used by the American Indians to heal wounds from poisoned arrows. It is used as a culture medium and as a medicine. In cosmetics, it is used to help moisturizers penetrate the skin.

ARSENIC COMPOUNDS • Arsenic is an element that occurs throughout the universe and is highly toxic in most forms. Its compounds are used in hair tonics and hair dyes and have been employed to treat spirochetal infections, blood disorders, and skin diseases. Ingestion causes nausea, vomiting, and death. Chronic poisoning can result in pigmentation of skin and kidney and liver damage. In hair tonics and dyes, it may cause contact dermatitis. The limit of arsenic in colors is 0.0002 percent. Arsenic can also cause the skin to be sensitive to light and break out in a rash or to swell. On the Canadian Hotlist (*see*). Banned in cosmetics by the EU and ASEAN (*see*).

ARTEMIA • Named for the Greek goddess of the forests and hills, this is a genus of crustaceans found in salt lakes and brines of saltworks.

ARTEMISIA ABROTANUM • *See* Artemisia Capillaris.

ARTEMISIA ABSINTHIUM • *See* Wormwood.

ARTEMISIA CAPILLARIS • Mugwort. Wormwood. A shrub native to the eastern United States. Hippocrates recommended this herb to aid in the delivery of the placenta after childbirth. One of the most commonly used herbal preparations to induce menstruation, the extract has been shown to stimulate uterine muscle. The Chinese dry mugwort and then burn it in a therapeutic technique, moxibustion, to treat a variety of ills. Contains volatile oils, tannin (*see*), and the sugar inulin.

ARTICHOKE EXTRACT • A tall herb, *Cynara scolymus,* that resembles a thistle. It is edible. It is used in cosmetics to "relax" the muscles as it is rubbed on the skin.

ARTIFICIAL • In the context of cosmetics, a substance not duplicated in nature. A scent, for instance, may have all-natural ingredients, but it must be called artificial if it has no counterpart in nature.

ARTIFICIAL NAIL REMOVER • Contains acetonitrile, also known as methyl cyanide. May cause skin irritation. Cyanide poisoning from ingestion of such products has been reported. On the Canadian Hotlist (*see*).

ARTIFICIAL NAILS • Plastics designed to be pasted or self-adhered to one's natural nails to give the appearance of long, lovely, undamaged fingernails. After application, the artificial nails are cut or filed to the desired length and shape. Artificial nails were developed from materials used by dentists to fill teeth. The basic ingredients include a vinyl compound (methyl methacrylate is one of the most commonly used vinyls), a catalyst, and a plasticizer. Allergy and irritation to the skin may develop from ingredients in the fake nails or in the adhesive. Artificial nails can be used to beautify as well as camouflage discolored, thickened, or malformed fingernails. Unfortunately, this group of cosmetics is responsible for both allergic contact dermatitis and nail damage. The most popular type of artificial nail is the preformed plastic nail. These come in press-on, preglued forms, and in forms requiring glue application. The acrylic glue used is typically methacrylate based and a possible cause of allergic contact dermatitis. Stronger nail adhesives are used to provide better adhesion but can cause the nail plate to separate from the nail bed. In addition, traumatic removal of artificial nails may result in the nail plate splitting into layers.

Preformed nails are not recommended if you have weak nails, congenital nail deformity, or nail plate irregularities, since a smooth nail surface is required for adhesion. Many have been opting for sculptured nails. The word *sculptured* is used since the custom-made artificial nail is sculpted on a template attached to the natural nail plate. The sculptured nail, if well done, can be hard to differentiate from a natural nail. The sculptured nail is made from acrylic and mixed with a number of substances in order to form the shape of each individual nail. Finished nail sculptures require more care than natural fingernails. After two to four months of wear, the natural nail plate becomes yellowed, dry, and thin. Most nail operators prefer to allow the natural nail to grow out and act as a support for the sculpture. However, typically the nails become thin, bendable, and weak. For this reason, dermatologists advise not wearing sculptured nails for more than three consecutive months and recommend you allow one month between applications. Silk or linen cloth wraps may be combined with nail sculptures to add additional strength to the artificial nail or to aid in covering nail defects. There are, however, problems associated with the application and wearing of nail sculptures. One is the skill, training, and licensing of the operator. Poorly trained operators may allow liquid acrylic to enter the nail fold, which may cause nail tissue damage. The failure to sterilize equipment or apply antifungal, antibacterial solutions to the nail plate may result in fungal, viral, or bacterial infections. Allergic contact dermatitis is also a problem. The chemicals typically used are strong sensitizers. It is very important that the nail operator be careful to avoid skin contact. *See* your dermatologist for patch testing if you suspect you are sensitive or allergic to these substances. Tearing the natural nail plate from the nail bed is a common problem since the bond between the sculpture and the natural nail plate is stronger than the adhesion between the natural nail and nail bed. This also occurs in individuals sensitive to the acrylic. Many are upset at the broken, thinned, yellowed appearance of their nails following sculpture removal. Nail adhesives are on the Canadian Hotlist (*see*).

ARUNIKA EKISU • *Arnica montana. A. montana* Flower Extract. A skin-conditioning ingredient.

ARUTEA EKISU • The extract of the roots and leaves of *Althaea officinalis*. A skin-conditioning ingredient.

ARYLALCANOIC • Rubefacient (*see*) used in Europe.

ASAFOETIDA EXTRACT • Asafetida. Devil's Dung. A gum or resin obtained from the roots or rhizome of *Ferula asa-foetida,* any of several plants grown in Iran, Turkestan, and Afghanistan. The soft lumps, or "tears," have a garlicky odor and are used as a natural flavoring. The gums have also been used medicinally as an expectorant and to break up intestinal gas. Also being used in skin lightener products because it has been shown to reduce the development of melanin (*see*).

ASARUM SIEBOLDI • Snakeweed. European Wild Ginger. The leaves contain a highly aromatic essential oil. It can cause profuse discharge of mucus from the nasal passages.

ASCOPHYLLUM NODOSUM • Knotted Wrack. A common large brown seaweed, dominant on sheltered rocky shores. The species has long, straplike fronds with large egg-shaped air bladders at regular intervals. Used in body care products. *See* Thalassotherapy.

ASCORBIC ACID • Vitamin C. A preservative and antioxidant widely used in cosmetic creams, particularly bleach and lemon creams and soaps, hair dyes and conditioners. Promoted in antiwrinkle products. Vitamin C is necessary for normal teeth, bones, and blood vessels. The white or slightly yellow powder darkens upon exposure to air. Reasonably stable when it remains dry in air, but deteriorates rapidly when exposed to air while in solution.

ASCORBYL METHYLSILANOL PECTINATE • An antioxidant. *See* Pectin.

ASCORBYL PALMITATE • A salt of ascorbic acid (*see*), it is used as a preservative and antioxidant in cosmetic creams and lotions to prevent rancidity.

ASCORBYL STEARATE • *See* Ascorbyl Palmitate.

ASEAN • Association of Southeast Asian Nations. A regional community of ten states with the aim of accelerating economic growth and social progress, and promoting peace and security.

ASEAN COLORS ALLOWED FOR USE IN COSMETIC PRODUCTS • Not all inclusive.

10006 Green allowed only in products briefly in contact with the skin.

10020 Green for all cosmetics except around eyes.

10316 (3) Yellow for all cosmetics except around eyes.

11680 Yellow for cosmetics except mucous membranes.

11710 Yellow for cosmetics except mucous membranes.

11725 Orange allowed only in products briefly in contact with the skin.

11920 Orange allowed in all cosmetic products.

12010 Red for cosmetics except mucous membranes.

12120 Red intended only for cosmetics briefly in contact with the skin.

12370 Red intended only for cosmetics briefly in contact with the skin.

12420 Red intended only for cosmetics briefly in contact with the skin.

12480 Brown intended only for cosmetics briefly in contact with the skin.

12490 Red allowed in all cosmetics.

12700 Yellow intended only for cosmetics briefly in contact with the skin.

13015. E 105. Fast Yellow. Allowed in all cosmetics.

15620 Red intended only for cosmetics briefly in contact with the skin.

18130 Red intended only for cosmetics briefly in contact with the skin.

18690 Yellow intended only for cosmetics briefly in contact with the skin.

14270. E103. Orange 6. Allowed in all cosmetics.

ASIATIC ACID • A carboxylic fatty acid that is used as a skin-conditioning ingredient.

ASIATICOSIDE • Derived from the plant *Centella asiatica,* known to possess wound-healing properties. Enhanced healing activity has been attributed to increased collagen formation and angiogenesis. Used as an antioxidant and skin-conditioning ingredient.

ASPALATHUS LINEARIS • A member of the pea family. Rooibos is the Afrikaans name for tea from this tree also known as "bushman" or "red-bush" tree. Actually, a South African shrub having flat acuminate leaves and yellow flowers; leaves are aromatic when dried and used to make an herbal tea. Extract contains tannin (*see*) and is used as a skin conditioner.

ASPARAGOPSIS ARMATA • Red Algae (*see*).

ASPEN • *Populus tremuloides.* Used in fragrances.

ASIMINA TRIOBA • *See* Pawpaw Extract.

ASPARAGINE • A nonessential amino acid (*see*). It is widely found in plants and animals both free and combined with proteins. It is used as a culture medium and as a medicine. In cosmetics, it is used to help moisturizers penetrate the skin.

ASPARAGUS ROOT EXTRACT • *Asparagus officinalis.* Sparrowgrass. The root is used in Chinese medicine as a tonic. In India, it is used as a hormonal tonic for the female reproductive system. It is prescribed for women to promote fertility, relieve menstrual pains, increase breast milk, and generally nourish and strengthen the female reproductive system. It is also used as a tonic for the lungs in consumptive diseases and for wasting in AIDS. Asparagus contains glycosides, asparagine, sucrose, starch, and mucilage. In 1992, the FDA proposed a ban on asparagus in oral menstrual drug products because it has not been shown to be safe and effective for its stated claims.

ASPARTAME • A compound prepared from aspartic acid (*see*) and phenylalanine, with about two hundred times the sweetness of sugar, discovered during routine screening of drugs for the treatment of ulcers. The G.D. Searle Company sought FDA approval in 1973. The FDA approved it in 1974, but objections that aspartame might cause brain damage led to a stay, or legal postponement, of that approval. Another problem arose. An FDA investigation of records of animal studies conducted for Searle drug approvals and for aspartame raised questions. The FDA arranged for an independent audit, which took more than two years and concluded that the aspartame studies and results were authentic. The agency then organized an expert board of inquiry and the members concluded that the evidence did not support the charge that aspartame might kill clusters of brain cells or cause other damage. However, persons with phenylketonuria, or PKU, must avoid protein foods such as meat that contain phenylalanine—one of two components of aspartame. The board did, however, recommend that aspartame not be approved until further long-term animal testing could be conducted to rule out a possibility that aspartame might cause brain tumors. The FDA's Bureau of Foods reviewed the study data already available and concluded that the board's concern was unfounded. Aspartame was approved for use as a tabletop sweetener in certain dry foods on October 22, 1981. It also was approved for breath mints, hard and soft; as a flavor enhancer in chewing gum and hard candy; instant coffee and tea beverages; ready-to-serve nonalcoholic beverages, fruit juice–based beverages and concentrates or syrup; as a flavor enhancer for malt beverages containing less than 3 percent alcohol; and in frostings, toppings, fillings, glazes, and icings for precooked baked goods. Used in cosmetics as a flavoring ingredient.

ASPARTIC ACID, DL & L FORMS • Aminosuccinate Acid. A nonessential amino acid (*see*) occurring in animals and plants, sugarcane, sugar beets, and molasses. It is usually synthesized for commercial purposes.

ASPERGILLUS • A genus of fungi. It contains many species of mold spores, which produce the antibiotic aspergillic acid. An *Aspergillus flavus*–Oryzae group of molds has been cleared by the U.S. Department of Agriculture's Meat Inspection Division to soften tissues of beef cuts, with: "Solutions containing water, salt, monosodium glutamate, and approved proteolytic enzymes applied or injected into cuts of beef shall not result in a gain of more than 3 percent above the weight of the untreated product." It is also used in bakery products such as bread, rolls, and buns. Toxicity is unknown but because of the use of the fungi-antibiotic and monosodium glutamate, allergic reactions would certainly be possible. Used in eye cosmetics.

ASPERULA ODORATA • *See* Woodruff.

ASPIRIN • Acetylsalicylic Acid. It is the most commonly taken drug in the United States. It is widely used as an analgesic, antifever, and anti-inflammatory. It produces allergic reactions in an estimated two persons per one hundred. Of the people with severe asthma, about 5 to 10 percent are aspirin sensitive. Allergy to aspirin occurs most frequently in people between the ages of forty and sixty who have a long history of sinusitis, nasal polyps, and high levels of eosinophils (a type of white blood cell). Allergy to aspirin can cause symptoms that range from rashes, hives, and swelling to asthmatic attacks that may be life-threatening. The onset of severe symptoms may come within fifteen minutes after ingesting aspirin, or it may not occur for hours. The exact mechanism of the aspirin reaction remains uncertain because no antibodies to aspirin have been found. However, those allergic to aspirin may also be sensitive to other salicylates (*see*) such as tartrazine, used in yellow and orange dyes.

ASTAXANTHIN • A yellow coloring found mostly in animal organisms, it is used in fish feed for salmon to increase their orange coloring. It is exempt from color certification. Used as a colorant and skin conditioner. Astaxanthin protects the skin against UV damage and is reputedly more efficient than other carotenoids (*see*). Research published in a 2008 edition of *Experimental Dermatology* compares the protection provided by astaxanthin (AX) to that of canthaxanthin (CX) and beta-carotene. Out of the three it was astaxanthin that provided the most effective protection when human dermal fibroblasts underwent UV radiation, concluded the scientists led by Emanuela Camera from San Gallicano Dermatology Institute in Rome. UVA radiation is known to both trigger the creation of reactive oxygen species (ROS) and deplete the antioxidant defense system of the fibroblasts by affecting antioxidant enzymes such as catalase and superoxide dismutase. For this reason, supplementing the system with antioxidants theoretically can help protect against UV damage, explained the authors.

ASTER TATARICUS • Species of aster. Extracts from the roots are used by herbalists to treat cold symptoms, pulmonary complaints, and fluid retention in the lungs and bronchial passages.

ASTRAGALUS EXTRACT • *See* Astragalus Membranaceus Extract.

ASTRAGALUS MEMBRANACEUS EXTRACT • This herb is the root of *Astragalus* of the family Leguminosae. It is produced mainly in the Chinese provinces of Shanxi, Gansu, Heilongjiang, and Inner Mongolia. It is dug in spring or autumn, sliced and dried in the sun, then used unprepared or stir-baked with honey. Sweet flavor. The Chinese believe it promotes pus discharge and tissue regeneration and acts to reduce swelling.

ASTRAGALUS SINICUS AND EXTRACT • Chinese Milk Vetch Extract. Derived from *Astragalus sinicus*. Used in skin cleansers. *See* Astragalus Membranaceus Extract.

ASTRINGENT • Usually promoted for oily skin. A clear liquid containing mostly alcohol, but with small amounts of other ingredients such as boric acid, alum, menthol, and/or camphor. A typical astringent formula: ethanol, 50 percent; sorbitol, 2.5 percent (*see both*); perfume oil, 0.1 percent; menthol, 0.1 percent; boric acid, 2.0 percent (*see both*); water, 44.9 percent. In addition to making the skin feel refreshed, it usually gives a tightened feeling from the evaporation of the ingredients. According to the American Medical Association, there is no evidence that astringents tighten or shrink the pores. Usually toxic when ingested because of denatured alcohol content. Botanical astringents include: stringent agrimony, alder, apple, avens, bayberry, bearberry, bethroot, betony (wood), birch, bistort, blackberry, bugle, burnet (greater), cassia, cedar, horse chestnut, chestnut, cinnamon, black cohosh columbine, comfrey, costmary, cudweed, dog-rose, elder, elecampane, elm, evening primrose, eyebright, fireweed, frostwort gale, goldenrod, hawthorn, horsetail, hound's tongue, houseleek, ivy, Jacob's ladder, knotgrass, lady's mantle, larch, lily, loosestrife, lungwort, red maple, matico, meadowsweet, mullein, myrrh, nettle, oak, olive, pipsissewa, plantain, poppy, quince, ragwort, raspberry, red root, rhubarb, rose (pale), rose (red), rosemary, rowan tree, rupturewort, sage, sassy bark, scullcap (Virginian), self-heal, St. John's wort, silverweed, Solomon's seal, speedwell strawberry, tag alder, tea, thistle (scotch), tree of heaven, vervain, vine, walnut, willow (white), wintergreen, witch hazel.

ASTROCARYUM MURUMURU • *See* Palm Oil.

ATELOCOLLAGEN • A collagen (*see*) that has been treated with enzymes to soften it.

ATHLETE'S FOOT • Tinea Pedis. A fungus infection in which the skin between and under the toes, especially the fourth and fifth toes, becomes irritated, red, flaky, and itchy. Sweat or water makes the top layer of the skin white and soggy. Other parts of the foot may also be affected.

ATOPIC DERMATITIS • A chronic, itching inflammation of the skin also called eczema (*see*).

ATRACTYLIS LYRATA • Byakujutsu. The FDA has it on its poison plant list, meaning there have been some scientific reports of toxicity.

ATRACTYLOIDES JAPONICA • Atractyloides. Japanese Honeysuckle. Used in Oriental medicine as a diuretic to eliminate excess moisture and sodium.

ATRIPLEX NUMMULARIA • Old Man Saltbush. Australian Saltbush. Saltbushes are extremely tolerant of salt content in the ground. Their name comes from the fact that they retain salt in their leaves. They thrive where summers are hot. Used as a skin conditioner.

ATROPA BELLADONNA AND ITS PREPARATIONS • Belladonna, or deadly nightshade (*Atropa belladonna* or its variety acuminata Royle ex Lindl), beladona, belladone, belladonnae herbae pulvis standardisatus, belladonna herbum, belladonna homaccord, belladonna injeel, belladonna leaf, belladonna pulvis normatus, belladonnae folium, belladonna radix, belladonne, devil's cherries, great morel, herba somniferum, strygium, stryshon. Belladonna is an herb that has been used through the ages for everything from headaches to inflammation and menstrual symptoms. Belladonna is known to contain active agents with anticholinergic (*see*) properties, such as atropine, hyoscine (scopolamine), and hyoscyamine. The drug atropine is produced from the foliage, which along with the berries are extremely toxic, with hallucinogenic properties. Some of the derivatives are used in medicine. Common adverse effects include dry mouth, urinary retention, flushing, pupillary dilation, constipation, confusion, and delirium. Because the compound made the pupils of the eyes dilated and that was thought to make women more beautiful, it was used as a cosmetic. Banned in cosmetics by the EU, UK, and ASEAN (*see*).

ATROPINE, ITS SALTS AND DERIVATIVES • Banned in cosmetics by the EU, UK, and ASEAN. *See* Atropa Belladonna.

ATTAPULGITE • *See* Fuller's Earth.

AUCOUMEA KLAINEANA • Tropical African tree. Yields fragrant oleo-gum resins from the bark. Used principally in incense manufacture and perfumery.

AVENA SATIVA MEAL • *See* Oat Bran and Oatmeal.

AVENS • *Geum urbanum.* Clove Root. Colewort. Herb Bennet. Wild Rye. A perennial herb that derives its name from the Spanish for "antidote." It contains essential oils (*see*), tannins (*see*), resin, and organic acids. It is used as an astringent tonic for stomach problems, diarrhea, and leukorrhea, and as a gargle for sore throats.

AVERRHOA CARAMBOLA • Derivative of an East Indian tree widely cultivated in the tropics. Has somewhat acid fruit and is used in Chinese cookery.

AVOBENZONE • 1-(4-methoxyphenyl)-3-(4-tert-butylphenyl)propane-1,3-dione, Butyl methoxy dibenzoylmethane, BMDBM, Parsol 1789, Eusolex 9020. An oil-soluble ingredient used in sunscreen products to absorb the full spectrum of UVA rays. Its ability to absorb ultraviolet light over a wider range of wavelengths than many organic sunscreen agents has led to its use in many commercial preparations marketed as "broad spectrum" sunscreens. Although there is little information about it being tested, avobenzone was patented in 1973 and was approved in the EU in 1978. It was approved by the FDA in 1988. Its use is permitted worldwide. Avobenzone has been shown to degrade significantly in light, resulting in less protection over time. The UVA light in a day of sunlight in a temperate climate is sufficient to break down most of the compound. This degradation can be reduced by using a photostabilizer, like octocrylene (*see*).

AVOCADAMIDOPROPALKONIUM CHLORIDE • A quaternary ammonium compound (*see*) made from avocados.

AVOCADO • *Persea gratissima.* The pulpy green fruit of the genus *Persea,* originating in South America and Mexico, it is also called alligator pear, and the tree has been nicknamed "the testicle tree," because of the shape of its fruit. The avocado is used in folk medicine as an aphrodisiac. An emollient, it is used in "organic" cosmetics for its high fat and vitamin A and C components. It is also used in shampoos. The CIR Expert Panel (*see*) concludes this is a safe ingredient in the present practices of use and concentration.

AVOCADOMIDE DEA • A mixture of the fatty acids (*see*) derived from avocado (*see*).

AVOIDANCE • Measures taken to avoid contact with allergy-producing substances. Since there are no cures for allergies, as of yet, avoiding allergens is the best way to combat them.

AWAPUHI EXTRACT • Wild Ginger. Hawaiians used the awapuhi rhizomes to scent their tapa. Medicinally it was used for bruises, cuts, and sores and for headaches, toothaches, ringworm, and other skin diseases, as well as achy joints and sprains.

AYURVEDIC EXTRACTS • Ayurvedic medicine is an ancient system of health care that is native to the Indian subcontinent and means the "knowledge of life." "Life" itself is defined as the "combination of the body, sense organs, mind, and soul, the factor responsible for preventing decay and death, which sustains the body over time, and guides the processes of rebirth."

AZELAIC ACID • Prepared by oxidation of ricinoleic acid, it occurs in rancid oleic acid. It is used in anti-acne preparations.

AZELAMIDE MEA • *See* Azelaic Acid.

AZELOYL DI(ETHYL SALICYLATE) • Nonanedioic Acid. Used as a skin conditioner. *See* Azelaic Acid and Salicylates.

AZO DYES • Used in nonpermanent hair rinses and tints. Azo dyes belong to a large category of colorings that are characterized by the way they combine with nitrogen. These are a very large class of dyes made from diazonium compounds and phenol. The dyes usually contain a mild acid, such as citric or tartaric. They can cause allergic reactions. People who become sensitized to permanent hair dyes containing para-phenylenediamine (*see* Phenylenediamine) also develop a cross-sensitivity to azo dyes. That is, a person who is allergic to permanent *p*-phenylenediamine dyes will also be allergic to azo dyes. There are reports that azo dyes are absorbed through the skin. Examples of azo dyes include: CI 11680; CI 11710; 12010; and CI 1805. *See* Acid Dyes, the name the United States uses; efforts are being made to harmonize dyes for all countries.

AZTEC MARIGOLD • Tagetes. Extract and Oil. The meal is the dried, ground flower petals of *Tagetes erecta,* a strong-scented, tropical American herb, mixed with no more than 0.3 percent ethoxyquin, a herbicide and antioxidant. The extract is taken from tagetes peels. Both the meal and the extract are used to enhance the yellow color of chicken skin and eggs. They are incorporated in chicken feed, supplemented sufficiently with yellow coloring xanthophyll. The coloring has been permanently listed since 1963 but is exempt from certification. The oil is extracted from the Aztec flower and used in fruit flavorings for beverages, ice cream, ices, candy, baked goods, gelatin, desserts, and condiments. Used in skin care products.

AZUKI BEANS • Used as an abrasive in scrub products.

AZULENE • A blue to greenish black hydrocarbon. Used as an antacid in cosmetics. It has shown anti-inflammatory effects, but the CIR Expert Panel (*see*) concludes there is insufficient data to support the safety of this ingredient in cosmetic products.

B

BABASSU • A nondrying edible oil expressed from the kernels of the babassu palm, *Orbignya barbosiana,* grown in Brazil. Used in foods and soaps, but it is expensive.

BABASSUAMIDE • A mixture of fatty acids derived from babassu (*see*). It is used as a hair conditioner, foam booster, and thickening ingredient.

BABASSUAMIDE DEA • Fatty acids derived from babassu (*see*).

BABASSUAMIDOPROPALKONIUM CHLORIDE • The quaternary ammonium (*see*) derived from babassu (*see*). Used as an antistatic ingredient in hair conditioners.

BABASSUAMIDOPROPYL BETAINE • A compound containing the fatty acids of babassu (*see*) and betaine (*see*). Used as an antistatic ingredient in hair and skin products.

BABIES • Baby products are products intended to be used on infants and children under the age of three. Specially formulated to be mild and nonirritating and use ingredients that are selected for these properties. Included are baby shampoos and baby lotions, oils, powders, and creams. Ingredients banned by the EU in products for youngsters under three years: boric acid, calcium salicylate, magnesium salicylate, MEA salicylate, potassium salicylate, salicyclic acid, sodium salicylate. Others not recommended for children include alpha hydroxy and botanical complexes, ammonium glycolate, citric acid, glycolic acid, glyomer in cross-linked-g-fatty acids, alpha natrium, depilatories containing hydroxide sulfide, thioglycolid acid, thioglycolate. The fewer "cosmetics" you use on babies, the better, but certainly don't use any on babies under three unless the label specifically says it is appropriate, and even then proceed with caution. For ingredient and safety information on baby products, Cosmeticsinfo.org, a trade group, says: "Six of the seven phthalates studied in this investigation are not used in infant shampoo, lotion, or powder. The presence of these phthalates in urine samples, if true, could not have been caused by use of infant personal care products. The phthalates either came from another source or were erroneously reported to be present. This uncertainty could have been avoided if the researchers had analyzed the infant personal care products to determine if these phthalates were present in the products before reporting a correlation." The only phthalate that is sometimes present in personal care products intended for use on children and infants is diethyl phthalate (DEP). However, when it is used in such products, the amount used is so low that it would be unlikely to yield metabolites that could be detected in the urine samples analyzed. A study by the U.S. Food and Drug Administration (FDA), http://www.cfsan.fda.gov/~dms/cos-phth.html, published in 2006, shows that DEP is the only phthalate present in lotions and shampoo and the one baby product analyzed in the study and that the levels in these products are very low.

The Cosmeticsinfo.org trade site also says about phthalates in cosmetics: "Is the DEP used in some baby care products safe?"

These are ingredients often found in baby products (*see all*):

- Botanicals
- Carbomer
- Cetyl Alcohol
- Citric Acid
- Colorants
- Dimethicone
- Dipropylene Glycol
- Fragrance
- Glycerin
- Glyceryl Stearate
- Isopropyl Palmitate
- Mineral Oil
- Myristyl Myristate
- PEG-80 Sorbitan Laurate
- PEG-100 Stearate
- PEG-150 Distearate
- Phthalates
- Polyquaternium-10 Tetrasodium EDTA
- Preservatives
- Sodium Laureth Sulfate
- Sodium Lauryl Sulfate
- Sorbitan Stearate
- Stearic Acid

- Stearyl Alcohol
- Synthetic Beeswax
- Talc
- Tocopheryl Acetate
- Water

BABY CREAM • Aimed at protecting babies' skin against irritation and soothing it, such formulas usually contain mineral oil, paraffin, lanolin, white beeswax, and ceresin. They may also contain many other ingredients, including petrolatum, mineral wax, glyceryl monostearate, methyl- and propylparabens, extract of lanolin, sterol, hydrogenated fatty oils, and spermaceti (*see all*). Lanolin, lanolin derivatives, beeswax, and the parabens are common allergens, and if your baby develops a rash, consult your physician.

BABY LOTION • Aimed at protecting, soothing, and cleansing the delicate skin of babies. Usually contains antimicrobials, emulsifiers, humectants to retain moisture, thickeners, and often some perfume. The product may also contain lanolin, mineral oil, cetyl alcohol, preservatives, and antioxidants (*see all*). Few problems are reported by consumers except for an occasional rash. However, a number of the ingredients used can cause allergic responses, particularly the perfumes and antimicrobials. If your baby develops a rash, read the label and check the product against ingredients listed in this book. Take the information to your physician, who can make the definitive diagnosis.

BABY OIL • Aimed at protecting and soothing baby skin. Usually contains mineral oil, palmitate, lanolin, vegetable oils, and lanolin derivatives (*see all*). Mineral oil or vegetable oil right from the pantry will do the same job and lessen the chances of allergic contact dermatitis. If you suspect the product is causing a rash, check the ingredients on the label and see if they may be allergens for your child. Take the information to your physician, who can make a definitive diagnosis.

BABY POWDER • Soothes, dries, and protects baby skin from irritation. Usually contains talc, kaolin, zinc oxide, starch, magnesium carbonate (*see all*), perfume oil, and—although there have been repeated warnings against it—boric acid (*see*). Cornstarch from your pantry shelf does not carry the problems of talc (*see*) and will work as well and less expensively.

BABY SHAMPOOS • Products that are intended to be used to cleanse the hair of infants and children under the age of three. According to Cosmeticsinfo.org, the trade group of the industry, these products are specially formulated to be nonirritating and mild to the eyes. Often, these products contain nonionic ingredients, which tend to be milder than ionic ingredients, which carry a slight negative charge. Adults who have sensitive hair or who are very sensitive to ordinary products may also use baby shampoos. The trade group says, "Manufacturers conduct extensive safety tests to ensure that these products are safe for use on young children. All products should be used only under close adult supervision. It is very important to read and follow the directions for use that are on the product. Any consumer having questions about the use of the product should call the number provided on the label of the product."

BABY SOAP • Usually a mild sodium soap of coconut and/or palm oil. Some are made of polyunsaturated vegetable oils. Baby soaps may contain colloidal oatmeal, a mild, soap-free sudsing ingredient, lanolin derivatives, and a germ killer such as chlorobutanol. If your baby is known to be allergic to any of the above, check with the company about the soap's ingredients and then check them in this book.

BACILLUS FERMENT • Used in producing a chemical change with the use of harmless bacteria. *See* Bacillus/Glutamic Acid Ferment Filtrate.

BACILLUS/GLUTAMIC ACID FERMENT FILTRATE • The filtered fermentation of glutamic acid (*see*) with the harmless bacteria, *Bacillus natto,* used as a skin-conditioning ingredient. *Bacillus natto* is often made into an edible product that smells like cheese.

BACILLUS/RICE BRAN EXTRACT/SOYBEAN EXTRACT FERMENT • Fermented soybean and rice bran with a harmless bacterial used as a humectant, antioxidant, hair- and skin-conditioning ingredient, and an emollient.

BACITRACIN • Bactine First Aid Antibiotic. Baciguent. Campho-Phenique Triple Antibiotic. Mycitracin. Aquaphor. Antibiotic Ointment. Neosporin. Polysporin. Introduced in 1948, it is used systemically to treat pneumonia or abscesses caused by staphylococci. It is used topically to treat staphylococcic and streptococcic infections of the skin, outer ear, and eyelids. It is combined with other drugs into ointments that have a wide spectrum of bacteria-killing action. It is used as a germ killer in cosmetics.

BACKHOUSIA CITRIODORA • Lemon Myrtle Oil. The species is known to have at least two chemical forms, and their respective aromatic essential oils (which give the aroma and flavor) are richer either in citral or its close chemical relative citronellal (*see*). The citral form seems to be much commoner, and this form is the one selected and grown for its sweet lemon-type perfume and flavor. When crushed, the leaves emit a very strong odor. The oil from the plant is used in flavorings and fragrances as well as a pesticide.

BACOPA • An Ayurvedic herb used in India for memory enhancement, epilepsy, insomnia, and as a mild sedative. This herb commonly grows in marshy areas throughout India. Studies show that bacopa has antioxidant properties, protects mental function in those with epilepsy who take the drug phenytion, while a study on rats showed bacopa administration improves learning skills. Two saponins, designated as bacopaside I and II, have been isolated from *Bacopa monnieri.* Recent human studies show bacopa has the ability to improve memory and mood. Extract of the plant is used as a skin-conditioning ingredient.

BACTERIAL CATALASE • A catalase is an enzyme in plant and animal tissues. It exerts a chemical reaction that converts hydrogen peroxide into water and oxygen. Derived from bacteria by a pure culture fermentation process, bacterial catalase may be used safely, according to the FDA, in destroying and removing the hydrogen peroxide that has been used in the manufacture of cheese—providing "the organism *Micrococcus lysodeikticus* from which the bacterial catalase is to be derived, is demonstrated to be non-pathogenic." The organism is removed from the bacterial catalase prior to the use of the catalase. The catalase is to be used in an amount not in excess of the minimum required to produce its intended effect. On the Canadian Hotlist (*see*). In Canada, catalases must carry a warning not to put the product on broken or abraded skin.

BACTRIS GASIPAES • Peach Palm. Tree grown in Hawaii and Central America. The fruit is rich in vitamin A and has a high protein and starch value. The fruit juice is used as a hair- and skin-conditioning ingredient.

BAK • *See* Benzalkonium Chloride.

BAKUCHIOL • Isolated from the seeds of *Psoralea corylifolia,* a tree native to China with various uses in traditional medicine, it has been reported to have antitumor activity. Used as a germicide in cosmetics.

BAKUMONDOU EKISU • An extract of the roots of *Ophiopogon japonicus* or other species of the lily family. Used as a skin-conditioning ingredient.

BALANITES ROXBURGHII • Desert Date, Lolab Tree. The fats and oils expressed from the seeds are used as a skin-conditioning ingredient.

BALM • A variation of the word *balsam*. Usually means a soothing ointment, especially a fragrant one, or a soothing application. *See also* Melissa Oil.

BALM MINT • *Melissa officinalis*. Balm of Gilead. The secretion of any of several small evergreen African or Asian trees with leaves that yield a strong aromatic odor when bruised. Known in ancient Palestine as a soothing medication for the skin. Used in cosmetics as an unguent that soothes and heals the skin. It is also used for its fragrance in perfumes.

BALM MINT OIL • A natural fruit and liquor flavoring ingredient for beverages, ice cream, candy, and baked goods. The balm leaves may also be used for flavorings in beverages and cosmetics. May cause allergic reactions.

BALM OF GILEAD EXTRACT • From the buds of *Commiphora opobalsamum*, a small evergreen grown in Africa and Asia. It has been valued since ancient times as an unguent that heals and soothes. Has a fragrant oil.

BALSAM • The natural exudate from tree or plant.

BALSAM CANADA • *Abies balsamea*. An oleoresin used in creams.

BALSAM COPAIBA • *Copaifera officinalis*. The oleoresin (*see*) from South American trees that yield a thick, brown liquid. It has a strong odor and is used in perfumes and soaps and as a film former.

BALSAM MECCA • Balsam of Gilead. Obtained from a twig. Insoluble in water, soluble in alcohol. Used to scent perfume.

BALSAM OREGON • *Pseudotsuga menziesii*. Douglas Fir Oil. Balsam Fir. Oregon Fir. Resin is used in perfumery.

BALSAM PERU • *Myroxylon pereirae*. A dark brown, viscous liquid with a pleasant lingering odor and a warm, bitter taste. It is used in face masks, perfumes, cream hair rinses, and astringents. Obtained from Peruvian balsam in Central America near the Pacific Coast. Mildly antiseptic and irritating to the skin; may cause contact dermatitis and a stuffy nose. It is one of the most common sensitizers and may cross-react with benzoin, rosin, benzoic acid, benzyl alcohol, cinnamic acid, essential oils, orange peel, eugenol, cinnamon, clove, balsam Tolu, storax, benzyl benzoate, and wood tars.

BALSAM TOLU • *Myroxylon balsamum*. An ingredient used in perfumery and soap. Extracted from a tree grown on elevated plains and mountains in South America. Yellowish brown or brown, thick fluid with a strong odor and taste. Its vapor has been used as an expectorant. *See* Balsam Peru for toxicity.

BAMBOO • A woody grass of *Bambusa arundinacea, B. vulgaris,* and related genera. Usually has a hollow stem. Young shoots are used as food. Employed in "organic" cosmetics. Used in bath products.

BAMBUSA ARUNDINACEA • *See* Bamboo.

BANANA • *Musa sapientum*. The common fruit, high in potassium (*see*), used for dry skin by organic cosmetic enthusiasts. A banana face mask formula: Mash 1 ripe banana and mix thoroughly with 1 tablespoon of almond meal (*see*) plus 2 tablespoons of yogurt. Spread mixture on face and neck. Leave on for 5 to 10 minutes. Remove with lukewarm water.

BAOBAB • *Adansonia digitata*. Monkey Bread Tree, the Cream of Tartar Tree, and the "Upside Down Tree." A member of the Bombacaceae family originally located in South Africa, Botswana, Namibia, Mozambique, and Zimbabwe but can be found in most countries within the African continent. Export by traders means the baobab tree is also common in America, India, Sri Lanka, Malaysia, China, Jamaica, and Holland. High in vitamin C, pectin, and calcium. Used to make soap and is being promoted for skin care. Besides moisturizing, it is included in exfoliating scrubs and hair care. The baobab has been approved recently by the UK for eating.

BAPTISIA TINCTORIA • Wild Indigo. The root contains alkaloids, glycosides, and resin (*see all*). It is used by herbalists to treat infections of the ear, nose, and throat. Taken both internally and as a mouthwash, it reputedly heals mouth ulcers and sore gums and helps to control pyorrhea. Internally, it is used by herbalists to aid in reducing fevers, constipation, and swollen glands. Externally, in an ointment, it is used to treat infected ulcers and soothe sore nipples. Used in a douche, herbalists say it helps relieve vaginal discharge. Toxic in large doses, it can cause severe diarrhea and violent vomiting and may affect the heart.

BARIUM HYDROXIDE • *See* Barium Sulfate.

BARIUM SALTS • The EU and ASEAN (*see*) banned barium in cosmetics with the exception of barium sulphate, barium sulphide, and lakes, salts, and pigments prepared from the coloring agents listed under the conditions specified above.

BARIUM SULFATE • Blanc Fixe. The salt of the alkaline earth metal, it is a fine, white, odorless, tasteless powder used as a white coloring and as a base for depilatories and other cosmetics. Barium hydroxide is also used in a similar manner. The barium products are poisonous when ingested and frequently cause skin reactions when applied. Only barium sulfate is permitted in Canadian cosmetics.

BARIUM SULFIDE • Used in depilatories as a base, it is a grayish white to pale yellow powder. A skin irritant, it causes rashes and chemical burns. Should never be applied to broken or inflamed skin. On the Canadian Hotlist (*see*).

BARLEY EXTRACT • *Hordeum vulgare.* Pearl Barley. Prelate. The seed is used by herbalists to treat diarrhea and bowel inflammation. Chinese herbalists use it as an anti-inflammatory diuretic for relieving gallbladder ailments, reducing swelling and tumors, and treating jaundice. It contains proteins, prolamines, albumen, sugars, starch, fats, B vitamins, and alkaloids (*see*).

BARLEY FLOUR • A cereal grass cultivated since prehistoric times. Used in the manufacture of malt beverages, as a breakfast food, and as a demulcent (*see*) in cosmetics.

BARM • A yeast formed during the fermentation of alcoholic beverages.

BAROSMA BETULINA • Buchu. From the leaves and roots of *Barosma betulina,* used as a skin-conditioning ingredient. *See* Buchu.

BARRIER INGREDIENT • A protective for hand creams and lotions, which acts as a barrier against irritating chemicals, including water and detergents. The water-repellent types deposit a film that acts as a barrier to water and water-soluble ingredients that irritate the skin; oil-repellent types act as barriers against oil and oil-soluble irritants. Silicones (*see*) are widely used as barrier ingredients. Other skin-protective ingredients in barrier ingredients include petrolatum, paraffin, ozokerite vegetables, beeswax, casein, various celluloses, alginic acid, zein, gum tragacanth, pectin, quince seed, bentonite, zinc oxide, zinc stearate, sodium silicate, talc, stearic acid, and titanium dioxide (*see all*).

BASE COAT • Similar to a nail polish (*see*) in form and formulation but does not contain pigment and has an increased amount of resin (*see*). Applied on the nail under nail polish to help prevent chipping and to allow smoother application of the nail enamel. *See* Nail Polish for toxicity.

BASIC BLUE 3 • A coal tar hair coloring. An oxazine color. *See* Coal Tar.

BASIC BLUE 6 • Medola's Blue. A phenol color. *See* Basic Dyes.

BASIC BLUE 7 • CI 42595. A triphenylmethane color (*see*) used in hair coloring.

BASIC BLUE 9 • Methylene Blue. CI 52015. Prepared from dimethylaniline and thiosulfuric acid. Dark green, odorless crystals used as a stain in bacteriology, as an ingredient for several chemicals, as a veterinary antiseptic, and as an antidote to cyanide poisoning. Also used in hair coloring.

BASIC BLUE 26 • CI 44045. A triphenylmethane color (*see*) used as a hair coloring.

BASIC BLUE 41 • CI 11154. Methylbenzothiazolium Chloride. *See* Basic Dyes.

BASIC BLUE 47 • A coal tar hair coloring. An anthraquinone color.

BASIC BLUE 99 • CI 56059. Arianor Steel Blue R. Used in hair dyes and tints and shampoos. May cause allergic reaction. The CIR Expert Panel (*see*) has listed this as top priority for review. *See* Basic Dyes.

BASIC BROWN 4 • CI 21010. Basic Brown R. Bismarck Brown 53. Prepared from toluene-2-4-diamine (*see* Toluene) with nitrous acid, it is a dark, solid brown, which turns reddish brown or violet in solution. Used in hair dyes. *See* Aniline for toxicity.

BASIC BROWN 1 • CI 12251. Arianor Sienna Brown R. An azo dye (*see*). A hair coloring.

BASIC BROWN 16 • CI 12250. Arianor Mahogany R. An azo dye (*see*) used as a hair coloring and in shampoos.

BASIC DYES • A group of dyes made from soluble salts, minerals, acids, and certain organic acids that form insoluble compounds with acidic fibers. They produce very bright colors but lack good fastness. *See* Aniline for toxicity.

BASIC GREEN 1 • CI 42040. Brilliant Green. A triphenylmethane group (*see*) color used as a hair coloring.

BASIC GREEN 4 • CI 42000 A coal tar color used in hair coloring.

BASIC ORANGE 1 • CI 11320. A coal tar color used in hair coloring. *See* Toluene.

BASIC ORANGE 2 • CI 11270. A coal tar hair coloring. *See* Benzene.

BASIC ORANGE 31 • An azo dye used in hair coloring. *See* Coal Tar.

BASIC RED 1 • CI 45160. An exanthene color used in hair coloring. *See* Coal Tar.

BASIC RED 2 • A phenazine color used in hair dyes.

BASIC RED 22 • CI 11055. A triazolium dye used as a hair coloring. *See* Azo Dyes.

BASIC RED 46 • A coal tar color used in hair coloring.

BASIC RED 51 • Ruby Red. A coal tar dye used in hair coloring.

BASIC RED 76 • CI 12245. *See* Azo Dyes.

BASIC RED 118 • CI 12251:1. A coal tar color used in hair coloring and in quaternary ammonium compounds. An amine color.

BASIC VIOLET 1 • CI 42535. Methyl Violet. A bright violet artificial coloring ingredient. On the Canadian Hotlist (*see*). *See* Aniline for toxicity.

BASIC VIOLET 2 • CI 42520. A triphenylmethane color used in hair coloring. *See* Coal Tar.

BASIC VIOLET 3 • CI 42555. (1- and 2-) Crystal Violet. Methyl Violet. Gentian Violet. A triarylmethane color. Dark green powder or greenish pieces with a metallic luster, it is used as an antiseptic and against worms as well as a coloring. The CIR Expert Panel (*see*) has listed this as top priority for review. On the Canadian Hotlist (*see*). Banned by the EU.

BASIC VIOLET 4 • CI 42600. A coal tar hair coloring.

BASIC VIOLET 10 • CI 45170. A xanthene (*see*) color. The salt of stearic acid is Solvent Red 49. The name can be used only when applied to batches of uncertified color. The CTFA adopted name for certified (*see*) batches is D & C Red No. 19, also called rhodamine B. A basic red dye, it is very soluble in water and alcohol and forms a bluish red fluorescent solution. Used as a dye for paper, wool, and silk, and as a biological stain as well as in cosmetics. On the Canadian Hotlist (*see*).

BASIC VIOLET 11:1 • CI 45174. A xanthene color used in hair coloring. *See* Coal Tar.

BASIC VIOLET 14 • CI 42510. Triphenylmethane color used in hair coloring. *See* Coal Tar.

BASIC VIOLET 16 • CI 48013. A coal tar color used in hair coloring.

BASIC YELLOW 11 • CI 48055. A triazolium dye. *See* Azo Dyes.

BASIC YELLOW 28 • CI 48054. A coal tar color used in hair coloring.

BASIC YELLOW 40 • A coal tar hair coloring.

BASIC YELLOW 57 • CI 1279. Arianor Straw Yellow. Hair coloring. *See* Basic Dyes.

BASIC YELLOW 87 • A hair coloring. *See* Pyridinium Compounds.

BASICOL T • A series of essential oils intended for replacement of oils of lavender, geranium, lemon, pine, ylang-ylang, neroli, and orris root (*see all*).

BASIL EXTRACT • The extract of the leaves and flowers of *Ocimum basilicum,* an herb having spikes of small white flowers and aromatic leaves used as a seasoning. A natural flavoring distilled from the flowering tops of the plant that has a slightly yellow-ish color and a spicy odor. GRAS

BASSIA LATIFOLIA • Llipe Butter. Seed Butter. Derived from a small family of European herbs that are also grown in North America. Used in skin conditioners.

BASSWOOD EXTRACT • Tilia. Extract of the flowers of *Tilia americana.*

BATH CAPSULES • Products intended to enhance the bathing experience by moistening, softening, and enhancing the cleaning of the skin. They usually have a pleasant aroma. There are nine ingredients (*see all*) commonly found in them:

- Botanicals
- Colors
- Fragrance
- Glycerin
- Hydrated Silica
- Preservatives
- Sodium Carbonate
- Sodium Chloride
- Sodium Dodecylbenzenesulfonate

BATH LOTION • For after a bath. Usually a cologne with some emollient oil. May also contain isopropyl myristate and fatty acids (*see both*). The emollient oil also acts as a carrier for the perfume. May cause allergic reactions depending upon your sensitivity and the ingredients used.

BATH OIL • Softens and protects the skin in a foaming or nonfoaming oil. The concentration of perfume in bath oil is usually quite high and may be a source of allergic reactions. The oil is usually a mineral or vegetable oil and includes a surfactant to cause the oil to spread on the surface of the water. A common ingredient of the foaming-type oil is TEA-lauryl sulfate, and sometimes foam stabilizers, such as saponin or methyl cellulose, are used to give the bubbles longevity; also the usual chemicals that are added are castor oil, isopropyl myristate, alcohol, lanolin, and certified colors (*see all*). A number of the ingredients may cause allergic contact dermatitis, so if you develop a rash, check the label.

BATH SALTS • May change the salinity of the bath water. Used to color, perfume, and chemically soften bath water, and to perfume the skin. Usually made from rock salt or sodium thiosulfate, which has been sprayed with alcohol, dye, or perfume. Rock salt is common table salt and has been used for treating inflammation of the skin. Sodium thiosulfate ("hypo") has been used to treat certain skin rashes and has a low toxicity. The effervescent type of bath salts are due to the added sodium bicarbonate and tartaric acid. The noneffervescent type may add trisodium phosphate and sodium chloride. Among other chemicals that may be in bath salts are borax, sodium hexylmetaphosphate, starch, sodium carbonate, and sodium sesquicarbonate (*see all*). Phosphate and borax may cause caustic irritation of the skin and mucous membranes; boric acid may be toxic when ingested or absorbed through the skin.

BATYL ALCOHOL • Derived from glycerin (*see*), it is isolated from shark oil, bone, and bone marrow. It is soluble in fat solvents. It is used as an emulsifier in skin creams.

BATYL ISOSTEARATE • An ester (*see*) of batyl alcohol and isostearic acid. *See* Glycerin.

BATYL STEARATE • An ester (*see*) of batyl alcohol (*see*).

BAY • *Pimenta acris.* Source of bay rum (*see*).

BAY LAUREL • *Laurus nobilis.* A tree of the laurel family, bay is native to southern Europe, where it can grow to a height of fifty feet. In Roman times, the aromatic quality of the leaves led the Romans to scatter it in buildings to ward off the plague. The bay was one of four hundred remedies used by Hippocrates, and through the centuries herbalists have used it to treat hysteria, ague, sprains, earache, and many other illnesses. Every part of the tree has healing properties, according to herbalists. It is used in "organic" cosmetics. *See also* Bay Oil. EU banned oil from the seed in cosmetics.

BAY OIL • Oil of Myrica. Astringent and antiseptic oil used in hair lotions and dressings, after-shave lotions, bay rum, and perfumes. Distilled from the leaves of the bayberry, it contains 40 to 55 percent eugenol (*see*). May cause allergic reactions and skin irritations.

BAY RUM • The alcoholic, aromatic oil distilled from the leaves of the bayberry and mixed with rum or made by mixing oil from the leaves with alcohol, water, and other oils. Widely used as an after-shave preparation and skin freshener. Also used in hair tonics. The basic formula for bay rum: bay oil, 0.20 percent; pimenta oil, 0.05 percent; ethyl alcohol, 50 percent; Jamaica rum, 10 percent; water, 39.75 percent; and caramel coloring. Can cause allergic reactions. *See* Eugenol for toxicity.

BAYBERRY • *Myrica cerifera.* Candleberry. Waxberry. Wax Myrtle. The bark contains volatile oil, starch, lignin, albumen, gum, tannic and gallic acids, astringent resins, and an acid resembling saponin. It is used by herbalists as a stimulant, astringent, and expectorant, and to induce sweating. It has been used to treat uterine prolapse and excessive menstrual bleeding and in a douche to treat vaginal infections. It has also been used to stop bleeding from the bowel and from the gums. A famous patent medicine containing bayberry, Dr. Thompson's Composition Powder, was used by many physicians to treat colds, coughs, and flu. There are several modern versions used by herbalists.

BAYBERRY WAX • Acrid and astringent resin from the dried root bark of the shrub that grows from Maryland to Florida and from Texas to Arkansas. It is used as an astringent in soaps and hair tonics. Formerly used to treat skin ulcers. May be irritating to the skin and cause an allergic reaction.

BEAN PALMITATE • The crushed beans of *Phaseolus* (beans) with palmitic acid (*see*) used in skin conditioners.

BEARBERRY EXTRACT • *See* Uva-Ursi.

BEAUTY MASKS • *See* Face Masks and Packs.

BEE BALM EXTRACT • An extract of the leaves of *Monarda didyma*. Contains bergamot (*see*). An orange flavoring extracted from a pear-shaped fruit whose rind yields a greenish brown oil. It is used in a tea for digestive problems and as a tonic. It can stain skin and may cause sensitivity to sunlight. *See also* Lemon Balm.

BEE POLLEN • A popular compound among naturalists, it contains nineteen amino acids, up to 35 percent protein, twelve vitamins, calcium, phosphorous, magnesium, iron, copper, manganese, sodium, potassium, chlorine, and sulfur. It is claimed that it increases stamina. Those who are allergic to bee stings may also be allergic to bee pollen. It is used in "organic" cosmetics.

BEEF • A number of cosmetic ingredients are derived from beef, including animal tissue extract; amniotic fluid; brain extract; calf blood extract; calf skin extract; calf skin hyolysate; collagen; elastin; embryo extract; glycoprotein; hemoglobin, hydrolysed; liver extract; mammarian hydrolysate; mammary extract; marrow extract; muscle extract; neatsfoot oil; omental lipids; placental enzymes, lipids, and proteins; serum albumin; serum protein; stomach extract; tallow; and udder extract (*see all*).

BEER • Used to rinse hair on the theory that it gives a feeling of increased body and manageability. The sugar and protein in the beer are probably responsible for the stiffening effect but, according to the American Medical Association, champagne would have the same effect. Beer leaves an odor on the hair that, unlike champagne, may, after a while, become quite unpleasant.

BEESWAX • From virgin bees and primarily used as an emulsifier. Practically insoluble in water. Yellow beeswax from the honeycomb is yellowish, soft to brittle, and has a honeylike odor. White beeswax is yellowish white and slightly different in taste but otherwise has the same properties as yellow beeswax. Used in many cosmetics, including baby creams, brilliantine hair dressings, cold cream, emollient creams, wax depilatories, eye creams, eye shadow, foundation creams, and makeup, lipstick, mascara, nail whiteners, protective creams, and paste rouge. Can cause contact dermatitis. The CIR Expert Panel (*see*) concludes this is a safe ingredient.

BEET EXTRACT • *Beta vulgaris*. The powdered stem base of the beet used for its reddish color in powders and rouges. No longer permitted as a colorant in the United States.

BEETROOT RED • Obtained from the roots of beets, this color is not approved in the United States but is used in European cosmetics.

BEHENALKONIUM CHLORIDE • *See* Quaternary Ammonium Compounds.

BEHENAMIDE • An amide (*see*) used as a thickening ingredient and an opacifier.

BEHENAMIDOPROPYL BETAINE • *See* Quaternary Ammonium Compounds and Betaine.

BEHENAMIDOPROPYL DIMETHYLAMINE • *See* Quaternary Ammonium Compounds.

BEHENAMINE OXIDE • *See* Behenic Acid.

BEHENETH-5, -10, -20, -30 • The polyethylene glycol ethers of behenyl alcohol. *See* Polyethylene Glycol and Behenyl Alcohol.

BEHENIC ACID • Docosanoic Acid. Colorless, water-soluble constituent of seed fats, animal fats, and marine animal oils. It is a fatty acid (*see*) used to opacify shampoos.

BEHENOXY DIMETHICONE • *See* Behenic Acid and Silicones.

BEHENOYL PG-TRIMONIUM • A quaternary ammonium compound (*see*).

BEHENTRIMONIUM CHLORIDE • *See* Quaternary Ammonium Compounds.

BEHENTRIMONIUM DIMETHICONE PEG-8 PHTHALATE • A quaternary ammonium compound (*see*) used as a hair-conditioning ingredient.

BEHENYL ALCOHOL • Docosanol. A mixture of fatty alcohols derived from behenic acid, a minor component of vegetable oils and animal fats. It is used in cosmetics as an opacifying ingredient, thickener, and emulsifier. Used also in synthetic fabrics and lubricants to prevent evaporation of water, and as an insecticide and antihistamine. Low toxicity.

BEHENYL BEESWAX • Skin conditioner. *See* Beeswax.

BEHENYL BEHENATE • The ester (*see*) of behenic acid (*see*).

BEHENYL BENZOATE • The ester (*see*) of behenyl benzoate. Used as a skin-conditioning ingredient. *See* Benzoic Acid.

BEHENYL BETAINE • *See* Behenic Acid and Betaine.
BEHENYL ERUCATE • Used in lipstick. *See* Behenic Acid and Erucic Acid.
BEHENYL HYDROXYETHYL IMIDAZOLINE • *See* Imidazoline.
BELAMCANDA CHINENSIS • Blackberry Lily. Freckle Face Leopard Flower. A plant material from China that grows in woods and creeks. It is used in Chinese medicine to treat sore throats and soothe mucous membranes.
BELLIS PERENNIS • Daisy Extract. The fresh or dried flowers of this plant, which is cultivated or grows wild all over North America, are used in an infusion or tincture. The flowers contain saponins, tannin, essential oil, flavones, bitter principle, and mucilage (*see all*). In cosmetics, it is used for skin lightening. *See* Melanin. Daisy also is used for coughs and inflammations of the mucous lining. It reputedly also helps arthritis, as well as liver and kidney problems.
BENINCASIA CERIFERA FRUIT AND SEED • Extract of wax gourd also called white pumpkin and winter melon. It is a vegetable and the wax is used in skin conditioners.
BENTONITE • A white clay found in the midwestern United States and in Canada. Used to thicken lotions, to suspend makeup pigments, and to emulsify oils, and used in makeup lotions, liquid makeup, and facial masks to absorb oil on the face and reduce shine. May clog the pores. Also used as a coloring. Inert and generally nontoxic, but if injected in rats, it can be fatal.
BENZALDEHYDE • Artificial Almond Oil. A colorless liquid that occurs in the kernels of bitter almonds. Lime is used in its manufacture. As the artificial essential oil of almonds, it is used in cosmetic creams and lotions, perfumes, soaps, and dyes. May cause allergic reactions. Highly toxic. The CIR Expert Panel (*see*) has listed this as top priority for review.
BENZALKONIUM BROMIDE • A quarternary ammonium compound (*see*) used as an antistatic ingredient, germicide, and deodorant. *See* Bromides, Potassium and Sodium.
BENZALKONIUM CHLORIDE • BAK. A widely used ammonium detergent (*see* Ammonium) in hair tonics, eye lotions, deodorants, mouthwashes, and after-shave lotions. It is a germicide with an aromatic odor and a very bitter taste. Used medicinally as a topical antiseptic and detergent. Allergic conjunctivitis has been reported when used in eye lotions. Lethal to frogs in concentrated oral doses. Highly toxic. In 1992, the FDA proposed a ban on the use of benzalkonium chloride to treat insect bites and stings and in astringent (*see*) drugs because it has not been shown to be safe and effective for stated claims in OTC products. It is a skin and eye irritant at concentrations greater than 0.1 percent. It is used in some cosmetic products at up to 5 percent. The CIR Expert Panel (*see*) concludes this is a safe ingredient if used at concentrations up to 0.1 percent. The EU advised that final hair care products should not exceed 3 percent, contact with the eyes should be avoided, and the hair products should be rinsed off. On the Canadian Hotlist (*see*).
BENZALKONIUM SACCHARINATE • A quarternary ammonium compound (*see*) used as an antistatic ingredient and germicide and deodorant. *See* Myristic Acid.
BENZALPHTHALIDE • Ultraviolet light absorber.
BENZAZEPINES AND BENZODIAZEPINES • Tranquilizing medications. *See* Benzene. Banned in Cosmetics by the EU and ASEAN (*see*).
BENZENE • A solvent obtained from coal and used in nail polish remover. Also used in varnishes, airplane glue, and lacquers, and as a solvent for waxes, resins, and oils. Highly flammable. Poisonous when ingested and irritating to the mucous membranes. Harmful amounts may be absorbed through the skin. Also can cause sensitivity to light

in which the skin may break out in a rash or swell. Inhalation of the fumes may be toxic. The Consumer Product Safety Commission voted unanimously in February 1978 to ban the use of benzene in the manufacture of many household products. The commission took the action in response to a petition filed by the Consumer Health Research Group, an organization affiliated with consumer advocate Ralph Nader. Earlier in the year, OSHA and the EPA both cited benzene as a threat to public health. For more than a century, scientists have known that benzene is a powerful bone-marrow poison, causing such conditions as aplastic anemia. Evidence has been mounting that it also causes leukemia. Derived from toluene or gasoline, it is used in the manufacture of detergents, nylon, and artificial leather; as an antiknock ingredient in gasoline; in airplane fuel, varnish, and lacquer; and as a solvent for waxes, resins, and oils. It has a chronic effect on bone marrow, destroying the marrow's ability to produce blood cells. Safety standards for cosmetic manufacturing workers and other workers have been set at 10 parts per million during an eight-hour day, but OSHA wants it reduced to 1 part per million. On the Canadian Hotlist (*see*). Banned in cosmetics by the EU and ASEAN (*see*).

1,2,4-BENZENETRIACETATE • Hair coloring. See Benzene.

BENZETHONIUM CHLORIDE • Widely used as an antistatic ingredient, deodorant, and cleansing ingredient in underarm deodorants, body and hand preparations, skin care products, and hair products. On the Canadian Hotlist (*see*) and is not permitted in products to be applied to mucous membranes. Permitted only at concentrations equal to or less than 0.2 percent in leave-on products and 0.3 percent in rinse-off products. *See* Quaternary Ammonium Compounds and Benzene.

BENZIDINE • A compound derived from nitrobenzene used mainly for dyeing textiles and paper that is a known human carcinogen (cancer-causing agent). Benzidine was one of the first chemicals for which an association of occupational exposure and increased incidence of urinary bladder cancer in humans was reported. Banned in cosmetics by the EU, UK and ASEAN (*see*).

BENZIMIDAZOL-2(3H)-ONE • *See* Benzene and Urea. Banned in cosmetics by the EU and ASEAN (*see*).

BENZOATES • There are many benzoates such as benzoic acid and sodium benzoate (*see both*) widely used in foods and cosmetics. They are antimicrobial preservatives. They have been associated with asthma and eczema. *See* Sodium Benzoate.

BENZOCAINE • Ethyl Aminobenzoate. A white, crystalline powder slightly soluble in water and a local anesthetic. Used in eyebrow-plucking creams and after-shave lotions. As an anesthetic, it is reported low in toxicity. However, there are reports of babies suffering from methemoglobinemia (lack of oxygen in the blood) due to absorption of benzocaine through the skin. But it is believed that the absorption was enhanced by inflamed skin or rectal fissures. Systemic central nervous system excitation has been reported in adults. However, scientists feel that the concentrations in most products have no toxic significance, though there are people who are allergic to benzocaine. On the Canadian Hotlist (*see*).

BENZODIHYDROPYRONE • Dihydrocoumarin. White to light yellow, oily liquid with a sweet odor. Prohibited. Should not be used as a fragrance ingredient based on its sensitizing potential. Banned by the UK and EU in fragrances.

BENZOIC ACID • A preservative that occurs in nature in cherry bark, raspberries, tea, anise, and cassia bark. First described in 1608, when it was found in gum benzoin. Used in chocolate, lemon, orange, cherry, fruit, nut, and tobacco flavorings. Also an antifungal ingredient in cosmetics such as hair rinses, cleansing products, and moisturizers. A mild irritant to the skin, it can cause allergic reactions. In 1992, the FDA proposed a ban on benzoic acid in astringent (*see*) drug products because it has not been shown to be safe and effective for its stated claims.

BENZOIN • Styrax benzoin. *See* Gum Benzoin.

BENZOPHENONES (1–12) • At least a dozen different benzophenones exist. They are used as fixatives (*see*) for heavy perfumes (e.g., geranium) and soaps (the smell of "new-mown hay"). Obtained as a white, flaky solid with a delicate, persistent, roselike odor, and soluble in most fixed oils and in mineral oil. Also used in the manufacture of hair sprays and in sunscreens. They help prevent deterioration of ingredients that might be affected by the ultraviolet rays found in ordinary daylight. May produce hives and contact sensitivity. In sunscreens they may cause immediate hives as well as other photoallergic reactions. Also may cause face and neck rashes when in shampoo. Toxic when injected. On the basis of the available information, the CIR Expert Panel (*see*) found it safe in the early 1980s but is considering new information to determine if the final safety assessment should be reaffirmed, amended, or have an addendum. The EU has banned benzophenone-3 in sunscreens. *See* Oxybenzone.

BENZOQUINE • *See* Oxyquinoline and Benzoic Acid.

BENZOTRIAZOLE • A preservative. *See* Benzene.

BENZOXONIUM CHLORIDE • A preservative. *See* Quaternary Ammonium Compounds.

BENZOXYQUINE • Benzoxiquine. 8-Hydroxyquinoline Benzoate. A water-soluble salt of benzoic acid (*see*). Used as an antiseptic. Also used medicinally in the treatment of dysentery. Toxic when ingested. The CIR Expert Panel (*see*) concludes the safety of this ingredient has not been documented and substantiated, and the Panel states that it cannot "conclude that this ingredient is safe for use in cosmetic products until the appropriate safety data have been obtained and evaluated."

BENZOYL BENZENE • A fixative for heavy perfumes such as geranium, especially when used in soaps. *See* Benzophenones.

BENZOYL CHLORIDE • A skin-conditioning ingredient. *See* Benzene.

BENZOYL PEROXIDE • A bleaching and drying ingredient in cosmetics. Toxic by inhalation. A skin allergen and irritant. The EU said in 2003 that its use in nail systems does not pose a risk due to the very low exposure to the consumer. It should be applied by professionals and skin contact should be avoided. Canada does not permit it in cosmetics intended to be applied to the skin, but it is permitted in artificial nail kits. On the Canadian Hotlist (*see*).

BENZYL ACETATE • A colorless liquid with a pear or flowerlike odor obtained from a number of plants, especially jasmine, for use in perfumery and soap. Can be irritating to the skin, eyes, and respiratory tract. Ingestion causes intestinal upset, including vomiting and diarrhea.

BENZYL ALCOHOL • A solvent in perfumes, a preservative in hair dyes, and a topical antiseptic. It is derived as a pure alcohol and is a constituent of jasmine, hyacinth, and other plants. It has a faint, sweet odor. Irritating and corrosive to the skin and mucous membranes. Ingestion of large doses causes intestinal upsets. In sensitive people, it may cross-react with balsam Peru (*see*).

BENZYL BENZOATE • Plasticizer in nail polishes, solvent, and fixative for perfumes. Occurs naturally in balsam Tolu and balsam Peru and in various flower oils. Colorless, oily liquid or white crystals with a light floral scent and sharp, burning taste.

BENZYL BENZOYLOXYBENZOATE • A fragrance ingredient. *See* Benzoic Acid.

BENZYL CINNAMATE • Sweet Odor of Balsam. Colorless prisms, used to give artificial fruit scents to perfumes. *See* Balsam Peru for toxicity.

BENZYL CYANIDE • Should not be used as or in fragrance ingredients. The recommendation is based on the absence of reports on the use of this material as a fragrance ingredient and/or inadequate evaluation of potential adverse effects resulting from its use in fragrances. Banned in fragrances by the UK and the EU. *See* Cyanide.

BENZYL ETHYL ETHER • Colorless, oily liquid; aromatic odor; insoluble in water; miscible in alcohol. Used in flavoring. Narcotic in high concentrations. May be a skin irritant.

BENZYL FORMATE • A synthetic flavoring ingredient used for its pleasant fruit odor in perfumery. No specific data for toxicity, but it is believed to be narcotic in high concentrations.

BENZYLHEMIOFORMAL • A germicide. *See* Gum Benzoin.

BENZYL HYALURONATE • A skin conditioner. *See* Hyaluronic Acid and Benzyl Alcohol.

3-BENZYLIDENE CAMPHOR • Bicyclo (2,2.1) Heptan-2-one. *See* Benzaldehyde.

BENZYL LAURATE • The salt of lauric acid (*see*).

BENZYL NICOTINATE • *See* Benzyl Alcohol and Niacin.

BENZYL PARABEN • A preservative. The CIR Expert Panel (*see*) concludes available data are insufficient to support the safety of benzyl paraben as used in cosmetics. *See* Parabens.

BENZYL PROPIONATE • Similar to benzyl acetate (*see*), but has a sweeter odor. Used in perfumes and as a flavoring.

BENZYL SALICYLATE • Salicylic Acid. A fixative in perfumes and a solvent in sunscreen lotions. It is a thick liquid with a light, pleasant odor and is mixed with alcohol or ether. May cause skin to break out in a rash and swell when exposed to sunlight. *See* Salicylates.

BENZYL TRIETHYL AMMONIUM CHLORIDE • An antistatic ingredient. *See* Quaternary Ammonium Compounds.

BENZYLTRIMONIUM HYDROLYZED COLLAGEN • The benzyl trimethyl ammonium salt of hydrolyzed animal protein. The word *animal* was taken out of the label listings. *See* Quaternary Ammonium Compounds and Surfactants.

BENZYL URSOLATE • Derivative of ursolic acid (*see*). An emollient and claimed as an anti-aging compound due to its photoaging inhibitor.

BERBERINE • Mild antiseptic and decongestant in eye lotions. Derived as yellow crystals from various plants. Relatively inactive physiologically, but ingestion of large quantities may cause fatal poisoning. Used as a dressing for skin ulcers.

BERBERIS • Holly-leafed Barberry. Oregon Grape Root. Mountain Grape. The dried roots of shrubs grown in the United States and British Columbia. Used medicinally to soothe skin ulcers and to break up intestinal gas. Used in creams as a mild antiseptic and decongestant. *See* Berberine for toxicity.

BERBERIS AQUIFOLIUM • Mountain Grape. Oregon Grape. An extract of a tall shrub native to the western section of the United States. Used medically to treat psoriasis and other skin problems. Used as a skin-conditioning ingredient in cosmetics.

BERGAMOT, RED • Oswego Tea. A pear-shaped orange whose rind yields a greenish brown oil much used in perfumery and brilliantine hairdressings. It can cause brown skin stains (berloque) when exposed to sunlight and is considered a prime photosensitizer (sensitivity to light). *See* Berloque Dermatitis.

BERLOQUE DERMATITIS • Some perfumes, which contain oil of bergamot (*see*) and other photosensitizers, may produce increased pigmentation (brown spots) in the area where the perfume has been applied, especially when it is immediately exposed to sunlight. There is no effective treatment, and the pigmentation generally persists for some time.

BERRY BARK • Myrica Oil. A yellow essential oil used in rum and other flavorings and fragrances. GRAS

BERTHOLLETIA EXCELSA • Extract of Brazil Nut. The oil is used as a skin conditioner.

BERYLLIUM AND ITS COMPOUNDS • Banned in cosmetics by ASEAN (see). EU authorities say there should be a substitute for it as soon as possible because it is a carcinogen, a mutagen, and toxic. The exception is aluminum beryllium, used as an abrasive (see).

BETA-CAROTENE • Provitamin A. Beta Carotene. Found in all plants and in many animal tissues. It is the chief yellow coloring matter of carrots, butter, and egg yolk. Extracted as red crystals or crystalline powder. It is used as a coloring in cosmetics. Also used in the manufacture of vitamin A. Too much carotene in the blood can lead to carotenemia, a pale yellow-red pigmentation of the skin that may be mistaken for jaundice. It is a benign condition, and withdrawal of carotene from the diet cures it. Beta-carotene has less serious side effects than vitamin A and was given to twenty-two thousand physicians as part of a five-year study to determine whether aspirin could protect against heart disease and beta-carotene against tumors. It is nontoxic. The Joint Expert Committee on Food Additives (JECFA) concluded that there was no objection to the use of vegetable extracts as coloring additives, providing the past specifications for carotenes were revised to include material derived from carrots, alfalfa, and palm oil, which are known to be used commercially. Beta-carotene is being studied for cancer-causing properties because it is positive as a mutagen in salmonella. GRAS

BETA-ENDORPHIN • A peptide hormone that normally works in human central nervous systems as a pain reliever. The most popular action of beta-endorphin is its creation of euphoria during exercise, which endurance athletes frequently refer to as "runner's high." Beta-endorphin is also produced outside of the central nervous system. Recently it was discovered that our skin cells produce beta-endorphin. From this discovery scientists believe that it has a role involved in the regulation of skin cell differentiation. In turn, beta-endorphin was shown to stimulate migration of keratinocytes and melanin production in melanocytes. Further to this, and most importantly for the cosmetics industry, it is also thought that beta-endorphin could have a potential in skin regeneration and wound healing.

BETA-GLUCANS • Polysaccharides (see) that yield sugars (glucose) on hydrolysis (when exposed to water treatment). Betaglucan is in cellulose and is found in edibles such as oat fiber and barley. Used as a thickener and as a skin conditioner.

BETA-HYDROXY ACIDS • Throughout the last decade, alpha-hydroxy acids (AHAs) have increasingly appeared as ingredients in cosmetics intended to reduce the signs of aging in the skin. Then beta-hydroxy acids (BHAs), or a combination of AHAs and BHAs, have appeared as ingredients in these skin-care products. While both AHAs and BHAs act as exfoliants, it has been claimed that BHAs are effective in reducing the appearance of fine lines and wrinkles and improving overall skin texture without the occasional irritation associated with the use of AHAs. BHA ingredients may be listed as salicylic acid (or related substances, such as salicylate, sodium salicylate, and willow extract).

BETAINE • Occurs in common beets and in many vegetables as well as animal substances. Used in resins, as emulsifiers, detergents, foam boosters, thickeners, and skin and hair conditioners. Has been used to treat muscle weakness. Coco-betaine (see) is an example.

BETA-NAPHTHOL • Used in hair dyes, skin-peeling preparations, and hair tonics. Prepared from naphthalene, which comes from coal tar. Also used in perfumes. Oral ingestion may cause kidney damage, eye injury, vomiting, diarrhea, convulsions, anemia, and death. Fatal poisoning from external applications has been reported. Local application may produce peeling of the skin, which may be followed by pigmentation, also contact dermatitis. On the Canadian Hotlist (*see*). *See* Naphthas.

BETA-SITOSTEROL • Common sterol (*see*) in plants. Isolated from wheat germ, rye germ, or cottonseed oils. Used medically to treat high cholesterol and prostate tumors. It is used in cosmetics as a skin conditioner.

BETA VULGARIS • *See* Beet Extract.

BETOXYCAINE, ITS SALTS AND ETHERS • Pain suppressors that also reportedly contribute to wound healing. Often cause sensitivity. They are banned in cosmetics by the EU and ASEAN (*see*).

BETULA • Obtained from the European white birch and a source of asphalt and tar, it is used as an antioxidant and fragrance ingredient in a wide variety of makeup and skin care products. In hair tonics, it reddens the scalp and creates a warm feeling due to an increased blood flow. Also used in moisturizing creams and astringents. Betula leaves were formerly used to treat rheumatism. *See* Salicylates.

BFE • Trade name for grapefruit extract.

BHA • *See* Butylated Hydroxyanisole.

BHT • *See* Butylated Hydroxytoluene.

BICARBONATE OF SODA • *See* Sodium Bicarbonate.

BICHLORIDE OF MERCURY • *See* Mercury Compounds.

BIDENS PILOSA • Beggar's Tick. Spanish Needle. Cobbler's Pegs. Extract of an erect annual or perennial herb, a major weed of vegetables and other crops; it is common in pastures, plantations, along roadsides, and on wasteland in the Pacific isles. Used as a skin-conditioning ingredient and humectant.

BIFIDA FERMENT LYSATE • A product of the fermentation of *Bifida*, a bacteria found in the digestive system. It is used as a skin conditioner. *See* Bifidus Factor.

BIFIDUS FACTOR • *Lactobacillus bifidus*. A bacteria found in the intestinal tract of breast-fed infants. It is prepared from the gastric mucosa of pigs and is used as a dietetic adjuvant in infant foods. It is also used in cosmetic emollients.

BILBERRY EXTRACT • Grown in the Alps and Scandinavia, this fruit is used by folk medicine practitioners to improve night vision. A number of modern studies have shown that bilberry anthocyanins (the blue-coloring chemicals) given orally improve vision in healthy people and also help treat people with eye diseases. The anthocyanins contained in bilberry act to prevent blood vessel fragility and inhibit blood clot formation. It has been reported that bilberry increases prostaglandin (*see*) release from arterial tissue, which dilates blood vessels. Bilberry also contains arbutin (*see*), a diuretic and antiinfective derived from the dried leaves.

BILE SALTS • The salts of bile acids are powerful cleansing ingredients and aid in the absorption of fats from the intestines.

BINDER • A substance, such as gum arabic, gum tragacanth, glycerin, and sorbitol (*see all*), which dispenses, swells, or absorbs water, increases consistency, and holds ingredients together. For example, binders are used to make powders in compacts retain their shape; binders in toothpaste provide for the smooth dispensing of the paste.

BIOCIDE • An ingredient to cleanse the skin and prevent odor by inhibiting the growth of bacteria, fungi, or yeast in a huge range of applications, from cosmetics and personal care products to laundry detergents, cleaning fluids, food and feed preservatives, and building materials. "However, the regular use of personal hygiene products (e.g., cosmetics, wipes), cleaning products, laundry detergents, pet disinfectants and general disinfectants are the major sources of exposure to biocides in home settings," experts explain. EU Directive 76/768/EEC (the so-called Cosmetics Directive) lists fifty-seven chemicals permitted, with the restrictions for the use as preservatives (i.e., antimicrobial substances with biocidal functions) in cosmetic products. Triclosan is among the most commonly used. The largest amount of triclosan in cosmetics was found in products for dental hygiene, including toothpaste. Besides cosmetics, triclosan is also used in cleaning products, paint, textiles, and plastic products. However, according to a Danish study, cosmetics would be the largest contributor to the amount of triclosan on the market, as they constituted 99 percent of the totally reported amount in the survey. Some mechanisms of resistance are common to both biocides and antibiotics (*see*). Biocides are believed to be invaluable as a means of preventing infection and enhancing hygiene.

BIOFLAVONOIDS • Vitamin P Complex. Citrus-flavored compounds needed to maintain healthy blood vessel walls. Widely distributed among plants, especially citrus fruits and rose hips. Usually taken from orange and lemon rinds and used as a reducing agent (*see*).

BIOLOGICAL ADDITIVES • The use of animal and plant ingredients has skyrocketed since the last edition of this book. *See* Aloe and Collagen as examples. Currently, human products are banned as well as those from endangered species or plants by the European Union. The EU also bans plants known to produce poisons such as belladonna (a nerve poison) and foxglove (a heart stimulant).

BIORESMETHRIN • An insecticide. *See* Pyrethrum.

BIOSACCHARIDE GUM-1 • A fermentation gum derived from sorbitol (*see*), used as a skin conditioner.

BIOTIN • Vitamin H. Vitamin B Factor. A whitish, crystalline powder used as a texturizer/moisturizer in cosmetic creams. Present in minute amounts in every living cell and in larger amounts in yeast and milk. Vital to growth. It acts as a coenzyme in the formation of certain essential fatlike substances and plays a part in reactions involving carbon dioxide. It is needed by humans for healthy circulation and red blood cells.

BIOTITE • Black Mica. A thickener. *See* Mica.

BIRCH FAMILY • Betulaceae. Used as an astringent in creams and shampoos, it is an ancient remedy. The medicinal properties of the plant tend to vary, depending upon which part of the tree is used. It has been used as a laxative, as an aid for gout, to treat rheumatism and dropsy, and to dissolve kidney stones. It is supposedly good for bathing skin eruptions. The oil is used in food flavorings. *See* Betula.

BISABOL • Oplopanax. A myrrh-type gum resin obtained from African trees. Widely used in cosmetics, including bath soaps, eye makeup removers, fragrances, deodorants, foundations, shaving creams, skin fresheners, baby lotions, powders, lipsticks, and aftershave lotions.

BISABOLOL • Dragosantol. Derived from chamomile (*see*) or made synthetically, it is an anti-irritant. The CIR Expert Panel (*see*) concludes this is a safe ingredient in the present practices of use and concentration.

BISAMINO PEG/PPG-41/3 AMINOETHYL PG-PROPYL DIMETHICONE • Occurs in sweat. Used to combat fungus in cosmetics and on the skin. Made by dissolving zinc oxide (*see*) in diluted undecylenic acid (*see*). Has an odor suggestive of perspiration. *See* Antiperspirants.

1,3-BIS(2,4-DIAMINOPHENOY)PROPANE HCL • A hair coloring. *See* Coal Tar.

BIS-DIGLYCERYL CAPRYLATE/CAPRATE/ISOSTEARATE/HYDROXY-STEARATE ADIPATE • A gel made from stearic acid and adipic acid (*see both*).

4,6-BIS (2-HYDROXYETHOXY)-*m*-PHENYLENEDIAMINE HCL • A coal tar hair coloring.

2,6-BIS (2-HYDROXYETHOXY)-3-5PYRIDINEDIAMINE HCL • A coal tar dye. An amine.

N,N-BIS-2-HYDROXYETHYL-*p*-PHENELENEDIAMINE SULFATE • It has produced strong sensitization in both guinea pigs and humans. The CIR Expert Panel (*see*) concludes this is a safe ingredient in the present practices of use and concentration. *See* Phenylenediamine.

BISHYDROXYETHYL BISCETYL MALONAMIDE • A fatty alcohol used as a skin conditioner. *See* Malonic Acid.

BIS-HYDROXYETHYL RAPESEEDMONIUM CHLORIDE • A quaternary ammonium compound (*see*) used as an antistatic ingredient.

BISMARK BROWN • Prepared from phenylenediamine (*see*) and nitrous acid, it is a basic brown color that is used in dyeing silk, wool, and leather. Can cause contact dermatitis.

BISMUTH CITRATE • Coloring restricted to hair dye only. *See* Bismuth Compounds.

BISMUTH COMPOUNDS • Subgallate, Subnitrate, Oxychloride. Bismuth is a gray-white powder with a bright metallic luster. It occurs in the earth's crust and for many years was used to treat syphilis. Bismuth subgallate, a dark gray, odorless, tasteless form, is used as an antiseptic and in dusting powder. Bismuth subnitrate is odorless and tasteless, and is used in bleaching and freckle creams and hair dyes. Bismuth oxychloride is sometimes called "synthetic pearl" and is used as a skin protective. Most bismuth compounds used in cosmetics have a low toxicity when ingested but may cause allergic reactions when applied to the skin. In 1992, the FDA proposed a ban on bismuth subnitrate in fever blister and cold sore treatment products and poison ivy, poison oak, and poison sumac OTC products because it has not been shown to be safe and effective for its stated claims.

BISMUTH OXYCHLORIDE • Permanently listed as a coloring in 1977. *See* Bismuth Compounds.

BIS-PEG-4-DIMETHICONE • Hair- and skin-conditioning ingredient. *See* Siloxanes and Silanes.

BISPHENOL A • BPA. Bisphenol A is used primarily to make polycarbonate plastics and resins and is integral to the manufacture of both materials. It is used in containers for some cosmetics. In 2003, researchers supported by the U.S. National Institute of Environmental Health Sciences reported in *Current Biology* that small amounts of the chemical had caused birth defects in mice. The substance was leached from plastic by inadvertent detergent use. In 1997, research at the University of Missouri–Columbia suggested that BPA has an estrogenlike activity. The Grocery Manufacturers Association came out fighting after the media publicity about this additive. They quote: "The Harvard Center for Risk Analysis convened a panel to evaluate the weight-of-evidence for the potential reproductive and/or developmental toxicity of BPA (Gray et al., 2004)." The panel stated the following conclusions: "No consistent affirmative evidence of low-dose BPA effects for any endpoint. . . . Lack of adverse effects in two multiple-generation reproductive and developmental studies casts doubt on suggestions of significant physiological or functional impairment. . . . Differences in the pattern of BPA responses compared to estradiol or diethylstilbestrol (DES) cast doubt on estrogenicity as a low-dose mechanism of action for BPA. . . . There is indirect evidence that humans may be less sensitive to possible estrogenic effects from BPA exposure due to pharmacodynamic factors." Banned by Canada and some U.S. states. *See* Phenols.

BISPHENYLHEXAMETHICONE • A silicone (*see*) used as an antifoaming ingredient, skin conditioner, and emollient.

BIS-PHENYLPROPYL DIMETHICONE • A hair conditioner. *See* Siloxanes.

BISPYRITHIONE • A germ killer. On the Canadian Hotlist (*see*). *See* Pyrethrum.

BISTORT EXTRACT • The extract of the roots of *Polygonum bistorta,* an herb found in Europe and North America. The roots are used as an astringent.

BISULFITES • Bisulfite straighteners or curl relaxers are used instead of the thioglycolates (*see* Thioglycolic Acid Compounds). They produce changes in the chemical bonds in the hair. The effectiveness of the bisulfite relaxers is similar to that of hot combing, but it is more permanent. The result is equivalent to the caustic alkali straighteners and superior to the thioglycolate method. Less irritating to the scalp and less damaging to the hair than other methods, but should not be used if the scalp or skin is sensitive, scaly, scratched, sore, or tender. Harmful effects frequently result from not following directions. *See also* Sodium Bisulfite.

BITHIONOL • Used as a germicide in cold creams, emollients, hair tonics, aftershave lotions, detergent bars, shampoos, creams, lotions, and bases to hide blemishes, and in medicated cosmetics. It is closely related to hexachlorophene, which has been banned by the FDA. Bithionol has been removed from many products sold in the United States because it causes a sensitivity to light; the skin breaks out with a rash and may swell. New evidence of clinical experience and photopatch tests indicate that bithionol is capable of causing photosensitivity in humans when used topically and that in some instances the photosensitization may persist for prolonged periods as severe reactions without further contact with sensitizing articles. Also, there is evidence to indicate that bithionol may produce cross-sensitization with other commonly used chemicals such as certain halogenated salicylanilides and hexachlorophene. It is, therefore, the view of the FDA that bithionol is a deleterious substance that may render any cosmetic product that contains it injurious to users. On the Canadian Hotlist (*see*). The EU and the FDA have now banned it in cosmetics.

BITTER ALMOND OIL • *Prunus amygdalus.* Almond Oil. Sweet Almond Oil. Expressed Almond Oil. A colorless to pale yellow, bland, nearly odorless essential and expressed oil from the ripe seed of the small sweet almond grown in Italy, Spain, and France. It has a strong almond odor and a mild taste. Used in the manufacture of perfumes and as an oil in hair creams, nail whiteners, nail polish removers, eye creams, emollients, soaps, and perfumes. Many users are allergic to cosmetics with almond oil. It causes stuffy nose and skin rashes.

BITTER CHERRY EXTRACT • *Prunus cerasus.* Used for its vitamin C component and as a flavoring and a scent.

BITTER ORANGE OIL • *Citrus aurantium* var. *amara.* Pale yellow volatile oil expressed from the fresh peel of a species of citrus and used in perfumes and flavorings. May cause skin irritation and allergic reactions.

BITTER PRINCIPLE • Any of a group of chemicals in plants that are very bitter tasting. They differ chemically but most belong to the iris or pine families. Bitter principles reputedly stimulate the secretion of digestive juices and stimulate the liver. They are being investigated scientifically today as antifungals and antibiotics as well as anticancer ingredients. The bitter principle in mallow plants is being investigated as a male contraceptive. Other bitter principles in herbs are used to combat coughs and as sedatives.

BITTERS • Usually refers to an alcohol prepared from parts of bitter herbs. Used as a mild tonic or stimulant to improve appetite. Also used as a flavoring ingredient.

BIXA ORELLANA • A solvent extraction of *Bixa orellana* seeds. Yellow carotenoid (*see*) solution or powder, it is a color additive in ink used for marking foods, and in oleomargarine, poultry, sausage casings, and shortening. May cause contact dermatitis (*see*).

BLACK • Carbon black (channel process) and bone black, previously commonly used, are no longer authorized for use. *See* Colors.

BLACK COHOSH • *Cimicifuga racemosa.* Snakeroot. Bugbane. Used in astringents, it is a perennial herb with a flower that is supposedly distasteful to insects. Grown from Canada to North Carolina and Kansas. It has a reputation for curing snakebite. It is used in ginger ale flavoring. A tonic and antispasmodic. *See also* Cohosh Root.

BLACK CURRANT EXTRACT • The extract of the fruit of *Ribes nigrum,* a European plant that produces hanging yellow flowers and black aromatic fruit.

BLACK LOCUST • Extract of *Robinia pseudoacacia.* Black Locust Extract. Acacia Glycolystat. The fragrant flowers can be smelled for hundreds of feet in the spring. The bruised foliage mixed with sugar attracts and kills flies.

BLACK MALVA • *Malva rotundafolia.* Flowering herb used in shampoos.

BLACK MUSTARD EXTRACT • *Brassica nigra. Sinapis alba.* A native of Europe and the Americas, it is cultivated in Holland, Italy, and Germany as a condiment. It is used medicinally to treat arthritis, sciatica, and other pains. It was also used as an emetic to counteract ingested poisons. Mustard seeds are used to stimulate appetite. Mustard plasters were a popular treatment for pains and swelling. It is used in footbaths and to treat colds. Mustard is rapidly absorbed and used as a counterirritant (*see*). It is irritating to the skin and can cause burns that are slow to heal.

BLACK PEPPER • *Piper nigra.* Used in body washes, conditioners, and shampoos. Reputedly analgesic and tonic.

BLACK POPLAR • *Populus nigra. See* Poplar Extract.

BLACK THORN • *Prunus spinosa.* A European tree or shrub that has hard wood and bears small white flowers and small purplish or blue-black astringent fruits. Used in astringents.

BLACK WALNUT EXTRACT • Extract of the leaves or bark of the black walnut tree, *Juglans nigra,* found in eastern North America. It produces nuts with a thick oil and is used as a black coloring.

BLACKBERRY • *Rubus fruiticosus.* The berries, leaves, and root bark are used to treat fevers, colds, sore throats, vaginal discharge, diarrhea, and dysentery. The berries contain isocitric and malic acids, sugars, pectin, monoglycoside of cyanidin, and vitamins C and A. The leaves and bark are said to lower fever; they are astringent and stop bleeding. The leaves are used in "organic" bath products to soothe and refresh the skin. *See* Malic Acid.

BLACKHEAD • An open, noninflammatory comedo. *See* Comedones.

BLACKSTRAP POWDER • Obtained from sugarcane in the processes of sugar manufacture. It is a natural flavoring ingredient.

BLADDER WRACK EXTRACT • *Fucus vesiculosus.* Fucus. Sea Wrack. A common black rockweed used in cosmetics such as tanning lotions.

BLANC FIXE • *See* Barium Sulfate.

BLEACH • *See* Hair Bleach and Skin Bleach.

BLEMISH COVER • Pimple and undereye covers come in stick or cream form based on oil, wax, and alcohol. Usually contain titanium dioxide (*see*) and pigments. Applied before makeup to cover marks, dark circles under the eyes, or other minor blemishes.

BLESSED THISTLE EXTRACT • *Cnicus benedictus.* Holy Thistle. The thistle contains tannin (*see*), lactone, mucilage (*see*), and essential oil. It is used by herbalists to treat stomach and liver complaints. It reputedly breaks up blood clots, relieves jaundice and hepatitis, and stops bleeding. It increases appetite and lowers fevers. The FDA issued a notice in 1992 that blessed thistle has not been shown to be safe and effective as claimed in OTC digestive aid products or in oral menstrual drugs.

BLETIA HYACINTHINA EXTRACT • Dai Chi (Baiji). *Bletilla striata.* The rhizomes are collected from August to November with a nonmetal cutting tool, cleaned, and dried. The medicine prepared from these tubers is used to treat tuberculosis, hemoptysis, gastric and duodenal ulcers, as well as bleeding, and cracked skin on the feet and hands. Other uses in China, Mongolia, and Japan include the introduction of euphoria, purification of blood, strengthening of lungs, as well as the treatment of pus, boils, abscesses, malignant swellings, ulcers, and breast cancer. Tubers have also been used as a demulcent for inflammation and chapped skin. The powdered roots mixed with oil have been used as an emollient for burns and skin diseases.

BLOODROOT • *Sanguinaria canadensis.* Redroot. Red Indian Paint Tetterwort. The root contains isoquinoline alkaloids, including sanguinaria and berberine. Herbalists use it to treat coughs, sore throats, skin eruptions, skin cancer, athlete's foot, and gum disease. The root is emetic and purgative in large doses. In smaller doses it is a stimulant, diaphoretic, and expectorant. *See also* Berberis.

BLUE 1 • CI 42090. A triphenylmethane color used in shampoos, skin care products, bath products, and dentifrices. *See* FD & C Colors.

BLUE 4 • CI 42090. Japan calls it AO205. A triphenylmethane color used in bath oils and salt, body and hand products, and shampoos. *See* D & C Blue No. 4.

BLUE ALGAE • A rich source of vitamin E, zinc, iron, and copper. It reportedly has a soothing effect on the skin. It is used in anti-aging products. *See* Haslea Ostrearia.

BLUEBERRY • *Vaccinium angustifolium.* Used to combat stretch marks and in conditioners. Gaining popularity in skin care products because of its vitamins, antioxidants, amino acids, and fatty acids.

BLUEBERRY EXTRACT • *Vaccinum myrtillus. See* Bilberry Extract.

BLUE COHOSH • *Caulophyllum thalictrioides.* Squawroot. Blueberry Root. Papooseroot. A tall herb of eastern North America and Asia, it has three-pointed leaves and a small, greenish yellow or purple flower. It produces large blue-berrylike fruits. Roots were used as an antiseptic. *See also* Cohosh Root.

BLUE FLAG • *Iris versicolor.* Flag Lily. Fleur-de-lis. Liver Lily. Poison Flag Wild Iris. The rhizome contains salicylic (*see*) and isophthalic acids, volatile oil, iridin, a glycoside (*see*), gum, resin, and sterols. Herbalists use it as a cathartic and emetic, and to treat liver complaints, swollen glands, hepatitis, jaundice, skin diseases, and loss of appetite. Promoted in herbal medicines as both relaxing and stimulating.

BLUE 1 LAKE • Acid Blue 9 Aluminum Lake. CI 42090. Japanese call it AO1. Used in lipsticks.

BLUE VIOLET • Ultramarine Blue. Ultramarine Violet. Used in ivory face powders. Originally made from lapis lazuli. *See* Ultramarine Blue.

BLUSHER • Used to put color on cheeks and on other parts of the face. Powder blushers are similar to pressed powder in composition but include lake colors (*see*). Stick blushers are similar in composition to lipsticks (*see*).

BODY BUTTERS • Added to many body care brand portfolios to entice women and men with "the new." Examples include Honey Olive Neroli massage body butter within the Boots Mediterranean range, Opal London's Water Lily & Almond Spa body butter, and Tisserand Aromatherapy Organic Lavender & Bergamot Body Butter. Oils are another upcoming format, ancient but made new by cosmetic marketers. Started in popularity in Germany and then quickly caught on as a versatile and less greasy alternative to body creams, butters, and balms. The Body Shop's Monoi Miracle Oil is a light, nongreasy coconut oil scented with gardenia flowers for use as a moisturizer on the body or even as a prewash on the hair. Bio-Oil, from the South African skin care company Union-Swiss, is claimed by the company to be one of the fastest-growing skin care products worldwide. The unique ingredient in Bio-Oil is PurCellin Oil, a rapidly absorbed "dry oil" that can be used to reduce the appearance of scars, stretch marks, and uneven skin tone and is recommended for dehydrated or aging skin.

BODY NOTE • The main and characteristic overall odor of a perfume. It has a much longer life than the top note (*see*) and usually contributes to the dryout (*see*).

BODY OIL • *See* Body Butters.

BOESENBERGIA PANDURATA • Finger Root. Root oil from a plant in the ginger family Zingiberaceae common to China and Southeast Asia. It is used as a flavoring, fragrance ingredient, and skin conditioner.

BOIS DE ROSE OIL • A fragrance from the chipped wood of the tropical rosewood tree obtained through steam distillation. The volatile oil is colorless or pale yellow, with a light camphor odor. It is also used as a food flavoring. There is reported use of the chemical; it has not yet been assigned for toxicology literature. GRAS. ASP

BOMBYX • Extract of the silk worm secretions. *See* Silk.

BONE BLACK • A coloring externally applied in cosmetics. As of 2003, the FDA has held the application for its use in abeyance (*see*) but lists it as unauthorized as a coloring. It is permitted by the EU.

BONE MARROW LIPIDS • *See* Marrow Lipids.

BORAGE EXTRACT • The extract of the herb *Borago officinalis*. Contains potassium and calcium. Widely used as an emollient and sometimes as a "tea" for sore eyes.

BORAGO • The extract of the herb *Borago officinalis*. Contains potassium and calcium and has emollient properties and is used in a "tea" for sore eyes. Used in cosmetics as a skin conditioner.

BORATES • Widely used as antiseptic ingredients and preservatives in cosmetics in spite of repeated warnings by medical scientists. Acute poisonings have followed ingestion, injection, enemas, lavage of body cavities, and application of powders and ointments to burned and abraded skin. Borates affect the central nervous system, gastrointestinal tract, kidneys, liver, and skin.

BORAX • Sodium Borate. A mild alkali found in the Far West, particularly in Death Valley, California. Used in cold creams, foundation creams, hair color rinses, permanent waves, and shaving creams. It is used as a water softener, as a preservative, and as a texturizer in cream products. Also used to prevent irritation of the skin by the antiperspirant aluminum chloride (*see*). *See* Boric Acid for toxicity.

BORIC ACID • An antiseptic with bactericidal and fungicidal properties used in baby powders, bath powders, eye creams, liquid powders, mouthwashes, protective creams, after-shave lotions, soaps, and skin fresheners. It is still widely used despite repeated warnings from the American Medical Association of possible toxicity. Severe poisonings have followed both ingestion and topical application to abraded skin. It is used to treat external ear canal infection by inhibiting bacteria present in the ear canal. It is used for temporary relief of chapped, chafed, or dry skin, diaper rash, abrasions, minor burns, sunburn, insect bites, and other skin irritations.

In 1992, researchers at the Developmental and Reproductive Toxicology Group, U.S. National Institute of Environmental Health Sciences, reported that developmental toxicity of boric acid in mice occurred below maternally toxic levels in rats and mice and adversely affected the fetuses. The Food and Drug Administration issued a notice in 1992 that boric acid has not been shown to be safe and effective for stated claims in OTC products, including astringent (*see*) drug products and fever blister and cold sore treatments and poison ivy, poison oak, and poison sumac drug products. The CIR Expert Panel (*see*) says based on available data, it is safe as a cosmetic ingredient at less than or equal to 5 percent; however, cosmetic formulations containing free sodium boric acid at this concentration should not be used on infant skin or injured skin. On the basis of the available information, the CIR Expert Panel found it safe in the early 1980s but is considering new information to determine if the final safety assessment should be reaffirmed, amended, or have an addendum. The EU has banned it for children under three years and said hair products containing borates should be well rinsed. Should also not be used on peeling or irritated skin. On the Canadian Hotlist (*see*). Warnings not required where boric acid is used as pH adjuster and concentration is under 0.1 percent. *See also* Tetraborates.

BORNELONE • UV Absorber-4. A compound that protects a cosmetic product from deterioration by ultraviolet light. *See* Borneol and Pentane.

BORNEOL • Used in perfumery, it has a peppery odor and a burning taste. Occurs naturally in coriander, ginger oil, oil of lime, rosemary, strawberries, thyme, citronella, and nutmeg. Toxicity is similar to camphor oil (*see*).

BORNYL ACETATE • A colorless liquid derived from borneol (*see*), it is used in perfumery and flavoring and as a solvent.

BORNYL FORMATE • Used in perfumes, soaps, and as a disinfectant. *See* Borneol.

BOROJOA PATINOI • Tree grown in southern Central America. It is cultivated in Colombia for its edible large fruits supposedly with aphrodisiac properties. Fruit juice is used as a hair and skin conditioner. *See* Botryocladia Occidentalis.

BORON • Occurs in the earth's crust in the form of its compounds, never as the element. It is used in dietary supplements up to 1 mg per day. Salts of boron are widely used as antiseptics even though toxicologists warn about possible adverse reactions. Borates are absorbed by the mucous membranes and can cause such symptoms as gastrointestinal bleeding, skin rash, and central nervous system stimulation. The adult lethal dose is one ounce. A preparation promoted as "anti-aging" contains 2 mg of boron in a vitamin and mineral supplement—it is claimed that it increases the production of testosterone.

BOSWELLIA CARTERII AND SERRATA • Olibanum. Frankincense Extract. The extract of *Boswellia carterii* of various species. The volatile, distilled oil from the gum resin of a plant found in Ethiopia, Egypt, and Arabia. It was one of the gifts of the Magi. It is used in cola, fruit, and spice flavorings for beverages, ice cream, ices, candy, and baked goods. Used in fragrances and skin products.

BOTANICAL GLYCERIN • Made from vegetables only, not animal fats. Used in soaps. *See* Glycerin and Botanicals.

BOTANICALS • Cosmetic ingredients derived directly from plants and that include extracts, juices, waters, distillates, powders, oils, waxes, gels, saps, tars, gums, proteins, starches, and resins. They have generally not undergone chemical processing. The FDA expressed concern about this category because many botanicals were showing up on the market about which little is known as far as effects on human physiology.

BOTRYOCLADIA OCCIDENTALIS • Borojo Red Seaweed. Used as a skin conditioner and as an anticoagulant.

BOUGAINVILLEA • A woody plant with ornamental tropical red or purple flowers. Used in "organic" cosmetics. May cause hives.

BOVINE • An animal of the family Bovidae, including cattle, buffalo, and bison; of, or pertaining to, cattle. The skull including the brain and eyes and tonsil and spinal cords aged twelve months banned in cosmetics by ASEAN. *See* Animal Parts.

BOXWOOD • *Cornus florida.* Dogwood. Green Ozier. A small tree found in all parts of the United States. The bark possesses astringent, stimulant, and tonic properties. The bark was used in the treatment of malaria, especially when the cinchona bark was unavailable.

BOYSENBERRY • *Rubus deliclosus.* A very large fruit. Used as a raspberry flavoring.

BRAIN EXTRACT and LIPIDS • The extract of bovine brains. Used in anti-aging creams. On the Canadian Hotlist (*see*). Must provide sourcing information on country of origin and supplier.

BRASENIA SCHREBERI • Water Shield. A floating-leaved plant, but the long leaf stalks reach all the way to the bottom where they attach to a long creeping root that is anchored in the mud. Occurs in lakes, ponds, and slow streams, and prefers water up to six feet deep. Sprinkled throughout the majority of the United States. Its submersed parts and undersides of leaves are covered with a viscous jellylike substance used in cosmetics.

BRASSICA • *See* Mustard Oil.

BRASSICA CAMPESTRIS (RAPESEED) ACID • *See* Rapeseed Acid.

BRASSICA GEMMIFERA • Extract of brussel sprouts used as a skin conditioner.

BRASSICA JUNCEA • Brown mustard extract.

BRASSICA NIGRA • Extract of black mustard.

BRASSICA OLERACEA BOTRYTIS EXTRACT • Extract of cauliflower used as an emollient.

BRASSICA OLERACEA CAPITATA JUICE • Extract of cabbage juice. Used in skin products.

BRASSICA RAPA (TURNIP) ROOT • *See* Turnip Extract.

BRAZIL NUT OIL • The oil expressed from the nuts of the Brazil nut tree, *Bertholletia excelsa*. Used in skin conditioners and as an emollient.

BRAZILWOOD • Redwood. Pernambuco Wood. Grown in Brazil. Used in the manufacture of red lake pigment, which produces warm brown shades in hair colorings. *See* Colors.

BREATH FRESHENERS • Most breath fresheners contain flavoring, artificial sweeteners, water, and alcohol. They are sold in glass or plastic bottles that measure out small amounts or are sprayed from aerosols. However, the propellants in the aerosols may be toxic when used in excess. The spray is really propelled mouthwash.

BREVOORTIA • *See* Menhaden Oil.

BREWER'S YEAST • Originally used by beer brewers, it is a good source of B vitamins and protein. It can cause allergic reactions.

BRIDEWORT • *See* Filipendula Rubra.

BRILLIANT BLACK 1 • CI 28440. A diazo (*see*) color.

BRILLIANTINES • Hairdressings that impart a shine to the hair. Cream brilliantines are usually made of mineral oil (25 percent), beeswax, triethanolamine stearate, and water (65 percent). Liquid brilliantine is composed of mineral oil (75 percent) and isopropyl myristate. Solid brilliantines are made of mineral oil, petrolatum, and paraffin. So-called two-layer dressings contain mineral oil, alcohol, and water. They also may contain antiseptics such as cetyl alcohol, cholesterol, gums such as tragacanth, lanolin, oil of bergamot, and other essential oils, olive oil, synthetic oils, synthetic thickeners, and tars. Toxicity depends upon ingredients.

BROMATES • A salt of bromic acid, used in permanent wave neutralizers. Bromates are used as maturing ingredients and conditioners in bread. Severe poisoning has followed ingestion and topical application to abraded skin.

BROMELAIN • Bromelin. A protein-digesting and milk-clotting enzyme found in pineapple. Used to peel top layers of skin. A search of the toxicology literature concerning this additive has not yet been performed by the FDA's data bank. Because it causes sloughing of the skin, it may cause irritation and an allergic reaction, especially if you are allergic to pineapple.

BROMELIA BALANSEA • A tropical American plant. *See* Pineapple Juice.

BROMIC ACID • Its salts, the bromates (*see*), are powerful oxidizing agents in the solid state. Used in making dyes and pharmaceuticals.

BROMIDES, POTASSIUM AND SODIUM • A group of sedative drugs now used only rarely. Potassium bromide has been used medically as a sedative and anticonvulsant. Sodium bromide has been used as a sedative and a sleep inducer. The bromides can cause skin rashes. Large doses of the bromides can cause central nervous system depression, and prolonged intake may cause mental deterioration. The use of sodium or potassium bromide in OTC sleep aids was determined to be ineffective in 1991, and manufacturers had to reformulate or have their products banned.

BROMINE • A dark, reddish brown liquid derived from seawater and natural brines by oxidation of bromine salts. Toxic by ingestion and inhalation. It reacts with many metals to form bromides (*see*). On the Canadian Hotlist (*see*). EU and ASEAN (*see*) banned it in cosmetics.

BROMO ACID • *See* D & C Red No. 21.

BROMOCHLOROPHENE • A germicide and deodorant ingredient.

BROMOCINNAMAL • A flavoring. *See* Cinnamon.

BROMOCRESOL GREEN • This coal tar coloring is not listed for use in the United States but is in Europe.

5-BROMO 5-NITRO-1,3-DIOXANE • Bronidox L. Preservative. May release formaldehyde (*see*). Significant skin and eye irritation has been observed in animal studies at concentrations higher than 0.1 percent. There is concern that it can form cancer-causing nitrosamines (*see*). The CIR Expert Panel (*see*) concludes this is "a safe ingredient at concentrations up to 0.1 percent except under circumstances where its action with amines or amides can result in the formation of nitrosamines." On the Canadian Hotlist (*see*). Permitted at a concentration equal to or less than 0.1 percent in Canada but not permitted in formulations that contain amines or amides.

2-BROMO-2-NITROPANE-1,3-DIOL • A preservative. The CIR Expert Panel (*see*) concludes this is "a safe ingredient at concentrations up to 0.1 percent except under circumstances where its action with amines or amides can result in the formation of nitrosamines." Has been linked to allergic reactions. *See* Bronopol.

BROMOTHYMOL BLUE • This coal tar color is not approved for use in the United States but is in Europe.

BRONOPOL • Bronosol. Odorless crystals from chloroform widely used as a preservative in cosmetics and toiletries. In European tests, the incidence of sensitization to this ingredient was considered to be lower than to parabens (*see*). Solvent used for nail polishes, fats, oils, and dyes. Also used as an intermediate (*see*) in the manufacture of cosmetics and as a propellant. It inhibits the growth of bacteria, fungi, and yeasts. It is used as a preservative for a wide variety of cosmetics, especially shampoos, creams, lotions, rinses, and eye makeup. It can form nitrosamine or nitrosamide when acting with amines or amides such as triethanolamine or its salts. Of 191 samples tested, 77 contained the powerful cancer-causing ingredient N-Nitrosodiethanolamine (NDELA).

The preservative also breaks down at neutral and alkaline pHs to produce formaldehyde and one or two or more bromo compounds. Formaldehyde is a suspected carcinogen. Therefore, if you see it listed as an ingredient with another compound ending in "amine" or "amide," don't purchase it. It is fifth on the list of preservatives that cause contact dermatitis, according to the American College of Dermatology Test Trays. The FDA said in 2008 that in the past, formation of nitrosamines in cosmetic products containing the preservative Bronopol TM (2-bromo-2-nitro 1,3-propanetiol) has been an issue. Bronopol TM is no longer widely used, and as a result of product reformulation the occurrence of nitrosamines has been significantly reduced. It is necessary, however, to monitor the use of Bronopol TM in cosmetic products to assure that a nitrosamine issue does not reoccur. If the ingredient Bronopol TM is encountered in a cosmetic product, include a complete list of the product ingredients in the EIR for submission to

CFSAN so the potential for nitrosamine formulation can be evaluated. The EU and the FDA have banned chloroform in cosmetics.

BRONZE POWDER • Any metal such as a copper alloy or aluminum in fine flakes and used as a pigment to give the appearance of a metallic surface. Used in hair coloring to give a shine and as a "frost" or "pearl" in other cosmetics. Permanently listed as a cosmetic coloring in 1977.

BRONZERS • Colored lotion that temporarily stains the skin tan.

BROOM OIL • *Cytisus scoparius. Sarothamnus scoparius.* Scoparius. Scotch Broom. Spartium. Witch's Broom. A shrub, it has long been used by herbalists as a diuretic and cathartic. It is emetic in large doses.

BROWN MUSTARD EXTRACT • *Brassica juncea. See* Mustard Oil.

BROUSSONETIA KAZINOKI • Kozo skin-conditioning ingredient from a Japanese tree. A fiber from the bark is used in making paper, cloth, and rope.

BROWN 1 • CI 20170. A diazo color. *See* D & C Brown No. 1.

BRUCINE SULFATE • Salt of the poison taken from the seeds of the strychnos shrub. It has a very bitter taste and is used primarily for denaturing alcohols and oils used in cosmetics, and has been patented. As poisonous as strychnine when ingested. On the skin, toxicity is unknown. On the Canadian Hotlist (*see*). Permitted in Canada at concentrations equal to or less than 0.1 percent. Banned in cosmetics by the EU and ASEAN (*see*).

BRUSHLESS LATHER • *See* Brushless Shaving Cream.

BRUSHLESS SHAVING CREAM • Not a soaplike lather shaving cream, but a vanishing or cold cream with additional lubricants added. Because lather creams soften the beard and brushless creams do not, one has to towel the face to effect some softening. Brushless creams usually contain 10 to 20 percent stearic acid (*see*), 3 to 13 percent mineral oil, 0.5 to 2 percent base, up to 5 percent lanolin, up to 0.5 percent gums and thickeners, 60 to 75 percent water, and 0.2 percent preservative.

BSE • Abbreviation for bovine spongiform encephalopathy or "mad cow disease." Fears that this disease can be passed on to humans via cosmetics derived from cattle, sheep, and goats caused the EU to regulate the use of certain parts of these animals in March 1981.

BUBBLE BATH • Foams, perfumes, and softens bathwater and generally makes bathing something of a special event. Liquid bubble bath may contain TEAdodecylbenzene sulfonate, fatty acid alkanolamides, perfume, water, and methylparaben. Powdered bubble bath may contain sodium lauryl sulfate, sodium chloride, and perfume. The products may also contain any of the following: alcohol, alkyl benzene sulfonate, various colorings, dioctyl sodium sulfosuccinate, propylene glycol, sodium hexametaphosphate, sodium sulfate, and sodium tripolyphosphate. Ingestion of bubble baths may cause gastrointestinal disturbances, and skin irritations have been reported, especially in children. Reports to the FDA concern skin irritation, urinary and bladder infections, toxic encephalopathy with brain damage, stomach distress, irritation and bleeding of the genital area, inflammation of the genitals, and eye injury. In 1977, the FDA required manufacturers to keep alkylarylsulfonate below 10 percent, preferably between 2 and 5 percent. Children should not take prolonged and/or unsupervised bubble baths. Adults may aggravate dryness or inflammation of the skin by taking bubble baths. The FDA says children's foaming detergent bath products such as bubble bath products are misbranded unless the labeling bears adequate directions for safe use and a precautionary statement.

BUBULUM • *See* Neatsfoot Oil.

BUCHU • Hottentot Tea. Zulu Bucu. The dried leaves of *Barosma betulina* or of *B. crenulata,* a citrus shrub grown in South Africa. It is widely used in that country for medicinal purposes. Herbalists use it worldwide to treat diseases of the kidney, urinary tract, and prostate. The leaves contain barosma camphor and essential oil. When given warm, it stimulates sweating. In 1992, the FDA proposed a ban on buchu powdered extract in oral menstrual drug products because it has not been shown to be safe and effective for its stated claims.

BUCKBEAN EXTRACT • *Menyanthes trifoliata.* Meyanthin. Bog-Bean. Water Shamrock. A common plant in bogs, it is used by herbalists as a tonic and to reduce fever. It is also used to treat skin diseases due to rheumatism. Depending on the strength and dosage, its action ranges from that of a bitter tonic and cathartic to a purgative and emetic. In folk medicine, buckbean was used to treat edema, scabies, and fever.

BUCKTHORN • Frangula. A shrub or tree grown on the Mediterranean coast of Africa, it has thorny branches and often contains a purgative in the bark or sap. Its fruits are used as a source of yellow and green dyes.

BUCKWHEAT • An herb of the genus *Fagopyrum.* Contains rutin, a pale yellow crystal found in many plants, particularly buckwheat. Used as a dietary supplement for capillary fragility.

BUDDLEJA • Extract of *Buddleja officinalis.* Used in skin conditioners.

BUFFALO FAT • The fat obtained from buffalo used as a skin-conditioning ingredient.

BUFFER • Usually a solution with a relatively constant acidity-alkalinity ratio, which is unaffected by the addition of comparatively large amounts of acid or alkali. A typical buffer solution would be hydrochloric acid and sodium hydroxide (*see*).

BUGLEWEED • Sweet Bugle. Extract of the various parts of *Lycopus virginicus,* grown in North America. Contains a volatile oil, resin, and tannin. Used in perfumery.

BUGLOSS EXTRACT • Extract of the various parts, including the roots, stems, leaves, and fruit of *Lycopsis arvensis.* Cultivated for its beautiful flowers. *See* Alkanet Root and Horehound.

BUMETRIZOLE • An absorbent. *See* Phenols.

BUPLEURUM FALCATUM • Hare's Ear Root. A perennial herb growing wild on the sunny sides of sedge thickets, it is one of the most important herbs used in Chinese herbalism. It is not reputedly a tonic herb, but it is claimed to be useful in the tonic system because of its ability to "relieve liver tension and digestive disturbances, and because it is detoxifying and anti-microbial." Bupleurum is said to have the ability, when combined with other herbs, to clear stagnation virtually anywhere in the body. It can be used to relieve spasms, muscle tension, lumps, bleeding due to heat and menstrual irregularity. In cosmetics, it is said to have anti-inflammatory properties.

BURDOCK ROOT EXTRACT • *Arctium lappa.* Cocklebur. Lapp. Bardane Beggar's Buttons. The roots, seeds, and leaves contain the essential oil of this common roadside plant. It contains nearly 45 percent inulin and many minerals. Herbalists use it for skin diseases, blood purification, urinary problems, and as a tonic. Cosmeticians use it to soothe the skin. Chinese burdock is used to eliminate excess nervous energy, and the root is considered to have aphrodisiac properties. It is sold in drugstores as an ointment to treat minor burns, cuts, or other skin traumas. It is used by gypsies in a pouch hung around the neck to ward off arthritis. It is also used to induce sweating in an effort to rid the body of toxins. In modern experiments, burdock root extract has been shown to have antitumor effects and to produce an increased flow of urine. Burdock fruit is the latest ingredient to join the fight against skin aging.

The *Arctium lappa* (active ingredient arctiin) extract can, according to a study published in the *Journal of Cosmetics Dermatology,* help protect against chronic tissue inflammation and at the same time stimulate the synthesis of connective tissues such as collagen.

BUROW'S SOLUTION • *See* Aluminum Acetate.

BUTADIENE/ACRYLONITRILE COPOLYMER • May cause eczema (*see*). Butadiene has been found to be carcinogenic in rubber plant workers. *See* Acrylates.

BUTADIENE/ISOPRENE COPOLYMER • A skin-conditioning ingredient. Butadiene has been found to cause leukemia in rubber plant workers by researchers at the University of Texas Medical Branch at Galveston. *See* Polymer and Butadiene/Acrylonitrile Copolymer.

BUTALBITAL COMPOUNDS • Used in the relief of tension or muscle contraction, headache, and other aches and pains. The active ingredients are aspirin, codeine or acetaminophen, caffeine, and the barbiturate butalbital. The most frequent adverse reactions are drowsiness and dizziness. Less frequent adverse reactions are light-headedness, nausea, vomiting, and gas. May also cause skin reactions.

BUTANE • n-Butane; iso-Butane. Methylsulfonal; Bioxiran; Dibutadiene Dioxide. Used in antiperspirant/deodorants for both men and women, styling mousse/foam; body spray; hair spray; fragrance for men; shaving cream (men's); sunless tanning; hair color and bleaching. A flammable, easily liquefiable gas derived from petroleum. A solvent, refrigerant, and food additive. Also used as a propellant or aerosol in cosmetics. The principal hazard is that of fire and explosion, but it may be narcotic in high doses and cause asphyxiation. It has been determined by the National Institute of Occupational Safety and Health to be an animal carcinogen. On the basis of the available information the CIR Expert Panel found it safe in the early 1980s and in 2002. GRAS. E

BUTANEDIOIC ACID • *See* Succinic Acid.

2,3-BUTANEDIOL • An alcohol used as a skin conditioner and humectant. *See* Butylene Glycol.

BUTCHER'S BROOM • *Ruscus aculeatus.* A shrub native to Europe, with stiff prickle-tipped, flattened stems resembling true leaves, used in cosmetics. Formerly used as a broom by butchers. In animal experiments, clinical trials have shown the effectiveness of butcher's broom extract in treating chronic blood clots of the lower limbs and varicose veins.

BUTETH-3 CARBOXYLIC ACID • *See* Carboxylic Acid and Propylene Glycol.

BUTOXY CHITOSAN • The derivative of chitosan (*see*) and acetoacetic acid. Used as a film former and thickening ingredient. *See* Chitin.

BUTOXYDIGLYCOL • An ether alcohol. *See* Diethylene Glycol.

BUTOXYETHANOL • Butyl Cellosolve. A solvent for nitrocellulose (*see*), resins, grease, oil, and albumen. It is used as a solvent in hair and nail products. Severe eye irritation occurs in undiluted forms in rabbits. Moderate and no corneal injury were observed at concentrations of 15 percent and 5 percent in liquids. The CIR Expert Panel (*see*) concludes this is safe as used in rinse-off and leave-on products at concentrations up to 10 percent. *See* Polyethylene Glycol for toxicity.

BUTOXYETHYL ACETATE • A solvent. *See* Ethylene Glycol.

BUTOXYETHYL NICOTINATE • An ester of niacin (*see*) used as a skin conditioner.

BUTTERS • Acids, Esters, and Distillate. In cosmetology, substances that are solid at room temperature but melt at body temperature are called butters. Butters are a group of natural fats. Butters may be used in stick or molded cosmetics such as lipsticks or to give the proper texture to a variety of finished products. All these butters contain 50 to 60 percent saturated fatty acids, mainly stearic acid, and up to 47 percent monounsaturated oleic acid. The plants are generally tropical and contain many ingredients used in hair and skin products. Butter acids are synthetic butter and cheese flavoring additives for beverages, ice cream, ices, candy (2,800 ppm), and baked goods. Butter esters are synthetic butter, caramel, and chocolate flavoring additives for beverages, ice cream, ices, baked goods, toppings, and popcorn (1,200 ppm). Butter starter distillate is a synthetic butter flavoring additive for ice cream, ices, baked goods, and shortening (12,000 ppm). Cocoa butter is one of the most frequently used in both foods and cosmetics. Newer butters are made from natural fats by hydrogenation (*see*), which increases the butter's melting point or alters its plasticity. *See* Fatty Acids.

BUTTERMILK • The fluid remaining after butter has been formed from churned cream. It can also be made from sweet milk by the addition of certain organic cultures. Used as an astringent right from the bottle. Apply liberally and let dry about 10 minutes. Rinse off with cool water. Also used as a freckle bleach. Apply 1 tablespoon of cooking oil or your favorite moisturizer. Mix 7 tablespoons of buttermilk with 1 tablespoon of grated fresh horseradish (keep it away from your eyes). Combine the ingredients and apply to your face. Leave on for 15 minutes and rinse off with cool water. Then reapply your moisturizer or oil.

BUTYL- • Derived from butane (*see*).

BUTYL ACETATE • Acetic Acid. Butyl Ester. A colorless liquid with a fruity odor used in perfumery, nail polish, and nail polish remover. Also used in the manufacture of lacquer, artificial leather, plastics, and safety glass. It is an irritant and may cause eye irritation (conjunctivitis). It is a narcotic in high concentrations and toxic to man when inhaled at 200 ppm. On the basis of available data, the CIR Expert Panel concludes that this ingredient is safe as presently used in cosmetics.

BUTYL ACETYL RICINOLEATE • *See* Ricinoleate.

BUTYLACRYLATE/HYDROXYETHYL METHACRYLATE • A film former. *See* Acrylates.

BUTYL ALCOHOL • A colorless liquid with an unpleasant odor, used as a clarifying ingredient (*see*) in shampoos; also a solvent for waxes, fats, resins, and shellac. It may cause irritation of the mucous membranes, headache, dizziness, and drowsiness when ingested. Inhalation of as little as 25 ppm causes pulmonary problems in man. It can also cause contact dermatitis when applied to the skin. The CIR Expert Panel (*see*) concludes this is a safe ingredient in nail products.

n-**BUTYL ALCOHOL** • Used as a solvent and denaturant.

t-**BUTYL ALCOHOL** • Denaturant and solvent. *See* Butyl Alcohol.

BUTYL AMINOETHYL METHYL ACRYLATE • Used in hair sprays. *See* Acrylates.

BUTYL BENZOIC ACID/PHTHALIC ANHYDRIDE/TRIMETHYLOETH-ANE COPOLYMER • A polymer (*see*) formed when the water is removed from the phthalic acid and the acid is combined with trimethyloethane monomers.

BUTYL BENZYL PHTHALATE • The aromatic ester that is used as a sanitizer and plasticizer. There are questions about phthalates (*see*), but the CIR Expert Panel (*see*) concludes this is a safe ingredient.

BUTYL ESTER OF ETHYLENE/MALEIC ANHYDRIDE COPOLYMER • A resin (*see*) made from ethylene and maleic anhydride (*see*). Used in hair sprays and setting lotions, and as a thickener in cosmetics.

BUTYL ESTER OF PVM/MA COPOLYMER • Butyl Ester of Poly (Methyl Vinyl Ether, Maleic Acid). Spirit Gum. Plastic material formed from vinyl methyl ether and maleic anhydride. Used in hair sprays and setting lotions, and as a thickener. On the basis of available data, the CIR Expert Panel concludes that this ingredient is safe as presently used in cosmetics.

BUTYL GLYCOLATE • A plasticizer in nail lacquers. *See* Butyl Acetate.

BUTYL GLYCOSIDE • Obtained by the condensation of butyl alcohol with glucose (*see both*). Used as an emulsifier.

t-**BUTYL HYDROQUINONE** • An antioxidant. A weak depigmenter at 1.0 and 5.0 percent but not at 0.1 percent. The CIR Expert Panel (*see*) concludes this is a safe ingredient if it does not exceed 0.1 percent. *See* Hydroquinone.

BUTYL *p*-HYDROXYBENZOATE • Butyl Paraben. Butyl *p*-Oxybenzoate. Almost odorless, small colorless crystals or a white powder used as an antimicrobial preservative.

BUTYL LACTATE • A synthetic butter, butterscotch, caramel, and fruit flavoring ingredient for beverages, ice cream, ices, candy, and baked goods. Used in cosmetics in creams, lotions, fragrances, and soaps as a solvent.

BUTYL METHOXYDIBENZOYLMETHANE • Used in the formulation of sun protection products, as well as bath, skin, cleansing, hair, nail, and fragrance products. The CIR Expert Panel (*see*) has deferred evaluation of this ingredient because the safety has been assessed by the FDA. This deferral of review is according to the provisions of the CIR procedures. In the United States, when this ingredient is used in sun protection products, it will be listed on the label as avobenzone (*see*).

4-TERT-BUTYL-3-METHOXY-2,6-DINOTROTOLUENE. • A synthetic fixative, it is widely used as a fragrance ingredient in perfumes, soaps, detergents, creams, lotions, and dentifrices in the United States at an estimated 100,000 pounds per year. It reportedly damages the myelin, the covering of nerve fibers. It can cause photosensitivity (*see*) and contact dermatitis. The problem is mostly with after-shave lotions. Musk tetralin, in use for twenty years as a fragrance ingredient, was identified as a neurotoxin and removed from the market in 1978. Musk ambrette has been generally recognized as safe as a food additive by the FDA, but see the introduction to this book. On the Canadian Hotlist (*see*). Banned by ASEAN in cosmetics. *See* Musk Ambrette.

BUTYL MYRISTATE • A fatty alcohol used in nail polishes and nail polish removers, lipsticks, and face and protective creams. It is derived from myristic acid (*see*) and butyl alcohol (*see*). More irritating than ethanol (*see*), but less so than some other alcohols.

BUTYL OLEATE • Light-colored liquid with a mild odor. The ester of butyl alcohol and oleic acid (*see both*), it is a plasticizer, particularly for polyvinyl chloride (*see*), and is used in waterproofing, as a solvent and lubricant, and in polishes. In cosmetics, it is used as a skin conditioner and emollient.

BUTYL PABA • The ester of butyl alcohol and para-aminobenzoic acid (*see both*).

BUTYL PALMITATE • Used in shampoos to leave a gloss on the hair. *See* Palmitic Acid.

BUTYL PHTHALYL BUTYL GLYCOLATE • *See* Butyl Glycolate.

BUTYL STEARATE • A synthetic antifoaming ingredient used in the production of beet sugar. Used as a binder and surfactant in cosmetics. Also a synthetic banana, butter, and liquor flavoring for beverages, ice cream, ices, candy, baked goods, chewing gum, and liqueurs. Used as a skin-conditioning ingredient. On the basis of the available animal and human data, the CIR Expert Panel (*see*) concludes that this ingredient is safe as used in cosmetics. However, it has been linked to promoting acne.

BUTYLATED • The introduction of the butyl group-carbon and hydrogen from butane into a compound to make it less susceptible to damage from oxygen.

BUTYLATED HYDROXYANISOLE • BHA. A preservative and antioxidant in cosmetics, foods, and beverages. White to slightly yellow, waxy solid with a faint characteristic odor. Can cause allergic reactions.

BUTYLATED HYDROXYTOLUENE • BHT. A preservative and antioxidant in cosmetics, foods, and beverages. A white crystalline solid with a faint characteristic odor.

Prohibited as a food additive in England. Chemically similar to BHA, it can cause allergic reactions.

BUTYLATED POLYOXYMETHYLENE • A compound from formaldehyde and urea (*see both*).

BUTYLATED POLYOXYMETHYLENE UREA • Formerly butylated ureaformaldehyde resin. A product of an amino resin mixed with urea and formaldehyde (*see both*). The word *formaldehyde* was taken out of the label listing for cosmetics.

BUTYLATED UREA-FORMALDEHYDE RESIN • *See* Butylated Polyoxymethylene Urea.

BUTYLATED XYLENONE • An antioxidant. *See* Phenols.

BUTYLCARBAMATE • The ester of carbamic acid, which occurs in the blood and urine of mammals. Used in sunblocks. *See* Urea.

BUTYLENE GLYCOL • This humectant is most resistant to high humidity and thus valuable in hair sprays and setting lotions. It retains scents and preserves against spoilage. It has a similar toxicity to ethylene glycol (*see*), which when ingested may cause transient stimulation of the central nervous system, then depression, vomiting, drowsiness, coma, respiratory failure, and convulsions; renal damage may proceed to kidney failure and death. One of the few humectants not on the GRAS list of the FDA, although efforts to place it there have been made through the years.

1,3-BUTYLENE GLYCOL • A clear, colorless, viscous liquid with a slight taste. A solvent and humectant most resistant to high humidity and thus valuable in foods and cosmetics. It retains scents and preserves against spoilage. It has a similar toxicity to ethylene glycol (*see*), which when ingested may cause transient stimulation of the central nervous system, then depression, vomiting, drowsiness, coma, respiratory failure, and convulsions; renal damage may proceed to uremia and death. One of the few humectants not on the GRAS list, although efforts to place it there have been made through the years. ASP

BUTYLENE GLYCOL MONTANATE • A mixture of esters of montan wax with ethyelene glycol and butylene glycol (*see all*). Used as a surfactant (*see*) and thickener.

BUTYLOCTYL BENZOATE • A plasticizer, skin conditioner, emollient, and solvent. The CIR Expert Panel (*see*) concludes this is a safe ingredient. *See* Benzoic Acid.

BUTYLOCTYL CANDELILLATE • A skin-conditioning ingredient and a cover-up. *See* Candelilla Wax.

BUTYLPARABEN • Widely used in cosmetics as an antifungal preservative, it is the ester of butyl alcohol and *p*-hydroxybenzoic acid.

BUTYLPHTHALIMIDE • A skin-conditioning ingredient. *See* Phthalic Acid.

4-BUTYLRESORCINOL • Antioxidant. *See* Resorcinol.

BUTYL-1,2,3-TRIMETHYL-4,6-DINITROBENZENE • *See* Musk Tibetene.

BUTYRALDEHYDE • A synthetic flavoring ingredient found naturally in coffee and strawberries. Used in butter, caramel, fruit, liquor, brandy, and nut flavorings for beverages, ice cream, ices, candy, baked goods, alcoholic beverages, and icings. Used also in the manufacture of rubber, gas accelerators, synthetic resins, and plasticizers. May be an irritant and a narcotic.

BUTYRIC ACID • *n*-Butyric Acid. Butanoic Acid. A clear, colorless liquid present in butter at 4 to 5 percent. It has a strong, rancid butter odor and is used in butterscotch, caramel, and fruit flavorings. It is used in chewing gums and margarines, as well as in cosmetics. It is found naturally in apples, geraniums, rose oil, grapes, strawberries, and wormseed oil. It has a low toxicity but can be a mild irritant. It caused tumors when applied to the skin of mice in 108-milligram doses per kilogram of body weight and cancer when injected into the abdomen of mice in 18-milligram doses per kilogram of body weight. A NIOSH review has determined it is a positive animal carcinogen. It has a low toxicity but can be a mild irritant. GRAS

BUTRYIS LAC • Buttermilk powder.

BUTYROLACTONE • Butanolide. Liquid lactone used chiefly as a solvent for resins. It is also an intermediate (*see*) in the manufacture of polyvinylpyrrolidone (*see*) and a solvent for nail polish. Human toxicity is unknown.

BUTYROSPERMUM PARKII • *See* Shea Butter.

BUTYRUM • The EU name for butter, the U.S. designation on a label.

BUXUS CHINENSIS • *See* Jojoba Oil.

BUXUS SEMPERVIRENS • *See* Boxwood.

C

C30-59 • *See* Carboxylic Acid.

C40-60 • Thickener. *See* Carboxylic Acid.

C18-36 ACID • A synthetic mixture of saturated, waxy fatty acids containing 18 to 36 carbons in the alkyl (*see*) chain. *See* Fatty Acids.

C29-70 ACID • C29–70 Carboxylic Acids. A mixture of synthetic aliphatic acids with 29 to 70 carbon atoms in the alkyl (*see*) chain. *See* Fatty Acids.

C18-36 ACID GLYCOL ESTER • *See* Fatty Acids.

C18-36 ACID TRIGLYCERIDE • *See* Fatty Acids.

C9-11 ALCOHOLS • A mixture of synthetic fatty alcohols with 9 to 11 carbons in the alkyl (*see*) chain. *See* Fatty Acids.

C12-15 ALCOHOLS BENZOATE • *See* C12–15 Alkyl Benzoate.

C12-15 ALCOHOLS LACTATE • *See* C12–15 Alkyl Lactate.

C12-15 ALCOHOLS OCTANOATE • *See* C12–15 Alkyl Octanoate.

C12-16 ALCOHOLS • A mixture of synthetic fatty acids.

C14-15 ALCOHOLS • Alkyls. A mixture of synthetic fatty alcohols with 14 to 15 carbons in the alkyl (*see*) chain. *See* Fatty Acids.

C9-16 ALKANES/CYCLOALKANES • Hydrocarbons (*see*) that are solvents, surfactants, and cleansing ingredients. These are substances of very high concern according to ECHA (*see*) because they are suspected of being persistent, bioaccumulative, and toxic.

C18-28 ALKYL ACETATE • Esters that are skin conditioners and emollients.

C18-38 ALKYL BEESWAX • Skin conditioner. *See* Beeswax.

C20-40 ALKYL BEHENATE • A skin conditioner. *See* Behenic Acid.

C12-15 ALKYL BENZOATE • Ester of benzoic acid (*see*) and C12–15 alcohols. Used in face creams. *See* Fatty Acids.

C12-15 ALKYL LACTATE • The ester of lactic acid and C12–15 alcohols. *See* Fatty Acids.

C12-15 ALKYL OCTANOATE • The ester of octanoic acid (*see*) and fatty alcohols.

C12-15 ALKYL SALICYLATE • A skin conditioner. *See* Salicylic Acid.

C16-40 ALKYL STEARATE • Skin conditioners and thickening ingredients for compounds.

C15-18 GLYCOL • The long-chain diol that has 13 to 16 carbons in the alkyl (*see*) chain. *See* Fatty Acids.

C18-20 GLYCOL ISOSTEARATE • The ester of isostearate with 16 to 18 carbons in the alkyl chain. *See* Fatty Acids.

C18-20 GLYCOL PALMITATE • *See* Fatty Acids.

C10-40 ISOALKYL ACID • Fatty acids used as a conditioner in hair and skin products.

C14-20 ISOALKYLAMIDOPROPYLETHYLDIMONIUM ETHOSULFATE • A quaternary ammonium compound (*see*).

C8-9, C9-11, C9-13, C9-14, C10-11, C10-13, C11-12, C11-13, C12-14, C13-16, AND C20-40 ISOPARAFFINS • Mixtures of aliphatic hydrocarbons with the number of carbons in the alkyl (*see*) chain given by the numbers. *See* Fatty Acids.

C7-8 ISOPARAFFIN • A hydrocarbon used as a solvent. *See* Paraffin.

C13-14 ISOPARAFFIN • A widely used solvent in moisturizers, shaving products, and moisturizers. *See* Paraffin.

C20-48 OLEFIN • Hydrocarbons used as skin-conditioning ingredients. *See* Oleic Acid.

C11-15 PARETH -3, -5, -7, -9, -12, -20, -30, -40 • Mixture of polyethylene glycols; the higher the number, the thicker the mixture. *See* Polyethylene Glycols.

C11-15 PARETH -7 CARBOXYLIC ACID • Polyethylene mixture of carboxylic acid (*see*).

C11-15 PARETH-12 STEARATE • The ester of pareth-15-12 and stearic acid (*see*).

C11-15 PARETH-40 • Polyethylene glycol ether (*see*) of a mixture of synthetic fatty alcohols. *See* Polyethylene Glycol and Fatty Alcohols.

C12-13 PARETH-3, -7 • Polyethylene glycol ether of a mixture of synthetic fatty alcohols and ethylene glycol (*see all*).

C12-15 PARETH-2, -3, -4, -5, -7, -9, -12 • The polyethylene glycol ethers of fatty alcohols with ethylene oxide. *See* Polyethylene Glycol, Ethers, and Fatty Alcohols.

C12-15 PARETH-2 PHOSPHATE • A mixture of the esters of phosphoric acid (*see*) and polyethylene glycol ethers (*see*).

C14-15 PARETH -7, -11, -13 • The polyethylene glycol ether of a mixture of synthetic fatty alcohols with ethylene oxide (*see all*).

C30-46 PISCINE OIL • A marine oil derived from fish. It is used as a thickener.

C10-18 TRIGLYCERIDES • A mixture of fatty acids and glycerin. Used as a thickener.

C20-40 ACID • *See* Fatty Acids.

CABBAGE EXTRACT • *Brassica oleracea capitata.* Kale. Used in skin masks.

CABBAGE ROSE • A fragrant garden rose, *Rosa centifolia,* with upright branches and large full white or pink flowers. Used in fragrances.

CACTUS • A family of prickly plants, Cactaceae, comprising over fifteen hundred species almost all of which are native to America. It has no leaves but stores a great deal of water. Cacti bear beautiful, short-lived flowers. They are the source of the drug mescaline and some species are edible. Extracts of cacti are used in "organic" cosmetics.

CADE OIL • *See* Juniper Tar.

CADMIUM CHLORIDE • A white powder, soluble in water, used in photography and in dye, particularly hair dye. Inhalation of the dust is highly toxic, and ingestion can cause death. Caused tumors when injected under the skin in rats and when given intravenously. It also caused cancer in mice when injected under the skin. NIOSH review determined that it was a positive animal carcinogen. On the Canadian Hotlist (*see*). EU has banned it in cosmetics.

CAFFEIC ACID • An antioxidant. *See* Carboxylic Acid.

CAFFEINE • Guaranine. Methyltheobromine. Theine. An odorless white powder with a bitter taste that occurs naturally in coffee, cola, guarana paste, tea, and kola nuts. Obtained as a by-product of caffeine-free coffee. It is used as a stimulant and flavoring in lipsticks, to aid ingredients to penetrate the skin, and to stimulate the skin. It is a central nervous system, heart, and respiratory system stimulant when ingested. Can alter blood sugar release and cross the placental barrier.

CAJEPUT • *Melaleuca leucadendra.* Cajuput. White Tea Tree. Tea Tree. The spicy oil contains, among other ingredients, terpenes, limonene, benzaldehyde, valeraldehyde, and dipentene. Native to Australia and Southeast Asia, it is used to treat fungus infections such as athlete's foot, and as a liniment for a wide variety of ailments. Herbalists use it to relieve itchy scalp, arthritic pains, and as an antiseptic for cuts.

CAJUPUT • *See* Cajeput.

CAKE MASCARA • Mascara based on fats or soap molded forms. It is applied with a brush dipped in water. A more liquid product is used in a cylinder into which a brush is inserted and pulled out, coated with mascara. A typical cake mascara formula: triethanolamine stearate, 54 percent; carnauba wax, 25 percent; paraffin, 12.5 percent; lanolin, 4.5 percent; carbon black, 3.8 percent; propylparaben, 0.2 percent; other, 1 percent (*see* ingredients above under separate listings). *See* Mascara for toxicity.

CAKILE MARITIMA • Sea Rocket. A plant of the genus *Cakile.* A succulent herb found along the sandy shore.

CALAMINE • Zinc oxide with about 5 percent ferric oxide that occurs as a pink powder. Used in protective creams, astringents, lotions, ointments, washes, and powders in the treatment of skin diseases; also to impart a flesh color. Some calamine formulations contain significant amounts of phenol (*see*), and ingestion or repeated applications over large areas of skin may cause phenol poisoning. The FDA proposed a ban in 1992 for the use of calamine to treat insect bites and stings and poison ivy, poison oak, and poison sumac because it has not been shown to be safe and effective for stated claims in OTC products. The FDA said calamine could be used as "a skin protectant" but not as an "external analgesic."

CALAMINTHA OFFICINALIS • *See* Mint.

CALAMUS ROOT EXTRACT • *Acorus calamus.* Sweet Flag. Sweet Sedge. The rhizome contains essential oil, mucilage, glycosides, amino acid, and tannins (*see all*). Calamus root is an ancient Indian and Chinese herbal medicine used to treat acid stomach, irregular heart rhythm, low blood pressure, lack of mental focus, and for coughs. Native Americans would chew the root to enable them to run long distances with increased stamina.

CALCIFEROL • Vitamin D.

CALCIUM • The adult body contains about three pounds of calcium, 99 percent of which provides hardness for bones and teeth. Approximately 1 percent of calcium is distributed in body fluids, where it is essential for normal cell activity.

CALCIUM ACETATE • Brown Acetate of Lime. A white amorphous powder that has been used medicinally as a source of calcium. Used cosmetically to solidify fragrances and as an emulsifier and firming ingredient. Also used as a corrosion inhibitor in metal containers.

CALCIUM ALGINATE • *See* Alginates.

CALCIUM ALUMINUM BOROSILICATE • A thickening ingredient. *See* Silicates.

CALCIUM ASCORBATE • *See* Ascorbic Acid.

CALCIUM BEHENATE • The calcium salt of behenic acid (*see*) used as a wax.

CALCIUM BENZOATE • *See* Benzoic Acid.

CALCIUM BROMIDE • *See* Bromides, Potassium and Sodium.

CALCIUM CARBONATE • Chalk. Absorbent that removes shine from talc. A tasteless, odorless powder that occurs naturally in limestone, marble, and coral. Used as a white coloring in cosmetics and food, an alkali to reduce acidity, a neutralizer and firming ingredient, and a carrier for bleaches. Also used in dentrifices as a tooth polisher, in deodorants as a filler, in depilatories as a filler, and in face powder as a buffer. A gastric antacid and antidiarrhea medicine, it may cause constipation. GRAS. ASP. E

CALCIUM CARRAGEENAN • *See* Carrageenan.

CALCIUM CASEINATE • Binder, thickener, hair- and skin-conditioning ingredient. The calcium salt of casein (*see*).

CALCIUM CHLORIDE • The chloride salt of calcium. Used in its anhydrous (*see*) form as a drying ingredient for organic liquids and gases. An emulsifier and texturizer in cosmetics and an antiseptic in eye lotions. Also used in fire extinguishers, to preserve wood, and to melt ice and snow. Employed medicinally as a diuretic and a urinary acidifier. Ingestion can cause stomach and heart disturbances.

CALCIUM CYCLAMATE • Artificial sweetening ingredient about thirty times as sweet as refined sugar, removed from the food market on September 1, 1969, because it was found to cause bladder cancer in rats. At that time 175 million Americans were swallowing cyclamates in significant doses in many products ranging from chewing gum to soft drinks. There has been a concerted effort to bring cyclamates back to the market, but as of this writing, they have not been approved. The FDA's Cancer Assessment Committee's review of all the evidence reportedly indicates that neither cyclamate nor its major metabolic end product cyclohexylamine cause cancer. Still listed for use in cosmetics.

CALCIUM DIHYDROGEN PHOSPHATE • A pH adjuster. *See* pH.

CALCIUM DISODIUM EDTA • Edetate Calcium Disodium. Calcium Disodium Ethylenediamine Tetraacetic Acid. A preservative and sequestrant (*see* Sequestering Ingredient). Used as a food additive to prevent crystal formation and to retard color loss.

CALCIUM DNA • The calcium salt of DNA (*see*) used as a skin conditioner.

CALCIUM DODECYLBENZENE SULFONATE • A cleansing ingredient. *See* Benzene.

CALCIUM FERRITE • A coloring. *See* Iron Oxides.

CALCIUM FLUORIDE • Oral hygiene product. The EU label says "Contains calcium fluoride." It is on the Canadian Hotlist (*see*). *See* Sodium Fluoride.

CALCIUM FRUCTOHEPTONATE • Used as a skin conditioner. *See* Fructose.

CALCIUM GLUCOHEPTONATE • An organic salt that is used in skin conditioners.

CALCIUM GLUCONATE • Odorless, tasteless, white crystalline granules, stale in air. Used as a buffer, firming ingredient, and sequestrant (*see* Sequestering Ingredient). May cause gastrointestinal and cardiac disturbances. The final report to the FDA of the Select Committee on GRAS Substances stated in 1980 that it should continue its GRAS status with no limitations other than good manufacturing practices. The FDA issued a notice in 1992 that calcium gluconate has not been shown to be safe and effective as claimed in OTC digestive aid products.

CALCIUM HYDROXIDE • Limewater. Lye. Used in cream depilatories; as a hair straightener; also in mortar, plaster, cement, pesticides, fireproofing, and as an egg preservative. Employed as a topical astringent and alkali in solutions or lotions. Accidental ingestion can cause burns of the throat and esophagus; also death from shock and asphyxia due to swelling of the glottis and infection. Calcium hydroxide also can cause burns of the skin and eyes. It can cause blindness. The EU says maximum allowance in product is 7 percent by weight.

CALCIUM HYPOCHLORITE • A germicide and sterilizing ingredient, it is the active ingredient of chlorinated lime and is used in the curd washing of cottage cheese, in sugar refining, as an oxidizing and bleaching ingredient, and as an algae killer, bactericide, deodorant, disinfectant, and fungicide. Under various names, dilute hypochlorite is found in homes as laundry bleach and household bleach. Household mildew removers contain 5 percent calcium hypochlorite, which is twice as toxic as common household sodium hypochlorite bleach. Industrial strength hypochlorite bleaches contain 15 to 20 percent solutions. Occasionally, cases of poisoning occur when people mix household hypochlorite solution with various other household chemicals, which causes the release of poisonous chlorine gas. As with other corrosive ingredients, calcium hypochlorite's toxicity depends on its concentration. It is highly corrosive to skin and mucous membranes. Ingestion may cause pain and inflammation of the mouth, pharynx, esophagus, and stomach, with erosion particularly of the mucous membranes of the stomach.

CALCIUM LACTATE • White, almost odorless crystals or powder used as a buffer and as such is a constituent of baking powders; also used in dentifrices. In medical use, given for calcium deficiency; may cause gastrointestinal and cardiac disturbances. In 1992, the FDA proposed a ban on calcium lactate in oral menstrual drug products because it has not been shown to be safe and effective for its stated claims.

CALCIUM LIGNOSULFONATE • *See* Lignoceric Acid.

CALCIUM MONOFLUOROPHOSPHATE • An inorganic salt used in oral care products. The EU calculates at 0.50 percent when mixed with other fluorine compounds. Fluorine concentration must not exceed 0.15 percent, and the EU label must say "Contains monofluorophosphate." See Fluorine Compounds and Fluoride.

CALCIUM MONTANATE • *See* Montan Wax.

CALCIUM MYRISTATE • An anticaking ingredient, stabilizer in emulsions, and thickening ingredient. *See* Myristic Acid.

CALCIUM NITRATE • *See* Nitrate.

CALCIUM OXIDE • Lime. Quicklime. White or gray crystals or powder commercially obtained from limestone. Used as an alkali in cosmetics, as an insecticide and fungicide, and for dehairing hides. A strong caustic that may cause severe irritation of the skin and mucous membranes and can cause both thermal and chemical burns.

CALCIUM PANTETHEINE SULFONATE • Organic salt used in skin conditioners. *See* Pantothenic Acid.

CALCIUM PANTOTHENATE • Pantothenic Acid Calcium Salt. Vitamin B_5. The calcium salt of pantothenic acid, found in liver, rice bran, and molasses, and essential for metabolism of carbohydrates, fats, and other important substances. Sweetish taste with a slightly bitter aftertaste, soluble in water, it is a member of the B-complex family of vitamins. It is also found in large amounts in the jelly of the queen bee, the so-called royal jelly of cosmetic advertising fame. It is used as an emollient and to enrich creams and lotions.

CALCIUM PARABEN • A preservative. *See* Parabens.

CALCIUM PEROXIDE • *See* Peroxide.

CALCIUM PHOSPHATE • White, odorless powder used as an anticaking ingredient in cosmetics and foods. Employed in toothpaste and tooth powder as an abrasive. Practically insoluble in water.

CALCIUM PROPIONATE • Propanoic Acid, Calcium Salt. White crystals or crystalline solid with the faint odor of propionic acid. It is used as a preservative in cosmetics and as an antifungal medication for the skin. The FDA has asked for further study for safety. GRAS. ASP. E

CALCIUM PYROPHOSPHATE • A fine, white, odorless, tasteless powder used as a nutrient, an abrasive in dentifrices, a buffer, and as a neutralizing ingredient in foodstuffs.

CALCIUM SACCHARATE • *See* Saccharin.

CALCIUM SACCHARIN • *See* Saccharin.

CALCIUM SALICYLATE • The European Union has banned this for use for children under three except in shampoos. *See* Salicylates.

CALCIUM SILICATE • Okenite. An anticaking ingredient, white or slightly cream-colored, free-flowing powder used in face powders because it has extremely fine particles and good water absorption. Also used as a coloring ingredient. Used in baking powder, in road construction, and in lime glass. Practically nontoxic orally, but inhalation may cause irritation of the respiratory tract.

CALCIUM SODIUM BOROSILICATE • A thickener. *See* Calcium and Silicates.

CALCIUM/SODIUM PVM/MA • A mixture of calcium and sodium salts with polyvinyl acetate and maleic acids (*see both*).

CALCIUM SORBATE • A preservative. *See* Sorbic Acid.

CALCIUM STEARATE • Prepared from limewater (*see*), it is an emulsifier used in hair-grooming products. Also used as a coloring ingredient, in waterproofing, and in paints and printing ink. On the basis of the available information, the CIR Expert Panel (*see*) found it safe in the early 1980s but is considering new information to determine if the final safety assessment should be reaffirmed, amended, or have an addendum.

CALCIUM STEAROYL LACTYLATE • The calcium salt of the stearic acid ester of lactyl lactate. Free-flowing powder used as a texturizer and to improve the flow of cosmetic powders.

CALCIUM SULFATE • Plaster of Paris. A fine, white to slightly yellow, odorless, tasteless powder used in toothpaste and tooth powders as an abrasive and firming ingredient. Also used as a coloring ingredient in cosmetics. Because it absorbs moisture and hardens quickly, its ingestion may result in intestinal obstruction. Mixed with flour, it has been used to kill rodents. GRAS. ASP. E

CALCIUM SULPHIDE • A yellow powder formed by heating gypsum with charcoal at 1000 degrees F. Employed in depilatories. Used in acne preparations. Also used as a food preservative and in luminous paints. It can cause allergic reactions.

CALCIUM TARTRATE • *See* Tartaric Acid.

CALCIUM THIOGLYCOLATE • Used in cream depilatories and permanent wave lotions. Odorless or with a faint odor. Also used to tan leather. Chronic application has led to thyroid problems in experimental animals. Some people develop skin problems on the hands or scalp with hemorrhaging under the skin.

CALCIUM TITANATE • A coloring. *See* Titanium Oxide and Calcium.

CALCIUM UNDECYLENATE • A fine, white powder used to kill bacteria and fungus. *See* Undecylenic Acid.

CALCIUM XYLENESULFONATE • The calcium salt of xylene (*see*). Used as a surfactant and to attract water.

CALENDULA EXTRACT AND OIL • Products from the flowers of pot marigolds grown in gardens everywhere. Formerly used to soothe inflammation of skin and mucous membranes, now used in "natural" creams, oils, and powders for babies. Use of this as a colorant is prohibited in the United States. It is widely used, however, in shampoos, soaps, skin fresheners, suntan gels, hair preparations, permanent waves, baby lotions, and face powders. GRAS.

CALF BLOOD EXTRACT • Used in anti-aging products.

CALF SKIN EXTRACT • An oil extracted from bovine skin. Used in anti-aging products.

CALF SKIN HYDROLYSATE • Hydrolysate (*see*) of calf skin derived by acid, enzyme, or other method of hydrolysis. Used in anti-aging products. Reportedly helps build collagen (*see*). A bright, greenish yellow gel used in hair-waving fluids, toothpastes, bath salts, soaps, and shampoos. It is a potential allergen. It is present in yellow Irish Spring, pink Dove, and Caress bath soap. It may cross-react with other quinoline colors used in drugs. The uncertified color is called Acid Yellow 3.

CALIFORNIA NUTMEG EXTRACT • Stinking Nutmeg Extract. Derived from *Torreya californica. See* Nutmeg.

CALLUNA VULGARIS • Heather. Ling Extract. A purple evergreen that grows in northern and alpine regions.

CALLUSES • Hard, rough skin on the sides and soles of the feet often caused by poor-fitting shoes or walking shoeless or sockless.

CALOMEL • Mercurous Chloride. A white, odorless, tasteless, heavy powder used in bleach and freckle creams. It slowly decays in sunlight into mercuric chloride and metallic mercury. Banned in July 1973, when the FDA ordered all mercury cosmetics (except for mercury preservatives in eye products) off the market. In 1996, the Texas Department of Health and the New Mexico Department of Health reported a mercury-containing beauty cream in stores and flea markets. It contained calomel with about 6 to 10 percent mercury by weight. In response to media announcements, 238 persons in the West and Midwest contacted their health department to report use of the cream, called Crema de Belleza-Manning. The health departments said that although the potential health risks associated with the product were recognized only in 1996, the cream has been produced since 1971 and the prevalence of its use in this country "cannot be accurately estimated."

CALOPHYLLUM OIL • Santa Maria Tree. Extract from a tropical tree having thick, shiny feather-veined leaves, clustered white flowers, aromatic resinous juice, and oily seeds. Used in moisturizing creams.

CAMELLIA KISS SEED OIL • Plant extract that has emollient properties for skin. There is some research showing it to have anti-inflammatory properties as well. *See* Camellia Oil.

CAMELLIA OIL • *Camellia oleifera. C. sinensis. C. japonica.* Green Tea. A tropical Asiatic evergreen shrub or small tree with reddish or white flowers. Used to scent perfumes and in antiwrinkle creams. Green tea has many beneficial effects and has reportedly anticholesterol, anti–high blood pressure properties. It also contains tannins (*see*). *See* Tea Tree Oil.

CAMOMILE • *See* Chamomile.

CAMPHOR OIL • *Cinnamomum camphora.* Used in emollient creams, hair tonics, eye lotions, preshave lotions, after-shave lotions, and skin fresheners as a preservative and to give a cool feeling to the skin. It is used as a spice flavoring for beverages, baked goods, and condiments. It is also used in horn-rimmed glasses, as a drug preservative, in embalming fluid, in the manufacture of explosives, in lacquers, as a moth repellent, and topically in liniments, cold medications, and anesthetics. It is distilled from trees at least fifty years old grown in China, Japan, Taiwan, Brazil, and Sumatra. It can cause contact dermatitis. In 1980, the FDA banned camphorated oil as a liniment for colds and sore muscles because of reports of poisonings through skin absorption and because of accidental ingestion. A New Jersey pharmacist had collected case reports and testified before the Advisory Review Panel on OTC Drugs to the FDA in 1980. On the Canadian Hotlist (*see*). Canada requires the inner and outer label of a cosmetic, in liquid form, that contains more than 30 percent camphor to carry a statement to the effect that it is for external use only and is poisonous if ingested.

CANADIAN BALSAM • Film former used in shampoos and hair conditioner. *See* Abies.

CANADIAN HOTLIST • Contains information about more than two hundred suspect cosmetic ingredients that have the potential for adverse affects or which have been restricted or banned. All the information contained on Cosmetic Notification Forms submitted to the Canadian Microbiology and Cosmetics Section, Product Safety Bureau, is entered into the Cosmetic Notification System (CNS). If an ingredient on the notification form also appears in the CNS "hotlist," that notification will be "flagged" by the system. Generally this involves advising the manufacturer by letter of concern regarding the "hotlist" ingredient. The hotlist is an ever-evolving document that is continually updated. It is expected to be completed in 2010. Check http://www.hc-sc.gc.ca/cps-spc/person/cosmet/info-ind-prof/_hot-list-critique/hotlist-liste-eng.php.

CANANGA OIL • A natural flavor extract obtained by distillation from the flowers of the tree. Light to deep yellow liquid with a harsh, floral odor. Used in cola, fruit, spice, and ginger ale flavoring for beverages, ice cream, ices, candy, baked goods. May cause allergic reactions.

CANARIUM • Essential oil used as a fragrance ingredient. *See* Olive Oil.

CANAVALIA ENSIFORMIS • Jack Bean. Sword Bean. Fast-growing, usually erect, sometimes shrubby twining annual. The seeds are edible but somewhat toxic if consumed in large quantities. Used as a skin conditioner.

CANDELILLA WAX • *Euphorbia cerifera.* Obtained from candelilla plants for use in lipsticks, solid fragrances, and liquid powders to give them body. Used in emollients to protect the skin against moisture loss. Also used in the manufacture of rubber, in waterproofing and writing inks, and to harden other waxes. The CIR Expert Panel (*see*) concludes this is a safe ingredient.

CANDIDA BOMBICOLA/SUCROSE/VEGETABLE ACID ESTER FERMENT • Esters of sunflower seed oil, palm kernel acids, and rapeseed oil (*see all*). Used in creams and oils.

CANDLENUT TREE • *See* Kukui Nut Oil.

CANEKUBA SATIVA • Gold of Pleasure. Derived from *Camelina sativa. See* Tea Tree Oil.

CANOLA OIL • A low erucic-acid rapeseed oil (*see*) used in salad oils because it contains 50 percent less saturated fat than other popular oils. GRAS

CANOLAMIDOPROPYL BETAINE • An antistatic ingredient used as a skin conditioner and a cover-up. Used in hand and face creams, soft soaps, and mud packs. Can cause acnelike skin eruptions.

CANOLAMIDOPROPYL ETHYLDIMONIUM ETHOSULFATE • A quaternary ammonium compound (*see*) used as an antistatic ingredient in hair products.

CANTHARIDES TINCTURE • *Cantharidis vesicatoria.* Spanish Fly. Obtained from blister beetles that thrive in southern and central Europe and powdered for use in hair tonics and lotions to stimulate the scalp. A powerful irritant to the skin and causes blistering. If ingested, it can cause severe intestinal upset, kidney damage, and death. Long reputed to have aphrodisiac effects. The EU has banned it in cosmetics.

CANTHARIDIN • Skin vesicant, rubefacient (*see*) in hair tonic. Can cause allergic reaction. On the Canadian Hotlist (*see*). The EU has banned it in cosmetics. *See* Cantharides Tincture.

CANTHAXANTHIN • A color additive derived from edible mushrooms, crustaceans, trout, salmon, and tropical birds. It produces a pink color. It is a synthetic non-provitamin A carotenoid that is easily absorbed by fat. It is taken for the purpose of skin "tanning" and may be provided by tanning salons or by mail order. It is not approved as a prescription or OTC drug. A report from Vanderbilt University's Department of Pharmacy cited the case of a healthy young woman who ingested canthaxanthin given to her by a commercial tanning salon. She developed aplastic anemia and died. The frequency of the adverse effects of this ingredient is unknown, the Vanderbilt researchers said, because there is no current way to monitor distribution. In the August 1993 issue of *American Pharmacy,* Darrell Hulisz, Pharm.D., and pharmacist Ginger Boles described this condition—called canthaxanthin-induced retinopathy—as "a common adverse effect associated with canthaxanthin use," adding, "The patient experiencing this form of retinopathy rarely is symptomatic, although decreased visual acuity has been reported." Oral intake, thus, may cause loss of night vision, since there is some evidence that high intakes of the substance lead to deposition on the retina. *See* Beta-Carotene.

CAPERS • *Capparis spinosa.* A natural flavoring from the spiny shrub. The pickled flower bud is used as a condiment for sauces and salads. GRAS

CAPPARIS SPINOSA • *See* Capers.

CAPRACYL BROWN 2R • *See* D & C Brown No. 1.

CAPRAE LAC • Goat's milk.

CAPRAMIDE DEA • *See* Capric Acid.

CAPRIC ACID • Obtained from a large group of American plants. Solid crystalline mass with a rancid odor used in the manufacture of artificial fruit flavors in lipsticks and to scent perfumes

CAPRINE • Goat. The spleen and ingredients derived therefrom are banned by ASEAN with the exception of tallow that has been used and strictly certified by the producer.

CAPROIC ACID • Hexanoic Acid. A synthetic flavoring that occurs naturally in apples, butter acids, cocoa, grapes, oil of lavender, oil of lavandin, raspberries, strawberries, and tea. Used in butter, butterscotch, fruit, rum, and cheese flavorings. Used also in the manufacture of "hexyl" derivatives such as 4-hexylresorcinol (*see*).

CAPROYL ETHYL GLUCOSIDE • A cleansing ingredient. *See* Capric Acid.

CAPROYLAMINE OXIDE • *See* Caprylic Acid and Capric Acid.

CAPRYL ALCOHOL • *See* Caprylic Acid and Alcohol.

CAPRYL BETAINE • *See* Caprylic Acid and Betaine.

CAPRYLCAPRAMIDOPROPYL BETAINE • An antistatic ingredient for hair products and a foam booster. *See* Betaines.

CAPRYL HYDROXYETHYL IMIDAZOLINE • *See* Imidazoline.

CAPRYLETH-4 CARBOXYLIC ACID • A cleansing ingredient. *See* Carboxylic Acid and Polyoxyethylene Compounds.

CAPRYLIC ACID • An oil liquid made by the oxidation of octanol for use in perfumery. Occurs naturally as a fatty acid in sweat, in the milk of cows and goats, and in palm and coconut oil.

CAPRYLIC ALCOHOL • *See* 1-Octanol.

CAPRYLIC/CAPRIC GLYCERIDES • Emollient. On the basis of the available information, the CIR Expert Panel (*see*) found it safe in the early 1980s but is considering new information to determine if the final safety assessment should be reaffirmed, amended, or have an addendum. *See* Capric Acid and Glycerin.

CAPRYLIC/CAPRIC/LAURIC TRIGLYCERIDE • A mixture of triester of glycerin with caprylic, capric, and lauric acids (*see all*). An oily mixture derived from coconut oil, it is used extensively in cosmetics as a vehicle for pigment dispersions in bath oils, hair sprays, and lipsticks. Also used as an emollient to prevent water loss from the skin. Low toxicity.

CAPRYLIC/CAPRIC TRIGLYCERIDE • An oily liquid made from coconut oil. In cosmetics and personal care products, caprylic/capric triglyceride is used in the formulation of lipstick, eye makeup, foundations, blushers, perfumes, moisturizers, suntan and sunscreen products and many other products, including in brown spot skin fade creams.

CAPRYLIC/CAPRIC/STEARIC TRIGLYCERIDE • A mixture of the triester of glycerin with caprylic, capric, and stearic acids (*see all*).

CAPRYLOYL COLLAGEN AMINO ACIDS • Caprylic acid (*see*) with amino acids from collagen (*see*).

CAPRYLOYL HYDROLYZED COLLAGEN • The condensation product of capric acid and hydrolyzed collagen (*see*). The word *animal* has been removed from this ingredient. Used as a hair conditioner, skin conditioner, and as a cleansing ingredient.

CAPRYLOYL HYDROLYZED KERATIN • The condensation product of caprylic acid and hydrolyzed keratin. Formerly called hydrolyzed animal keratin. Hair-conditioning and -cleansing ingredient.

CAPRYLYL GLYCOL • An alcohol that is used in hair conditioners and emollients. *See* Capric Acid and Glycol.

CAPRYLYL HYDROXYETHYL IMIDAZOLINE • *See* Imidazoline.

CAPRYLYUCAPRYL GLUCOSIDE • A carbohydrate that acts as a cleansing ingredient in shampoos and cold cream, and in pads. *See* Capric Acid.

CAPSAICIN • The prinicipal pungent constituent of hot peppers. It is being studied for use as an analgesic and as an anti-inflammatory medication. It is in many anti-arthritis creams.

CAPSANTHIN/CAPSORUBIN • A hair coloring that is used in European products but is banned from American colors. It is a coal tar color.

CAPSELLA BURSA • Shepherd's Heart. Shepherds Purse. Extract of the herb *Capsella bursa-pastoris,* a member of the mustard family. Pungent and bitter, it was valued for its astringent properties by early American settlers. Cotton moistened with its juice was used to stop nosebleed. In an oil-in-water emulsion, it is used as a base for skin preparations. Among its constituents are saponins, choline, acetylcholine, and tyramine (*see all*). These preparations are used in modern medicine to stimulate neuromuscular function. The herb also reduces urinary tract irritation and has been shown to contract the uterus and lower blood pressure.

CAPSICUM • The dried, ripe fruit of the capsicum or African chili plant used in hair tonics to stimulate the scalp and medicinally to soothe irritated skin and as an internal gastric stimulant. May cause skin irritation and allergic reaction.

CAPTAN • N-(Trichloromethylthio)-4-cyclohexene-1,2-dicarboximide. A preservative used in cosmetics. It is a fungicide of low toxicity, but in large doses can cause diarrhea and weight loss. No human poisonings are known. It is mutagenic and has produced cancer in mice following oral administration. The CIR Expert Panel (*see*) concludes that the available data are insufficient to support the safety of captan as used in cosmetics. On the Canadian Hotlist (*see*). The EU has banned captan in cosmetics.

CARAMEL • Used as a coloring in cosmetics and a soothing ingredient in skin lotions. Burnt sugar with a pleasant, slightly bitter taste. Made by heating sugar or glucose and adding small quantities of alkali or a trace mineral acid during heating.

CARAPA GUAIANENSIS OIL • A denaturant (*see*).

CARAWAY SEED AND OIL • *Carum carvi.* The dried, ripe seeds of a plant common to Europe and Asia and cultivated in England, Russia, and the United States. A volatile, colorless to pale yellow liquid, it is used in liquor flavorings for beverages, ice cream, baked goods, and condiments; also used as a spice in baking. The oil is used in grape licorice, anisette, kummell, liver, sausage, mint, caraway, and rye flavorings for beverages, ice cream, ices, candy, baked goods, chewing gum, meats, condiments, and liquors. The oil is used to perfume soap. Can cause contact dermatitis.

CARBAMATE • A compound based on carbamic acid, which is used only in the form of its numerous derivatives and salts. Carbamates are used in pesticides. Among the carbamate pesticides are aldicarb, 4-benzothienyl-N-methyl carbamate, bufencarb (BUX), carbaryl, carbofuran, isolan, 2-isopropyl phenyl-N-methyl carbamate, 3-isopropyl phenylmethyl carbamate, maneb, propoxur, thiram, zectran, zineb, and ziram. Carbamic acid, which is colorless and odorless, causes depression of bone marrow and degeneration of the brain, nausea, and vomiting. It is moderately toxic by many routes.

CARBAMIDE • *See* Urea.

CARBENIA BENEDICTA • *Cnicus benedictus.* Blessed Thistle. Holy Thistle. The thistle contains tannin (*see*), lactone, mucilage (*see*), and essential oil. Used by herbalists to treat stomach and liver complaints. It increases appetite, lowers fevers, and reputedly breaks up blood clots, relieves jaundice and hepatitis, and stops bleeding. In 1992, the FDA issued a notice that blessed thistle had not been shown to be safe and effective as claimed in OTC digestive-aid products or oral menstrual drugs.

CARBITOL • Carbide. Carbon. A solvent for nail lacquers and enamels. Absorbs water from the air and is mixable with acetone, benzene, alcohol, water, and ether. More toxic than polyethylene glycol (*see*).

CARBOCYSTEINE • *See* Carbon and Cysteine, L-Form.

CARBOHYDRATES • Starches and sugars contain a high proportion of carbohydrates. These are chemicals that contain carbon, hydrogen, and oxygen. Gums and mucilages are complex carbohydrates and are ingredients in many soothing cosmetics.

CARBOMER -934, -940, -941 • Carbopol. Carboxypolymethylene. A white powder, slightly acidic, that reacts with fat particles to form thick, stable emulsions of oils in water. Used as thickening, suspending, dispersing, and emulsifying ingredients in the cosmetics field. On the basis of the available information, the CIR Expert Panel (*see*) found it safe in the early 1980s but is considering new information to determine if the final safety assessment should be reaffirmed, amended, or have an addendum.

CARBON • A nonmetallic element occurring as diamond and graphite and forming a constituent of coal, petroleum, and asphalt, of limestone and other carbonates, and of all organic compounds and also obtained artificially in varying degrees of purity such as carbon black, charcoal, and coke.

CARBON BLACK • Several forms of artificially prepared carbon or charcoal, including animal charcoal, furnace black, channel (gas) black, lamp black, activated charcoal. Animal charcoal is used as a black coloring in confectionery. Activated charcoal is used as an antidote for ingested poisons, and as an adsorbent in diarrhea. The others have industrial uses. Carbon black, which was not subject to certification (*see*) by the FDA, was reevaluated and then banned in 1976. It was found in tests to contain a cancer-causing by-product that was released during dye manufacture. It can no longer be used in candies such as licorice and in jelly beans or in drugs or cosmetics. Banned.

CARBON DIOXIDE • Colorless, odorless, noncombustible gas with a faint acid taste. Used as a pressure-dispensing ingredient in gassed creams. Also used in the carbonation of beverages and as dry ice for refrigeration in the frozen food industry. Used onstage to produce harmless smoke or fumes. May cause shortness of breath, vomiting, high blood pressure, and disorientation if inhaled in sufficient amounts.

CARBON DISULFIDE • The EU has banned it in cosmetics.

CARBONIC ACID • Forms carbonate and bicarbonate salts by reaction with an alkali. It is produced in the fermentation of liquors, and by the combustion and decomposition of organic substances, or other substances. Combined with lime it constitutes limestone, or common marble and chalk. Plants imbibe it for their nutrition and growth, the carbon being retained and the oxygen given out.

CARBOPOL • *See* Carbomer.

CARBOWAX • Solid polyethylene glycols used in cosmetics and pharmaceuticals. May cause an allergic reaction. *See* Polyethylene Glycol.

CARBOXYBUTYL CHITOSAN • A film former and hair- and skin-conditioning ingredient. *See* Chitin.

CARBOXYLIC ACID • A broad group of organic acids that includes the fatty acids as well as the amino acids, benzoic acids, and salicylic acids.

CARBOXYMETHYL CELLULOSE • Sodium. A synthetic gum used in bath preparations, beauty masks, dentifrices, hair-grooming aids, hand creams, rouge, shampoos, and shaving creams. As an emulsifier, stabilizer, and foaming ingredient, it is a barrier ingredient (*see*) made from cotton by-products, and it occurs as a white powder or in granules. Employed as a stabilizer in ice cream, beverages, and other foods and medicinally as a laxative or antacid. It has been shown to cause cancer in animals when ingested. Its toxicity on the skin is unknown.

CARBOXYMETHYL CHITIN • *See* Chitin.

s-CARBOXYMETHYL CYSTEINE • Used in astringents and lotions. *See* Cysteine, L-Form.

CARBOXYMETHYL DEXTRAN • A film former and thickener. *See* Dextran.

CARBOXYMETHYL HYDROXETHYLCELLULOSE • A binder and emulsifier. *See* Cellulose and Ethylene Glycol.

CARBOXYMETHYL HYDROXYPROPYL GUAR • A gum used as a binder and stabilizer. *See* Guar Gum.

CARBOXYPOLYMETHYLENE • *See* Carbomer.

CARBROMAL • Sedative. Banned in cosmetics by most regulatory agencies.

CARCINOGEN • A cancer-causing ingredient.

CARCINOGENIC • A substance that is capable of causing cancer.

CARDAMOM OIL • *Elettaria cardamomum.* Grains of Paradise. A natural flavoring and aromatic ingredient from the dried, ripe seeds of trees common to India, Ceylon, and Guatemala. Used in perfumes and soaps, in butter, chocolate, and other food flavoring. As a medicine, it breaks up intestinal gas. May be mutagenic. ASP. GRAS

CARMINE • Cochineal. Ponceau Red 4 *Coccus catil.* A crimson pigment derived from a Mexican and Central American species of a scaly female insect that feeds on various cacti. Carmine and cochineal extracts are permanently listed, but cochineal alone is not authorized for use. The colorings are used in red applesauce, confections, baked goods, meats, and spices. Cochineal was involved in an outbreak of salmonellosis (an intestinal infection) that killed one infant in a Boston hospital and made twenty-two patients seriously ill. Carmine used in the diagnostic solution to test the digestive organ was found to be the infecting additive. Also used in cosmetics. University of Michigan medical researchers said this color additive extracted from dried bugs and used in candy, yogurt, fruit drinks, and other foods can cause life-threatening allergic reactions. It is often just listed as a "natural" ingredient on the label. The British and European Parliament at this writing are seeking to ban this coloring because it reportedly affects hyperactivity in young children. *See* Cochineal. ASP

CARMINIC ACID • Natural Red No. 4. Used in mascaras, liquid rouge, paste rouge, and red eye shadows. It is the glucosidal coloring matter from a scaly insect (*see* Carmine). Color is deep red in water and violet to yellow in acids. May cause allergic reactions. Banned by the FDA. *See* Colors.

CARNATION • The essential oil of a double-flowered variety of clove pink. Pale green solid that does not have the characteristic odor of carnations until diluted. Used in fragrances.

CARNAUBA WAX • *Copernicia cerifera.* The exudate from the leaves of the

Brazilian wax palm tree used as a texturizer in foundation makeups, mascara, cream rouge, lipsticks, liquid powders, depilatories, and deodorant sticks. It comes in a hard, greenish to brownish solid and rarely causes allergic reactions. The CIR Expert Panel (*see*) concludes this is a safe ingredient.

CARNITINE • Vitamin BT. A thyroid inhibitor found in muscle, liver, and meat extracts. It stimulates fatty-acid oxidation and manufacture. Muscles that contain approximately 98 percent of carnitine must take it up from the blood. When carnitine is deficient, muscles become weak, and the person is intolerant of exercise. Used in skin creams and primarily promoted as an anti-aging ingredient. It is an amino acid, a building block of protein, so whether it works or not has not been evaluated by the FDA. It does cause a rash in some sensitive people. Other potential adverse reactions include nausea, vomiting, cramps, diarrhea, and body odor. ASP

CAROB EXTRACT • *Ceratonia siliqua. See* Locust Bean Gum.

CAROTENE • *See* Beta-Carotene.

CAROTENOIDS • Found in parsley, carrots, sweet potatoes, and most green, red, and yellow vegetables and fruits, these are vitamin A precursors that are antioxidants and cell-differentiation ingredients (cancer cells are undifferentiated). There are hundreds of carotenoids in nature.

CARRAGEENAN and SALT • *Chondrus crispus.* Irish Moss. A stabilizer and emulsifier, seaweedlike in odor, derived from Irish moss, used in oils in cosmetics and foods. It is completely soluble in hot water and not coagulated by acids. Used medicinally to soothe the skin. The use of Irish moss in food and medicine has been known in India for hundreds of years. Its use in the United States began in 1935 but really became common during World War II as a replacement for agar-agar. Sodium carrageenan is on the FDA list for further study. Carrageenan stimulated the formation of fibrous tissue when subcutaneously injected into guinea pigs. When a single dose of it dissolved in saline was injected under the skin of rats, it caused sarcomas after approximately two years. Its cancer-causing ability may be that of a foreign body irritant, because upon administration to rats and mice at high levels in their diet, it did not appear to induce tumors, although survival of the animals for this period was not good. Its use as a food additive is being studied. Salts of carrageenan, such as calcium, ammonium, potassium, or sodium, are used as a demulcent to soothe mucous membrane irritation. It is used for producing gels.

The final report to the FDA of the Select Committee on GRAS Substances stated in 1980 that while no evidence in the available information demonstrates it is a hazard to the public at current use levels, uncertainties exist, requiring that additional studies be conducted. Carrageenan is at this writing on the FDA lists for cancer study since it is a carcinogen in animals. The JECFA (see abbreviations list) requested in 2003 that based on laboratory results, carrageenan should be restricted in infant formulas but that it is acceptable for use as a food additive for adults. ASP. E

CARRIBEAN SEA-WHIP EXTRACT • Used in anti-aging products, it is said to soothe inflammation and act as a natural sunscreen based upon the adaptations of shallow-water marine life.

CARROT JUICE POWDER • *See* Carrot Oil.

CARROT OIL • Either of two oils from the seeds of carrots, *Daucus carota sativus.* A light yellow essential oil, which has a spicy odor and is used in liqueurs, flavorings, and perfumes. Rich in vitamin A, it is also used as a coloring. Has been permanently listed since 1964. A skin irritant. When heated to decomposition, it emits acrid smoke and irritating fumes. GRAS. ASP

CARROT SEED EXTRACT • Extract of the seeds of *Daucus carota sativus.*

CARUM CARVI • *See* Caraway Seed and Oil.

CARVEOL • A synthetic mint, spearmint, spice, and caraway flavoring ingredient for beverages, ice cream, ices, candy, and baked goods. Found naturally in caraway and grapes, and baked fruit.

CARVONE (D or L) • Oil of Caraway. D-Carvone is usually prepared by distillation from caraway seed and dill seed oil. It is colorless to light yellow with an odor of caraway. L-Carvone occurs in several essential oils. It may be isolated from spearmint oil or synthesized commercially from *d*-limonene. It is colorless to pale yellow with the odor of spearmint. D-Carvone is a synthetic liquor, mint, and spice flavoring ingredient for beverages, ice cream, ices, candy, and baked goods. Used also in perfumery and soaps. It breaks up intestinal gas and is used as a stimulant. GRAS.

CARVYL ACETATE • A synthetic mint flavoring for beverages, ice cream, ices, candy, and baked goods.

CARVYL PROPIONATE • A synthetic mint flavoring for beverages, ice cream, ices, candy, and baked goods.

CARVYLOPHYLLENE ACETATE • A general fixative that occurs in many essential oils, especially in clove oil. Colorless, oily, with a clovelike odor. Used for beverages, ice cream, ices, candy, baked goods, and chewing gum. Practically insoluble in alcohol.

CARYA ILLINOINENSIS • Pecan. A coloring ingredient used in cosmetics. It is the nut from a hickory of the south-central United States with rough bark and hard but brittle wood. Employed medicinally by the American Indians.

CASCARA • *Rhamnus purshianus.* A natural flavoring derived from the dried bark of a plant grown from northern Idaho to northern California. Cathartic. Used in butter, caramel, and vanilla flavorings. Used to soothe skin in lotions and creams.

CASCARILLA BARK • Sweet Bark, Sweetwood Bark. Family: Euphorbiaceae. A natural flavoring ingredient obtained from the bark of a tree grown in Haiti, the Bahamas, and Cuba. Used as a flavoring and softener in cosmetics. As a flavoring in food, it is GRAS.

CASEARIA SYLVESTRIS • A plant that contains analgesic, antacid, anti-inflammatory, and styptic properties. Herbalists use it to treat burns, wounds, and small skin injuries. It is also used in South America in dental-care products as an antiseptic.

CASEIN • The principal protein of cow's milk used in protective cream and as the "protein" in hair preparations to make the hair thicker and more manageable. It is a white, water-absorbing powder without noticeable odor and is used to make depilatories less irritating and as a film former in beauty masks. It is also used as an emulsifier in many cosmetics and in special diet preparations.

CASHEW NUT OIL • Oil expressed from the seeds of *Anacardium occidentale.*

CASHMERE • Cosmetic companies have adapted the softness of the keratin fibers in cashmere wool to develop makeup leave-on and rinse-off products for skin, hair, and nail care. The functional ingredient is an amino acid complex produced by the water treatment of the keratin (*see*) fibers in cashmere.

CASSIA OIL • Cloves. Chinese Oil of Cinnamon. Darker, less agreeable, and heavier than true cinnamon. Obtained from a tropical Asian tree and used in perfumes, poultices, and as a laxative. It can cause irritation and allergy such as a stuffy nose. EAF

CASSIE FLOWERS • Flavoring. Cassie perfume is distilled from the flowers. Cassie absolute is employed in preparation of violet bouquets, extensively used in European perfumery. Trees used as ingredient in Ivory Coast for arrow poison. The seeds, containing an unnamed alkaloid, are used to kill rabid dogs in Brazil. Bark is astringent and demulcent, and along with leaves and roots is used for medicinal purposes. Woody branches used in India as toothbrushes. The gummy roots are also chewed for sore throat. Said to be used for alterative, antispasmodic, aphrodisiac, astringent, demulcent, diarrhea, febrifuge, rheumatism, and stimulant. It is also used for dyspepsia and neuroses. Mexicans sprinkle powdered dried leaves onto wounds. The flowers are added to ointment, rubbed on the forehead for headache. Costa Ricans decoct the gum from the trunk for treating diarrhea, vaginal discharge, and uterine bleeding. Panamanians and Cubans use the pod to treat conjunctivitis. Cubans use the pod decoction for sore throat. For rheumatic pains, West Indians bind bark strips to the afflicted joint. The root decoction has been suggested as a folk remedy for tuberculosis and cancer.

CASTANEA SATIVA • *Castanea vulgaris.* Chestnut. Spanish Chestnut. Sweet Chestnut. Horse Chestnut. Nut from a tree of the beech family, used as a remedy for piles, backaches, and for coughs. An astringent, the bark and leaves were used to make a tonic, which also was useful, reportedly, in the treatment of upper respiratory ailments such as coughs, particularly whooping cough. The bark of Spanish chestnut contains tannin (*see*).

CASTILE SOAP • A fine, hard, bland soap, usually white or cream-colored, but sometimes green, named for the region of Spain where it was originally made from olive oil and sodium hydroxide (*see*).

CASTOR • *Ricinus communis* Oil. See Castor Oil.

CASTOR OIL • Palm Christi Oil. The seed of the castor-oil plant. After the oil is expressed from the beans, a residual castor pomace remains, which contains a potent allergen. This may be incorporated in fertilizer, which is the main source of exposure, but people who live near a castor-bean processing factory may also be sensitized. Used in bath oils, nail polish removers, solid perfumes, face masks, shaving creams, lipsticks, and many men's hairdressings. It is also used as a plasticizer in nail polish. It forms a tough, shiny film when dried. More than 50 percent of the lipsticks in the United States use a substantial amount of castor oil. Ingestion of large amounts may cause pelvic congestion. Soothing to the skin.

CASTOREUM • Castor. Used in perfumes as a fixative (*see*). A creamy, orange-brown substance with a strong, penetrating odor and bitter taste that consists of the dried perineal glands of the beaver and their secretion. The glands and secretions are taken from the area between the vulva and the anus in the female beaver and from the scrotum and the anus in the male beaver. Professional trappers use castor to scent bait.

CATALASE • An enzyme from bovine liver used in milk, for making cheese, and for the elimination of peroxide. It is used also in combination with glucose oxidase for treatment of food wrappers to prevent oxidative deterioration of food and cosmetics. The EU banned it in cosmetics.

CATALYST • A substance that causes or speeds up a chemical reaction but does not itself change.

CATECHOL • Catechin. A modifier in hair colorings used as a drabber. It is phenol alcohol found in catechu black (*see*). Determined by Proposition 65 (*see*) in 2003 to cause cancer.

CATECHOLAMINES • A group of self-made chemicals such as neurotransmitters and hormones, which can be made synthetically. Among the major catecholamines are dopamine, norepinephrine, and epinephrine. The catecholamines are involved in the regulation of blood pressure, heart rate, muscle tone, metabolism, and central nervous system function.

CATECHU BLACK • A preparation from the heartwood of *Acacia catechu,* used in toilet preparations and for brown and black colorings. Used as an astringent. May cause allergic reactions.

CATECHU EXTRACT • Black Cutch Extract. Cachou Extract. Cashoo Extract. Pegu

Catechu extract. A preparation from the heartwood of the *Acacia catechu* (*see* Acacia) grown in India, Sri Lanka, and Jamaica.

CATIONIC • A group of synthetic compounds employed as emulsifiers, wetting ingredients, and antiseptics in special hand creams. Their positively charged ions (cations) repel water. Any class of synthetic detergents usually consisting almost entirely of quaternary ammonium compounds (*see*) with carbon and nitrogen. Used also as wetting and emulsifying ingredients in acid to neutralize solutions or as a germicide or fungicide. Toxicity depends upon ingredients used.

CATNIP • *Nepeta cataria.* Catnep. Catnip. An aromatic plant of the mint family common to North America and Europe, it was said in folk medicine that the root, when chewed, made the quietest person fierce and quarrelsome. In modern medicine, it is used as a digestive herb, prescribed for stomach pains and flatulence. The leaves contain essential oils and tannins. Herbalists use it in a tea as a sedative, for insomnia, fever, colds, and diarrhea. It has been reported effective in treating iron-deficiency anemia, menstrual and uterine disorders, and dyspepsia. The FDA issued a notice in 1992 that catnip has not been shown to be safe and effective as claimed in OTC digestive aid products.

CATTLE PRODUCTS • Vegetarians, animal activists, and members of certain religions may not want to use cosmetic products from cattle. These include animal tissue extract; amniotic fluid; brain extract; calf blood extract; calf skin extract; calf skin hydrolysates; collagen; elastin; embryo extract; glycoprotein; hemoglobin, hydrolysed; liver extract; liver hydrolysates; mammarian hydrolysates; mammary extract; marrow extract; muscle extract; neatsfoot oil; omental lipids; placental enzyme; placental lipids; placental protein; serum albumin; serum protein; stearin; stomach extract; sodium cocoate; tallow; and udder extract.

CAULERPA TAXIFOLIA • *See* Algae.

CAULIFLOWER UNSAPONIFIABLES • *Brassica oleracea botrytis.* The portion of cauliflower oil that is not saponified (*see* Saponification) during the refining recovery of cauliflower fatty acids.

CAUSTIC SODA • *See* Sodium Hydroxide.

CAVIAR EXTRACT • The extract of eggs of the sturgeon.

CAYENNE • *Capsicum annum.* Red pepper. Green pepper. Derived from the pungent fruit of a plant, it originated in Central and South America. It contains capsaicin (*see*), carotenoids, flavonoids, essential oil, and vitamin C. Cayenne is a stimulant, an astringent (*see*), and an antispasmodic. Herbal scientists used it as a rub for inflamed joints or to stop external bleeding. *See* Capsicum.

CD • The abbreviation for completely denatured alcohol, meaning a poison has been added so that it is not drinkable.

CD ALCOHOL 19 • A denatured alcohol used as a solvent. *See* Denaturant.

CDER • FDA Center for Drug Evaluation and Research.

CEANOTHUS EXTRACT • The extract of the herb *Ceanothus americanus.* Also called New Jersey tea.

CEDAR • *Cedrus atlantica.* Cedar Wood Oil. The oil from white, red, or various other cedars obtained by distillation from fresh leaves and branches. It is often used in perfumes, soaps, and sachets for its warm, woodsy scent. Used frequently as a substitute for oil of lavender. There is usually a strong camphor odor that repels insects. Cedar oil can be a photosensitizer, causing skin reactions when the skin is exposed to light.

CEDRENOL • *See* Cedar.

CEDRO OIL • *See* Lemon Oil.

CEDROL • *See* Cedar.

CEDRUS ATLANTICA • *See* Cedar.

CEDRYL ACETATE • Colorless liquid having a light cedar odor. Used in fragrances. *See* Cedar. ASP

CEKUR • *Kaempferia galanga.* Kencur. Orodary Roots. A very short herb with leaves spreading horizontally and lying flat on the ground. In spite of its name and the fact that it is a member of the ginger family, it does not taste at all like ginger, but has a distinctive flavor of its own. In India, a perfume used in hair washes, powders, and other cosmetics is made from rhizomes and leaves and worn by women for fragrance and also used for protecting clothes against insects.

CELANDINE EXTRACT • *Chelidonium majus.* Swallow wort. This tall herb contains alkaloids, choline, histamine, tyramine, saponins, chelidoniol, chelidonic acid, carotene, and vitamin C. Herbalists use it for the treatment of hepatitis, jaundice, cancer, psoriasis, eczema, corns, and warts. Used for more than two thousand years to soothe the eyes, it also reputedly detoxifies the liver and relieves muscle spasms and bronchospasms.

CELERY • *Apium graveolens.* The root, leaves, and seed are used for medicinal purposes. It grows wild in ditches and salt marshes and has a coarse texture. The seed was one of the first condiments to reach the country of the Gauls and Franks. It was introduced into Europe by military men upon returning home from Roman conquests. Celery seed is used by herbalists as a diuretic, blood cleanser, and to treat arthritis. It is used in "organic" cosmetics. Celery seed may cause a sensitivity to light, and some people are allergic to it.

CELLULAR COMMUNICATORS • Claimed "to help reduce the appearance of wrinkles and age related skin damage."

CELLULAR MEMBRANE COMPLEX • A fluid in the shaft that binds the hair. The difference between coarse and fine hair has a physiochemical basis: All hairs have a tough, shell-like casing (the cuticle) and a soft, fibrous inner cortex. In coarse hair, the cuticle makes up 10 percent of the volume and the cortex 90 percent. In fine hair, the proportion is 40 percent cuticle and 60 percent cortex. Hair product manufacturers claim cellular membrane complex can benefit from a "conditioner." Hair is dead. Active growth of the hair is only within the bulb.

CELLULOID • A nail finish composed essentially of cellulose nitrate and camphor (*see* Camphor Oil) or other plasticizers. Also used for brushes and combs as well as for photographic films and various household products.

CELLULOSE • Chief constituent of the fiber of plants. Cotton contains about 90 percent. It is the basic material for cellulose gums (*see*). Used as an emulsifier in cosmetic creams.

CELLULOSE GUMS • Any of several fibrous substances consisting of the chief part of the cell walls of plants. Ethylcellulose is a film former in lipstick. Methylcellulose (Methocel) and hydroxy ethylcellulose (Cellosize) are used as emulsifiers in hand creams and lotions. They are resistant to bacterial decomposition and give uniform viscosity to products. On the basis of the available animal and human data, the CIR Expert Panel (*see*) concludes that this ingredient is safe as used in cosmetics. Some are ASP and others EAF.

CENTAUREA CYANUS • Cornflower. European plant with blue, pink, or white flowers.

CENTAURY • *Erythraea centaurium.* A small, pretty annual native to the United Kingdom, it is used by herbalists for jaundice. A tisane (*see*) made as a tonic, to stimulate appetite and digestion. It is a strong antiseptic and good for cuts and scratches and is also used as a mouthwash. Legend has it that its medicinal properties were discovered by a centaur. Used in "organic" cosmetics.

CENTELLA • Asiaticoside. A member of the Umbelliferae family like celery, the active principle is asiaticoside. It has wound-healing properties.

CENTURY EXTRACT • Centuaury. Agave American. A succulent perennial native to tropical America. The leaves and juice contain saponins, volatile oil, gums, and proteins. It is used in cosmetics as an astringent and to soothe. It is promoted to even out skin tones and help fade freckles and other discolorations. Used by herbalists as a diuretic, antiseptic, and to induce menstrual flow. It is also used for skin diseases and to treat burns and cuts. It may be toxic in large doses. It can cause irritation of the mucous membranes of the stomach, nausea, vomiting, and hemorrhage. Large and frequent doses can lead to liver damage.

CEPHAELIS IPECACUANHA • *See* Ipecac.

CEPHALINS • Central nervous system tissue used in skin conditioners and anti-aging creams.

CERAALBA • *See* Beeswax.

CERAMICROCRISTALLINA • *See* Microcrystalline Wax.

CERAMIDES • Naturally occurring skin fats rarely found at greater than trace levels in tissues, although they can exert important biological effects. Depending on the particular layer of the skin (epidermis, stratum corneum, etc.), the composition can vary. These lipids obviously have a role in the barrier properties of the skin, limiting loss of water and solutes and at the same time preventing ingress of harmful substances. Ceramide B-lactoside is from the spinal cord and Ceramide dihexoside Spleen from animals. Some ceramides can be extract from plants such as sunflowers and cranberries. Synthetic fatty alcohols are used in hair conditioners and skin conditioners.

CERCLA • The Comprehensive Environmental Response, Compensation, and Liability Act (CERCLA), as amended by the Superfund Amendments and Reauthorization Act (SARA), requires ATSDR (U.S. Agency for Toxic Substances and Disease Registery) and the Environmental Protection Agency (EPA) to prepare a list, in order of priority, of substances that are most commonly found at facilities on the National Priorities List (NPL) and that are determined to pose the most significant potential threat to human health due to their known or suspected toxicity and potential for human exposure at these NPL sites. CERCLA also requires this list to be revised periodically to reflect additional information on hazardous substances. It should be noted that this priority list is not a list of "most toxic" substances, but rather a prioritization of substances based on a combination of their frequency, toxicity, and potential for human exposure at NPL sites.

CEREBROSIDES • Fatty acids and sugars found in the covering of nerves. *See* Animal Parts.

CERESIN • Ceresine Earth Wax. Used in protective creams. It is a white or yellow, hard, brittle wax made by purifying ozokerite (*see*), found in the Ukraine, Utah, and Texas. It is used as a substitute for beeswax and paraffin (*see both*); also used to wax paper and cloth, as a polish, wax, and paraffin; in dentistry for taking wax impressions. May cause allergic reactions.

CEREUS GRANDIFLORUS • *See* Cactus.

CERIA/SILICA • An ultraviolet light absorber. *See* Silica.

CERIA/SILICA TALC • Ultraviolet light absorber. *See* Talc.

CERIUM OXIDE • An opacifying ingredient.

CEROTIC ACID • Hexacosanoic Acid. A fatty acid obtained from beeswax, carnauba wax, or Chinese wax. White, odorless crystals or powder soluble in alcohol, benzene, ether, and acetone. *See* Beeswax.

CERTIFIED • Each batch of coal tar or petrochemical colors, with the exception of those used in hair dyes, must be certified by the FDA as "harmless and suitable for use."

The manufacturer must submit samples of every batch for testing and the lot test number accompanies the colors through all subsequent packaging.

CETALKONIUM CHLORIDE • Derived from ammonium, it is an antibacterial ingredient used in cosmetics. Soluble in water, alcohol, acetone, and ethyl acetate. *See* Quaternary Ammonium Compounds.

CETEARALKONIUM BROMIDE • The quaternary ammonium salt that is a blend of cetyl and stearyl radicals.

CETEARETH-3 • CetylStearyl Ether. An oily liquid distilled from a combination of cetyl alcohol made from spermaceti (*see*) and stearyl alcohol made from sperm whale oil. The compound is used as an emollient, an emulsifier, an antifoam ingredient, and a lubricant in cosmetics.

CETEARETH-4, -6, -8, -10, -12, -15, -17, -27, -30 • *See* Ceteareth-3.

CETEARETH-5 • Emollient and emulsifier from cetyl alcohol and ethylene oxide. *See* Cetyl Alcohol and Ceteareth-3.

CETEARETH-20 • Widely used polyethylene glycol ether of cetearyl alcohol (*see*) as a surfactant, cleansing ingredient, and solubilizer. Used in hair conditioners and dyes, body and hand preparations, moisturizers, indoor tanning and suntan products, and mud packs. The CIR Expert Panel (*see*) cautioned that this ingredient enhances skin absorption of drugs and that care should be taken when creating formulations, especially those products intended for use on infants.

CETEARETH-25 • Widely used polyethylene glycol ether of cetearyl alcohol that is used as a surface-active ingredient, cleansing ingredient, and a solubilizer.

CETEARYL ALCOHOL • Cetostearyl Alcohol. Emulsifying wax. A mixture chiefly of the fatty alcohols—cetyl and stearyl (*see both*)—and used primarily in ointments as an emulsifier. Very widely used in hair tints, cleansing lotions, skin care preparations, night skin care, shampoos, hair straighteners, suntan preparations, lipsticks, permanent waves, eye makeup, makeup bases, and foot powders and sprays. The CIR Expert Panel (*see*) concludes this is a safe ingredient.

CETEARYL GLUCOSIDE • Made from cetearyl alcohol and glucose (*see both*) and used as an emulsifier in fragrances, cleansers, and body and hand preparations.

CETEARYL OCTANOATE • *See* Caprylic Acid.

CETEARYL STEARATE • A skin-conditioning ingredient.

CETETH-1 • *See* Ceteth-2.

CETETH-2 • Polyethylene (2) Cetyl Ether. A compound of derivatives of cetyl, lauryl, stearyl, and oleyl alcohols (*see all*) mixed with ethylene oxide, a gas used as a fungicide and a starting material for detergents. Oily liquids or waxy solids. Used as a surface-active ingredient (*see*) and an emulsifier to allow oil and water to mix to form a smooth cosmetic lotion or cream. *See* individual alcohols for toxicity.

CETETH-4, -6, -10, -12, -30 • The CIR Expert Panel (*see*) concludes this is a safe ingredient. *See* Ceteth-2.

CETETH-20 • Polyethylene glycol ether of cetyl alcohol (*see*) widely used in hair products, skin-care preparations, cleansing products, and moisturizers. Also used in shaving preparations and depilatories. May irritate the skin and scalp.

CETETHYL MORPHOLINIUM ETHOSULFATE • The CIR Expert Panel (*see*) concludes there is insufficient data to support the safety of this ingredient for use in cosmetics.

CETRARIA ISLANDICA • Iceland Moss. Iceland Lichen. So named because Icelanders reputedly were the first to discover its benefits. It is high in mucilage, with some iodine, traces of vitamin A, and usnic acid. Herbalists use the lichen as a gentle laxative and to relieve upper respiratory problems associated with degenerative wasting.

CETRIMONIUM BROMIDE • A cationic (*see*) detergent and antiseptic, disinfectant, and cleansing ingredient in skin-cleaning products and shampoos. It masks or decreases perspiration odors. Can be fatal if swallowed. Toxic to mice embryos when given intravenously and in food. Can be irritating to the skin and eyes. The CIR Expert Panel (*see*) concludes on the basis of animal studies this ingredient is safe for use in rinse-off products, and for use at concentrations of up to 0.25 percent in leave-on products.

CETRIMONIUM CHLORIDE • The CIR Expert Panel (*see*) concludes on the basis of animal studies this ingredient is safe for use in rinse-off products, and for use at concentrations of up to 0.25 percent in leave-on products. *See* Quaternary Ammonium Compounds.

CETRIMONIUM TOSYLATE • A quaternary ammonium compound (*see*).

CETYL- • Means derived from cetyl alcohol (*see*).

CETYL ACETATE • The ester (*see*) of cetyl alcohol and acetic acid (*see both*). Used in hand lotions.

CETYL ACETYL RICINOLEATE • *See* Oleic Acid and Cetyl Acetate.

CETYL ALCOHOL • An emollient and emulsion stabilizer used in many cosmetic preparations including baby lotion, brilliantine hairdressings, deodorants and antiperspirants, cream depilatories, eyelash creams and oils, foundation creams, hair lacquers, hair straighteners, hand lotions, lipsticks, liquid powders, mascaras, nail polish removers, nail whiteners, cream rouges, and shampoos. Cetyl alcohol is waxy, crystalline, and solid, and found in spermaceti (*see*). It has a low toxicity for both skin and ingestion and is sometimes used as a laxative. Can cause hives.

CETYL AMMONIUM • An ammonium compound, germicide, and fungicide used in cuticle softeners, deodorants, and baby creams. Medicinally an antibacterial ingredient. *See* Quaternary Ammonium Compounds for toxicity.

CETYL ARACHIDATE • An ester produced by the reaction of cetyl alcohol and arachidic acid. The acid is found in fish oils and vegetables, particularly peanut oil. A fatty compound used as an emulsifier and emollient in cosmetic creams.

CETYL BETAINE • Occurs in the common beet and many vegetable and animal substances. Colorless, deliquescent crystals with a sweet taste. *See* Quaternary Ammonium Compounds.

CETYL ESTERS • The CIR Expert Panel (*see*) concludes on the basis of animal studies this ingredient is safe for use in rinse-off products, and for use at concentrations of up to 0.25 percent in leave-on products. *See* Synthetic Spermaceti.

CETYL HYDROXYETHYLCELLULOSE • An emulsifier and stabilizer. *See* Methylcellulose and Cetyl Alcohol.

CETYL LACTATE • Emollient to improve the feel and texture of cosmetic and pharmaceutical preparations. Produced by reaction of cetyl alcohol and lactic acid (*see both*).

CETYL MYRISTATE • Produced by the reaction of cetyl alcohol and myristic acid (*see both*).

CETYL OCTANOATE • The ester of cetyl alcohol and 2-ethylhexamonic acid. A moisturizer used in creams and lipsticks. *See* Cetyl Alcohol and Caproic Acid.

CETYL OLEATE • The ester of cetyl alcohol and oleic acid (*see both*).

CETYL PALMITATE • Produced by the reaction of cetyl alcohol and palmitic acid. Used in the manufacture of soaps and lubricants. Widely used in skin care preparations, eye shadows, foundations, mud packs, after-shave lotions, and eye lotions. On the basis of the available information, the CIR Expert Panel (*see*) found it safe in the early 1980s but is considering new information to determine if the final safety assessment should be reaffirmed, amended, or have an addendum.

CETYL PHOSPHATE • A mixture of esters of phosphoric acid and cetyl alcohol (*see both*).

CETYL PYRROLIDONYLMETHYL DIMONIUM CHLORIDE • A quaternary ammonium (*see*) product.

CETYL RICINOLEATE • Salt derivative of castor oil used in tanning preparations. *See* Ricinoleic Acid.

CETYL STEARATE • An emollient used as a skin-conditioning ingredient. On the basis of the available animal and human data, the CIR Expert Panel (*see*) concludes that this ingredient is safe as used in cosmetics.

CETYL STEARYL GLYCOL • A mixture of cetyl glycol and stearyl glycol fatty alcohols that are used as emulsifiers and emollients in cosmetic creams.

CETYLAMINE HYDROFLUORIDE • An organic salt of fluoride. *See* Fluoride.

CETYLARACHIDOL • Suds and foam stabilizer used in hair and body shampoos and in various types of household detergents. It also has mild conditioning properties, and in some instances it may be used as an emulsifier. *See* Quaternary Ammonium Compounds for toxicity.

CETYLPYRIDINIUM CHLORIDE • CPC. A white powder soluble in water and alcohol. The quaternary salt of pyridine (*see*) and cetyl chloride. A white powder used as an antiseptic and disinfectant in mouthwashes and topical antiseptics and as a deodorant. *See* Quaternary Ammonium Compounds for toxicity.

CETYLTRYMETHYLAMMONIUM BROMIDE • An antimicrobial preservative that helps destroy and prevent growth of germs. *See* Quaternary Ammonium Compounds.

CFR • FDA Code of Federal Regulations for drug and biologic manufacturers revised through April 1, 2008.

CFSAN • Center for Food Safety and Applied Nutrition.

CHAENOMELES JAPONICA • *See* Quince Seed.

CHALK • Purified calcium carbonate (*see*) used in nail whiteners, powders, and liquid makeup to assist in spreading and to give the characteristic smooth feeling. A grayish white, amorphous powder usually molded into cones for the cosmetic industry. Used medicinally as a mild astringent and an antacid.

CHAMAECYPARIS OBTUSA • Cypress. An essential oil used in fragrances.

CHAMAZULENE • A hydrocarbon used in skin conditioners.

CHAMOMILE • *Anthemis nobilis. Ormenis multicaulis.* Roman, German, and Hungarian Chamomile. The daisylike white and yellow heads of these flowers provide a coloring ingredient known as apigenin. The essential oil distilled from the flower heads is pale blue and is added to shampoos to impart the odor of chamomile. Powdered flowers are used to bring out a bright yellow color in the hair. Also used in rinses and skin fresheners. Roman and English chamomiles are used as flavorings. Chamomile contains sesquiterpene lactones, which may cause allergic contact dermatitis and stomach upsets.

CHAMOMILLA RECUTITA • Camomile Oil. Wild Chamomile Extract. The volatile oil distilled from the dried flower heads or extract of the flower heads of *Matricaria chamomilla*. Used internally as a soothing tea and tonic and externally as a soothing medication for contusions and other inflammation. *See* Tannic Acid and Chamomile.

CHAPARRAL EXTRACT • The extract of the desert plant chaparral, Larrea mexicana. The leaves of this dwarf evergreen contain antioxidants and are considered by herbalists as an antibiotic. The leaves are ground and may be used in a tea or in capsules. It is used for blood purification, cancer and tumors, antioxidants, arthritis, colds and flu, diarrhea, and urinary tract infections. The American Indians used it to treat arthritis. A modern Argentine study showed that the primary constituent of chaparral, NDGA (nordihydroguaiaretic acid), an antioxidant, possesses pain-relieving properties and blood-pressure-lowering properties. Two cases of chaparral-induced toxic hepatitis were reported in 1992 by the FDA.

CHARCOAL • Formerly widely used as a black coloring. The FDA no longer authorizes its use.

CHAULMOOGRA OIL • *Taraktagenos kurzii.* An East Indian tree, the oil has long been used to treat leprosy and skin diseases. The soft fat from the seeds is composed chiefly of glycerides (*see*).

CHECKERBERRY EXTRACT • *See* Wintergreen Oil.

CHECKERBERRY OIL • *See* Wintergreen Oil.

CHEILITIS • Dermatitis of the lips attributed to lipsticks. The symptoms are dryness, chapping, and cracked and peeling lips. Sometimes this is accompanied by swelling and blistering. About 95 percent of the symptoms have been found to be caused by the indelible dyes used in most lipsticks. The lips are more susceptible to irritation and allergic problems than other parts of the body due to the absence of the horny or dead layer of skin that protects the rest of the body. Even minute amounts of lipstick can cause gastrointestinal problems such as gastritis, enteritis, and colitis in susceptible women. Many allergic women are able to solve the problem of cheilitis merely by changing brands of lipsticks. Others may be able to use hypoallergenic brands that do not contain the most common sensitizers—lanolin and perfumes or the staining dye dibromofluorescein (*see*).

CHELATING INGREDIENT • Any compound, usually one that binds and precipitates metals, such as ethylenediamine tetraacetic acid (EDTA), which removes trace metals. *See* Sequestering Ingredient.

CHELIDONIUM MAJUS • Swallowwort. Devil's Milk. Rock Poppy. This tall herb contains alkaloids, choline, histamine, tyramine, saponins, chelidoniol, chelidonic acid, carotene, and vitamin C. Herbalists use it for the treatment of hepatitis, jaundice, cancer, psoriasis, eczema, corns, and warts. Used for more than two thousand years to soothe the eyes, it also reputedly detoxifies the liver and relieves muscle spasms and bronchospasms. The plant can cause miscarriage when ingested and therefore should not be used during pregnancy. Sanguinarine found in this plant produces glaucoma in experimental animals and also cancer.

CHEMICAL PEEL • A treatment that consists of applying a chemical solution that causes the aged or damaged skin to "peel off" and new skin regenerates in its place. Stronger solutions are applied by physicians than those available in OTC products.

CHENOPODIUM • Essential Oil. Should not be used as or in fragrance ingredients. The recommendation is based on the absence of reports on the use of this material as fragrance ingredient and/or inadequate evaluation of potential adverse effects resulting from its use in fragrances. On the Canadian Hotlist (*see*). The EU banned it in cosmetics. *See* Quince Seed.

CHERIMOYA • A small, widely cultivated American tree, *Annona cherimola,* with three-petaled, yellowish flowers. Used in "organic" cosmetics.

CHERRY LAUREL WATER • *Runus laurocerasus.* Banned in cosmetics by ASEAN.

CHERRY PIT OIL • A natural lipstick flavoring and fragrance extracted from the pits of sweet and sour cherries. Also a cherry flavoring for beverages, ice cream, and condiments. ASP

CHERRY PLUM • Source of purplish red color. *See* Anthocyanins.

CHESTNUT • *Castanea vulgaris.* Spanish Chestnut. Sweet Chestnut. Horse Chestnut. Nuts from a European tree used as a remedy for piles, backaches, and for coughs. An astringent, the bark and leaves were used to make a tonic, which was also reportedly useful in the treatment of upper respiratory ailments such as coughs, and particularly whooping cough.

CHESTNUT LEAVES EXTRACT • Contains natural herbicides that the tree uses to inhibit the growth of neighboring plants. Horse chestnut leaves have been used by herbalists as a cough remedy and to reduce fevers. The leaves were also believed to reduce pain and inflammation of arthritis and rheumatism. Extract contains minerals, tannins, free amino acids, and vitamins B_1, B_2, and PP. It reportedly has antimicrobial, antiinflammatory, and healing properties. EAF

CHIA OIL • Oil expressed from the seed of *Salvia hispanica* used in skin conditioners.

CHICHOPHEN AND ITS SALTS • Used to treat skin problems but has been found to cause liver damage and ulcers. Banned cosmetics by ASEAN (*see*) and the UK.

CHICKWEED • *Stellaria media.* Starweed. Herbal Slim. The herb contains saponins, which exert an anti-inflammatory action similar to cortisone, but according to herbalists, it is much milder and without the side effects. Chickweed is also used for weight loss, for skin irritations, itches, and rashes and to soothe sore throat and lungs.

CHICORY EXTRACT • *Cichorium intybus.* Wild Succory. Related to dandelion; in ancient times, it was used as a narcotic, sometimes administered before operations. On the Continent, chicory is much cultivated, not only as a salad and vegetable, but also for fodder and more especially for the sake of its root, which though woody in the wild state, under cultivation becomes large and fleshy, with a thick rind, and is employed extensively when roasted and ground, for blending with coffee. An infusion of the herb is useful for skin eruptions connected with gout. Herbalists consider that the leaves when bruised make a poultice for swellings, inflammations, and inflamed eyes.

CHIMYL ALCOHOL • Obtained from shark liver oil and other fish oils. Used as skin conditioners and emollients.

CHINA CLAY • *See* Kaolin.

CHINESE ANGELICA ROOT • *Aralia chinensis.* An Asiatic shrub with prickly skin and a long inflorescence. Used in "organic" cosmetics.

CHINESE HIBISCUS EXTRACT • From the leaves and flowers of *Hibiscus rosa-sinensis.*

CHINESE MAGNOLIA EXTRACT • From the flowers and buds of *Magnolia biondii* or other species of magnolia.

CHINESE TEA EXTRACT • From the leaves of *Thea sinensis* or the seeds of *Camelia oleifera abal.* Contains tannin, which is soothing to the skin.

CHITIN • A white powder similar in structure to cellulose (*see*), it is the principal constituent of the shells of crabs, lobsters, and beetles. It is also found in some fungi, algae, and yeasts. It is used in wound-healing emulsions and in tanning products.

CHITOSAN • A derivative of chitin (*see*) used to aid coloring.

CHITIN-GLUCAN • A copolymer (*see*) found in the cell wall of several fungi including *Aspergillus niger.* Research that was published in the December 2008 issue of the *International Journal of Cosmetics Science* suggests that chitin-glucan has moisturizing properties and can help fight against some of the signs of skin aging. The authors note that, previously, chitin-based ingredients were often sourced from shellfish, and therefore could not be used in cosmetics products trying to avoid animal-derived ingredients. Chitin-glucan ingredient is extracted from the vegetative part (mycelium) of a microscopic fungi, *Aspergillus niger.*

CHITOSAN • A derivative of chitin (*see*) used to aid coloring.

CHLORACETAMIDE • A preservative that was used in cold cream, cleansing lotions, body and hand preparations, mud packs, shampoos, and hair preparations. In 1999, the CIR Expert Panel (*see*) established by the Cosmetic, Toiletry, and Fragrance Association found this ingredient unsafe for use because it caused allergic reactions. It is on the Canadian Hotlist (*see*). *See* Acetamide and Quaternary Ammonium Compounds.

4-CHLORO–2-AMINOPHENOL • A coal tar and an amine color. *See* Coal Tar.

CHLORAL HYDRATE • Knockout Drops. Transparent, colorless crystals with a slightly acrid odor and bitter taste, it is used in hypnotic drugs, in the manufacture of liniments, and in hair tonic. It may cause contact dermatitis, gastric disturbances, and when ingested it is narcotic. The lethal human dose is 10 grams. On the Canadian Hotlist (*see*).

CHLORAMINE-T • Sodium *p*-Toluenesulfonchloramide. A preservative and antiseptic used in nail bleaches, dental preparations, and mouthwashes. White crystals fairly soluble in water, which lose moisture at 100 degrees F. It is a powerful antiseptic and is used for washing wounds. May be irritating to the skin and cause allergic reactions. On the Canadian Hotlist.

CHLORAMPHENICOL • An antibiotic derived from the soil bacterium *Streptomyces venezuelae* or produced synthetically and effective against a broad spectrum of microorganisms. Serious side effects may include: unusual bleeding or bruising; fever or chills, sore throat; mouth sores; unusual weakness or tiredness; skin rash, itching; confusion; blurred vision and gray syndrome (blue-gray skin color, low body temperature, uneven breathing, bloated stomach).

CHLORATES OF ALKALI METALS. Used as a tooth whitener in toothpaste. The EU says it should not exceed 5 percent.

CHLORELLA • Green Algae. Cheap source of vitamin B complex and used in anti-aging products.

CHLORELLA FERMENT • Extract of the rust of the fermentation of chlorella (*see*) by yeast. Used for astringents, hair tonics, and moisturizers.

CHLORHEXIDINE • A white, crystalline powder used as a topical antiseptic and skin-sterilizing ingredient in liquid cosmetics and in European feminine hygiene sprays. May cause contact dermatitis. Strongly alkaline. The CIR Expert Panel (*see*) concludes on the basis of present data, chlorhexidine and its salts are safe for use in cosmetic products at concentrations of up to 0.14 percent as chlorhexidine; 0.19 percent as chlorhexidine diacetate (*see*); 0.20 percent as chlorhexidine digluconate; and 0.16 percent as chlorhexidine dihydrochloride. It is on the Canadian Hotlist (*see*).

CHLORHEXIDINE DIACETATE • The salt of chlorhexidine and acetic acid. Derived from methanol and acetic acid (*see*), which are derived from fruits. It is used as an antiseptic. It is on the Canadian Hotlist (*see*). *See* Chlorhexidine.

CHLORHEXIDINE DIGLUCONATE • *See* Chlorhexidine.

CHLORHEXIDINE DIHYDROCHLORIDE • Salt of chlorhexidine and hydrochloric acid. Derived from methanol (*see*). Used as a solvent. *See* Chlorhexidine.

CHLORINATED HYDROCARBONS • Hydrocarbons in which one or more of the hydrogen atoms have been replaced by chlorine (*see*). Many members of the group have been shown to cause cancer in animals and some in humans. Among the designated carcinogens: chloroform, vinyl chloride, trichloroethylene, and carbon tetrachloride (*see all*). Concern about the potential hazard of certain chlorinated hydrocarbons is based on their ubiquity; their persistence in the environment; their capacity to accumulate in living organisms, including humans and the human fetus; and the experimental evidence of a potential carcinogenic effect.

CHLORINE • A nonmetallic element, a diatomic gas that is heavy, noncombustible, and greenish yellow, it is found in the earth's crust and has a pungent, suffocating odor. In liquid form it is a clear amber color with an irritating odor. It does not occur in a free state but as a component of the mineral halite (rock salt). Toxic and irritating to the skin and lungs, it has a tolerance level of one part per million in air. It is used in the manufacture of carbon tetrachloride and in flame-retardant compounds; and in processing fish, vegetables, and fruit. It is used in the manufacture of carbon tetrachloride, trichloroethylene, shrinkproofing wool, in special batteries, and in the manufacture of ethylene dichloride (*see*). The chlorine used to kill bacteria in drinking water may contain carcinogenic carbon tetrachloride, a contaminant formed during the production process. Chlorination has also been found to sometimes form undesirable "ring" compounds in water, such as toluene, xylene, and the suspected carcinogen styrene—they have been observed in both drinking water and waste-water plants in the Midwest. Chlorine is a powerful irritant and can be fatal upon inhalation. In fact, it is stored in military arsenals as a poison gas. A National Cancer Institute study published in 1987 linked bladder cancer to people who had been drinking chlorinated surface water for forty or more years. On the Canadian Hotlist (*see*). The EU has banned it in cosmetics.

CHLORINE DIOXIDE (CIO2) • Japanese researchers found that it can help to combat bad breath for up to four hours when used in a mouthwash.

CHLORO- • Signifies a substance contains chlorine (*see*).

CHLOROACETIC ACID • Made by the chlorination of acetic acid (*see*) in the presence of sulfur or iodine. Used in the manufacture of soaps and creams. It is irritating to the skin and mucous membranes and can be toxic and corrosive when swallowed.

CHLOROBUTANOL • A white, crystalline alcohol used as a preservative in eye lotions and as an antioxidant in baby oils. It has a camphor odor and taste. Formerly used medicinally as a hypnotic and sedative; today it is employed as an anesthetic and antiseptic. A central nervous system depressant, it is used as a hypnotic drug.

***p*-CHLORO-*m*-CRESOL** • A preservative in skin care and suntan cosmetic formulations. Prohibited for use in products in contact with mucous membranes. A solution as low as 0.05 percent caused eye irritation in rabbits. A chronic feeding study caused kidney damage in male rats and an increase in adrenal tumors. Some evidence of skin irritation and sensitization was found in animal studies. The CIR Expert Panel (*see*) concludes that the available data are insufficient to support the safety of this ingredient in cosmetic products. ASEAN prohibits in products intended to come into contact with mucous membranes. *See* Cresols.

CHLOROETHANE • On the Canadian Hotlist (*see*). The EU banned it in cosmetics. *See* Ethyl Chloride.

CHLOROFLUOROCARBON PROPELLANTS • The use of chlorofluorocarbon propellants (fully halogenated chlorofluoroalkanes) in cosmetic aerosol products intended for domestic consumption is prohibited. The following are fully halogenated chlorofluorocarbons: chlorofluorocarbon 11 (trichlorofluoromethane), chlorofluorocarbon 12 (dichloro-difluoromethane), chlorofluorocarbon 113 (trichlorotrifluoroethane), chlorofluorocarbon 114 (dichlorotetra-fluoroethane), and fluorocyclobutane C318 (octofluoro-cyclobutane). The FDA said in 2008 that chlorofluorocarbon-containing cosmetic aerosol products may continue to be manufactured for export provided there is no diversion of products into domestic commerce. The use of chlorofluorocarbons in cosmetics as propellants in self-pressurized containers is prohibited by the FDA in the United States.

CHLOROFORM • Used in products to clean wool or synthetic fabrics, and as a solvent for fats, oils, waxes, resins, and as a cleaning ingredient. Chloroform has many serious side effects and is considered a carcinogen. Exposure to it may also cause respiratory and skin allergies. Complaints received by the FDA about blisters and inflammation of the gums caused by toothpaste were found to be due to the amount of chloroform in the product. The manufacturer was asked to reduce the amount of the substance. Large doses may cause low blood pressure, heart stoppage, and death. In April 1976, the FDA determined that chloroform may cause cancer and asked drug and cosmetics manufacturers who have not already done so to discontinue using it immediately, even before it was officially banned. The National Cancer Institute made public in June 1976 the finding that chloroform was found to cause liver and kidney cancers in test animals. On the Canadian Hotlist (*see*). The European Union and the United States banned it in cosmetics. *See* Bronopol.

CHLOROGENIC ACIDS • Isolated from coffee beans, used as an antioxidant.

5-CHLORO-8-HYDROXYQUINOLONE • *See* Oxyquinoline Sulfate.

CHLOROMETHOXYPROPYLMERCURIC ACETATE • A preservative. *See* Mercury Compounds.

2-CHLORO-5-NITRO-N-HYDROXYETHYL-*p*-PHENYLENEDIAMINE • A coal tar hair coloring. *See* Coal Tar and Phenylenediamine.

CHLOROPHENE *o*-BENZYL-*p*-CHLOROPHENOL • Prepared from benzyl chloride and phenoxide followed by chlorination. Used in Lysol disinfectant. *See* Phenols for toxicity.

***p*-CHLOROPHENOL** • A bacteria killer. Can cause ear, nose, and throat irritations, skin rashes, and reproductive problems. Chlorophenol compounds are on the Community Right-to-Know List (*see*). Caused tumors and birth defects in laboratory animals.

2-CHLORO-*p*-PHENYLENEDIAMINE • *See* p-Phenylenediamine.

2-CHLORO-*p*-PHENYLENEDIAMINE SULFATE • *See* p-Phenylenediamine.

CHLOROPHYLL • The green coloring matter of plants, which plays an essential part in the plant's photosynthesis process. Used in antiperspirants, dentifrices, deodorants, and mouthwashes as a deodorizing ingredient. It imparts a greenish color to certain fats and oils, notably olive and soybean oil. Can cause a sensitivity to light.

CHLOROPHYLLIN • Copper derivative, used as a deodorant ingredient in mouthwashes, breath fresheners, and body deodorants. Derived from chlorophyll, the green coloring matter of plants. Banned by the FDA. *See* Chlorophyll.

CHLOROPHYLLIN COPPER COMPLEX • Banned by the FDA as a coloring. *See* Chlorophyllin.

CHLOROPROPIONIC ACID AND SALTS • Prepared from cyanohydrin and hydrochloric acid. It absorbs water.

4-CHLORORESORCINOL • *See* Resorcinol.

CHLOROTHYMOL • A chloro derivative of thymol (*see*) and a powerful germicide used in mouthwashes, hair tonics, and baby oils. It kills staph germs and is used topically as an antibacterial. Can be irritating to the mucous membranes and can possibly be absorbed through the skin.

CHLOROXYLENOL • A white, crystalline solid used as an antiseptic, germicide, and fungicide in hair tonics, shampoos, contraceptive douches, deodorants, bath salts, vaginal deodorants, and brushless shaving creams. Penetrates the skin but has no apparent irritating effects when diluted at 5 percent. May cause greenish discoloration of the hair when swimming in chlorinated water. Active ingredient in germicides, antiseptics, and antifungal preparations. Toxic by ingestion. May be irritating to and absorbed by the skin. The CIR Expert Panel (*see*) concludes, on the basis of animal studies, this ingredient is safe.

CHLORPHENESIN • An alcohol used as a germicide. The UK restricts it to 0.3 percent in all products.

CHLORPHENIRAMINE • An antihistamine recategorized first in low dosage from RX to OTC in 1976 and in stronger strengths in 1981. It is used to counteract tooth-whitening processes and other potentially allergenic cosmetics. It is used to treat stuffy nose and other allergy symptoms. The FDA issued a notice in 1992 that chlorpheniramine maleate has not been shown to be safe and effective for stated claims in OTC products for poison ivy, poison oak, and poison sumac drug products.

CHLORZOXAZONE • Crystals from acetone (*see*). Used to relieve muscle aches and spasms. May adversely affect the liver and have an adverse reaction with other chemicals. On the Canadian Hotlist (*see*). The EU banned it in cosmetics.

CHOCOLATE. *See* NanoCocoa.

CHOLESTEROL • A fat-soluble, crystalline steroid alcohol (*see*) occurring in all animal fats and oils, nervous tissue, egg yolk, and blood. Used as an emulsifier and lubricant in brilliantine hairdressings, eye creams, shampoos, and other cosmetic products. It is important in metabolism but has been implicated as contributing to clogging of the arteries.

CHOLESTERYL ACETATE • An ester (*see*) of cholesterol (*see*) used as a skin conditioner.

CHOLESTERYL ISOSTEARATE • A skin-conditioning ingredient. *See* Cholesterol.

CHOLESTERYL MACADAMIATE • Fatty acids obtained from macadamia nuts and used as a skin-conditioning ingredient.

CHOLESTERYL OLEYL CARBONATE • A skin-conditioning ingredient used in anti-aging products. *See* Cholesterol and Oleic Acid.

CHOLESTERYL/BEHENYL/OCTYL-DODECYL/LAUROYL SURFACTANT • A skin-conditioning ingredient. *See* Cholesterol.

CHOLESTERYL/OCTYLDODECYL LAUROYL GLUTAMATE • A skin-conditioning ingredient. *See* Cholesterol and Glutamate.

CHOLETH-10–24 • The polyethylene glycol ether (*see*) of cholesterol (*see*). Used in hand creams. On the basis of the available information, the CIR Expert Panel (*see*) found it safe in the early 1980s but is considering new information to determine if the final safety assessment should be reaffirmed, amended, or have an addendum.

CHOLIC ACID • A colorless or white, crystalline powder that occurs in the bile of most vertebrates and is used as an emulsifying ingredient in dried egg. Bitter taste, sweetish aftertaste. The final report to the FDA of the Select Committee on GRAS Substances stated in 1980 that it should continue its GRAS status with no limitations other than good manufacturing practices in food.

CHOLINE • A syrupy liquid included in the B-complex vitamins. It is a base widely distributed among plant and animal products. It is either free or in combination with lecithin. It is essential to the metabolism of fat, especially in the liver, and it is used in the form of salts to treat liver disease. On the Canadian Hotlist (*see*). Choline salts and their esters are banned by the EU in cosmetics.

CHOLINE BITARTRATE • A dietary supplement included in the B-complex vitamins and found in the form of a thick syrupy liquid in most animal tissue. It is necessary to nerve function and fat metabolism and can be manufactured in the body but not at a sufficient rate to meet health requirements. Dietary choline protects against poor growth, fatty liver, and renal damage in many animals. GRAS. ASP

CHOLINE CHLORIDE • Ferric Choline Citrate. A dietary supplement with the same function as choline bitartrate (*see*). The final report to the FDA of the Select Committee on GRAS Substances stated in 1980 that it should continue its GRAS status with no limitations other than good manufacturing practices in food.

CHOLINE HYDROCHLORIDE • Colorless to white, water-absorbing crystals used as a fungicide on various feeds. On the Community Right-to-Know List (*see*). Moderately toxic to humans if ingested. May be mutagenic.

CHONDROITIN • A major constituent of cartilage in the body.

CHONDRUS • *See* Carrageenan.

CHROMIC ACID AND ITS SALTS • Brownish flakes used in chromium plating and as a pigment. On the Canadian Hotlist (*see*). *See* Chromium Compounds.

CHROMIUM COMPOUNDS • Chromium occurs in the earth's crust. Chromic oxide is used for green eye shadow and chromium oxide for greenish mascara. Inhalation of chromium dust can cause irritation and ulceration. Ingestion results in violent gastrointestinal irritation. Application to the skin may result in allergic reaction. The most serious effect of chromium is lung cancer, which may develop twenty to thirty years after exposure. The EU banned it as well as chromic acid and its salts. Chromium is poisonous in large amounts. Ingestion can result in violent gastrointestinal irritation. Chromium can be carcinogenic according to Environmental Defense. It is number 18 on the CERCLA (*see*) Priority List of Hazardous Substances.

CHROMIUM HYDROXIDE GREEN • Coloring, permanently listed for use as a cosmetic coloring in 1977. *See* Chromium Compounds.

CHROMIUM OXIDE GREENS • Widely used coloring in eyeliners, mascara, eyebrow pencils, eye makeup, face powders, makeup bases, dusting powders, and cleansing products. *See* Chromium Compounds.

CHROMIUM SULFATE • Violet or red powder used in the textile industries, in green paints and varnishes, green ice, ceramics, in tanning, and in green eye shadows. Can cause contact dermatitis.

CHRONOLINE • A biomimetic tetrapeptide that boosts the production of key components like collagen and fibronectin (*see all*) aimed at skin structural support. The manufacturer claims ChroNOline provides reduction in the appearance of fine lines and wrinkles after only twenty-eight days.

CHRYSANTHELLUM INDICUM • *See* Chrysanthemum.

CHRYSANTHEMUM • *Chrysanthemum sinense.* Ye Ju. Corn Marigold. A large family of perennial herbs thought to originate in Asia. A tea made from this flower is used to treat conjunctivitis and skin diseases. Taken internally, it is used to lower blood pressure. A number of medicines and the insecticidal pyrethrins (*see*) are derived from this family.

CHYMOSIN • Enzyme prepared from calf stomach. Used as a stabilizer and thickener. GRAS. EAF

CHYMOTRYPSIN • Catarase. Chymar. Zolyse. A pancreatic enzyme. *See* Enzyme.

CHYPRE • A nonalcoholic type of perfume containing oils and resins.

CI 10006–CI 77947 • Color Index Inorganic colors used mostly in hair dyes. They are listed by number in the European Union but are not permitted to be listed that way on U.S. labels. Most of them are designated D & C colors or by ingredient name (such as Manganese Violet instead of CI 77742) if they are permitted in U.S. products approved for use in the United States.

CI 12140 • Banned by the EU and on the Canadian Hotlist.

CI 13065 • On the Canadian Hotlist (*see*).

CI 42640 • Banned by ASEAN. Also on the Canadian Hotlist. It is an established fact that the coloring agent CI 42640 is a substance that produces carcinogenic effects. This substance should therefore be prohibited in cosmetic products.

CI 42051 • The European Union's name for the triphenylmethane color (*see*) also called Acid Blue 3, Calcium Salt, and Food Blue 5. Not approved for use in the United States.

CI 62045 • The European Union's name for the anthraquinone color (*see*). Also called Acid Blue 62. Not approved for use in the United States.

CI 69800 • The European Union's name for the anthraquinone color (*see*) also called Pigment Blue 60 and Vat Blue 4. Not approved for use in the United States.

CI 69825 • The European Union's name for the anthraquinone color (*see*) also called Pigment Blue 64 and Vat Blue 6. Not approved for use in the United States.

CI 71105 • The European Union's name for the indigoid color also called Vat Orange 7 and Pigment Orange 43. Not approved for use in the United States.

CI 73000 • The European Union's name for the indigoid color also called Pigment Blue 66 and Vat Blue 1. Not approved for use in the United States.

CI 73015 • The European Union's name for the indigoid color also called Blue No. 2 and Japan Blue 2.

CI 73360 • The European Union's name for the thioindigoid color also called Vat Red 1 and Japan Red 226.

CI 73385 • The European Union's name for the thioindigoid color also called Vat Violet 2 and pigment Violet 36. Not approved for use in the United States.

CI 73900 • The European Union's name for the quinacridone color also called Pigment Violet 19. Not approved for use in the United States.

CI 73915 • The European Union's name for the indigoid color also called Pigment Red 22. Not approved for use in the United States.

CI 74100 • The European Union's name for the phthalocyanine color also called Heliogen Blue G and Pigment Blue 16. Not approved for use in the United States.

CI 74160 • The European Union's name for the phthalocyanine color also called Copper and Pigment Blue 15.

CI 74180 • The European Union's name for the phthalocyanine color also called Direct Blue 86 and Acid Blue 87. Not approved for use in the United States.

CI 74260 • The European Union's name for this phthalocyanine color. It is also called Pigment Green 7 and Heliogen Green G. Not approved for use in the United States.

CI 75100 • A botanically derived color also called Crocetin and Natural Yellow 6. Not approved for use in the United States.

CI 75120 • The European Union's name for this color from *Bixa orellana*. Also called Natural Orange 4 and Norbixin.

CI 75125 • The European Union's name for a botanical color beta-carotene also called Natural Yellow 27 and Violaxanthin. Not approved for use in the United States.

CI 75130 • The European Union's name for the carotenoid color also called Beta-Carotene, Natural Brown 5, and Natural Yellow 26.

CI 75135 • The European Union's name for a botanically derived color also called Rubixanthin. Not approved for use in the United States.

CI 75170 • The European Union's bane fir, a natural purine. Also called Natural White 1 or Pearl Essence.

CI 75300 • The European Union's name for the botanically derived color from curcumin (*see*). Also called Natural Yellow 3 or Turmeric Yellow.

CI 75470 • The European Union's name for the naturally derived color carmine also called Natural Red 4 or Cochineal.

CI 75810 • The European Union's name for copper derivative from green plants. Also called Natural Green 3 or Potassium Sodium Copper Chlorophyllin.

CI 77000 • The European Union's name for finely powdered aluminum. Also called Aluminum Powder or Pigmental Metal 1.

CI 77002 • The European Union's name for aluminum hydroxide. Also called Pigment White 24 or Aluminum Hydroxide.

CI 77004 • The European Union's name for this hydrated aluminum silicate. Also called Bentonite (*see*) or Pigment White 19.

CI 77007 • The European Union's name for sodium aluminum sulfosilicates. Also called Ultramarine or Pigment Blue 29.

CI 77015 • The European Union's name for aluminum silicated with ferric oxide. Also called Pigment Red 102. Not approved for use in the United States.

CI 77120 • The European Union's name for barium sulfate color. Also called Pigment White 21. Not approved for use in the United States.

CI 77163 • The European Union's name for bismuth oxychloride. Also called Pigment White 14.

CI 77220 • The European Union's name for calcium carbonate. Also called Pigment White 18 or Synthetic Chalk. Not approved for use in the United States.

CI 77231 • The European Union's name for gypsum (*see*) derived color. Also called Calcium Sulfate and Pigment White 25.

CI 77266 • The European Union's name for the carbon black color. Also called Pigment Black 6. Not approved for use in the United States.

CI 77267 • The European Union's name for the bone charcoal coloring. Also called Bone Black (*see*) or Pigment Black 9. Not approved for use in the United States. Made from animal bones.

CI 77268:1 • The European Union's name for this carbon coloring. Also called Food Black 3 and Carbo Medicinalis Vegetalis. Not approved for use in the United States. Black bone carbon made from animal bones.

CI 77288 • The European Union's name for chromium-derived green. Also called Pigment Green 17 or Chromic Oxide.

CI 77289 • The European Union's name for the chromic hydroxide green. Also called Pigment Green 18.

CI 77346 • The European Union's name for the color derived from cobalt. Also called Cobalt Blue or Pigment Blue 28. Not approved for use in the United States. Banned in the EU.

CI 77400 • The European Union's name for the mixture of copper and zinc with a small amount of aluminum or tin. Also called Bronze Powder or Copper Powder.

CI 77480 • The European Union's name for the color derived from gold. Also called Gold Leaf.

CI 77489 • The European Union's name for the iron-derived color. Also called iron oxide (*see*).

CI 77491, CI 77492, CI 77499, CI 77510 • The European Union's name for iron oxide colors. Also called Ferric Oxide, Pigment Brown 7, Pigment Yellow 42, and Prussian Blue among others.

CI 77713 • The European Union's name for the magnesium carbonate color. Not approved for use in the United States.

CI 77742 • The European Union's name for the color derived from ammonium manganese pyrophosphate. Also called Mango Violet, Manganese Violet, and Pigment Violet 16.

CI 77745 • The European Union's name for the manganese orthophosphate color. Also called Manganous Phosphate. Not approved for use in the United States.

CI 77820 • The European Union's name for the silver color.

CI 77891 • The European Union's name for the color derived from titanium dioxide. Also called Pigment White 6.

CI 77947 • The European Union's name for the zinc oxide color. Also called Pigment White 4 or Flowers of Zinc.

CIBOTIUM BAROMETZ • Pengawar. A genus of oriental tree ferns with gracefully drooping flowers. Used in fragrances.

CICHORIUM INTYBUS • Chicory. Wild Succory. *See* Chicory Extract.

CICLOPIROX OLAMINE • A germicide. *See* Pyridine.

CIMICIFUGA RACEMOSA • Black Cohosh. Snakeroot. Bugbane. Black Snakeroot. Rattleroot. Used in astringents, perennial herb with a flower that is supposedly distasteful to insects. Grown from Canada to North Carolina and Kansas. It has a reputation for curing snakebites. It is used in ginger ale flavoring. A tonic and antispasmodic. The root contains various glycosides (*see*) including estrogenic substances and tannins. Herbalists have used it to relieve nerve pains, menstrual pains, and the pain of childbirth. Also used to speed delivery and to reduce blood pressure. Black cohosh is also believed to have sedative properties. In 1992, the FDA proposed a ban on black cohosh in oral menstrual drug products because it had not been shown to be safe and effective as claimed.

CINCHONA EXTRACT • The extract of the bark of various species of *Cinchona* cultivated in Java, India, and South America. Quinine is derived from it.

CINNAMAL • Cinnamaldehyde. Cinnamic Aldehyde. A synthetic, yellowish, oily liquid with a strong odor of cinnamon isolated from a wood-rotting fungus. Occurs naturally in cassia bark extract, cinnamon bark, and root oils. Used for its aroma in perfume and for flavoring in mouthwash and toothpaste. Also to scent powder and hair tonic. It is irritating to the skin and mucous membranes, especially if undiluted. One of the most common allergens. The CIR Expert Panel (*see*) has listed this as top priority for review.

CINNAMALDEHYDE • Cinnamic Aldehyde. A synthetic yellowish oily liquid with a strong odor of cinnamon isolated from a wood-rotting fungus. Occurs naturally in cassia bark extract, cinnamon bark, and root oils. Used in cola, apple, cherry, liquor, rum, nut, pecan, spice, cinnamon, vanilla, and cream soda flavorings for beverages, ice cream, ices, candy (700 ppm), baked goods, chewing gum (4,900 ppm), condiments, and meats. It is estimated that eaters' only exposure is 0.099 mg/kg per person per day. Also used in perfume industry, to flavor mouthwash and toothpaste, and to scent powder and hair tonic. It is irritating to the skin and mucous membranes, especially if undiluted. University of Illinois researchers reported in 2004 that chewing gum containing it reduced bacteria in the mouth and bad breath. Can cause inflammation and erosion of the gastrointestinal tract. One of the most common allergens. It cross-reacts with balsam Peru and benzoin. May cause depigmentation and hives. GRAS. ASP

CINNAMATES • Salts or esters of cinnamic acid (*see*). In sunscreens include octyl methoxycinnamate and cinoxate, the most frequently used UVB absorbers in the United States. They are often found in color cosmetics that have an SPF factor, with a potent UVB absorber (*see* Absorbent) and when combined with other ingredients helps make them more water resistant and stable. However, people with sensitivities to balsam Peru, balsam Tolu, coca leaves, cinnamic aldehyde, and cinnamic oil can also be sensitive to the cinnamates (*see all*).

CINNAMIC ACID • Used in suntan lotions and perfumes. Occurs in storax, balsam Peru, cinnamon leaves, and coca leaves. Usually isolated from wood-rotting fungus. It may cause allergic skin rashes. ASP

CINNAMIC ALCOHOL • Fragrance ingredient. One of the most common allergens in fragrances and flavorings. Used in mouthwashes, toilet soaps, toothpastes, and sanitary napkins. *See* Cinnamic Aldehyde.

CINNAMIC ALDEHYDE • Found in cinnamon oil, cassia oil, cinnamon powder, patchouli oil, flavoring ingredients, toilet soaps, and perfumes. It cross-reacts with balsam Peru and benzoin. May cause depigmentation and hives. It is used in synthetic jasmine and may be the cause of a reaction to that compound.

CINNAMOMUM CAMPHORA • Camphor Bark Oil. Obtained from the bark of the tree and used in hand products. *See* Cinnamon and Camphor Oil.

CINNAMOMUM LOUREIRRII BARK EXTRACT • *See* Cinnamon.

CINNAMOMUM CASSIA • *See* Cinnamon Oil.

CINNAMOMUM ZEYLANICUM • *See* Cinnamon.

CINNAMON • *Cinnamomum cassia*. Used to flavor toothpaste and mouthwash and to scent hair tonic and powder. Obtained from the dried bark of cultivated trees. Extracts have been used to break up intestinal gas and to treat diarrhea, but can be irritating to the gastrointestinal system. When used as a flavoring in toothpaste, it can cause mouth irritation if users are sensitive to cinnamon.

CINNAMON BARK • Extract and Oil. From the dried bark of cultivated trees, the extract is used in cola, eggnog, root beer, cinnamon, and ginger ale for beverages, ice cream, baked goods, condiments, and meats. The oil is used in berry, cola, cherry, rum, root beer, cinnamon, and ginger ale flavorings for beverages, condiments, and meats. Can be a skin sensitizer in humans and cause mild sensitivity to light. GRAS. ASP

CINNAMON LEAF OIL • *See* Cinnamon Oil.

CINNAMON OIL • Oil of Cassia. Chinese Cinnamon. Yellowish to brown, volatile oil from the leaves and twigs of cultivated trees. About 80 to 90 percent cinnamal. It has the characteristic odor and taste of cassia cinnamon and darkens and thickens upon aging or exposure to air. Cinnamon oil is used to scent perfumes and as a flavoring in dentifrices. Can cause contact dermatitis.

CINNAMYL ACETATE • A synthetic flavoring ingredient; colorless to yellow liquid with a sweet floral odor. Occurs naturally in cassia bark. Used in apricot, cherry, grape, peach, pineapple, cinnamon, and vanilla flavorings. *See* Cinnamyl Alcohol and Acetic Acid.

CINNAMYL ALCOHOL • Occurs in storax, balsam Peru, cinnamon leaves, and hyacinth oil. A crystalline alcohol with a strong hyacinth odor used in synthetic perfumes and in deodorants for flavoring and scent. Can cause allergic reactions.

CINNAMYL ANTHRANILATE • A synthetic flavoring ingredient and fragrance ingredient used since the 1940s as an imitation grape or cherry flavor. It is used as a fragrance in soaps, detergents, creams, lotions, and perfumes. United States sales equaled more than two thousand pounds in 1976. The National Cancer Institute reported, December 20, 1980, that it caused liver cancer in male and female mice and caused both kidney and pancreatic cancers in male rats in feeding studies. Earlier studies showed it increased lung tumors in mice. The FDA banned the use of it in food in 1982. Most companies voluntarily stopped using it in cosmetics after publication of the NCI information.

CINNAMYL ESTERS • Used in perfumery. *See* Cinnamic Acid and Esters.

CINOXATE • A sunscreen. 2-Ethoxyethyl *p*-methoxycinnamate. Permitted in the United States and Austria. Has not been tested by their federal agencies. *See* Cinnamic Acid.

CIR • Abbreviation for the Cosmetic Ingredient Review.

CIR EXPERT PANEL • Established in 1976 by the Cosmetic, Toiletry, and Fragrance Association (CTFA) (now called the Personal Care Products Council), the CIR Expert Panel reviews in a public forum the safety of ingredients used in cosmetics. The CIR Expert Panel's formal decision regarding the safety of an ingredient, and the basis for that decision, is made publicly available in its final reports. In addition to making reports directly available to the public, CIR submits its safety assessments for publication in the *International Journal of Toxicology.*

CIS- • Latin meaning "on the side." When a certain atom is positioned on one side of a group of carbons, it is called cis- as in cis-jasmone.

CIS-3-HEXEN-1-OL • *See* Cis- and Hexanol.

CIS-3-HEXENYL ACETATE • *See* Cis- and Hexanol.

CIS-3-HEXENYL SALICYLATE • *See* Salicylates and Hexanol.

CIS-JASMONE • A substance found in jasmine (*see*). Used in perfumery.

CISTUS LABDANIFERUS OIL • Native to Spain and Greece, this is the "rockrose" grown in some North American gardens. Possibly the Bible's onycha and "rose of

Sharon," it often replaces ambergris. It has long been popular in Spain, which remains the major producer today. Shepherds in ancient Crete would drive their herds through the plants so the sticky gum would collect on the animal's coats; after combing it out, they'd take the gum to market. Don't confuse this plant with laudanum, an old-time pain remedy made of opium. The essential oil is used in fragrances and shampoos. *See* Rockrose.

CISTUS MONSPELIENSIS EXTRACT • From *Cistus monspeliensis.* Used as a fragrance ingredient. *See* Rockrose.

CITRAL • A flavoring used in foods and beverages. Used in perfumes, soaps, and colognes for its lemon and verbena scents. Found also in detergents and furniture polish. Occurs naturally in grapefruit, orange, peach, ginger, grapefruit oil, oil of lemon, and oil of lime. A light oily liquid isolated from citral oils or made synthetically. The compound has been reported to inhibit wound healing and tumor rejection in animals. Vitamin A counteracts its toxicity, but in commercial products to which pure citral has been added, vitamin A may not be present.

CITRAL DIMETHYL ACETAL • *See* Citric Acid and Acetic Acid.

CITRATES • The salts or esters of citric acid (*see*) used as softening ingredients. Citrates may interfere with the results of laboratory tests including tests for pancreatic function, abnormal liver function, and blood alkalinity and acidity.

CITRIC ACID • One of the most widely used acids in the cosmetic industry, it is derived from citrus fruit by fermentation of crude sugars. Employed as a preservative and sequestering ingredient (*see*) to adjust acid-alkali balance and as a foam inhibitor and plasticizer. It is also used as an astringent alone or in astringent compounds. Among the cosmetic products in which it is frequently found are freckle and nail bleaches, bath preparations, skin fresheners, cleansing creams, depilatories, eye lotions, hair colorings, hair rinses, and hair-waving preparations. The clear, crystalline, water-absorbing chemicals are also used to prevent scurvy, a deficiency disease, and as a refreshing drink with water and sugar added. Removes trace metals and brightens color in various commercial products. It has been used to dissolve urinary bladder stones. *See* Alpha-Hydroxy Acids. GRAS. ASP. E

CITRONELLA OIL • *Cymbopogon nardus.* A natural food flavoring extract from fresh grass grown in Asia. Used in perfumes, toilet waters, and perfumed cosmetics; also an insect repellent. May cause allergic reactions such as stuffy nose, hay fever, asthma, and skin rash when used in cosmetics. GRAS. ASP

CITRONELLAL • A fragrance ingredient. The chief constituent of citronella oil (*see*). Also found in lemon and lemongrass oils. Colorless liquid with an intense lemon-rose odor. Used in citrus, lemon, cherry, and spice flavorings for beverages, ice cream, ices, candy, baked goods, chewing gum, and gelatin desserts. A skin irritant. *See* Citronella Oil for toxicity. ASP

CITRONELLOL • Used in perfumes. It has a roselike odor. Occurs naturally in citronella oil, lemon oil, lemongrass oil, tea, rose oil, and geranium oil. A mild irritant.

CITRONELLYL ESTERS • *See* Citronella Oil and Esters.

CITRULLINE • An amino acid used as a skin-conditioning ingredient.

CITRULL • *See* Cucumber.

CITRULLUS COLOCYNTHIS • Coloc. From the family of Cucurbitaceae, colocynthis is a trailing plant that grows in sandy places. Homeopaths mix the powdered, dried fruit with alcohol and allow the compound to sit for a week. This is one of the main colic remedies used by homeopaths. *See* Colocynth.

CITRULLUS VULGARIS • A skin-conditioning ingredient. *See* Watermelon.

CITRUS AURANTIUM-AMARA (BITTER ORANGE) FLOWER EXTRACT • Extract from *Citrus aurantium-amara* used as a skin conditioner. *See* Bitter Orange Oil.

CITRUS BIOFLAVONOIDS • Vitamin P complex nutrient supplement up to one gram per day. Occurs naturally in plant coloring and in the tonka bean; also in lemon juice. High concentrates can be obtained from all citrus fruits, rose hips, and black currants. Commercial methods extract rinds of oranges, tangerines, lemons, limes, kumquats, and grapefruit. P vitamin is related to healthy blood vessels and skin. Any claim for bioflavonoids renders the product illegal, according to FDA rules.

CITRUS CLEMENTINA JUICE • From the pulp of *Citrus clementina* used as a skin conditioner. Has a fresh green odor and is used in fragrances.

CITRUS GRANDIS • Widely used in cleansing and skin care products. Grapefruit.

CITRUS JUNOS FRUIT EXTRACT • Extract from the fruit of *Citrus junos,* a sour orange also known as Yuza. Used as a skin conditioner, antioxidant, and chelating ingredient (*see*).

CITRUS LIMONUM • Lemon.

CITRUS MEDICA VULGARIS FRUIT EXTRACT • Fo Shou Gan. *See* Lemon Oil.

CITRUS NOBILIS • Mandarin Orange. A small orange, with easily separable rind. It is thought to be of Chinese origin and is counted a distinct species.

CITRUS OILS • Eugenol, eucalyptol, anethole, orris, and menthol (*see all*). Used in flavoring food products and cosmetics and as odorants in special soaps.

CITRUS × PARADISI • Grapefruit.

CITRUS PEEL EXTRACT • A natural flavor extract from the peel or rind of grapefruit, lemon, lime, orange, and tangerine. Used as flavoring additives in bitters, lemon, lime, orange, vermouth, beer, and ginger ale flavorings for beverages, ice cream, ices, candy, and baked goods. Attempts are being made at this writing to develop antibacterial and antifungal ingredients from citrus fruit. An Israel-based company has created an extraction method to harness the preservative from citrus peel and solve the shelf life problems facing natural and organic manufacturers. GRAS. ASP

CITRUS TANGERINA • Tangerine.

CITRUS UNSHIU • Japanese Orange Peel. Fragrance ingredient.

CIVET • Civet, Absolute • Zibeth. Zibet. Zibetum. Essential oil used as a fixative in perfumery. It is the civet cat's unctuous secretion from between the anus and genitalia of both male and female civet cat. Semisolid, yellowish to brown mass, with an unpleasant odor, it is also used as raspberry, butter, caramel, grape, and rum flavorings for beverages, ice cream, ices, candy, baked goods, gelatin desserts, and chewing gum. GRAS. There is reported use of the chemical; it has not yet been assigned for toxicology literature search by the FDA. EAF

CLARIFICATION • Removal from liquid of small amounts of suspended matter; for example, the removal of particles and traces of copper and iron from vinegar and certain beverages.

CLARIFYING INGREDIENT • A substance that removes small amounts of suspended matter from liquids. Butyl alcohol, for instance, is a clarifying ingredient for clear shampoos.

CLARY • *Salvia sclarea.* Clary Sage. A fixative (*see*) for perfumes. A natural extract of an aromatic herb grown in southern Europe and cultivated widely in England. A well-known spice in food and beverages. GRAS. EAF

CLAVICEPS PURPUREA • Fungus. On the Canadian Hotlist (*see*). The EU bans it in cosmetics. *See* Ergot.

CLAY PACK • *See* Face Masks and Packs.

CLAYS • Bentonite. Veegum. China Clay. Kaolin. Used for color in cosmetics, as a clarifying ingredient (*see*) in liquids, as an emollient, and as a poultice.

CLEANSING CREAMS AND LOTIONS • Used to dissolve sebum (*see*), loosen particles of grime, and to facilitate the removal of dirt. They usually contain mineral oil, triethanolamine stearate, and water. Among other ingredients commonly used are alcohol, alkanolamines, allantoins, antibacterials, and preservatives, methyl and propyl parabens, fatty alcohols, lanolin, perfumes, glycerol, propylene glycol, fatty oils, thickeners, and waxes. A well-known hypoallergenic cold cream contains water, mineral oil, waxes, borax, and depollenized beeswax. The American Medical Association and dermatologists say that soap and water will serve the same purpose as cleansing creams and lotions, is less expensive, and offers less risk of allergy. (However, soap can be more drying to the skin.) Antibacterials, preservatives, parabens, lanolin, thickeners, and perfumes are all common causes of allergic contact dermatitis (*see all*).

CLEAVERS • *Galium aparine.* Catchweed. Goosegrass. Clives. A native of Europe, Asia, and North America, the Greeks called it philantropon because they considered its clinging habit showed a love of mankind. It was also used by dieters to keep them lean and lank. Used in homeopathic medicine for skin diseases such as psoriasis and scurvy. The whole herb is used by herbalists to treat kidney and bladder problems and gallstones. It has diuretic properties. It is used in "organic" cosmetics.

CLEMATIS EXTRACT • Old Man's Beard Extract. The extract obtained from the leaves of *Clematis vitalba.* A red or violet herb or woody vine. It is used in "organic" cosmetics.

CLIMBAZOLE • Germicide.

CLINTONIA BOREALIS • Lily of the Valley. May Blossom. The wildflower, which grows in woodlands, causes vomiting. The flower was believed to stimulate secretions of the nasal mucous membranes. Contains certain cardiac glycosides similar to those of digitalis. It is used in cosmetics as an anti-irritant, and there is some research to show that it increases cell proliferation.

CLOFLUCARBAN • *See* Aniline Dyes.

CLORTRIMAZOLE • A germicide.

CLOVE OIL • *Eugenia caryophyllus.* Used as an antiseptic and flavoring in tooth powders and as a scent in hair tonics and to flavor postage stamp glue; as a toothache treatment; as a condiment; and as a flavoring in chewing gum. It is 82 to 87 percent eugenol (*see*) and has the characteristic clove oil odor and taste. Strongly irritating to the skin and can cause allergic skin rashes. Its use in perfumes and cosmetics is frowned upon by regulating authorities, although in very diluted forms it is allegedly innocuous. In 1992, the FDA proposed a ban on clove oil in astringent (*see*) drug products because it has not been shown to be safe and effective for its stated claims.

CLOVER • *Trifolium* subspecies. An herb; a natural flavoring extract from a plant characterized by three leaves and flowers in dense heads. Used in fruit flavorings. May cause sensitivity to light. ASP.

CLOVER BLOSSOM EXTRACT • The extract of the flowers of *Trifolium pratense.* Used in fruit flavorings. May cause sensitivity to light.

CLOVERLEAF OIL • *Eugenia caryophyllus.* Leaf Oil. The volatile oil obtained by steam distillation of the leaves. It consists mostly of eugenol (*see*).

CLUB MOSS • *Lycopodium clavatum.* American Indians sprinkled a powder made from this herb on wounds to stop bleeding. The powder is used today for minor skin wounds.

CMR • Abbreviation for Carcinogenic, Mutagenic, or Toxic effect to Reproduction based upon the evaluation of a substance of "very high concern" by the European Chemical Agency (ECHA) .

CNIDIUM OFFICINALE • A Chinese herb long used for kidney problems, impotence, vaginal infections, and fungus. Used in cosmetics as a fragrance ingredient and skin conditioner.

COAL TAR • Used in adhesives, creosotes, insecticides, phenols, woodworking, preservation of food, and dyes to make colors used in cosmetics, including hair dyes. Thick liquid or semisolid tar obtained from bituminous coal, it contains many constituents including benzene, xylenes, naphthalene, pyridine, quinoline, phenol, and creosol. The main concern about coal tar derivatives is that they cause cancer in animals, but they are also frequent sources of allergic reactions, particularly skin rashes and hives. It is a substance included in many topical preparations for the treatment of psoriasis and dandruff. Coal tar OTC products for dandruff, seborrheic dermatitis, and psoriasis have to state the concentrations of coal tar contained in any coal tar solution, derivative, or fraction used in the source of the coal tar product, the FDA ruled in 1992. The FDA then issued a notice in 1992 that coal tar has not been shown to be safe and effective for stated claims in OTC products. On the Canadian Hotlist (*see*). In Canada, hair dye products must carry a caution: "This product contains ingredients that may cause skin irritation on certain individuals and a preliminary test according to accompanying directions should first be made. This product must not be used for dying the eyelashes or eyebrows. To do so, may cause blindness." When permitted in shampoos or conditioners, which are to be washed off after less than twenty minutes, provided the product is not represented as therapeutic (for control of dandruff, psoriasis, etc.), the coal tars do not pose a hazard or safety concern at the concentration present in the product, and in Canada "no reference to their presence is made on the product labeling, other than a complete ingredient declaration without undue emphasis. May cause acne." Crude and refined coal tars have been banned in cosmetics by ASEAN. Coal tar is number 23 on the CERCLA (*see*) Priority List of Hazardous Substances.

COBALT ACETYLMETHIONATE • The metal cobalt mixed with methionine (*see*). The EU bans cobalt in cosmetics.

COBALT ALUMINUM • Coloring.

COBALT BENZENESULPHONATE • Banned in cosmetics by the EU and on the Canadian Hotlist. *See* Benzene.

COBALT CHLORIDE • A metal used in hair dye. Occurs in the earth's crust; gray, hard, and magnetic. Excess administration can produce an overproduction of red blood cells and gastrointestinal upset. The EU bans cobalt in cosmetics. *See* Metallic Hair Dyes.

COBALT NAPHTHTHENATE • *See* Cobalt Chloride.

COCA • Theobroma cacao. *See* Cocoa.

COCAINE AND SALTS • From the leaves of *Erythroxylon coca* and other species of *Erythroxylon,* it is a controlled substance. It is used in cosmetics as a topical anesthetic.

COCAMIDE (DEA, MEA) • Widely used fatty acid of coconut oil. Used as a thickener and foam booster. Formation of nitrosamines (*see*) are a problem with these ingredients. Based on the available data, the CIR Expert Panel (*see*) concludes that cocamide DEA is safe as a cosmetic ingredient in concentrations up to 10 percent; however, it should not be used in cosmetic products containing nitrosating ingredients. Has been linked to allergic reactions. *See* Coconut Oil.

COCAMIDE BETAINE • May form nitrosamines (*see*). Based on the available data, the CIR Expert Panel (*see*) concludes that this ingredient is safe as a cosmetic ingredient. However, it should not be used in cosmetic products containing nitrosating ingredients. Has been linked to allergic reactions. *See* Quaternary Ammonium Compounds and Coconut Oil.

COCAMIDE MIPA • May cause allergies. *See* Coconut Oil.

COCAMIDOPROPYL BETAINE • Widely used salt of fatty acids, it is used in hair conditioners. It is antistatic and a cleanser. It is also a foam booster and a thickener. *See* Coconut Oil.

COCAMIDOPROPYL DIMETHYLAMINE • An antistatic ingredient. *See* Coconut Oil.

COCAMIDOPROPYL DIMETHYLAMINE HYDROLYZED COLLAGEN • A hair and skin conditioner. *See* Hydrolyzed Collagen and Coconut Oil.

COCAMIDOPROPYL DIMETHYLAMINE LACTATE • A hair-conditioning ingredient. *See* Lactic Acid and Coconut Oil.

COCAMIDOPROPYL DIMETHYLAMMONIUM C8–16 ISOALKYLSUC-CINYL LACTOGLOBULIN SULFONATE • Used as a hair- and skin-conditioning ingredient. *See* Lactic Acid and Coconut Oil.

COCAMIDOPROPYL HYDROXYSULTAINE • Widely used as an antistatic ingredient in hair and skin creams. It is also used to increase foaming and thickening ingredients in shampoos and bath preparations. *See* Coconut Oil.

COCAMIDOPROPYL OXIDE • *See* Coconut Oil.

COCAMIDOPROPYL SULTAMINE • *See* Coconut Oil.

COCAMIDOPROPYLAMINE OXIDE • *See* Coconut Oil.

COCAMINE OXIDE • *See* Coconut Oil.

COCAMINOBUTYRIC ACID • *See* Coconut Oil and Butyric acid.

COCAMINOPROPIONIC ACID • *See* Coconut Oil.

COCAMPHODIPRIOPIONATE • *See* Coconut Oil.

COCAMPHODIPROPIONIC ACID • *See* Coconut Oil.

CO-CARCINOGEN • A substance that works together with a cancer-causing substance to produce cancer.

COCCINIA INDICA • From the fruit of *Coccinia indica.*

COCETH-6 • *See* Coconut Oil.

COCETH-10 • A derivative of coconut alcohol, it is used as an emulsifying ingredient.

COCHINEAL • Ponceau Red 4R. The European Union calls it CI 75470. A deep crimson dye is extracted from the female cochineal insects. Cochineal is used to produce scarlet, orange, and other red tints. The coloring comes from carminic acid. Cochineal extract's natural carminic-acid content is usually 19–22 percent. The insects are killed by immersion in hot water (after which they are dried) or by exposure to sunlight, steam, or the heat of an oven. Each method produces a different color, which results in the varied appearance of commercial cochineal. Because it is an azo dye, it may elicit intolerance in people allergic to salicylates (aspirin). University of Michigan medical researchers said this color additive extracted from dried bugs and used in candy, yogurt, fruit drinks, and other foods can cause life-threatening allergic reactions. Additionally, it is a histamine liberator and may intensify symptoms of asthma. It is considered carcinogenic in some countries, including the United States, Norway, and Finland, and it is currently listed as a banned substance by the U.S. Food and Drug Administration (FDA). Since 2000 the FDA has seized Chinese-produced haw flakes (a fruit candy) on numerous occasions for containing Ponceau 4R. Possible cause of hyperactivity. On September 6, 2007, the British Food Standards Agency revised advice on certain artificial food additives, including this. Cochineal or Ponceau Red 4R is often listed as a "natural" ingredient on the label. A paper on the subject was published as long ago as 1997 in the November issue of *Annals of Allergy, Asthma & Immunology.* At this writing, the British and European Parliament and the UK are seeking to ban this coloring because it reportedly affects hyperactivity in young children, and, under a new FDA ruling, food and drink manufacturers that color their products with cochineal extract and carmine must declare the ingredients on the label. The FDA said it has revised its requirements for these color additives in response to reports of severe allergic reactions, including anaphylaxis, to food containing cochineal extract and food and cosmetics containing carmine. ASP. *See* Carmine. E

COCHLEARIA ARMORACIA and C. OFFICINALIS • *Armoracia lapathifolia gilib.* Horseradish. Scurvy Grass. Contains ascorbic acid (*see*) and acts as an antiseptic in cosmetics. It contains vitamin C and is used by herbalists to treat arthritis pain by stimulating blood flow to inflamed joints. Potential adverse reactions include diarrhea and sweating if taken internally in large amounts. GRAS

COCILLANA BARK • Dried bark of *Guarea rusbyi,* grown in Bolivia. Contains resins, fat, and tannin. Used in emollients.

COCKSCOMB EXTRACT • Gallus Extract. Obained from the enzymatic decomposition of rooster (gallus) cockscomb used as a moisturizer and skin conditioner.

COCKSCOMB FLOWER • *Celosia cristata.* Ji Guan Hua. *See* Amaranthus Caudatus.

COCO PROTEIN • Used in "organic" shampoos. *See* Coconut Oil.

COCOA • A powder prepared from the roasted and cured kernels of ripe seeds of *Theobroma cacao* and other species of *Theobroma.* A brownish powder with a chocolate odor, it is used as a flavoring. May cause wheezing, rash, and other symptoms of allergy, particularly in children. A nanoemulsion of the cocoa bean extract is a newer ingredientt in skin care. *See* NanoCocoa.

COCOA BUTTER • Theobroma Oil. Softens and lubricates the skin. A solid fat expressed from the roasted seeds of the cocoa plant that is used in eyelash creams, lipsticks, nail whiteners, rouge, pastes, soaps, and emollient creams as a lubricant and skin softener. Frequently used in massage creams and in suppositories because it softens and melts at body temperature. May cause allergic skin reactions. EAF

COCOA BUTTER SUBSTITUTE FROM COCONUT OIL • GRAS. EAF

COCOA BUTTER SUBSTITUTE FROM HIGH OLEIC SAFFLOWER • Good substitute for olive oil and shea butter (*see both*). EAF

COCOA BUTTER SUBSTITUTE FROM PALM KERNEL OIL • Coating material for vitamins, citric acid, succinic acid, and spices. Used in lieu of cocoa butter in sweets. It is also used to cover vitamins. There is reported use of the chemical; it has not yet been assigned for toxicology literature. GRAS. EAF

COCOA EXTRACT • Extract of *Theobroma cacao. See* Cocoa Butter.

COCOALKONIUM CHLORIDE • A quaternary ammonium compound (*see*).

COCOAMIDOETHYL BETAINE • A surfactant, cleansing ingredient, and foam booster. *See* Betaines and Coconut Oil.

COCOAMIDOPROPYL BETAINE • Made from coconut oil and beets, it is used in eye makeup remover. Found in baby and adult shampoos. May cause facial or neck dermatitis, even if it doesn't cause scalp problems. The face and neck are more sensitive than the scalp. May cause an eyelid rash.

COCOAMINDOPROPYL AMINE OXIDE • Widely used hair conditioner, bath ingredient, lotion, and tonic ingredient in hair-grooming products. Based on the available data, the CIR Expert Panel (*see*) concludes that there is insufficient data to support the safety of this ingredient in cosmetic products. *See* Quaternary Ammonium Compounds and Coconut Oil.

COCOAMPHOACTATE • *See* Coconut Oil.

COCOAMPHOCARBOXYMETHYLHYDROXYPROPYLSULFONATE • *See* Coconut Oil.

COCOAMPHOCARBOXYPROPIONIC ACID • *See* Coconut Oil.

COCOAMPHODIACETATE • Widely used in cosmetics in the manufacture of toilet soaps, creams, lubricants, chocolate, and suppositories. *See* Coconut Oil.

COCOAMPHOHYDROXYPROPYLSULFONATE • *See* Coconut Oil.

COCOAMPHODIPROPIONATE • *See* Coconut Oil.

COCO-BETAINE • *See* Coconut Oil.

COCO-CAPRYLATECAPRATE • An emollient. *See* Coconut Oil.

COCO-GLUCOSIDE • Cleansing ingredient. *See* Coconut Oil and Carbohydrates.

COCO-GLYCERIDES • Skin-conditioning ingredient and emollient. *See* Coconut Oil and Glycerides.

COCO-RAPESEEDATE • An ester of coconut oil and rapeseed oil (*see both*) used as an emollient ingredient.

COCO-SULTAINE • An antistatic ingredient in hair products and a skin-conditioning ingredient. Also a foam booster. *See* Coconut Oil and Betaines.

COCODIMONIUM-HYDROXYPROPYL HYDROLYZED COLLAGEN • *See* Quaternary Ammonium Compounds.

COCODIMONIUM HYDROXYPROPYL HYDROLYZED HAIR KERATIN • Hydrolyzed (*see*) hair keratin. Used as an antistatic ingredient and as a skin conditioner.

COCODIMONIUM HYDROXYPROPYL SILK AMINO ACID • Quaternary ammonium compound (*see*) used as antistatic ingredient in hair and skin products. *See* Coconut Oil and Silk.

COCOMORPHOLINE OXIDE • *See* Coconut Oil.

COCONUT • The fruit of the coconut palm. The coconut consists of an outer fibrous husk enclosing a large nut that contains a white edible layer. Coconut is often dried and grated and used extensively in cooking and confectionery. The coconut also produces a valuable oil that has been used for thousands of years. Sap from the coconut tree can be fermented and used to produce a palm wine, which is similar to the Turkish arrack or arak spirit. Coconut aroma and flavor is often found in red wines and is a quality that is attributed to the use of certain oak barrels.

COCONUT ACIDS • Surfactants and cleansing ingredients used in bath soaps and detergents, shaving creams, cold creams, and shampoos. *See* Coconut Oil.

COCONUT ALCOHOLS • *See* Coconut Oil.

COCONUT FATTY ACIDS • *See* Coconut Oil and Fatty Acids.

COCONUT OIL • *Cocos nucifera*. The white, semisolid, highly saturated fat expressed from the kernels of the coconut. Widely used in the manufacture of baby soaps, shampoos, shaving lathers, cuticle removers, preshaving lotions, hairdressings, soaps, ointment bases, and massage creams. Stable when exposed to air. Lathers readily and is a fine skin cleanser. Usually blended with other fats. May cause allergic skin rashes.

COCONUT PROTEIN • Derived from coconut, it is used in shampoos, particularly in "natural" products.

COCOTRIMONIUM CHLORIDE • Coconut Trimethyl Ammonium Chloride. *See* Quaternary Ammonium Compounds.

COCOYL HYDROLYZED COLLAGEN • Formerly called cocoyl hydrolyzed animal protein. *See* Hydrolyzed and Proteins.

COCOYL HYDROLYZED SOY PROTEIN • Used as a hair- and skin-conditioning ingredient. *See* Coconut Oil and Soy Acid.

COCOYL HYDROXYETHYL IMIDAZOLINE • *See* Coconut Oil and Imidazoline.

COCOYL IMIDAZOLINE • Heterocyclic compound used as a detergent emulsifier. *See* Cocoa Butter and Ethylenediamine.

COCOYL SARCOSINAMIDE DEA • Diethanolamine Cocoyl Sarcosinamide. Used as a detergent emulsifier. *See* Cocoa Butter.

COCOYL SARCOSINE • Formed from caffeine by decomposition with barium hydroxide. Used to make antienzyme ingredients for toothpastes that help to prevent decay.

COCOYLDIMONIUM HYDROXYPROPYL HYDROLYZED COLLA-GEN • A hydrolyzed animal protein used in emollients. *See* Coconut Oil and Proteins.

COCOYL-POLYGLYCERYL-4-HYDROXYPROPYL DIHYDROXYETHY-LAMINE • *See* Coconut Oil and Surfactants.

COD-LIVER OIL • The fixed oil expressed from fresh cod livers used in skin ointments and special skin creams to promote healing. Pale yellow, with a bland, slightly fishy odor. Contains vitamins A and D, which promote healing of wounds and abscesses.

CODIUM TOMENTOSUM • Extract of *Codium tomentosum,* a green seaweed used as a food in Asia. Used as a moisturizer in cosmetics.

CODONOPSIS • Extract from the root of *Codonopsis tangshen.* Codonopsis is a fast-growing vine that blooms during the summer and fall. The roots of codonopsis are harvested during its third or fourth year of growth and are used medicinally. The chief chemical components of codonopsis include saccharides such as fructose and inulin. It also contains glycosides (such as syringin and tangshenoside I), alkaloids (such as choline and perlolyrine), and seventeen kinds of amino acids and microelements. Codonopsis is known as the "poor man's ginseng." There are scientific studies concerning its use in bolstering immunity. It is used in massage products.

COENZYME A • Participant in a variety of biochemical reactions, including the breakdown of carbohydrates and fats. Coenzyme A is derived from adenine, ribose, and pantothenic acid (a vitamin of the B complex). Used in skin conditioners.

COENZYME Q10 • *See* COQ10.

COFFEA ARABICA • Extract of coffee. Used as a fragrance ingredient and skin-conditioning ingredient.

COFFEA ROBUSTA EXTRACT • Extract of green coffee.

COFFEE OIL • Used as a flavoring.

COGNAC OIL • Wine Yeast Oil. The volatile oil obtained from distillation of wine, with the characteristic aroma of cognac. Green cognac oil is used as a flavoring for beverages, ice cream, ices, candy, baked goods, chewing gum, liquors, and condiments. White cognac oil, which has the same constituents as green oil, is used in berry, cherry, grape, brandy, and rum flavorings. It is used in cosmetics as a flavoring and for its aroma. GRAS

COHOSH ROOT, BLACK AND BLUE • Black cohosh is *Cimicifuga racemosa.* Black Snakeroot. Bugbane. Rattleroot. The root contains various glycosides (*see*), including estrogenic substances and tannins. Herbalists use it to relieve nerve pains and to relieve menstrual pains and the pain of childbirth. It is also used to speed delivery to reduce blood pressure. Black cohosh is also believed to have sedative properties. In 1992, the FDA proposed a ban on black cohosh in oral menstrual drug products because it has not been shown to be safe and effective for its stated claims. Blue cohosh is *Caulophyllum thalictrioides.* Papoose root. Squaw root. The rhizome contains fungicidal saponin, glycosides, gum, starch, salts, phosphoric acid, and a soluble resin. Herbalists use it for menstrual irregularities and pain and to ease the pain of childbirth. It is also used to treat worms.

COIX LACRYMA-JOBI • Extract of Job's Tears. Asiatic flowers and seeds. *See* Job's Tears.

COLA ACUMINATA • Kola nut extract. Guru Nut. A natural extract from the brownish seed, about the size of a chestnut, produced by trees in Africa, the West Indies, and Brazil. Contains caffeine (*see*). Cola nuts are chewed for the stimulating effect of the alkaloids caffeine and theobromine they contain. Used in flavorings and skin stimulants. GRAS

COLA NITIDA • *See* Cola Acuminata.

COLCHICINE • Colabid. ColBenemid. Colsalide. Novo colchicine. A drug introduced in 1763 prepared from roots of the meadow saffron (*see*), which is specific in relieving gout, but why it works is unclear. It impairs the absorption of vitamin B_{12}. Its salts and derivatives are banned in cosmetics by the EU.

COLCHICUM AUTUMNALE • On the Canadian Hotlist (*see*). *See* Cochicine and Meadow Saffron. Banned in cosmetics by the EU.

COLD CREAM • Originally developed by the Greek physician Galen, the original formula consisted of a mixture of olive oil, beeswax, water, and rose petals. The product was called cold cream because after it was applied to the skin, the water evaporated and gave a feeling of coolness. Cold cream is still used, although the olive oil has been replaced with mineral or other oils that do not so easily become rancid. Beeswax (*see*) can cause allergic contact dermatitis, as can rose petals, perfume, or other additives added to the original formula. *See also* Cleansing Creams and Lotions.

COLETH-24 • Emulsifier and emollient derived from cholesterol and ethylene oxide.

COLEUS BARBATUS EXTRACT • An extract of the roots of an herb with large blue flowers, a member of the mint family. Used as a humectant (*see*) in oral care products and skin conditioners. May be irritating.

COLEUS OIL • Coleus oil is an essential oil extracted from the roots of *Coleus forskohlii,* a plant from the Natural Order Labiatae (Lamiaceae), a family of mints and lavenders. This species is a perennial herb with fleshy, fibrous roots that grows wild in the warm subtropical temperate areas in South Asia. The roots are eaten as a condiment or pickle in India. In recent years *C. forskohlii* has gained pharmacological importance as the only known plant source of the biologically active compound forskolin, and coleus oil is a useful by-product of forskolin extraction. The newly discovered antimicrobial properties of the oil (of specific composition obtained using a proprietary extraction process) render it useful in topical preparations. Has a pleasing spicy aroma.

COLIPA • The European Cosmetic, Toiletry, and Perfumery Association. Colipa is the European trade association representing the interests of the cosmetics, toiletry, and perfumery industries and was set up in 1962 to act as a voice for the multibillion-dollar industry. Colipa's membership consists of the national associations of the fifteen EU member states, twenty-three major international companies, and thirteen associate or corresponding members—a total of more than two thousand companies ranging from major international firms to small family-run organizations, often operating in niche markets. The cosmetics industry employs over five hundred thousand people in the European Union and claims it is committed to the "on-going development of safe, innovative and effective products and to continuously meeting the demands of consumers through intensive market research and enhanced product information."

COLLAGEN • Protein substance found in connective tissue. In cosmetics, it is usually derived from animal tissue. The collagen fibers in connective tissues of the skin undergo changes from aging and overexposure to the sun that contribute to the appearance of wrinkles and other outward signs of aging. Cosmetics manufacturers have heralded collagen as a new wonder ingredient, but according to medical experts, it cannot affect the skin's own collagen when applied topically. However, it is being used to fill out acne scars and other depressions, including wrinkles, by injection. Allergic reactions are not infrequent, and test spots are supposed to be done first to see whether an allergic response is provoked. Derived from animal skin and ground-up chicken feet, it has been alleged that these ingredients form films that may smother and overmoisturize the skin.

COLLAGEN AMINO ACIDS • Formerly called animal collagen amino acids. The major protein of the white fibers of connective tissue, cartilage, and bone that is insoluble in water but is easily altered to gelatins by boiling in water, dilute acids, or alkalis. *See* Collagen and Amino Acids.

COLLINSONIA CANADENSIS • Stone Root. A member of the mint family. Among the Iroquois and other nations in the east, the roots of this plant have a tradition of use as a stimulating remedy for ailments of the heart and kidneys, as well as for general listlessness. The leaves and root of the plant have been applied externally as an anti-inflammatory, while the leaves have been taken internally to induce vomiting. *See* Stoneroot.

COLLODION • A mixture of nitrocellulose, alcohol, and ether in a syrupy liquid, colorless or slightly yellow. It is used as a skin protectant, in clear nail polish, as a corn remover, in the manufacture of lacquers, artificial pearls, and cement. May cause allergic skin reactions.

COLLOIDAL OATMEAL • Meal obtained by grinding oats. Soothing to the skin. In 1992, the FDA proposed a ban on colloidal oatmeal in astringent (*see*) drug products because it had not been shown to be safe and effective as claimed.

COLLOIDAL SULFUR • A pale yellow mixture of sulfur and acacia (*see*) used as an emulsifier. *See* Sulfur.

COLLYRIUM • A commercial preparation for local application to the eye, usually a wash or lotion. *See* Boric Acid.

COLOCASIA ANTIQUORUM • A small family of Asiatic herbs. *See* Taro.

COLOCYNTH • *Citrullus colocynthis.* Bitter Apple. A denaturant used in alcohols for cosmetics. Derived from the dried pulp of a fruit grown in the Mediterranean and Near East regions. It is a super cathartic if ingested and has caused deaths. Has also caused allergic problems in cosmeticians.

COLOGNE • Scented liquid products typically made of alcohol and various fragrant oils. They are also called eau de cologne. Named originally after the city in Germany, it is usually limited to citrus and floral bases. It has a higher alcohol content than perfume, usually is applied more generously, and leaves a cooling, refreshing feeling on the skin. It is also made as a paste or semisolid stick. May cause allergic reactions depending on ingredients. Those allergic to citrus and floral bases should avoid colognes and try perfumes made of wood or animal scents. There are nineteen ingredients commonly found in colognes (*see all*):

- Alcohol Denat.
- Beeswax
- Botanical Ingredients
- Butane
- Butylene Glycol
- Colorants
- Diethyl Phthalate
- Diisopropyl Adipate
- Dimethicone
- Dipropylene Glycol
- Fragrance
- Glycerin

- Glyceryl Stearate
- PEG-4 Dilaurate
- PEG-100 Stearate
- Petrolatum
- Polysorbate 20
- Propylene Glycol
- UV Filter Ingredients

COLOGNE, SOLID • Solid colognes are used in sticks or in small containers. Such products consist of 80 percent alcohol, about 10 percent sodium stearate, some sorbitol, cologne essence, and water. Gel colognes consist of 60 to 70 percent alcohol, perfume oils, emulsifiers, and about 30 percent water.

COLOPHONY • *See* Rosin and Pine Resin.

COLORS • Food colors of both natural and synthetic origin are extensively used in cosmetics. When the letters FD & C precede a color, it means the color can be used in a food, drug, or cosmetic. When D & C precede the color, it signifies that it can only be used in drugs or cosmetics, but not in food. Ext. D & C before a color means that it is certified for external use only in drugs and cosmetics and may not be used on the lips or mucous membranes. No coal tar colors are permitted for use around the eyes. In fact, the FDA does not allow any color additive to be applied around the area of the eye unless specifically approved for that purpose. There is still a great deal of controversy about the use of coal tar colors because almost all have been shown to cause cancer when injected into the skins of mice. Furthermore, many people are allergic to coal tar products. The bulk of the colors are derived from coal tar. Aniline, a coal tar derivative, is poisonous in its pure state.

A provisional listing is a category that is supposed to be abolished. It consists of colors whose safety has not been proven or even studied; in some cases this dates back to when the list was enacted in 1960. Permanent listing means the FDA is convinced that the dye is safe to use as it is now employed in cosmetics. Batch-by-batch certification is used to determine how well the concoction matches the FDA standards—the chemical formula approved. The color additives for which certification is not required are mostly dyes or pigments of vegetable, animal, or mineral origin, and generally require less processing. Many of the colors are vegetable compounds—beet powder, caramel, beta-carotene, grape skin extract. A few are of animal origin—cochineal extract, taken from the dried bodies of certain insects. Among the natural colors used are annatto, carotene, chlorophyll, saffron, and turmeric. The big problem with coal tar colors, of course, is their potential as carcinogens, but they are also potential sensitizers. Each batch of a coal tar color has to be certified as "safe." F & C Red No. 40 is one of the most widely used coal tar colorings. *See also* Yellow No. 5, Tartrazine, Coal Tar, Catechu Black, and Carmine. The word *pigment,* however, usually means a colored or white chemical compound that is insoluble in a particular solvent. The word *dye* generally refers to a chemical compound, most often of coal tar origin, which is soluble.

Cosmetic manufacturers have unique problems with coloring their products. They must choose a color substance that is not only safe and stable in a product, but one that will psychologically entice the customer into buying the product. For instance, most hand lotions are either white, pink, cream, or blue. Research sponsored by cosmetic companies has shown that women over twenty-five years of age want pink shades while teenagers prefer blue hand lotions.

Many natural colors derived from plants and animals have been in use since humans first started trying to make themselves look better with makeup. Examples of such naturally derived colors are annatto, saffron, chlorophyll, and beta-carotene (*see all*). Inorganic colors used in cosmetics include iron oxides, bronze powder, ultramarines, chromium oxide greens, and a number of white products such as titanium dioxide, barium sulfate, and zinc oxide (*see all*). However, widely used and under FDA scrutiny are the coal tar colors. In 1900, there were more than eighty dyes in use in cosmetics, foods, and drugs. There were no regulations and the same dye used to color clothes could also be used to color candy or cosmetics. In 1906, the first comprehensive legislation for food colors was passed. There were only seven colors that, when tested, were shown to be composed of known ingredients that demonstrated no harmful effects. A voluntary system of certification for batches of color dyes was set up. In 1938, new legislation was passed, superseding the 1906 act. The colors were given numbers instead of chemical names and every batch had to be certified. The manufacturers must submit to the government samples from every batch of coal tar color. Each sample is analyzed for purity. The lot test number must then accompany the colors through all subsequent packaging. The manufacturer must pay 15 cents a pound and not less than $100 for each batch tested. Each petition for listing of a new color additive must be accompanied by a deposit of $2,600 for cosmetics. To amend a listing asking for a new use of a color, the government requires a check of $1,800. If you want to object or request public hearings on a color, it will cost you $250.

What is considered a safe color? According to the FDA: "Safety for external color additives will normally be determined by tests for acute oral toxicity, primary irritation, sensitization, subacute skin toxicity on intact or abraded skin and carcinogenicity (cancer causing) by skin application." The FDA commissioner may waive any such tests if data before him established otherwise that such a test is not required to determine safety. Here are the certified colors classified into the following categories according to their chemical ancestry:

1. Nitro Dyes. Containing one atom of nitrogen and two of oxygen, there are only a few certified because they can be absorbed through the skin and are toxic. Ext. D & C Yellow is one. *See* Nitro-.

2. Azo (monoazo). This includes the largest number. They are all characterized by the presence of the azo bond. *See* Azo Dyes.

3. Triphenylmethane. FD & C Blue No. 1 is the most popular dye of this group and is widely used. *See* Triphenylmethane Group.

4. Xanthene. This group contains very brilliant, widely used lipstick colors. D & C Orange is one. *See* Xanthene.

5. Quinoline. There are only two certified in this category, D & C Yellow No. 10 and No. 11. They are bright greenish yellows. *See* Quinoline.

6. Anthraquinone. Widely used in cosmetics because it is not affected by light. Ext. D & C Violet No. 2 is one. *See* Anthraquinone.

7. Indigo. These dyes have been in use a long time. D & C Blue No. 6 is an example. *See* Indigo. There are a few other miscellaneous dyes.

In 1950, children were made ill by certain coloring used in candy and popcorn. These incidents led to the delisting of FD & C Orange No. 1 and Orange No. 2 and FD & C

Red No. 32. Since that time, because of experimental evidence of possible harm, Red 1, Yellow 1, 2, 3, and 4 have also been delisted. Violet 1 was removed in 1973. In 1976, one of the most widely used of all colors, FD & C Red No. 2, was removed because it was found to cause tumors in rats. In 1976, Red No. 4 was banned for coloring maraschino cherries (its last use), and carbon black was also banned at the same time because it contains cancer-causing ingredients. Earlier, in 1960, scientific investigations were required by law to determine the suitability of all colors in use for permanent listing. Citrus Red No. 2 (limited to 2 ppm) for coloring orange skins has been permanently listed; Blue No. 1, Red No. 3, Yellow No. 5, and Red No. 40 are permanently listed but without any restrictions. In 1959, the Food and Drug Administration approved the use of "lakes," in which the dyes have been mixed with alumina hydrate to make them insoluble. *See* FD & C Lakes. The other food, drug, and cosmetic coloring additives remained on the "temporary list." The provisional list permitted colors then in use to continue on a provisional, or interim, basis pending completion of studies to determine whether the colors should be permanently approved or terminated. FD & C Red No. 3 (erythrosine) is permanently listed for use in food and ingested drugs and provisionally listed for cosmetics and externally applied drugs. It is used in foods such as gelatins, cake mixes, ice cream, fruit cocktail cherries, bakery goods, and sausage casings.

The FDA postponed the May 2, 1988, closing date for three provisionally listed color additives—FD & C Red No. 3, D & C Red No. 33, and D & C Red No. 36—to allow additional time to study "complex scientific and legal questions about the colors before deciding to approve or terminate their use in food, drugs and cosmetics." The Agency asked for sixty days to consider the impact of the October 1987 U.S. Court of Appeals ruling that there is no exception to the Delaney Amendment (*see*), which says that cancer-causing ingredients may not be added to food.

On July 13, 1988, the Public Citizens Health Research Group announced that the FDA agreed to revoke by July 15, 1988, the permanent listing of four color additives used in drugs and cosmetics—D & C Red No. 8, D & C Red No. 9, D & C Red No. 19, and D & C Orange No. 17. In a unanimous decision in October 1987, the U.S. Court of Appeals for the District of Columbia said the FDA lacked legal authority to approve two of the colors, D & C Orange No. 17 and D & C Red No. 19, since they had been found to induce cancer in laboratory animals. The Supreme Court ruled against an appeal on April 18, 1988. Meanwhile, Public Citizens Health Group also brought a similar suit, challenging the use of D & C Red No. 8 and D & C Red No. 9, which was before the U.S. Circuit Court of Appeals in Philadelphia. Under an agreement between the FDA and Public Citizens, the case was sent back to the FDA, and the agency delisted these colors as well as D & C Orange No. 17 and D & C Red No. 19.

Other countries, as well as the World Health Organization, maintain there are inconsistencies in safety data and in the banning of some colors, which, in turn, affects international commerce. As of this writing, there is still a great deal of confusion about the colors, with the FDA maintaining that the cancer risk is minimal—as low as one in a billion—for the colors; and groups such as Ralph Nader's Public Citizens Health Group maintaining that any cancer risk for a food additive is unacceptable. In 1990, the lakes (*see*) of Red No. 3 were removed for all uses from the approved list. The color itself was also removed in 1990 for cosmetic and external drug use. It is still, as of this writing, approved for food and ingested drugs.

COLORS, NATURAL • Lycopene, caramel, annatto, red beet juice, turmeric, paprika, chlorophlly green, anthocyan (*see all*). There is controversy over whether cochineal (*see*) is a natural color.

COLOSTRUM • A thin, white, opalescent fluid, the first milk secreted at the end of pregnancy. It differs from milk secreted later because it contains more protein and albumen. It is also rich in antibodies, which confer passive immunity to the newborn. Used in skin-conditioning ingredients.

COLTSFOOT • *Tussilago farfara.* Wild Ginger. Used for its soothing properties in shampoos and astringents. From an herb used historically to fight colds and asthma, it reputedly opens pores and allows sweating. It has been used as a soothing ointment.

COMBRETUM MICRANTHUM • Germicide in cosmetics used medically against herpes. A tropical shrub rich in tannins (*see*).

COMEDOGEN • A substance that promotes acne and blackheads. Usually oily or greasy ingredients that block hair follicles, which subsequently become filled with products of glands and skin, causing bacteria to breed and lead to a localized inflammation or infection.

COMEDONES • Acne lesions. Plugs of sebaceous (oil) matter that obstruct the hair follicle. They are called whiteheads if the top of the follicle remains narrow, and blackheads if the follicle is stretched wide.

COMFREY • *Symphytum officinale.* Knitbone. Blackwort. Healing Herb. The leaf and root contain allantoin, mucilage, tannins, starch, inulin (*see*), steroidal saponins, and pyrrolizine alkaloids. It has been reported to be toxic when taken internally and to cause liver damage. Herbalists recommend comfrey for rapid wound and bone healing and use a decoction for diarrhea, hemorrhage, and bleeding. Potential adverse reactions include liver dysfunction. Pyrrolizidine alkaloids have been found to cause cancer in laboratory rats. Formerly regarded as safe, reports of toxic effects surfaced when its use became popular. Symptoms of poisoning appear after a few months of use. It is a strong liver toxin. Comfrey was banned in Canada in 1989. Widely used in cosmetics in eye makeup, bath soaps, skin fresheners, foundations, cold creams, and cleansing lotions.

COMFREY EXTRACT • The extract of the roots and rhizomes of *Symphytum officinale.* Used for centuries by monks as a healer of bruises, a mouthwash and gargle, and as a compress for eye injuries.

COMMIPHORA ABYSSINICA • Myrrh Gum. *Commiphora molmol* or myrrh or Guggul. One of the gifts of the Magi, it is a yellowish to reddish brown, aromatic, bitter gum resin that is obtained from various myrrh trees, especially from East Africa and Arabia. The gum resin has been used to break up intestinal gas and as a topical stimulant. The Chinese, for centuries, used the herb to treat menstrual problems and bleeding. In Asia and Africa, it was used as an antiseptic for mucous membranes. It is also used as a stimulant tonic; there are constituents in myrrh that stimulate gastric secretions and relax smooth muscles. In modern studies, myrrh has been shown to inhibit gram-positive bacteria such as *Staphylococcus aureus.* The herb contains volatile oils, including limonene, eugenol, and pinene, which have been found helpful in easing breathing during colds, and increasing circulation. It also contains tannin, which is thought to be the reason that myrrh allays the pain and speeds the healing of mouth ulcers and sore gums. In 1992, the FDA issued a notice that myrrh fluid extract had not been shown to be safe and effective as claimed in OTC digestive aid products.

COMMUNITY RIGHT-TO-KNOW LIST • Manufacturers that employ toxic chemicals while making products must respond, under the law, to inquiries from employees and citizens in the area. Cyanide, which is used in the manufacture of pesticides and some food additives, is an example of a chemical on this list compiled by the U.S. Environmental Protection Agency.

CONCHIORIN POWDER • A protein found in the pearl oyster. Used as a skin-conditioning ingredient.

CONCRETES • Waxlike substances prepared from natural raw materials, almost exclusively vegetable in origin, such as bark, flower, herb, leaf, and root and used in perfumes and stick deodorants.

CONDITIONERS • Applied to the hair after shampooing to improve its sheen, feel, and controllability. Usually rinsed off, but many stay-on products have come on the market that coat the hair. *See* Hair Conditioners and Emollients.

CONDITIONING CREAMS • See Emollients.

CONDURANGO EXTRACT • Eagle Vine. *Marsdenia condurango.* An American vine. The dried bark contains glycosides, resin, tannin (*see all*), and oils. A bitter-tasting herb, it is used to treat digestive and stomach problems, stimulate appetite, and relax nerves. Used in herbal makeups.

CONEFLOWER EXTRACT • *See* Echinacea.

CONEFLOWERS • *See* Echinacea.

CONIUM MACULATUM • Hemlock. Poison Hemlock. Poison Parsley. Found in many parts of Europe and the Americas, hemlock is related to parsnip, carrot, celery, fennel, and parsley. It is famed as the poison used to execute Socrates and other ancient Greeks; it was mixed with opium and used as a suicide drink for old, frail Roman philosophers. The narcotic drug, conium, comes from the dried, unripe fruit of hemlock. Herbalists once used it is a sedative, antispasmodic, and an antidote to other poisons. Hemlock is poisonous. On the Canadian Hotlist (*see*). The EU banned it in cosmetics.

CONJUGATED GLYCOPROTEINS • A composition made up of carbohydrates and simple proteins. Used in tanning creams.

CONJUNCTIVITIS • Pink Eye. An infection of the membrane that lines the eyelids and covers the white portion of the eye.

CONNECTIVE TISSUE • Extract of animal connective tissue used in anti-aging products.

CONTACT DERMATITIS • *See* Allergic Contact Dermatitis.

CONTACT DERMATITIS OF THE EYELIDS • *See* Eyelids.

CONVALLARIA MAJALIS • Lily of the Valley. Fragrance from the roots and bulbs of *Convallaria majalis.* Perennial herb from a slender rhizome; two or three leaves, basal. Poisonous if ingested. Causes irregular and slow pulse, abdominal pain, and diarrhea. *See* Lily of the Valley.

CONVALLATOXIN • Toxic glycoside isolated from lily of the valley (*Convallaria majalis*); used as a radiotonic agent and for its digitalis-like actions. Banned in cosmetics by the EU.

COPAIBA BALSAM • *Balsam capivi.* Jesuit's balsam. Oleoresin from South American species of *Copaifera leguminosae* found in Brazil, Venezuela, Colombia, and the Amazon valley. A transparent, thick, yellowish liquid with a strange odor and bitter, acrid taste, it is used in the manufacture of paper and to remove oil.

COPAIFERA OFFICINALIS • *See* Copaiba Balsam.

COPAL • A resin obtained as a fossil or as an exudate from various species of tropical plants. Must be heated in alcohol or other solvents. Used in nail enamels. May cause allergic reactions, particularly skin rashes.

COPERNICIA CERIFERA • *See* Carnauba Wax.

COPOLYMER • Result of polymerization (*see* Polymer), which includes at least two different molecules, each of which is capable of polymerizing alone. Together they form a new, distinct molecule. They are used in the manufacture of nail enamels, face creams, and masks.

COPPERCEUTICALS • The use of copper in compounds to prevent scarring of the skin and as a proposed anti-aging ingredient. Reportedly, safety tests of skin regenerative copper peptides have failed to find any toxicity problem. Extremely small amounts penetrate the skin, and no rise in blood copper has been reported in animals or humans treated with copper peptides.

COPPER, METALLIC POWDER, AND VERSENATE • Used as a coloring ingredient in cosmetics. One of the earliest known metals. An essential nutrient for all mammals. Naturally occurring or experimentally produced copper deficiency in animals leads to a variety of abnormalities including anemia, skeletal defects, and muscle degeneration. Copper itself is nontoxic, but soluble copper salts, notably copper sulfate, are highly irritating to the skin and mucous membranes and when ingested cause serious vomiting. Copper metallic powder was permanently listed as a cosmetic coloring in 1977.

COPPER GLUCONATE • An odorless, light blue, fine powder. Used as a feed additive, dietary supplement, and mouth deodorant. *See* Copper.

COPPER-8-HYDROXYQUINOLATE • *See* Copper and Oxyquinoline Sulfate.

COPPER PCA • A humectant. *See* Copper.

COPPER POWDER • A color additive that is exempt from certification (*see* Certified). *See* Copper.

COPTIS JAPONICA • A small herb with white flowers.

COQ10 • Coenzyme Q10. Ubiquinone. Discovered in 1957, it belongs to a class of compounds called quinones. Its name also comes from the word *ubiquitous,* which means "found everywhere." CoQ10 is found in every cell in your body. Some foods, notably pork and beef heart, contain small amounts of CoQ10. An antioxidant nutrient involved in the production of energy within cells, it is widely used in this country for various cardiac conditions, especially congestive heart failure (CHF) and for health food products for athletes. It is being added to cosmetics to scavenge free radicals (*see*) and "fight signs of aging skin." *See* Ubiquinones.

CORALLINA OFFICIALIS • A West Indian climbing plant with bright fruit. Used in skin toners.

CORCHORUS CAPSULARIS • A Japanese vegetable with large leaves and yellow flowers.

CORIANDER OIL • *Coriandrum sativum.* The volatile oil from the dried ripe fruit of a plant grown in Asia and Europe. Used as a flavoring ingredient in dentifrices. Colorless or pale yellow liquid with a taste and odor characteristic of coriander, which is also used as a condiment. Can cause allergic reactions, particularly of the skin. It smells similar to the seed oil but is stronger, greener, and not as sweet. Coriander oil is a natural deodorant and is frequently used in perfumery and as a flavoring. EAF

CORIANDRUM SATIVUM • The colorless, or pale yellow, volatile oil from the dried ripe fruit of a plant grown in Asia and Europe; the name means "buglike odor." The ancient Egyptians used it for headaches. In the seventeenth century, it was used to dispel "wind." It still is used today as a laxative and to aid digestion. Coriander is used (up to 1 gram) to break up intestinal gas. It also is employed as a flavoring ingredient in dentifrices. Can cause allergic reactions, particularly of the skin.

CORN • *Zea mays.* Corn Sugar. Dextrose. The genus name *Zea* means "cause of life," and the species name *mays* means "mother." Used in maple, nut, and root beer flavorings for beverages, ice cream, ices, candy, and baked goods. The oil is used in emollient creams and toothpastes. The syrup is used as a texturizer and carrying ingredient in cosmetics. It is also used for envelopes, stamps, sticker tapes, ale, aspirin, bacon, baking mixes and powders, beers, bourbon, breads, cheeses, cereals, chop suey, chow mein, confectioners' sugar, cream puffs, fish products, ginger ale, hams, jellies, processed meats, peanut butters, canned peas, plastic food wrappers, sherbets, whiskeys, and American wines. It may also be found in capsules, lozenges, ointments, suppositories, vitamins, fritters, Fritos, frostings, canned or frozen fruit, graham crackers, gravies, grits, gum, monosodium glutamate, Nescafé, oleomargarine, pablum, paper, tortillas, vinegar, yeasts, bologna, baking powders, bath powders, frying fats, fruit juices, laxatives. May cause allergic reactions including skin rashes and asthma. ASP

CORN ACID • *See* Corn Oil.

CORN COB MEAL • The milled powder prepared from the cobs of *Zea mays*. Used as a thickener and an abrasive in cosmetics.

CORN FLOUR • A finely ground powder. Used in face and bath powder. *See* Corn Oil.

CORN GERM EXTRACT • The extract of the germ of *Zea mays*.

CORN GLYCERIDES • Triglycerides derived from corn used as a skin-conditioning ingredient, humectant, and emulsifier. *See* Corn.

CORN OIL • Used in emollient creams and toothpastes. Obtained as a by-product by wet milling the grain for use in the manufacture of cornstarch, dextrins, and yellow oil. It has a faint, characteristic odor and taste and thickens upon exposure to air, but it can cause skin reactions in the allergic. Human skin irritant and allergen. Has caused birth defects in experimental animals. ASP. GRAS

CORN OIL PEG-6 ESTERS • *See* PEG and Esters.

CORN POPPY EXTRACT • The extract obtained from the petals of the *Papaver rhoeas*.

CORNFLOWER • The dried flowers of *Centaurea cyanus*.

CORNFLOWER EXTRACT • The extract obtained from the flowers of *Centaurea cyanus*. Used as a blue dye.

CORN SILK EXTRACT • *Zea mays*. The stigmas from the female flowers of maize, fine soft threads 10–20 cm long. When fresh, they are like silk threads of a light green or yellow-brown color; when dry, they resemble fine, dark, crinkled hairs. Corn silk reputedly clears toxins, catarrh, deposits, and irritants out of the kidneys and bladder and has a gentle antiseptic and healing action. Corn silk has been used as a remedy for frequency of urination and bedwetting due to irritation or weakness of the urinary system and has been used for urinary stones and gravel. By reducing fluid retention in the body, corn silk may help reduce blood pressure, and by aiding elimination of toxins and wastes from the body, corn silk may relieve gout and arthritis and act as a gentle detoxifying remedy. Corn silk's healing and soothing properties are touted as helpful for relieving skin irritation and inflammation and for healing wounds and ulcers. May inhibit tumors. GRAS. ASP

CORNSTARCH • Many containers are powdered with cornstarch to prevent sticking. It is also used in dusting powder and as a demulcent for irritated colons. May cause allergic reactions, including skin rashes and asthma.

CORN SYRUP • Corn Sugar. Dextrose. A sweet syrup prepared from cornstarch. Used as a texturizer and carrying ingredient in cosmetics. Also used for envelopes, stamps, and sticking tapes, aspirin, and many food products. May cause allergic reactions.

CORNUS OFFICINALIS • Japanese Dogwood Cornel. Sour Mountain Date. A slender tree. Produces attractive bright yellow flowers on bare wood and autumn-toned leaves. Its fruit is reputed to have aided the longevity and exceptional health of Emperor Qian Long of the Manchu Dynasty (1644–1911). These fruits have been much celebrated in Chinese herbal medicine. Used as a skin-conditioning ingredient.

CORTHELLUS SHIITAKE • A Japanese mushroom that has long been used for therapeutic purposes. May lower blood pressure and blood cholesterol, according to recent studies.

CORTICOSTEROIDS • A class of compounds comprising steroid hormones secreted by the adrenal cortex and their synthetic analogs. In pharmacologic doses introduced in 1948, corticosteroids are used primarily for their anti-inflammatory and/or immunosuppressive effects. Topical corticosteroids, such as betamethasone dipropionate, are effective in the treatment of corticosteroid-responsive skin problems primarily because of their anti-inflammatory, anti-itching, and vasoconstrictive actions. The absorption through the skin of topical corticosteroids involves many factors including the vehicle, the condition of the skin, and the use of covering dressings. Topical corticosteroids can be absorbed from normal, intact skin.

CORYLUS AMERICANA and C. ROSTRATA • Hazelnut. An ornamental tree with a sweet gum. Used for brown coloring and as a skin-conditioning ingredient.

CORYLUS AVELLANA • *See* Hazel Extract.

CORYNEBACTERIUM FERMENT • Used in the production of treatment creams and oils.

COSMETICS • One of the most common causes, if not the most common cause, of allergic contact dermatitis, and frequently the cause of nasal and lung symptoms, particularly scented products. Until fairly recently, it was believed that cosmetics could not be absorbed through the skin. It is now known that many things can be absorbed through the skin, some chemicals to a greater degree than others depending upon composition and upon the part of the anatomy to which they are applied. Many cosmetics manufacturers promote their products as "hypoallergenic." A nonallergenic product is impossible because there is always someone who will be allergic to something. There are sixty known ingredients in past or present cosmetics known to cause allergic reactions in many people. Included in this list are such common substances as acacia, benzaldehyde, cornstarch, gum arabic, spearmint oil, and wheat starch (*see all*). By leaving the sixty offenders out of cosmetics or by reducing the number of ingredients altogether, particularly perfumes, manufacturers then claim their products are "hypoallergenic." The FDA has wrestled for years with the claim and has asked manufacturers to prove that their products are unlikely to cause an allergic reaction. As the mandate stands now, it is up to the manufacturer to decide the testing method used to determine the hypoallergenicity of the product. Throughout this book there are ingredients that often cause allergic reactions when in cosmetics. If you read the labels and check the book, you will be able, in most instances, to avoid those products that may be causing you a problem.

COSMETICITY • A term used to describe a consumer's "experience" of a cosmetic from the packaging to the effect of the ingredient.

COSTUS • A fixative in perfumes. The volatile oil is obtained by steam distillation from dried roots of an herb. Light yellow to brown viscous liquid, with a persistent violetlike odor. Used also as a food flavoring. EAF

COTTON • *Gossypium*. A soft, white, cellulosic substance composed of the fibers surrounding the seeds of various plants of the mallow family.

COTTONSEED • *Gossypium herbaceum*. The water-soluble, protein material in cottonseed contains one of the most powerful allergens for humans. Used in sunscreens, eyeliners, emollients, moisturizers, and emulsifiers.

COTTONSEED ACID • *See* Cottonseed Oil.

COTTONSEED FLOUR • Cooked, partly defatted, and toasted flour used for pale yellow color and to make gin. Can cause allergic skin reactions and asthma.

COTTONSEED OIL • The fixed oil from the seeds of the cultivated varieties of the plant. Pale yellow, oily, odorless liquid used in the manufacture of soaps, creams, baby creams, nail polish removers, and lubricants. Known to cause many allergic reactions but because of its wide use in cosmetics, foods, and other products, it is hard to avoid.

COUCH GRASS ROOT EXTRACT • *Agropyron repens*. Dog Grass. Twitch Grass. A weed that herbalists use to cool fevers and soothe and heat internal irritation or inflammation. Dogs and cats, when they have upset stomachs, will seek out and eat this plant. The roots possess both diuretic and demulcent properties and have been used by herbalists for centuries to treat bladder problems in humans. Couch grass contains high concentrations of mucilage, which gives the plant its soothing effect on mucous membranes. The plant is also reported to have antibiotic activity. In 1992, the FDA proposed a ban on couch grass in oral menstrual drug products because it has not been shown to be safe and effective for its stated claims.

COUMARINS • Tonka Bean. Cumarin. A fragrant ingredient of tonka beans, sweet woodruff, cramp bark, and many other plants. It is made synthetically as well. Used in over three hundred products in the United States, including acne preparations, antiseptics, deodorants, "skin fresheners," hair dyes, and shampoos. It has been widely used as a fragrance in soaps, detergents, perfumes, and sunscreens. May produce allergic contact dermatitis (*see*) and photosensitivity (*see*). It has anti-blood-clotting effects and anticlotting ingredients are derived from it. Coumarin is prohibited in foods because it is toxic by ingestion and carcinogenic on the skin.

COUNTERIRRITANT • An ingredient applied locally to produce superficial inflammation with the object of reducing existing inflammation in deeper adjacent structures. Iodine (*see*) is an example of a counterirritant.

C-PARETHS • Emulsifiers from carboxylic acid or phosphoric acid (*see both*).

CRANBERRY • Several low, berry-bearing shrubs related to the blueberry, native to northern Eurasia and North America. The American cranberry, *Vaccinium macrocarpon*, is cultivated in Massachusetts, New Jersey, and Wisconsin. Used in "organic" cosmetics.

CRANESBILL EXTRACT • The extract of wild geranium, *Geranium maculatum*, or other native geranium species. *See* Geranium Oil.

CRATAEGUS • The extract of the berries, flowers, and/or leaves of the English hawthorn, *Crataegus oxyacantha*. Used in dyes and skin tonics and to relieve inflammation and acne. Can cause dilation of blood vessels. *See* Hawthorn Berry.

CREAM • The thick, yellow part of cow's milk that contains 18 to 40 percent butterfat. Used as a skin-conditioning ingredient.

CREAM OF TARTAR • A white, crystalline salt in tartars from winemaking, prepared especially from argols and also synthetically from tartaric acid (*see*). Has a pleasant acid taste. Used as a thickening ingredient and in certain treatment of metals.

CREAM RINSE • Creme Rinse. Hair conditioners (*see*) that are poured on the hair after shampooing and then rinsed with water. A typical formula for a cream rinse: lanolin, 10 percent; mineral oil and lanolin esters, 5 percent; cholesterol, 0.25 percent; sorbitan stearate, 3 percent; preservative, 0.15 percent; distilled water, 78.60 percent; and perfume.

CREAMS • *See* Emollients, Hand Creams and Lotions, Cold Cream, and Hormone Creams.

CREATININE • A waste product of protein breakdown.

CREMER • A new vegetable substitute for petroleum jelly (*see*).

CREOSOTE • On the Canadian Hotlist (*see*). *See* Coal Tar.

o-**CRESOL** • A phenol (*see*) used as a preservative.

p-**CRESOL** • Used as a preservative and as a synthetic nut and vanilla flavoring ingredient. Obtained from coal tar. It occurs naturally in tea, and is used in cosmetics, beverages, ice cream, ices, candy, and baked goods. It is more powerful than phenol (*see*) and less toxic.

p-**CRESYL ACETATE** • *See p*-Tolyl Acetate.

CRITHMUM MARITIMU • Sea Fennel. Crest Marine. Zas. Sanpetra. Crithmus. Strong smell like furniture polish. Used in "firming creams." Has high levels of vitamin C. Used as a diuretic to cleanse toxins and improves digestion.

CROCUS SATIVUS • Saffron Crocus. Used in perfumery and coloring in cosmetics. It is the dried stigma of the crocus cultivated in Spain, Greece, France, and Iran. Used also in bitters, liquors, and spice flavorings. Homeopathic physicians use it to induce menstruation, and as an antispasmodic. Excessive doses can cause miscarriage. Severe poisoning causes bleeding from the skin, a severe lowering of the heart rate, and collapse. Fatal cases have been reported when 5 to 10 grams of saffron have been ingested.

CROSCARMELLOSE • The absorbent, cross-linked polymer of cellulose gum (*see*).

CROSS-REACTIVITY • When the body mistakes one compound for another of similar chemical composition.

CROTONATES • Combining crotonic acid (*see*) and esters (*see*). *See* Croton Tiglium.

CROTON GLABELLUS • *Croton tiglium.* A small shrub or tree, the seeds of which are used in Chinese and homeopathic medicines as a strong cathartic, rubefacient, and vesicant. It is very toxic and is a potential cancer promoter. On the Canadian Hotlist (*see*). Banned by the EU in cosmetics.

CROTON TIGLIUM • On the Canadian Hotlist (*see*). The EU banned the oil in cosmetics. *See* Croton Glabellus.

CROTONIC ACID • Found in the clay soil of Texas. It is used in the manufacture of vitamin A and in lacquers.

CRUELTY-FREE • Implies that products have not been tested on animals. Most ingredients have been at some point tested on animals, so you may want to look for "no new animal testing" to get a more accurate designation.

CRYPTOCARYA • The bark of this East Indian tree yields a volatile oil fragrance ingredient and pesticide.

CRYSTALLINS • The protein found in the fiber cells of vertebrate eye lenses. It is used as a hair- and skin-conditioning ingredient.

CTFA • Abbreviation for the former name of the Cosmetic, Toiletry, and Fragrance Association.

CUBEB BERRIES • *Piper cubeba.* Tailed Pepper. Java Pepper. The mature, unripe dried fruit of a perennial vine grown in South Asia, Java, Sumatra, the Indies, and Sri Lanka. Java pepper was formerly used to stimulate healing of mucous membranes. It has a strong, spicy odor. The fruit has been used as a stimulant and diuretic and sometimes is smoked in cigarettes. The oil is used for chronic bladder troubles and is reputed to increase the flow of urine.

CUBEB OIL • *See* Cubeb Berries.

CUCUMBER • *Cucumis sativus.* The juice of the cucumber was reputedly used by Cleopatra to preserve her skin. It imparts a cool feeling to the skin. By ingestion, it is said by herbalists to be a good diuretic and to prevent constipation. Researchers are now studying its effect on cholesterol. The juice is soothing to the skin.

CUCUMIS MELO • Melon.

CUCUMIS SATIVUS • Used as an emollient and skin-conditioning ingredient in a wide number of cosmetics, including skin fresheners, cleansing lotions, eye makeup, bath products, and bubble baths. *See* Cucumber.

CUCURBITA PEPO • Pumpkin Seed Oil. Skin-conditioning ingredient.

CUCURBITACEAE • Gourd Extract.

CUDWEED EXTRACT • *Gnaphalium ulginosum.* The plant is used by herbalists to treat upper-respiratory inflammation including laryngitis, tonsillitis, and bronchitis. Grown widely in North America.

CUMIN • *Cuminum cyminum.* A fragile plant cultivated in Asia and the Middle East, it contains cuminic aldehyde, which may have some antiviral properties, and cumene, which is narcotic in high doses and potentially toxic by ingestion. The seed was used in medicine in ancient times as a stimulant and remedy for stomach ailments. It is used by herbalists to treat sore eyes. In cosmetics, it is used as an essential oil for flavoring and fragrances.

CUMINALDEHYDE • Used to make perfumes. Colorless to yellowish, oily, with a strong, lasting odor. It is a constituent of eucalyptus, myrrh, cassia, cumin, and other essential oils, but often is made synthetically for fragrances.

CUMINUM CYMINUM • *See* Cumin.

CUPRESSUS SEMPERVIRENS • Cypress. An astringent. *See* Cedrol.

CUPRIC ACETATE • The copper salt of acetic acid and copper (*see both*).

CUPRIC CHLORIDE • Copper Chloride. A copper salt used in hair dye.

CUPRIC SULFATE • Copper sulfate occurs in nature as hydrocyanite. Grayish white to greenish white crystals. Used as an agricultural fungicide, herbicide, and in the preparation of azo dyes (*see*). Used in hair dyes as coloring. Very irritating if ingested and is used medicinally as a skin fungicide.

CURARE • Muscle relaxant used in anesthesia (and, in the past, in arrow poisons by South American Indians). Curaine is any of a group of alkaloids derived from curare. Curare competes with acetylcholine, a chemical that carries information between nerve and muscle cells and blocks transmission of the information. Banned in cosmetics by the EU.

CURCUMA LONGA • Derived from an East Indian herb with an aromatic pepper-like, but somewhat bitter, taste. The cleaned, boiled, sun-dried, pulverized root is used in flavorings. Both turmeric and its oleoresin have been permanently listed for coloring food since 1966. It is exempt from certification. *See* Turmeric. GRAS

CURCUMA ZEDOARIA • Zedoary Oil. A bark extract from the East Indies, *Curcuma zedoaria* is used as bitters and ginger ale flavorings for beverages. GRAS

CURCUMIN • Turmeric. Orange-yellow colorant derived from the roots of *Curcuma longa* (*see*) and used as a natural food coloring and as an antioxidant. It does not require certification because it is a natural product, but the Expert Committee on Food Additives of the FDA recommended that the acceptable daily intake of curcumin (and turmeric) be limited to 0 to 0.5 milligrams per kilogram of body weight. A skin irritant. The JECFA (*see* abbreviations list), however, concluded in June 1998 that reproductive toxicity studies and more information concerning the solvents used in the manufacturing processes of this additive are needed. Eating curcumin, a natural ingredient in the spice turmeric, may reduce the chance of developing heart failure, researchers at the Peter Munk Cardiac Centre of the Toronto General Hospital in Canada reported in 2008. E

CURLED DOCK • Sour Dock. A weed with coarse leaves that is a member of the sorrel family and contains a sour juice. An extract of *Rumex crispus*.

CURRANT EXTRACT • From the berries of the red currant, *Ribes rubrum*.

CURRY RED • CI 16035. A color classed as a monoazo, the name can be used only when applied to uncertified batches of color. The CTFA-adopted name for certified (*see*) batches is FD & C Red No. 40 (*see*). Widely used in cosmetics such as lipsticks, hair products, in care preparations, mouthwashes, bath products, cold creams, cleansing lotions, and moisturizers.

CUSTARD APPLE • *Annona reticulata. See* Pawpaw Extract.

CUTANEOUS • Pertaining to the skin.

CUTANEOUS LYSATE • The end product of the controlled bacterial degradation of animal skin. It consists of a complex mixture of proteins and amino acids.

CUTICLE REMOVERS • Cuticle is the dead skin that covers the base of the nail.

Chemicals are used to either plasticize or dissolve the cuticle. Alkalis, such as lye, are used as cuticle softeners and removers. A typical cuticle remover contains coconut oil, potassium phosphate, potassium hydroxide, triethanolamine, and water. Contact dermatitis may occur. Potassium phosphate, potassium hydroxide, and triethanolamine can be irritants. Coconut oil (*see*) can cause allergic reactions.

CUTTLEFISH EXTRACT • An extract of the glands of *Sepia officinali.*

CYAMOPSIS TETRAGONOLOBA • *See* Guar Gum.

CYANIDE • Prussic Acid. Hydrocyanic Acid. An inorganic salt that is one of the most rapid poisons known. Poisoning may occur when any compound releases cyanide. Cyanide is used as a fungistat, insecticide, and rodenticide and is used in metal polishes, especially for silver, and in electroplating solutions, art materials, photographic processes, and metallurgy. It has been reported to reduce oxygen availability in the blood even in low doses. Hydrogen cyanide and its salts have been banned by the EU in cosmetics.

CYANO-, CYAN- • From the Greek *kyanos,* meaning a dark blue. The prefix is commonly used to signify compounds containing the cyanide group CN. If the cyanide is not released from the compound, its presence is presumed not harmful.

CYANOCOBALAMIN • Vitamin B_{12}. Used as a skin-conditioning ingredient.

CYANOPSIS TETRAGONOLOBA • *See* Guar Gum.

CYANOTIS ARACHNOIDEA • Spider Plant. Extractives and their physically modified derivatives such as tinctures, concretes, absolutes, essential oils, oleoresins, terpenes, terpene-free fractions, distillates, residues, used in cosmetics, especially in emollients.

CYATHEACEAE • Pengawar. A family of tropical tree ferns.

CYCLAMATES • Artificial sweetening ingredients about thirty times as sweet as refined sugar, removed from the U.S. food market on September 1, 1969, because they were found to cause bladder cancer in rats.

CYCLAMEN • A small genus of widely cultivated Eurasian plants of the family Primulaceae. Cyclamens have nodding white or pink flowers. Used as a fragrance ingredient.

CYCLAMEN ALCOHOL • Used as a stabilizer. Banned in fragrances by the UK. *See* Cyclamen.

CYCLAMEN ALDEHYDE • A colorless liquid aldehyde (*see*) having a lily-of-the-valley odor, made synthetically, and used in perfumes, especially for soap.

CYCLAMIC ACID • Fairly strong acid with a sweet taste. It is the acid from which cyclamates (*see*) were derived.

CYCLOCARBOXYPROPYLOLEIC ACID • Acrylinoleic Acid. C 29–70 Carboxylic Acid. Thickening, suspending, dispersing, and emulsifying ingredient in cosmetics.

CYCLODEXTRIN • A sweet compound. An absorbent and chelating ingredient (*see both*). *See* Dextrin.

a-CYCLODEXTRIN • Cyclohexa-Amylose, Cyclomalto-Hexose or Alpha-Dextrin. Liquefied starch is treated with the enzyme cyclodextringlycosyltransferase. Used as a carrier or stabilizer for flavors (flavor adjuvant), as a carrier or stabilizer for colors, vitamins, and fatty acids.

CYCLOETHOXYMETHICONE • A solvent used in skin conditioners.

CYCLOHEPTASILOXANE • Widely used as an anticaking ingredient, in powders, moisturizers, and hairsprays. *See* Siloxane.

CLOHEXANE • A hydrocarbon (*see*) used as a solvent.

CYCLOHEXANOL • Obtained from phenol, it is used as a solvent for resins. It has a narcoticlike action and has caused severe kidney problems in experimental animals.

CYCLOHEXANONE • Obtained from cyclohexanol (*see*), it has a combination peppermint and acetone odor. The vapor is harmful. It is used as a solvent for cellulose and in the preparation of resins. It is a colorless, oily liquid used in organic synthesis, particularly in the production of adipic acid, caprolactam, polyvinyl chloride, and methacrylate ester polymers. Also used as a solvent for natural and synthetic resins, waxes, and fats. The JECFA (see abbreviations list) says that consumer exposure may occur when it is used as a solvent. Eye, skin, and respiratory irritant. May cause dermatitis. Irritating to skin and eyes. Derived from phenol (*see*), it is used in many chemical products including fragrances and pharmaceuticals. It is being tested as a stimulant for nerve cells. It is also used in toxic herbicides. EAF

CYCLOHEXYLAMINE • A buffering ingredient used in hair sprays.

CYCLOMENOL AND ITS SALTS • Anti-male hormone. Banned by the EU in cosmetics.

CYCLOMETHICONE • A widely used silicone (*see*) in hair and skin conditioners. It is also used in deodorants, after-shave lotions, suntan gels, eye-makeup removers, lipsticks, dusting powders, skin freshener, and blushers.

CYCLOPENTANE • A colorless liquid derived from benzene and used as a solvent and in distillation.

CYCLOPENTASILOXANE • Hair and skin conditioner. *See* Cyclomethicone.

N-CYCLOPENTYL-*m*-AMINOPHENOL • Coal tar hair coloring. *See* Coal Tar.

CYCLOTRISILOXANE • A high-production chemical used to make silicone and silicone oils. Considered hazardous.

CYMBIDIUM GRANDIFLORUM • Orchid extract used in fragrances.

CYMBOPOGON MARTINI • Palmarosa. Geranium Oil. The volatile oil obtained by steam distillation from a variety of partially dried grass, grown in East India and Java. Used in rose, fruit, and spice flavorings for ice cream, ices, candy, and baked goods. Believed as toxic as other essential oils, causing illness after ingestion of a teaspoonful and death after ingestion of an ounce. A skin irritant. GRAS

CYMBOPOGON NARDUS • *See* Citronella Oil.

CYMBOPOGON SCHOENANTHUS • *See* Lemongrass Oil.

***p*-CYMENE** • A synthetic flavoring, a volatile hydrocarbon solvent that occurs naturally in star anise, coriander, cumin, mace oil, oil of mandarin, and origanum oil. Used in fragrance, also in citrus and spice flavorings for beverages, ice cream, candies, and baked goods. Its ingestion in pure form may cause a burning sensation in the mouth, and nausea, salivation, headache, giddiness, vertigo, confusion, and coma. Contact with the pure liquid may cause blisters of the skin and inflammation of mucous membranes.

***o*-CYMEN-3-OL** • See *p*-Cymene

***o*-CYMEN-5-OL** • Based on the available data, the CIR Expert Panel (*see*) concludes that the safety of this ingredient has not been documented for use in cosmetics. *See* Quaternary Ammonium Compounds.

CYNARA SCOLYMUS • Artichoke. A tall herb that resembles a thistle. Used as a flavoring.

CYNOMORIUM COCCINEUM EXTRACT • Red Thumb. It is collected and eaten by some people. The underground part of this strange parasite is cooked as if it were asparagus. It is used in Chinese products and others as a hormonelike compound for the skin.

CYPERUS • Sedge Root. A common wayside weed, it is closely related to the Egyptian papyrus plant. The root contains essential oils (*see*), including pinene and sesquiterpenes. It is used by herbalists to treat stomach cramps, colds, flu, menstrual irregularities, and depression. Used in cosmetics as a fragrance ingredient.

CYPRESS EXTRACT • An extract derived from the leaves and twigs of the cypress tree, *Cupressus sempervirens*. The oil has been used in folk medicine to treat whooping cough.

CYPRIPEDIUM PUBESCENS • Lady's Slipper. Herbalists use it to treat anxiety, stress, insomnia, neurosis, restlessness, tremors, epilepsy, and palpitations. It contains volatile oils, resins, glucosides, and tannin (*see all*).

CYSTAMINE BIS-LACTAMIDE • An amide (*see*) that is used as a skin-conditioning ingredient.

CYSTEAMINE • MEA. Mercamine. 2-Aminoethanethiol. A compound with an unpleasant odor that has many biological effects. It is used as an antidote to acetaminophen and experimentally as a radio protective ingredient. Used as an antioxidant in cosmetics.

CYSTEAMINE HCL • An organic salt used in hair-waving and -straightening products.

CYSTEINE, L-FORM • An essential amino acid (*see*), it is derived from hair and used in hair products and creams. Soluble in water, it is used in bakery products as a nutrient. It has been used to promote wound healing. On the list of FDA additives to be studied.

CYSTINE • A nonessential amino acid (*see*) found in urine and in horsehair. Colorless, practically odorless, white crystals, it is used as a nutrient supplement and in emollients and hair products.

CYTOCHROME C • A protein found in animal cells. It is used as a skin-conditioning ingredient.

D

D & C • Abbreviation for drug and cosmetic.

D & C BLUE NO. 1 ALUMINUM LAKE • Brilliant Blue Lake. Insoluble pigment prepared from FD & C Blue No. 1 (*see*). A coal tar derivative, this brilliant blue is used as a coloring in hair dyes and powders, among other cosmetics; also used in soft drinks, gelatin desserts, and candy. May cause allergic reactions. It will produce malignant tumors at the site of injection in rats. On the FDA permanent list of color additives. Rated 1A for toxicology by the World Health Organization, meaning it is completely acceptable for use in foods and cosmetics. *See* Colors.

D & C BLUE NO. 2 ALUMINUM LAKE • Acid Blue 74. Indigotine 1A. Indigo Carmine. An indigo (*see*) dye. Acid Blue No. 1 is the uncertified counterpart of FD & C Blue No. 1.

D & C BLUE NO. 4 • Acid Blue 9 (Ammonium Salt). Bright, greenish blue. A coal tar, triphenylmethane color used primarily in hair rinses. Permanently listed by the FDA, January 3, 1977. The name Acid Blue No. 4 can be used only when applied to batches of color that have been certified. The CTFA-adopted name for noncertified batches of this color is Acid Blue 9 Ammonium Salt. *See* Colors.

D & C BROWN NO. 1 • Resorcin Brown. Capracyl Brown. Acid Orange 24. Light orange-brown. A diazo color (*see* Colors) permitted for use only in preformed hair colors. The cosmetics industry has petitioned the FDA to allow wider use. Resorcin is irritating to the skin and mucous membranes. Absorption can cause depletion of oxygen in the body and death. Also used as an antiseptic and fungicide. Permanently listed for external use only in 1976. D & C Brown No. 1 can be used only when applied to certified colors. The CTFA name for noncertified batches of this color is Acid Orange 24.

D & C GREEN NO. 3 ALUMINUM LAKE • Food Green 3. The aluminum salt of FD & C Green No. 3. A brilliant, but not fast, dye. Fast Green FCF is the name for uncertified batches of this color. *See* Aniline Dyes for toxicity.

D & C GREEN NO. 5 • Acid Green 25. Dullish blue-green. Classed chemically as an anthraquinone color (*see* Colors). Used in suntan oils, bath salts, shampoos, hair rinses, toothpastes, soaps, and hair-waving fluids. Low skin toxicity but may cause skin irritation and sensitivity. Permanently listed by the FDA in 1982. The CTFA adopted name for uncertified batches of this color is Acid Green 25.

D & C GREEN NO. 6 • Solvent Green 3. Dull blue-green. Classified chemically as an anthraquinone color. Used in hair oils and pomades. Permanently listed by the FDA in 1982. The name for uncertified batches of this color is Solvent Green 3. *See* Colors.

D & C GREEN NO. 8 • Solvent Green 7. Yellowish green. Classed chemically as a pyrene color. Permanently listed by the FDA in 1976. The name for uncertified batches of this color is Solvent Green 7. *See* Colors.

D & C ORANGE NO. 4 • Acid Orange 7. Bright orange. Transparent orange used in lipsticks and face powders. Classed chemically as a monoazo color. Permanently listed in 1977. The name for uncertified batches of this color is Acid Orange 7. *See* Colors.

D & C ORANGE NO. 4 ALUMINUM LAKE • Persian Orange. Insoluble pigment prepared from D & C Orange No. 4 (*see*). *See* Colors and Lakes.

D & C ORANGE NO. 5 • Acid Orange 11. Solvent Red 72. Dibromofluorescein (*see*). Reddish orange. An orange stain used in lipsticks, face powders, and talcums. Permanently listed for use in lipsticks, mouthwashes, and dentifrices in 1982. Permanently listed for externally applied drugs and cosmetics in 1984. The name for uncertified batches of this color is Acid Orange 11.

D & C ORANGE NO. 5 ALUMINUM LAKE • Dawn Orange. Manchu Orange. Insoluble pigment prepared from D & C Orange No. 5 (*see*). *See* Colors and Lakes.

D & C ORANGE NO. 5 ZIRCONIUM LAKE • Petite Orange. Dawn Orange Acid Red 26. Ponceau R. *See* Lake and Zirconium. A monoazo dye. *See* Azo Dyes.

D & C ORANGE NO. 10 • Solvent 73. Diiodofluorescein. Reddish orange. Classed chemically as a fluoran color. Orange-red powder used in lipsticks and other cosmetics. The name for uncertified batches of this color is Solvent Red 73. *See* Colors.

D & C ORANGE NO. 10 ALUMINUM LAKE • Solvent Red 73. Erythrosine G. A xanthene (*see*) color.

D & C ORANGE NO. 11 • Acid Red 95. Clear red. Classed chemically as a xanthene color. It is the conversion product of D & C Orange No. 10 (*see*) to the sodium or potassium salt. The name for uncertified batches of this color is Acid Red 95. *See* Colors.

D & C ORANGE NO. 17 • Permanent Orange. Pigment Orange 5. Bright orange. Classed chemically as a monoazo color. The FDA permanently listed Orange No. 17, but its ruling was reversed by the U.S. Court of Appeals in 1987 for the District of Columbia, which said the FDA lacked legal authority to approve it since it was found to induce cancer. The court's ruling was in response to a lawsuit by Public Citizens Health Research Group, a consumer advocacy group. The color is no longer authorized for use. *See* Colors.

D & C RED NO. 4 ALUMINUM LAKE • Food Red 1. A monoazo color. The aluminum salt of FD & C Red No. 4 or Ponceau SX, the uncertified counterpart of FD & C Red No. 4 may be used to prepare this lake. *See* Azo Dyes.

D & C RED NO. 6 • Lithol Rubin B. Medium red. Classed chemically as a monoazo color. It is the calcium salt of D & C Red No. 7 (*see*). Lithol is a topical antiseptic. Permanently listed in 1983. The CTFA-adopted name for uncertified batches of this color is Pigment Red 57. *See* Colors.

D & C RED NO. 6 ALUMINUM LAKE • Pigment Red 57. Lithol Rubine. A monoazo color. *See* Azo Dyes.

D & C RED NO. 6 BARIUM LAKE • Rubine Lake. Pigment Red 57. Lithol Rubine B. A monoazo dye. An insoluble pigment prepared from D & C Red No. 6 (*see*) and barium. The CTFA name for uncertified batches of this color is Pigment Red 57:2 Barium Lake. *See* Colors and Azo Dyes.

D & C RED NO. 6 BARIUM/STRONTIUM LAKE • An insoluble pigment prepared by mixing barium and strontium salts of D & C Red No. 6.

D & C RED NO. 6 POTASSIUM LAKE • An insoluble pigment composed of the potassium salt of D & C Red No. 6. *See* D & C Red No. 6.

D & C RED NO. 6 STRONTIUM LAKE • An insoluble pigment prepared by mixing strontium with D & C Red No. 6.

D & C RED NO. 7 • Lithol Rubine B Ca. Bluish red. Classed chemically as a monoazo color. Used in nail lacquers and lipsticks. Lithol is a topical antiseptic. Permanently listed in 1987 for ingested drug and cosmetic lip products, amount not to exceed 5 mg per daily dose of drug. For general cosmetic use according to good manufacturing practices. This color is the salt of D & C Red No. 6. Uncertified batches of this color must be called Pigment Red 57. *See* Colors.

D & C RED NO. 7 ALUMINUM LAKE • Pigment Red 57. *See* Azo Dyes.

D & C RED NO. 7 BARIUM LAKE • Insoluble pigment prepared from D & C Red No. 7 (*see*). *See also* Colors and Lakes.

D & C RED NO. 7 CALCIUM LAKE • Pigment Red 57. Lithol Rubine B. A monoazo dye. An insoluble pigment prepared from D & C Red No. 7 (*see*) and calcium. *See* Colors and Azo Dyes.

D & C RED NO. 7 ZIRCONIUM LAKE • Pigment Red 57. Lithol Rubine B. A monoazo color. Carcinogenic in animals. *See* Colors. Ruling postponed.

D & C RED NO. 8 • Lake Red C. Pigment Red 53. Orange. Classed chemically as a monoazo color. Carcinogenic in animals. Permanently listed in 1987 for ingested drug and cosmetic lip products, amount not to exceed 0.1 percent by weight of finished product. The FDA permanent listing of D & C Red No. 8 has been challenged by a lawsuit by Public Citizens Health Research Group, a consumer advocacy group. This color is no longer authorized for use. *See* D & C Red No. 19 and Colors.

D & C RED NO. 9 • Lake Red C Ba. Scarlet coloring. It is the barium salt of D & C Red No. 8 (*see*). Used in face powders. Carcinogenic in animals. Permanently listed in 1987 for ingested drug and cosmetic lip products, amount not to exceed 0.1 percent of finished product. The permanent listing of this color, which has shown to be carcinogenic in animals, was challenged in 1988 by the Public Citizens Health Research Group, a consumer advocacy organization. This color is no longer authorized for use. *See* D & C Red No. 19 and Colors.

D & C RED NO. 10 • Litho Red. Yellowish red. No longer authorized for use.

D & C RED NO. 17 • Toney Red. Classed chemically as a diazo color. It is used in soaps, suntan oils, hair oils, and pomades. Carcinogenic in animals. No longer used much in lipsticks because of reports of ill effects. The FDA permanently listed D & C Red No. 17 in 1988, but its ruling was reversed by the U.S. Court of Appeals for the District of Columbia, which said the FDA lacked legal authority to approve it since D & C Red No. 17 was found to induce cancer. The court's ruling was in response to a lawsuit by Public Citizens Health Research Group, a consumer advocacy group. The uncertified name of this color is Solvent Red 23. *See* Colors.

D & C RED NO. 19 • Rhodamine B. Mingredienta. Classed chemically as a xanthene color. Its greenish crystals or yellow powder turns violet in solution. Used in lipsticks, rouges, soaps, bath salts, nail enamel, toothpaste, hair-waving fluids, and face powders. The FDA permanently listed D & C Red No. 19 in 1988, but its ruling was reversed by the U.S. Court of Appeals for the District of Columbia, which said the FDA lacked legal authority to approve D & C Red No. 19 since it was found to induce cancer. The court's ruling was in response to a lawsuit by Public Citizens Health Research Group, a consumer advocacy group. No longer authorized for use. *See* Colors.

D & C RED NO. 21 • Solvent Red 43. Tetrabromofluorescein (*see*). Classed chemically as a fluoran color. A bluish pink stain used in lipsticks, rouges, and nail enamels. Insoluble in water but used to color oils, resins, and lacquers. Permanently listed in 1982. The uncertified name for batches of this color is Solvent Red 43. *See* Colors.

D & C RED NO. 21 ALUMINUM LAKE • Insoluble pigment prepared from D & C Red No. 21 (*see*) and aluminum. The uncertified name for this color is Pigment Red 90:1 Aluminum Lake. *See* Colors and Lakes.

D & C RED NO. 21 ZIRCONIUM LAKE • Solvent Red 43. Merry Pink. Xanthene (see) dye.

D & C RED NO. 22 • Eosine YS. Yellowish pink. Classed chemically as a xanthene color. It is used in soaps, hair rinses, lipsticks, and nail polishes. Red crystals with bluish tinge or brownish red powder. Lethal dose in animals is quite small. Permanently listed in 1982. The CTFA name for uncertified batches of this color is Acid Red 87. *See* Colors.

D & C RED NO. 27 • Solvent Red 48. Philoxine B. Veri Pink. A xanthene (*see*) dye. Classed chemically as a fluoran color. A deep, bluish red stain used in lipsticks and rouges. Permanently listed in 1982. The uncertified name for this color is Solvent Red 48. The toxicological data reviewed by FDA prior to approval of D & C Red No. 27 did not include studies of acute phototoxicity or chronic phototoxicity (i.e., photocarcinogenesis). The FDA said in 2000, "Our current knowledge of the photochemistry and photobiology of D&C Red No. 27 raises new concerns about its long-term safety." The FDA has requested further testing. In the meantime, try to avoid this color. *See* Colors.

D & C RED NO. 27 ALUMINUM LAKE • Tetrabromo Tertrachloro Fluorescein Lake. Insoluble pigment prepared from D & C Red No. 27 (*see*) and aluminum. *See* Colors.

D & C RED NO. 27 BARIUM LAKE • Solvent Red 48. Petite Pink. A xanthene (*see*) dye.

D & C RED NO. 27 CALCIUM LAKE • An insoluble pigment composed of the calcium salt of D & C Red No. 27.

D & C RED NO. 27 ZIRCONIUM LAKE • Solvent Red 48. A xanthene (*see*) dye, deep, bluish red. Used in lipsticks and rouges.

D & C RED NO. 28 • Phloxine B. Acid Red 92. Classed chemically as a xanthene color. It is the conversion product of D & C Red No. 27 (*see*) to the sodium salt. Permanently listed in 1982. The name for uncertified batches of this color is Acid Red 92. *See* Colors. The toxicological data reviewed by FDA prior to approval of D & C Red No. 28 did not include studies of acute phototoxicity or chronic phototoxicity (i.e., photocarcinogenesis). The FDA said in 2000, "Our current knowledge of the photochemistry and photobiology of D & C Red No. 28 raises new concerns about its long-term safety. D & C Red No. 28 is now known to be an extremely efficient photodynamic sensitizer whose photo-excitation results in the formation of free radicals [*see*]. These highly reactive species attack cellular components such as fats, proteins and DNA. Investigators have shown that the genetic damage sensitized by D & C Red No. 28 is mutagenic in bacterial assays." The FDA has requested further testing. In the meantime, try to avoid this color.

D & C RED NO. 30 • Helindone Pink CN. Vat Red 1. Bluish pink. Classed chemically as an indigoid color. It is used in face powders, talcums, lipsticks, rouges, and soaps. The uncertified name for this color is Vat Red 1. *See* Colors.

D & C RED NO. 30 ALUMINUM LAKE • Vat Red 1. Thioindigoid Pink R. A thioindigoid color. A red vat dye made from indigo and sulfur. *See* Vat Dyes and Indigo.

D & C RED NO. 30 CALCIUM LAKE • Permanent Pink. Vat Red 1 Thioindigo Pink R. A thioindigo dye. *See* Vat Dyes and Indigo.

D & C RED NO. 30 LAKE • Insoluble pigment prepared from D & C Red No. 30 (*see*) with an approved metal. *See* Colors and Lakes.

D & C RED NO. 31 • Brilliant Lake Red R. Classed chemically as a monoazo color. It is used in lipsticks and nail enamels. *See* Colors.

D & C RED NO. 31 CALCIUM LAKE • Brilliant Lake Red R. Monoazo color used in lipsticks and nail enamels. *See* Azo Dyes.

D & C RED NO. 33 • Acid Red 33. Dull, bluish red. Classed chemically as a monoazo color. It is used in lipsticks, rouges, soaps, bath salts, and hair rinses. Was to be permanently listed in 1988, but the ruling has been postponed to allow the FDA "additional time to study complex scientific and legal questions about it." The uncertified name for this color is Acid Red 33. *See* Azo Dyes and Colors.

D & C RED NO. 34 • Fanchon Maroon. Deep Maroon. Classed chemically as a monoazo color. It is used in face powders, talcums, nail lacquers, lipsticks, rouges, toothpastes, and soaps. The uncertified name for this color is Pigment Red 63:1. *See* Colors.

D & C RED NO. 34 CALCIUM LAKE • Insoluble pigment prepared from D & C Red No. 34 (*see*). *See* Colors and Lakes.

D & C RED NO. 36 • Pigment Red 4. Tiger Orange. A monoazo dye. It is a bright orange used in lipsticks, rouges, face powders, and talcums. Was to be permanently listed in 1988, but the ruling has been postponed to allow the FDA "additional time to study complex scientific and legal questions about it." The uncertified name for this color is Pigment Red 4. *See* Colors and Azo Dyes.

D & C RED NO. 36 BARIUM LAKE • Pigment Red 4. Permanent Red 12. Orange hue. A monoazo color. *See* Azo Dyes.

D & C RED NO. 36 LAKE • Chlorinated Para Lake. Tang Orange. Insoluble pigment prepared from D & C Red No. 36 (*see*). *See* Colors and Lakes.

D & C RED NO. 36 ZIRCONIUM LAKE • Pigment Red 4. *See* D & C Red No. 36 Barium Lake.

D & C RED NO. 37 • Rhodamine B-Stearate Solvent. Banned in 1988. *See* Colors.

D & C RED NO. 40 ALUMINUM LAKE • Bluish pink. Classed chemically as a xanthene (*see*) color. Used in soaps. An insoluble color prepared from FD & C Red No. 40 (*see*).

D & C VIOLET NO. 2 • Alizurol Purple SS. Solvent Violet 13. Classed chemically as an anthraquine color. It is a dull, bluish violet used in suntan oils, pomades, and hair colors. The uncertified batch of this color must be called Solvent Violet 13. The request to provide listing of Ext. D & C Violet No. 2 for safe use in coloring externally applied drug products was held in abeyance (*see*) by the FDA in 2003.

D & C YELLOW NO. 5 ALUMINUM LAKE • Greenish yellow. Insoluble pigment prepared from FD & C Yellow No. 5 (*see*) and aluminum. *See* Colors and Lakes.

D & C YELLOW NO. 5 ZIRCONIUM LAKE • An insoluble pigment prepared from FD & C Yellow No. 5 (*see*) and zirconium. *See* Colors and Lakes.

D & C YELLOW NO. 6 ALUMINUM LAKE • Insoluble pigment prepared from FD & C Yellow No. 6 (*see*) and aluminum. *See* Colors and Lakes.

D & C YELLOW NO. 7 • Acid Yellow 73. Fluorescein. Classed chemically as a fluoran color. It is a water-absorbing, yellowish red powder freely soluble in water. The fluorescence disappears when the solution is made acid and reappears when it is made neutral. No toxic action on fish and believed to be nontoxic to humans. An uncertified batch of this color must be called Acid Yellow 73. *See* Colors.

D & C YELLOW NO. 8 • Uranine. Sodium fluorescein. Naphthol Yellow S. Classed

184 D & C YELLOW NO. 10

chemically as a xanthene color. It is the sodium salt of D & C Yellow No. 7 (*see*). Light yellow or orange-yellow powder soluble in water. The uncertified color is called Acid Yellow 73 Sodium Salt. *See* Colors.

D & C YELLOW NO. 10 • Acid Yellow 3. Classed chemically as a quinoline color. It is a bright, greenish yellow used in hair-waving fluids, toothpastes, bath salts, soaps, and shampoos. It is a potential allergen. It is present in yellow Irish Spring, pink Dove, and Caress bath soap. It may cross-react with other quinoline colors used in drugs. The uncertified color is called Acid Yellow 3. The UK has moved to phase out quinoline yellow because of its reported effect on hyperactivity in children.

D & C YELLOW NO. 10 ALUMINUM LAKE • Insoluble pigment prepared from D & C Yellow No. 10 (*see*) and aluminum. The uncertified version of this color is Pigment Yellow 115. *See* Colors and Lakes.

D & C YELLOW NO. 11 • Solvent Yellow 33. Classed chemically as a quinoline color. It is a bright, greenish yellow used in soaps, shampoos, suntan oils, hair oils, and pomades. The uncertified version of this color is Solvent Yellow 33. *See* Colors.

DAFFODIL EXTRACT • *Narcissus pseudonarcissus.* Narcissus Extract. A brilliant yellow, trumpetlike flowered plant of the narcissus family.

DAIDA • This is the term the Japanese use to list colors on cosmetic labels. It is followed by the color's number.

DAIDA1201 • CI 45370. Eosinic Acid. A class of rose-colored stains or dyes. *See* Eosine.

DAIDA1203 • A monoazo (*see*) orange coloring. Not approved for use in the United States but is approved in Japan.

DAIDA1204 • CI 21110. A diazo (*see*) color approved for use in Japan but not in the United States or the European Union.

DAIDA1205 • CI 15510. Acid Orange 7. A monoazo color (*see*) approved for use in Japan.

DAIDA1206 • CI 45425. Orange 10. Solvent Red 73. A xanthene (*see*) color.

DAIDA1207 • Japanese name for certified Acid Red 95.

DAIDA1401 • CI 11725. Japanese name for Pigment Orange. Not approved for use in the United States.

DAIDA1402 • CI 14600. Japanese name for a monoazo color (*see*) for Acid Orange 20. Not approved for use in the United States or the European Union.

DAIDA1403 • The Japanese name for a monoazo color (*see*) not approved for use in the United States or the European Union.

DAIDAI PEEL OIL • Japanese Bitter Orange Oil. The essential oil derived from the dried peel of immature fruit, Neroli bigarade oil is made from the peel of nearly ripe fruit by cold expression. These oils are widely used in perfumery and cosmetics. All parts of the sour orange are more aromatic than those of the sweet orange. The flowers are indispensable to the perfume industry and are famous not only for the distilled Neroli oil but also for "orange flower absolute" obtained by fat or solvent extraction. Petitgrain oil is distilled from the leaves, twigs, and immature fruits, especially from the Bergamot orange. Both petitgrain and the oil of the ripe peel are of great importance in formulating scents for perfumes and cosmetics. Petitgrain oil is indispensable in fancy eau-de-cologne. The seed oil is employed in soaps. EAF

DAIDZEIN • An isoflavone, which is a hormonelike substance found in soybeans. It is the second most plentiful isoflavone in soy, after genistein (*see*). Numerous studies have shown that, like genistein, daidzein is both a phytoestrogen and antioxidant, and it is most often used to treat conditions affected by estrogen levels in the body.

DAISY • *Bellies perennis.* It is used in cosmetics as a skin lightener. This extract along with ferulic acid, sodium gluconate, and citrates is marketed as a whitening complex with a strong capacity to inhibit melanin (*see*). *See also* Bellies Perennis.

DAISY EXTRACT • Extract of Daisy. Extract of the flowers of the English daisy, *Bellis perennis*. Certain plants of the daisy family may cause blisterlike eruptions when crushed on the skin. Used in sachets. Also included in love potions by ancient herbalists.

DALEA SPINOSA • Indigo Bush Oil. Probably the oldest known dye. Prepared from various *Indigofera* plants native to Bengal, Java, and Guatemala. Dark blue powder with a coppery luster. No known skin irritation.

DAMAR • Dipterocarp. Resin used to produce a gloss and adhesion in nail lacquer. It is a yellowish white, semitransparent exudate from a plant grown in the East Indies and the Philippines. Comes in varying degrees of hardness. It has a bitter taste. Also used for preserving animal and vegetable specimens for science laboratories. May cause allergic contact dermatitis.

a-DAMASCONE • A fragrance ingredient. EAF

DAMIANA LEAVES • The dried leaves of a plant of California and Texas used as a flavoring. Formerly used as a tonic and aphrodisiac. It has not yet been assigned for a toxicology literature search. GRAS. EAF

DANDELION LEAF AND ROOT • Lion's Tooth. *Taraxacum officinale.* Used as a skin-refreshing bath additive. Obtained from *Taraxacum* plants, which grow abundantly in the United States. The common dandelion weed eaten as a salad green was used by the Indians for heartburn. Rich in vitamins A and C, it is also used as a flavoring. ASP

DANDRUFF, HUMAN • The allergen in human skin flakes has been recognized for a long time and has been used as a test to determine a general tendency toward allergy. In one study, more than 90 percent of asthma patients had a positive skin test reaction in contrast to normals, who showed no reaction to the test. The reaction rate is even higher in those with allergic contact dermatitis or eczema. The subject of dandruff is a matter of controversy among allergists. Some point out that it is a self-produced antigen; others say it is part of the allergenic house-dust antigen; and still others say it is not a true allergen. Nevertheless, dandruff shampoos are among the top OTC sellers in pharmacies.

DANDRUFF SHAMPOOS • Usually shampoos that combine detergents with dry skin dissolvers. They contain sulfur, salicylic acid, resorcinol, and hexachlorophene. There are also after-shampoo dandruff rinses that contain quaternary ammonium compounds. And there are scalp lotions with antiseptics and stimulants such as resorcinol and/or chloral hydrate or tincture of capsicum. Hairdressings with zinc and cetalkonium chloride are also used to treat dandruff. Among other ingredients in dandruff products are allantoin for its healing properties and salicylanilide. A typical antidandruff formulation contains zinc pyrithione and a detergent. Another contains salicylic acid, sulfur, lanolin, cholesterol, and petrolatum. Certain ingredients such as sulfur, tar, lanolin, and salicylic acid are common allergens and may cause allergic contact dermatitis. The EU has banned pyrithione sodium and hexachlorophene in cosmetics.

DASHEEN EXTRACT • *See* Taro.

DATE • *Phoenix dactylifera.* The fruit from a tall palm tree cultivated in Asia and Africa. Used in organic cosmetics.

DATEM • A hair- and skin-conditioning ingredient as well as an emollient and emulsifying ingredient. *See* Fatty Acids.

DATURA STRAMONIUM • On the Canadian Hotlist (*see*). *See* Stramonium.

DAUCUS CAROTA • *See* Carrot Oil.

DAVANA OIL • *Artemesia pallens wall.* A plant extract used in fruit flavoring for cosmetics, beverages, ice cream, ices, candy, baked goods, and chewing gum. ASP

DBP • *See* Dibutyl Phthalate.

DEA • The abbreviation for diethanolamine (*see*).

DEA-C12-15 ALKYL SULFATE • *See* Alcohol and Sulfate.

DEA-CETEARETH-2 PHOSPHATE • A phosophorous compound used as a cleansing and emulsifying ingredient. Used in foundations and moisturizers. *See* Phosphorous.

DEA-COCOAMPHODIPROPIONATE • *See* Coconut Oil and Quaternary Ammonium Compounds.

DEA-CYCLOCARBOXYPROPYLOLEATE • The diethanolamine (*see*) salt of acrylinoleic acid.

DEA-DODECYLBENZENESULFONATE • *See* Quaternary Ammonium Compounds.

DEA-HYDROLYZED LECITHIN • *See* Hydrolyzed and Lecithin.

DEA-ISOSTEARATE • *See* Diethanolamine and Isostearic Acid.

DEA-LAURAMINOPROPIONATE • The diethanolamine salt of propionic acid (*see both*).

DEA-LAURETH SULFATE • *See* Quaternary Ammonium Compounds.

DEA-LAURYL SULFATE • *See* Quaternary Ammonium Compounds.

DEA-LINOLEATE • *See* Linoleic Acid.

DEA-METHOXYCINNAMATE • The diethanolamine salt of methoxycinnamic acid. *See* Diethanolamine and Cinnamic Acid.

DEA-METHYL MYRISTATE SULFONATE • Biterge. *See* Quaternary Ammonium Compounds.

DEA-MYRETH SULFATE • The diethanolamine salt of ethyoxylated myristyl sulfate. *See* Quaternary Ammonium Compounds.

DEA-MYRISTATE • The diethanolamine salt of myristic acid. Also called diethanolamine myristate. *See* Quaternary Ammonium Compounds.

DEA-OLETH-3 • *See* Oleth-20.

DEA-OLETH-10 PHOSPHATE • The diethanolamine salt of a mixture of esters of phosphoric acid and Oleth-10. Has been linked to allergic reactions. *See* Quaternary Ammonium Compounds.

DEA-STYRENE/ACRYLATES/DVB COPOLYMER • The diethanolamine salt of a polymer of styrene, divinylbenzene, and two or more monomers consisting of acrylic acid, methacrylic acid, or their esters. Used as an opacifier. *See* Acrylates, Styrene, Vinyl Polymers, and Benzene.

DEANOL • One of the newer ingredients, it is being promoted to increase the appearance of skin firmness in "anti-aging creams." Found in anchovies and sardines. Small amounts of it are also naturally produced in the human brain. Health-food outlets sell it in capsule form to "boost brain power." The EU, UK, and ASEAN (*see*) have banned deanol aceglumate in cosmetics.

DECANAL • An aldehyde (*see*) used as a fragrance ingredient.

DECANE • A hydrocarbon (*see*) used as a plasticizer, solvent, and thinner.

DECANOIC ACID • A synthetic flavoring ingredient that occurs naturally in anise, butter acids, oil of lemon, and oil of lime and is used in cosmetic fragrances. Also used to flavor butter, coconut, fruit, liquor, and cheese.

DECENAL • An aldehyde (*see*) used as a fragrance ingredient. ASP

DECENE • A hydrocarbon (*see*) used as a solvent and thinner.

DECENE/BUTENE COPOLYMER • Synthetic polymer (*see*) used as a thickener.

9-DECEN-1-OL • *See* Decylene. ASP

DECETH-4 • *See* Polyethylene Glycol and Decyl Alcohol.

DECETH-6 • The polyethylene glycol ether of decyl alcohol (*see*).

DECETH-7-CARBOXYLIC ACID • *See* Myristic Acid.

DECETH-4-PHOSPHATE • A mixture of polyethylene glycol, phosphoric acid esters, and decyl alcohol (*see all*).

DECETH-6-PHOSPHATE • A mixture of polyethylene glycol, phosphoric acid esters, and polyoxyethylene (*see all*).

DECYL ALCOHOL • An intermediate (*see*) for surface-active ingredients, an antifoam ingredient, and a fixative in perfumes. Occurs naturally in sweet orange and ambrette seed. Derived commercially from liquid paraffin (*see*). Colorless to light yellow liquid. Used also for synthetic lubricants and as a synthetic fruit flavoring. Low toxicity in animals for the skin.

DECYL BETAINE • *See* Betaine.

DECYL COCOATE • *See* Coconut Oil.

DECYL EVENING PRIMROSE ESTERS • Esters from evening primrose and decyl alcohol used as a skin-conditioning ingredient.

DECYL GLUCOSIDE • *See* Decyl Alcohol and Glucose.

DECYL HEMPSEEDATE • The ester of decyl aclohol and fatty acids derived from *Cannabis sativa* seed oil used as an emulsifier, emollient, and skin-conditioning ingredient.

DECYL ISOSTEARATE • *See* Decyl Alcohol and Isostearic Acid.

DECYL MERCAPTOMETHYLIMIDAZOLE • *See* Imidazole.

DECYL MYRISTATE • An ester of myristic acid (*see*) used as a skin-conditioning ingredient. It is opaque.

DECYL OLEATE • Widely used in hand creams, hair colorings, moisturizers, cold creams, makeup, and suntan products as a skin conditioner. On the basis of the available information, the CIR Expert Panel (*see*) found it safe in the early 1980s but is considering new information to determine if the final safety assessment should be reaffirmed, amended, or have an addendum. Has been linked with acne. *See* Decyl Alcohol.

DECYL POLYGLUCOSE • *See* Decyl Alcohol and Glucose.

DECYL SUCCINATE • Decyl Hydrogen Succinate. Produced by the reaction of decyl alcohol and succinic acid (*see both*). Used in the manufacture of perfumes and in cosmetics.

DECYL SWEET ALMOND ESTERS • A skin conditioner. *See* Almond Oil.

DECYL TETRADECANOL • *See* Decanoic Acid.

DECYLAMINE OXIDE • Capric Dimethylamine Oxide. *See* Capric Acid.

DECYLENE • A colorless liquid used in the manufacture of flavors, perfumes, pharmaceuticals, and dyes.

2-DECYLFURAN • Fragrance. Colorless solid; spicy, fatty aroma. EAF

DECYLTETRADECETH-30 • *See* Polyethylene Glycol and Decanoic Acid.

DEDM • Abbreviation for diethylol dimethyl.

DEDM HYDANTOIN • A preservative. *See* Hydantoin.

DEDM HYDANTOIN DILAURATE • A preservative. *See* Hydantoin and Lauric Acid.

DEER FAT • The fatty tissue obtained from deer used as a skin-conditioning ingredient.

DEER'S TONGUE LEAVES • Liatris. Vanilla Plant. Leaves of *Trilisa odoratissima,* found from Virginia to Florida and Louisiana. Contains the volatile oil coumarin (*see*). Used in perfumery and to make tobacco smell better.

DEHP • Di(2-ethylhexyl) phthalate. Di-octyl phthalate (DOP). One of the world's most commonly used plasticizers. In western Europe it accounts for 30 percent of all plasticizer usage. It is the phthalate ester of the alcohol 2-ethyl hexanol, which is normally manufactured from butyraldehyde. It is used in some fragrances. The FDA says exposure to

DEHP has produced a range of adverse effects in laboratory animals, but of greatest concern are effects on the development of the male reproductive system and production of normal sperm in young animals. The agency said it had not received reports of these adverse events in humans, but there have been no studies to rule them out. However, in view of the available animal data, precautions should be taken to limit the exposure of the developing male to DEHP. The CTFA (*see*) expressed concern about this finding in 2003. On the California list of potential cancer-causing agents. The EU banned DEHP in 2004.

DEHYDRATED • With the water removed.

DEHYDROACETIC ACID • DHA. Sodium Dehydroacetate. A weak acid that forms a white, odorless powder with an acrid taste. Used as an antienzyme ingredient in toothpastes to prevent tooth decay and as a preservative for shampoos. Also used as a fungi and bacteria-destroying ingredient in cosmetics. The presence of organic matter decreases its effectiveness. In the form of a mist or spray in commercial spray "tanning" booths to achieve the appearance of a tan worries the FDA. "Externally applied" cosmetics are those "applied only to external parts of the body and not to the lips or any body surface covered by mucous membrane" with a few exceptions such as mascara. When using DHA-containing products as an all-over spray or mist in a commercial spray "tanning" booth, it may be difficult to avoid exposure in a manner for which DHA is not approved, including the area of the eyes, lips, or mucous membrane, or even internally, the FDA says. It recommends consumers should request measures to protect their eyes and mucous membranes and prevent inhalation. DHA is not reportedly irritating or allergy causing, but it is a kidney-blocking ingredient and can cause impaired kidney function. Large doses can cause vomiting, imbalance, and convulsions.

7-DEHYDROCHOLESTEROL • *See* Cholesterol.

DEIONIZED AND DEMINERALIZED WATER • Water treated to remove components that could interfere with a cosmetic's stability and performance.

DELANEY AMENDMENT • Written by Congressman James Delaney, the amendment was part of a 1958 law requested by the Food and Drug Administration. The law stated that food and chemical manufacturers had to test additives before they were put on the market and the results had to be submitted to the FDA. Delaney's amendment specifically states that "no additive may be permitted in any amount if the tests show that it produces cancer when fed to man or animals or by other appropriate tests."

DELAYED HYPERSENSITIVITY • Manifested primarily as contact dermatitis due to drugs such as neomycin or to parabens (*see both*), a common preservative in topical medications. Certain multiple allergic reactions to drugs such as penicillin, nitrofurantoin, and hydantoin may also fall into this category.

DELESSERIA SANGUINEA • *See* Sanguinaria.

DELTA CADINENE • A sesquiterpene occurring in essential oils from juniper species and cedars (oil of cade). Used in perfumery. *See* Sesquiterpene Lactones.

DEMULCENT • A soothing, usually thick, oily, or creamy substance used to relieve pain in inflamed or irritated mucous surfaces. The gum acacia, for instance, is used as a demulcent.

DENATONIUM BENZOATE • A denaturant for alcohol that is to be used in cosmetics. It is intended to make alcohol unpalatable for drinking purposes and, therefore, is unpleasant to smell and taste. *See* Denatured Alcohol.

DENATONIUM SACCHARIDE • A denaturant for alcohol. *See* Denatonium Benzoate.

DENATURANT • A poisonous or unpleasant substance added to alcoholic cosmetics to make them undrinkable. It is also considered a substance that changes another substance's natural qualities or characteristics.

DENATURED ALCOHOL • Ethyl alcohol must be made unfit for drinking before it can be used in cosmetics. Various substances such as denatonium benzoate (*see*) are added to alcohol to make it malodorous and obnoxious in order to completely prevent its use or recovery for drinking purposes.

DENTAL BLEACH • Promoted greatly since the last edition of this book. These are products that are put on by your dentist or by toothpaste or products you apply yourself. Usually containing a strong peroxide compound (see Peroxide). Eight out of ten dentists now offer bleaching as an esthetic treatment for their patients. The American Dental Association has published the following statement: "Dentist-prescribed, home-applied bleaching made by a reputable manufacturer and used under the supervision of a dentist in a relatively short-term treatment duration is safe and recognized as most effective in lightening the color of teeth. Bleaching materials that have received the ADA Seal of Acceptance are recommended." Many toothpaste companies are now advertising bleaching in their products. In all cases, bleaching benefits vary. The only common adverse effect reported, if bleaching is done carefully, is apparently temporary tooth sensitivity. Mild thermal sensitivity (sensitivity to cold) is a common side effect associated with most in-office and dentist-prescribed home bleaching methods. However, no long-term irreversible tissue effects have been demonstrated in relevant clinical studies as yet.

DENTIFRICES • Their primary purpose is to clean accessible surfaces of the teeth with a toothbrush. Such cleansing is important to the appearance of teeth and to gum health, and it prevents mouth odor. Dentifrices usually come in the form of a paste or powder. Despite the brand claims, most dentifrices contain similar ingredients: binders, abrasives, sudsers, humectants, flavors, unique additives, and liquids. Binders include karaya gum, bentonite, sodium alginate, methylcellulose, carrageenan, and magnesium aluminum silicate. Among the abrasives are calcium carbonate, dibasic calcium phosphate, calcium sulfate, tricalcium phosphate, and sodium metaphosphate hydrated alumina. Sudsers include hard soap and the detergents sodium lauryl sulfate, sodium lauryl sulfoacetate, dioctyl sodium sulfosuccinate, sulfolaurate, and sodium lauryol sarcosinate. Humectants include glycerin, propylene glycol, and sorbitol. The most popular flavors are spearmint, peppermint, wintergreen, and cinnamon, but there are also such odd ones as bourbon, rye, anise, clove, caraway, coriander, eucalyptus, nutmeg, and thyme. Fluorides are added to reduce decay; also added are antienzyme ingredients (sodium dehydroacetate) and tooth whiteners (sodium perborate). Still other ingredients in dentifrices are sodium benzoate, ammonium antiseptics, sodium coconut monoglyceride sulfonate, sodium copper chlorophyllin, chloroform, starch, sodium chloride, calcium sulfate, strontium chloride, *p*-hydroxybenzoate as a preservative, and sodium dehydroacetate. Toothpastes promoted for sensitive teeth are questionable, according to the American Dental Association. The most popular toothpaste contains sodium fluoride, calcium pyrophosphate, glycerin, sorbitol, and a blend of anionic surfactants (*see*); its competitor contains sodium *n*-lauryol sarcosinate and sodium monofluorophosphate. Complaints to the FDA about dentifrices include sore mouth and gums, tooth enamel worn away, sore tongue, and sloughing of mucous membranes. Some toothpastes contained too much chloroform, which was reduced by the manufacturer upon the FDA's request. Tartar control became the "buzzword" in the 1980s, and most toothpastes promoted it. Since the 1990s, as the population grows older, manufacturers are promoting toothpastes for sensitive teeth and bicarbonate of soda and other ingredients for healthy gums as well as tartar removal.

DEODORANTS • Includes antiperspirants. It is not the normal secretions of the skin that produce an objectionable odor but the action of bacteria and chemicals on sweat that creates the unpleasant smell. The difference between deodorants and antiperspirants is in sequence. Deodorants control perspiration odors, but antiperspirants retard the flow of perspiration. Deodorants inhibit the growth of microorganisms, which produce the malodors; antiperspirants, which contain a hydrolyzing metal salt, develop a low pH (increased acidity) and inhibit moisture. The inhibiting action may be enhanced by antiseptics that deodorize. Aluminum salts are the most widely used for inhibiting perspiration; urea (see) may be added to neutralize the fabric-damaging acidity of the metal. Antiseptics may be incorporated into deodorant soaps. Deodorants, formerly called "unscented toilet waters" and "sanitary liquid preparations," once contained formaldehyde or benzoic acid, which have been replaced with quaternary ammonium compounds (see). Deodorant-action, liquid antiperspirants today usually contain aluminum chloride, urea, propylene glycol, and about 75 percent water. Deodorant-action, cream antiperspirants contain aluminum chlorhydroxide, sorbitan monostearate, poloxamers, stearic acid, boric acid, petrolatum, perfume, propylene glycol, and water. Spray deodorants have the same ingredients as liquid ones but are mixed with a propellant. The aluminum, alcohol, and zinc salts in deodorants and antiperspirants can cause skin and gastrointestinal irritations. Deaths from intentional inhalation of deodorant sprays have been reported. Vision has been affected by spray in the eyes. With all deodorants there can be stinging and burning, itching, sebaceous cysts, enlarged sweat glands, pimples under the arms, and lung and throat irritation. Seven cases of lung tumors attributed to underarm deodorant sprays were reported at the 1971 American Thoracic Society meeting in Los Angeles. See Vaginal Deodorants.

DEODORIZED KEROSENE • Deo-Base. Derived from petroleum, it is a mobile, water-white transparent liquid that has been deodorized and decolorized by washing kerosene with fuming sulfuric acid. It is a solvent used in brilliantines and emulsified lotions and creams, and as a constituent of hand lotions. It is a skin irritant, and dermatitis often occurs. Because of its solvent action on fats, it can cause a defatting and drying of the skin. In cosmetics, however, when it is used with fatty substances, its fat-solvent action is minimized and it is considered innocuous.

DEOXYRIBONUCLEASE • An enzyme that hydrolyzes (see) DNA (see).

DEPILATORIES • The most effective chemical hair removers yet discovered are the sulfides (see), particularly hydrogen sulfide, but they have an unpleasant odor that is hard to mask. Most sulfides have been replaced with salts of thioglycolic acid (see), which take more time to act but smell better and are not as irritating as sulfides. However, persons who have difficulty with detergent hands, ammonia, or strong soaps often have difficulty with thioglycolic depilatories. Also, ingestion of thioglycolic depilatories may cause severe gastrointestinal irritation. Cream depilatories that act by dissolving the hair usually contain calcium thioglycolate, calcium carbonate, calcium hydroxide, cetyl alcohol, sodium lauryl sulfate (a detergent), water, and a strong perfume (so as to remain stable in an alkali medium). Another type of depilatory made of wax acts by hardening around the hair and pulling it out. Such products usually contain rosin, beeswax, paraffin, and petrolatum. (See above ingredients under separate listings.) Among injuries recently reported to the FDA concerning depilatories were skin irritation, headaches, scars on the legs, skin burns, and rash. It can cause allergic reactions. See Flaxseed.

DEPROTEINATED YEAST • See Proteins and Yeast.

DEPROTEINIZED SERUM • Fluid portion of the blood from which protein has been removed.

DEQUALINIUM CHLORIDE • See Quaternary Ammonium Compounds.

DEQUALIUM ACETATE • See Quaternary Ammonium Compounds.

DERMATAN SULFATE • Chondroitin Sulfate. Chondroitin Sulfuric Acid. Occurs in both skeletal and soft connective tissue. It is abundant in skin, arterial walls, and heart valves.

DERMATITIS • Inflammation of the skin.

DERMIS • The lower layer of skin, overlying subcutaneous fat and composed of blood vessels, lymph sacs, sensory nerve endings, hair follicles, and oil and sweat glands.

DERMOLECTINE • Ingredient from potatoes. Acts similar to a hormone. Supposedly "wakes up the skin" and is promoted as a wrinkle fighter.

DESAMIDO COLLAGEN • Animal collagen that has been modified to change the amide group into carboxylic acid groups to change its texture and odor for use in "youth creams." The word *animal* was removed from the label.

DESOXYCHOLIC ACID • An emulsifying ingredient, white, crystalline powder, almost insoluble in water. Used in dried egg whites up to 0.1 percent. The final report to the FDA of the Select Committee on GRAS Substances stated in 1980 that it should continue its GRAS status with no limitations other than good manufacturing practices. Moderately toxic by ingestion. Has caused tumors in animals.

DESOXYEPHEDRINE HYDROCHLORIDE • Epinine. Desoxyephedrine. Obtained from laudanosine, or papaverine, which are both derived from the poppy. It is a blood vessel constrictor.

DESOXYRIBONUCLEIC ACID • DNA. A chain of molecules that contains the genetic code (blueprint) of cells.

DESQUAMATE • Normal shedding of the skin.

DETERGENTS • Any of a group of synthetic, organic, liquid, or water-soluble cleansing ingredients that, unlike soap, are not prepared from fats and oils and are not inactivated by hard water. Most of them are made from petroleum derivatives but vary widely in composition. The major advantage of detergents is that they do not leave a hard water scum. They also have wetting ingredient and emulsifying ingredient properties. Quaternary ammonium compounds (*see*), for instance, through surface action, exert cleansing and antibacterial effects. pHisoderm is an example of a liquid detergent, and Dove is an example of a solid detergent. Toxicity of detergents depends upon alkalinity. Dishwasher detergents, for instance, can be dangerously alkaline while detergents used in cosmetic products have an acidity-alkalinity ratio near normal skin, 5 to 6.5 pH.

DETOXOPHANE • An extract of cress sprouts that contains sulforaphane, a well-known activator of phase II enzymes of the cellular detoxification system. Claimed to protect skin against pollutants and "prevent visible signs of aging."

DEXAMETHASONE • A steroid drug used to treat allergies or inflammation. Among its side effects are muscle weakness, impaired wound healing, and increased blood sugar levels.

DEXTRAN • A term applied to polysaccharides produced by bacteria growing on sugar. Used as a thickening ingredient in cuticle removers, it is also employed as a foam stabilizer in beer. Injection into the skin has caused cancer in rats.

DEXTRAN SULFATE • The sulfuric acid ester of dextran (*see*).

DEXTRIN • British Gum. Starch Gum. White or yellow powder produced from starch and used as a diluting ingredient for dry extracts and emulsions and as a thickener in cream and liquid cosmetics. May cause an allergic reaction.

DIACETIN • A mixture of the diesters (*see*) of glycerin (*see*) and acetic acid (*see*), used as a plasticizer, softening ingredient, or as a solvent for cellulose derivatives, resins, and shellacs.

DIACETONE ALCOHOL • Used as a solvent for nail enamels, fats, oils, waxes, and resins. Also used as a preservative. Prepared by the action of an alkali such as calcium hydroxide on acetone (*see*). Highly flammable with a pleasant odor, it mixes easily with other solvents. May be narcotic in high concentrations and has caused kidney and liver damage, as well as anemia, in experimental animals when given orally.

DIACETYL • A catalyst (*see*) in the manufacture of fake nails. It occurs naturally in cheese, cocoa, pears, coffee, raspberries, strawberries, and cooked chicken but is usually prepared by a special fermentation of glucose. It is a yellowish green liquid. Also used as a carrier of aroma of butter, vinegar, and coffee, and to flavor oleomargarine. Diacetyl compounds have been associated with cancer when ingested by experimental animals.

DIACETYLMORPHINE • Diacetyl-N-allyl-N-morphine. A derivative of poppies, it has been banned in cosmetics by the EU and ASEAN (*see*).

DI-C-12-15 ALKYL ADIPATE • *See* Alcohol and Adipic Acid.

DI-C-12 ALKYL FUMARATE • An ester (*see*) of alcohol and fumaric acid (*see*). Used as a skin-conditioning ingredient.

DIAMINO- • A prefix meaning two amine atoms from ammonia.

3,4-DIAMINOBENZOIC ACID • *See* Benzoic Acid.

4,5-DIAMINO-1-((4-CHLOROPHENYL)METHYL)-1H-PYRAZOLESULFATE • A hair coloring. *See* Coal Tar.

2,4-DIAMINODIPHENYLAMINE • A hair coloring. *See* Coal Tar and Ammonia.

2,4-DIAMINO-5-METHYLETHIOXYPHENOL HCL • *See* Phenols and Ammonia.

4,5-DIAMINO-1-METHYLPYROZOLE HCL • *See* Ammonia and Pyrazole.

DIAMINONAPHTHALINE • A black dye. *See* Coal Tar.

DIAMINOPHENOL • A brown hair dye. Irritant for the sensitive. Must carry this warning: "Can cause an allergic reaction. Do not use to dye eyelashes or eyebrows." Salon or home applicators must wear suitable gloves. Approved by the EU and FDA. *See* Phenols.

2,4-DIAMINOPHENOL • Manufactured from aniline (*see*) and used in hair dye. The CIR Expert Panel (*see*) concluded that its use in hair dyes at concentrations up to 0.2 percent was safe. For toxicity, *see p*-Phenylenediamine. The EU says it can cause an allergic reaction and should not be used to dye eyelashes. Should be applied by professionals. *See* Phenols.

DIAMINOPHENOL HYDROCHLORIDE • A black-brown dye. The CIR Expert Panel (*see*) concluded that its use in hair dyes at concentrations up to 0.2 percent was safe. Has been linked to allergies. *See* Phenols.

2,4-DIAMINOPHENOXYETHANOL HCL • An aromatic amine salt used as a fixative, bactericide, and insect repellent. Slightly irritating to the skin. *See* Quaternary Ammonium Compounds.

4,4-DIAMINOPHENYLAMINE • *See* Ammonia and Phenylene Diamine.

2,6-DIAMINOPYRIDINE • *See* Pyridine.

DIAMMONIUM CITRATE • Ammonium salt of citric acid, dibasic. *See* Citric Acid.

DIAMMONIUM DITHIODIGLYCOLATE • Acetic acid, 2,2′-dithiobis-diammonium salt used in hair removal and hair waving. *See* Thioglycolic Acid Compounds.

DIAMMONIUM LAURYL SULFOSUCCINATE • The ammonium salt of lauryl alcohol. *See* Quaternary Ammonium Compounds.

DIAMMONIUM OLEAMIDO-PEG-2-SULFOSUCCINATE • An ammonium soap used as an emulsifying ingredient. *See* Quaternary Ammonium Compounds.

DIAMMONIUM PHOSPHATE • *See* Phosphate, Ammonia, and Surfactants.

DIAMMONIUM SODIUM SULFOSUCCINATE • The sodium salt of the diester of amyl alcohol and sulfosuccinic acid. A wetting ingredient and emulsifier. *See* Surfactants.

DIAMOND POWDER • A crystallized carbon used as an abrasive.

DIAMYLHYDROQUINONE • Santovar A. An antioxidant for resins and oils and a polymerization inhibitor. *See* Hydroquinone.

DIANTHUS CARYOPHYLLUS • A name given to several plants of the caryophyllaceous genus *Dianthus,* and to their flowers, which are sometimes very fragrant. Carnations belong to this family. Used as a fragrance ingredient.

DIAPER RASH • Ammonia Dermatitis. Skin irritation caused by urine and feces, and also by soap or detergents left in diapers if they are not thoroughly rinsed. The skin becomes red, spotty, sore, and moist.

DIAPER RASH PRODUCTS • The FDA issued a notice in 1992 that any diaper rash products with ingredients labeled with claims or directions for the use in the treatment or prevention of diaper rash have not been shown to be safe and effective as claimed in OTC products.

DIASTASE • A mixture of enzymes from malt. It converts at least fifty times its weight of potato starch into sugars in thirty minutes. Used to convert starch into sugar. In 1992, the FDA ruled that diastase and diastase malt aluminum hydroxide have not been shown to be safe and effective as claimed in OTC digestive aid products.

DIATALLOWETHYL HYDROXYETHYLMONIUM METHOSULFATE • *See* Quaternary Ammonium Compounds.

DIATOMACEOUS EARTH • Kieselguhr. A porous and relatively pure form of silica formed from fossil remains of diatoms—one-celled algae with shells. Inert when ingested. Used in pomades, dentifrices, nail polishes, face powders, as a clarifying ingredient, and as an absorbent for liquids because it can absorb about four times its weight in water. The dust can cause lung damage after long exposure to high concentrations. Not recommended for use on teeth or skin because of its abrasiveness.

DIAZO • A compound containing two nitrogen atoms, such as diazolidinyl urea (*see*), one of the newer preservatives, or diazepam, a tranquilizer and popular muscle relaxant.

DIAZO DYES • Coloring ingredients that contain two linked nitrogen atoms united to an aromatic group and to an acid radical. *See* Heliotropin.

DIAZOLIDINYL UREA • Oxymethurea. 1,3-Bis(hydroxymethyl) Urea. Crystals from alcohol, very soluble in water. Used in the textile industry in cotton; as a pesticide and in cosmetics as an antiseptic in hair care and nail preparations. May release formaldehyde (*see*). At concentrations up to 0.4 percent it was a mild cumulative skin irritant in humans. The CIR Expert Panel (*see*) concluded that on the basis of animal and clinical data, it is safe as a cosmetic ingredient up to a maximum concentration of 0.5 percent. The EU limits it to 2 percent and prohibits the hair preparations in aerosol dispensers, and the pH of the nail product applied must be less than 4. *See* Imidazolidinone. *See also* Urea.

DIBA • The abbreviation for dihydroxyisobutylamine.

DIBEHENHYL FUMARATE • Made from fumaric acid and behenyl alcohol (*see both*) it is used as a thickener.

DIBEHENYL METHYLAMINE • Methyl Dibenehenylamine. *See* Behenic Acid.

DIBEHENYL/DIARACHIDYL DIMONIUM CHLORIDE • *See* Quaternary Ammonium Compounds.

DIBEHENYLDIMONIUM CHLORIDE • *See* Quaternary Ammonium Compounds.

DIBEHENYLDIMONIUM METHOSULFATE • *See* Quaternary Ammonium Compounds.

DIBENZOTHIOPHENE • Thioxanthene. Diphenylene Sulfide. Prepared from thioxanthrone, it gives a green fluorescence. Used in dandruff treatment shampoos, and to add a green fluorescence. Also used in acne products. Colorless crystals made from alcohol, chloroform, and sulfur. Used as a psychopharmaceutical to treat mental disorders. When ingested can affect central nervous system, the blood, and blood pressure. Not approved by the FDA for acne or by the Italian government cosmetic overseers.

DIBENZOXAZOYL NAPHTHALENE • An ultraviolet light absorber. *See* Benzoic Acid and Naphthalene.

DIBENZYL ETHER • A synthetic fruit and spice flavoring ingredient for beverages, ice cream, ices, candy, baked goods, and chewing gum. The Flavor and Extract Manufacturer's Association evaluated the safety of this additive. High-dose female rats had increased liver weights. A no-effect level was achieved at 196 mg/kg/day. In a 60-kg human (about 132 pounds), this would be equivalent to approximately 11.8 grams a day.

DIBENZYLIDENE SORBITOL • *See* Sorbitol.

DIBROMO-2,4-DICYANOBUTANE • 2-Bromo-2-(bromoethyl)pentanedinitrile. 2-Bromo-2-(bromoethyl)glutaronitrile. Metacide 38. Tektamer 38. Various trade names. Used as a pesticide, preservative in cosmetics. The EU ruled in 2003 that its use should be restricted to rinse-off products at the current maximum permitted at 0.1 percent.

DIBROMOFLUORESCEIN • Used in indelible lipsticks, it is made by heating resorcinol and phthalic anhydride (*see both*) to produce fluorescent orange-red crystals. Ingestion can cause gastrointestinal symptoms. Skin application can cause skin sensitivity to light, inflamed eyes, skin rash, and even respiratory symptoms. *See* Colors.

DIBROMOPROPAMIDINE DIISETHIONATE • The salt of isethionic acid mixed with propane. It is used as an antiseptic and antimicrobial. May be irritating to the skin.

DIBROMOSALAN • 4,5-Dibromosalicylanilide. An antibacterial ingredient used as an antiseptic and fungicide in detergents, toilet soaps, creams, lotions, and powders. The FDA prohibited it in cosmetics in 2000 because it may cause sensitivity to light resulting in rash and swelling.

DIBUCAINE • Nupercaine. Bitter, water-absorbing crystals. Used as a local anesthetic for the skin, particularly in wax depilatories to prevent pain. Similar to cocaine when applied to the skin. Highly toxic when injected into the abdomens of rats; only one part per kilogram of body weight is lethal.

DIBUTYL ADIPATE • The diester of butyl alcohol and adipic acid (*see both*). A thickener in cosmetic products. A reduction in weight gain occurred in rabbits whose skin was painted with this substance. It was also mildly irritating to their skin and eyes. A significant increase in fetal abnormalities also occurred. The CIR Expert Panel (*see*) concludes that the available data are insufficient to support the safety of this ingredient in cosmetics.

DIBUTYL LAUROYL GLUTAMIDE • Gelling ingredient. *See* Lauric and Glutamic Acids.

DIBUTYL OXALATE • A plasticizer and solvent. Chelating ingredient. Toxic. Maximum allowed is 5 percent and it is restricted to professional use only. *See* Butyl Alcohol and Oxalic Acid.

DIBUTYL PHTHALATE • DBP. The ester of the salt of phthalic acid (*see*), which is isolated from a fungus. The colorless liquid is used as a plasticizer in nail polish and as a perfume solvent, fixative, shampoo, and antifoam ingredient. It is also an insect repellent. Has a low toxicity but if ingested can cause gastrointestinal upset. Linked to gene and hormone changes in rodents and genital abnormalities in human infants. This is a high-volume chemical with production exceeding 1 million pounds annually in the United States. Employed in at least three industries. Used in pesticide products. Suspected by the EPA and the National Toxicology Program of being toxic to development, the endocrine and gastrointestinal systems, and the liver, nerves, and kidneys. It has been linked to testicular cancer. Toxicant. Phthlates. The vapor is irritating to the eyes and mucous membranes. On the basis of the available information, the CIR Expert Panel (*see*) found it safe in the early 1980s to use on the skin but are considering new information to determine if the final safety assessment should be reaffirmed, amended, or have an addendum. It is on California Proposition 65's list of substances known to cause cancer or reproductive harm. At this writing, large cosmetic companies such as Procter & Gamble and Estée Lauder are reformulating their nail polishes to eliminate this chemical. The European Union has voted to ban this chemical in nail polishes. It has been labeled a "Substance of Very High Concern." Unilever, however, another big cosmetics manufacturer, indicated in 2004 it doesn't intend to change its formula for the U.S. market, despite the EU ban. The European Chemicals Agency stated the apparently increasing incidence of the testicular dysgenesis syndrome (TDS) in men is cause of concern.

DIBUTYL SEBACATE • Sebacic Acid. A synthetic fruit flavoring usually obtained from castor oil. Used in fruit-fragrance cosmetics. Mildly toxic by ingestion. Oral doses in rats cause reproductive effects. ASP

DIBUTYLENE TETRAFURFURAL • Derived from bran, rice hulls, or corncobs, it is used in the manufacture of medicinals and as a solvent and flavoring in cosmetics and food. Toxic when absorbed by the skin. Irritating to the eye.

DI-*t*-BUTYLHYDROQUINONE • A yellow powder used as an antioxidant. Animal studies show that this ingredient as low as 10 percent can cause redness of the skin and in feeding, it caused the deaths of all rats in the study within two weeks. The CIR Expert Panel (*see*) concluded that the available data for this ingredient are insufficient to support its safety as a cosmetic ingredient. *See* Hydroquinone.

DICALCIUM PHOSPHATE • Tooth polisher for dentifrices. *See* Calcium Phosphate.

DICALCIUM PHOSPHATE DIHYDRATE • Dicalcium phosphate (*see*) in powder form.

DICAPRYL ADIPATE • The diester of capryl alcohol and adipic acid (*see both*).

DICAPRYUDICAPRYLYL DIMONIUM CHLORIDE • *See* Quaternary Ammonium Compounds.

DICAPRYL ETHER • A skin-conditioning ingredient. *See* Caproic Acid.

DICAPRYLOYL CYSTINE • *See* Caprylic Acid and Cystine.

DICAPRYLSODIUM SULFOSUCCINATE • The sodium salt of the diester of capryl alcohol and sulfosuccinic acid. *See* Quaternary Ammonium Compounds.

DICETEARETH-10 PHOSPHATE • *See* Phosphoric Acid and Stearic Acid.

DICETYL ADIPATE • The diester of cetyl alcohol and adipic acid (*see both*).

DICETYL PHOSPHATE • A mixture of cetyl alcohol and phosphoric acid (*see both*).

DICETYL THIODIPROPIONATE • The diester of cetyl alcohol and thiodipropionic acid (*see both*).

DICETYLDIMONIUM CHLORIDE • *See* Quaternary Ammonium Compounds.

DICHLOROBENZYL ALCOHOL • An insecticide. *See* Benzyl Alcohol.

DICHLORODIMETHYL HYDANTOIN • *See* Hydantoin.

DICHLOROETHANES • Solvents no longer permitted in cosmetics by the EU.

DICHLOROMETHANE • Solvent. Harmful vapors. Harmful by skin absorption Has caused cancer in animal tests. The EU says it should not exceed 35 percent. Banned in the United States.

2,3-DICHLORO-2-METHYLBUTANE • Banned in cosmetics by the EU and ASEAN (*see*).

DICHLOROPHEN • *See* Dichlorophene.

DICHLOROPHENE • Dichlorophen. Antiphen. Hyosan. Crystals from toluene (*see*). A fungicide and bactericide used in dentifrices, shampoos, antiperspirants, deodorant creams, powder, and toilet waters. It is a potent allergen and is closely related to hexachlorophene (*see*). The EU says it must be printed on ingredient label.

DICHLOROPHENYL IMIDAZOLDIOXOLAN • A preservative. See Imidazole.

DICHLORO-*m*-XLENOL • A phenol used as a bactericide in soaps and as a mold inhibitor and preservative. *See* Phenols.

DICOCAMINE • *See* Coconut Acids.

DICOCODIMETHYLAMINE DILINOLEATE • The diamine salt of dimer acid and dimethyl cocamine (*see both*) used as a plasticizer. *See* Coconut Acids.

DICOCODIMETHYLAMINE DIMERATE • *See* Dicocodimethylamine Dilinoleate.

DICOCODIMONIUM CHLORIDE • *See* Quaternary Ammonium Compounds.

DICOCOYL PENTAERYTHRITYL DISTEARYL CITRATE • Fatty acids derived from coconut oil (*see*).

DICOCOYLETHYL HYDROXYETHYLMONIUM METHOSULFATE • *See* Quaternary Ammonium Compounds.

DICYCLOHEXYL SODIUM SULFOSUCCINATE • *See* Quaternary Ammonium Compounds.

DICYCLOPENTADIENE • Cyclopentadiene. Obtained from coal, it is used in the manufacture of resins and in camphors.

DIDECENE • A hydrocarbon (*see*) used as a skin-conditioning ingredient.

DIDECYLDIMONIUM CHLORIDE • *See* Quaternary Ammonium Compounds.

DIERUCIC ACID • A skin-conditioning ingredient and cover-up. See Erucic Acid.

DIESTER • A compound containing two ester groupings. An ester is formed from an alcohol and an acid by eliminating water. Usually employed in fragrant liquids for artificial fruit perfumes and flavors.

DIETHANOLAMIDOOLEAMIDE DEA • *See* Quaternary Ammonium Compounds.

DIETHANOLAMINE • Abbreviated as DEA. Colorless liquid or crystalline fatty acids from soybeans or coconut oils. It is used as a solvent, emulsifying ingredient, and detergent. Also employed in emollients for its softening properties and as a dispersing ingredient and humectant in other cosmetic products. It may be irritating to the skin and mucous membranes. The FDA became aware of a National Toxicology Program (NTP) study showing an association between the topical application of diethanolamine and certain DEA-related ingredients and cancer in laboratory animals. For the DEA-related ingredients, the NTP study suggests that the cancer response is linked to possible residual levels of DEA. Although DEA itself may be used in few products, DEA-related ingredients such as oleamide DEA, lauramide DEA, and cocamide DEA are widely used as emulsifiers or foaming ingredients and generally used at levels of 1 to 5 percent. The FDA is studying the problem and is going to consider legal options at this writing. *See* Ethanolamines.

DIETHANOLAMINE BISULFATE • *See* Ethanolamines.

DIETHOXYETHYL SUCCINATE • *See* Succinic Acid.

DIETHYL ASPARTATE • The diester of ethyl alcohol and aspartic acid (*see both*).

DIETHYL GLUTAMATE • *See* Glutamate.

DIETHYL KETONE • 3-Pentanone. Liquid with an acetone odor used as an emulsifier.

DIETHYL MALEATE • Banned in fragrances by the UK.

DIETHYL MALONATE • 2-Butanedioic acid, diethyl ester. Used in the manufacture of chemicals. *See* Malic Acid.

DIETHYL OXALATE • Chelating ingredient. Toxic. Restricted to professional use by the EU and the FDA.

DIETHYL PALMITOYL ASPARTATE • *See* Aspartic Acid.

DIETHYL PHTHALATE • Made from ethanol and phthalic acid (*see both*). Used as a solvent, a fixative for perfume, and a denaturant (*see*) for alcohol. It has a bitter and unpleasant taste. Irritating to mucous membranes. Produces central nervous system depression when absorbed through the skin. On the basis of the available information, the CIR Expert Panel (*see*) found it safe in the early 1980s but is considering new information to determine if the final safety assessment should be reaffirmed, amended, or have an addendum. Allowed in cosmetics by the EU and FDA.

DIETHYL SEBACATE • *See* Sebacic Acid.

DIETHYL SUCCINATE • The diester of ethyl alcohol and succinic acid (*see both*).

DIETHYL TOLUAMIDE • DEET. Made from *m*-toluoyl chloride and diethylamine in benzene or ether. A liquid soluble in water, it is used as an insect repellent. Irritating to the eyes and mucous membranes but not to the skin. Ingestion can cause central nervous system disturbances. On the Canadian Hotlist (*see*). EU. FDA

DIETHYLAMINE LAURETH SULFATE • *See* Surfactants.

DIETHYLAMINOETHYL COCOATE • Derived from coconut oil. *See* Surfactants.

DIETHYLAMINOETHYL METHYLCRYLATE • *See* Acrylates.

DIETHYLAMINOETHYL PEG-5 COCOATE • Derived from coconut oil (*see*). *See* Surfactants and Polyethylene Glycol.

DIETHYLAMINOETHYL PEG-5-LAURATE • *See* Polyethylene Glycol and Lauric Acid.

DIETHYLAMINOETHYL STEARAMIDE • *See* Diethanolamine.

DIETHYLAMINOETHYL STEARATE • *See* Stearic Acid and Amines.

DIETHYLAMINOMETHYL COUMARIN • *See* Coumarins.

N,N-DIETHYL-*m*-AMINOPHENOL • *See* Phenols.

N,N-DIETHYL-*m*-AMINOPHENOL SULFATE • *See* Phenols.

DIETHYLENE GLYCOL • Made by heating ethylene oxide and glycol. A clear, water-absorbing, almost colorless liquid; it is mixable with water, alcohol, and acetone. Used as a solvent, humectant, and plasticizer in cosmetic creams and hairsprays. A wetting ingredient (*see*) that enhances skin absorption. Can be fatal if swallowed. Not usually irritating to the skin, but can be absorbed through the skin and the use of glycols on extensive areas of the body is considered hazardous.

DIETHYLENE GLYCOL DIBENZOATE • The polyethylene glycol diester of benzoic acid (*see*).

DIETHYLENE GLYCOLAMINE/EPICHLOROHYDRIN PIPERAZINE COPOLYMER • A polymer formed by the reaction of a mixture of diethylene glycolamine and piperazine with epichlorohydrin, used as a solvent. See Epichlorohydrin.

DIETHYLENE TRICASEINAMIDE • Made from milk protein and casein (*see*).

DI(2-ETHYLHEXYL) PHTHALATE • *See* DEHP.

DIETHYLHEXYLCYCLOHEXAMINE • Derived from petroleum, it is used as a conditioner in hand and body preparations. *See* Hydrocarbons.

DIETHYLHEXYL PHTHALATE • A fragrance ingredient and solvent. *See* Phthalic Acid.

DIETHYLHEXYL SEBACATE • A fragrance ingredient and solvent used in aerosol hair sprays and other hair-grooming products.

DIETHYLSTILBESTROL • DES. Stilbestrol. A synthetic estrogen fed to cattle and poultry to "fatten them." A proven carcinogen, hormonal in nature, according to the

FDA, which has given top priority to the study of the safety of DES. The FDA stipulates a zero tolerance for the compound after a proper withdrawal period. In 1971, three Harvard scientists linked DES to a rare form of vaginal cancer in the daughters of women who had taken DES during pregnancy. The European Common Market, Italy, and Sweden have forbidden the use of DES in cattle. Can be absorbed through the skin. It is offered for sale to cosmetics manufacturers, so presumably some may be using it in hormone creams.

DIFFUSIVE • A term used to describe a perfume compound odor that spreads quickly and widely. This quality is good in perfumes but may be disliked in other products, such as hair sprays and deodorants.

DIGALLOYL TRIOLEATE • From digallic acid and oleic acid. An oily sunscreen ingredient devoid of anesthetic properties and stable under long periods of ultraviolet radiation. It may cause the skin to break out and redden when exposed to light.

DIGENEA SIMPLEX • Kainic Acid. Dried red algae that is used as a preservative. It is used to combat worms.

DIGITOXIN • Crystodigin. Purodigin. The main ingredient in digitalis, digitoxin is found in the leaves of the foxglove plant. It is used to treat congestive heart failure and irregular heartbeat and flutter. It works by strengthening the force of the heart's contractions and by regulating abnormal heart rhythms, especially fast irregular heartbeats. It is used in cosmetics. It is banned by the EU in cosmetics.

DIGLYCERIN • A humectant (*see*) derived from glycerin (*see*).

DIGLYCERYL STEARATE MALATE • The mixed ester of stearic acid and malic acid and glycerin polymer (*see all*).

DIHEPTYL SODIUM SULFOSUCCINATE • Available as a waxlike solid. Used as a wetting ingredient in bath oil preparation.

DIHEPTYLUNDECYL ADIPATE • *See* Adipic Acid.

DIHEXYL ADIPATE • A low-temperature plasticizer and skin-conditioning ingredient, emollient, and solvent in a wide variety of cosmetics such as makeup, moisturizers, makeup bases, blushers, and skin care products. *See* Adipic Acid.

DIHEXYL SODIUM SULFOSUCCINATE • Used in bath products. *See* Quaternary Ammonium Compounds.

DIHEXYL SODIUM SULFOSUCCINATE • *See* Quaternary Ammonium Compounds.

DIHEXYLDECYL LAUROYL GLUTAMATE • An amino acid used as an emollient ingredient. *See* Glutamate.

DIHYDROABIETYL ALCOHOL • *See* Abietic Acid and Abietyl Alcohol.

DIHYDROABIETYL METHACRYLATE • *See* Abietyl Alcohol.

DIHYDROACETIC ACID • Used in tanning creams. *See* Acetic Acid.

DIHYDROANISOLE • *See* Anisole.

DIHYDROCHALCONES • Abbreviated DHC. A class of intensely sweet compounds obtained by a simple chemical modification of naturally occurring bioflavonoids.

DIHYDROCHOLESTEROL • *See* Cholesterol.

DIHYDROCHOLESTERYL MACADAMIATE • Fatty acids (*see*) derived from macadamia nuts. *See* Macadamia Nut Oil.

DIHYDROCHOLESTERYL OCTYLDECANOATE • *See* Cholesterol and Octyldecanoic Acid.

DIHYDROCHOLETH-15 • The polyethylene glycol (*see*) ether of dihydrocholesterol. *See* Cholesterol.

DIHYDROCHOLETH-30 • The polyethylene glycol (*see*) ether of dihydrocholesterol. *See* Cholesterol.

DIHYDROCOUMARIN • Fragrance ingredient. Added to food as a flavoring. ASP. Banned in the UK in fragrances. *See* Coumarin.

DIHYDROGENATED TALLOW BENZYLMONIUMCHLORIDE • *See* Quaternary Ammonium Compounds.

DIHYDROGENATED TALLOWAMIDOETHYL HYDROXYETHYLMO-NIUM METHOSULFATE • Fatty acids (*see*) derived from hydrogenated tallow. *See* Tallow.

DIHYDROGENATED TALLOWETHYL HYDROXYETHYLMONIUM METHOSULFATE • A quaternary ammonium compound made from tallow (*see*).

DIHYDROGENATED TALLOW METHYLAMINE • *See* Tallow and Hydrogenated.

DIHYDROGENATED TALLOW PHTHALATE • A surfactant made from tallow alcohol and phthalic acid (*see*). Used as a surfactant and skin-conditioning ingredient. *See* Tallow.

DIHYDROGERANIOL • Banned in fragrances by the UK. *See* Geraniol.

DIHYDRONOOTKATONESynthetic, fruity, citruslike aroma of grapefruit used in flavors and fragrances. A derivative is used to repel termites. EAF

DIHYDRO-JASOMONE • *See* Jasomone.

DIHYDROPHYTOSTERYL OCTYLDECANOATE • *See* Octadecanoic Acid.

DIHYDROSTREPTOMYCIN • An antibiotic active against streptococcal bacteria. Used as a preservative.

DIHYDROXYACETONE • Permanently listed in 1973. Also used as an emulsifier, humectant, and fungicide. The Food and Drug Administration declared in 1973 that this color additive is safe and suitable for use in cosmetics or drugs that are applied to color the skin (suntan). A white powder that turns colorless in liquid form, it colors the skin an orange-brown shade, giving it a suntanned appearance. It is an ingredient in some suntan lotions for use indoors without sunlight. Obtained by the action of certain bacteria on glycerol, it has a sweet taste and characteristic odor. It is a strong reducing agent (*see*). It is converted by alkali to the fruit sugar fructose. Lethal when injected in large doses into rats. No known skin toxicity, and the FDA has exempted it from color additive certification, which means there is no need to test each batch as a means of protecting consumers as there is with coal tar colors. However, it can cause allergic contact dermatitis (*see*).

DIHYDROXYCOUMARIN • Possible skin sensitizer. Banned in fragrances by the UK. *See* Coumarins.

2,6,DIHYDROXY-3,4-DIMETHYLPYRIDINE • A hair coloring. *See* Coal Tar.

DIHYDROXYETHYL C9-11 ALKOXYPROPYLAMINE OXIDE • *See* Quaternary Ammonium Compounds.

DIHYDROXYETHYL C12-15 ALKOXYPROPYLAMINE OXIDE • *See* Thioglycolic Acid Compounds.

DIHYDROXYETHYL COCAMINE OXIDE • *See* Coconut Oil.

DIHYDROXYETHYL SOY GLYCINATE • *See* Quaternary Ammonium Compounds.

DIHYDROXYETHYL SOYAMINE DIOLEATE • The diester of oleic acid and dihydroxyethyl soyamine. *See* Thioglycolic Acid Compounds.

DIHYDROXYETHYL STEARAMINE OXIDE • *See* Stearic Acid.

DIHYDROXYETHYL STEARYL GLYCINATE • *See* Quaternary Ammonium Compounds.

DIHYDROXYETHYL TALLOWAMINE OLEATE • *See* Oleic Acid and Tallow.

DIHYDROXYETHYL TALLOWAMINE OXIDE • *See* Tallow.

2,5-DIHYDROXYETHYLAMINOTOLUENE • An amine hair coloring. *See* Coal Tar.

DIHYDROXYETHYLOLEYL GLYCINATE • *See* Glycine.

DIHYDROXYINDOLE • *See* Indole and Hydroxylation.

DIHYDROXYINDOLINE • A hair coloring. *See* Coal Tar.

DIIODOMETHYLTOLYLSULFONE • A preservative. *See* Toluene

DIISOBUTYL SODIUM SULFOSUCCINATE • The sodium salt of the diester of isobutyl alcohol and sulfosuccinic acid, used as an alkalizer. *See* Succinic Acid.

DIISOCETYL ADIPATE • Diester of hexadecyl alcohol and adipic acid. *See* Adipic Acid.

DIISODECYL ADIPATE • Made from adipic acid and decyl alcohol (*see both*).

DIISOPROPANOLAMINE • Widely used ingredient in fragrances, tonics, hair-grooming aids, permanent waves, hair dyes, and colors. Requires a patch test. Corrosion inhibitor and acid-alkali adjuster in cosmetic compounds. The CIR Expert Panel (*see*) concludes that this ingredient is safe in the present practices of use and concentrations in cosmetics. However, it should not be used in products containing nitrosating ingredients lest it form nitrosamines (*see*). *See* Isopropanolamine.

DIISOPROPYL ADIPATE • Widely used ingredient. An emollient that helps prevent dryness and protect the skin by softening and lubricating it to minimize moisture loss. Used in bath products, colognes, and toilet waters, after-shave lotions, skin fresheners, and suntan gels. On the basis of available data, the CIR Expert Panel concludes that this ingredient is safe as presently used in cosmetics. *See* Adipic Acid.

DIISOPROPYL DIMER DILINOLEATE • Skin-conditioning ingredient. The CIR Expert Panel (*see*) concludes that there is insufficient data available to support the safety of this ingredient in cosmetics. *See* Dilinoleate.

DIISOPROPYL DIMERATE • *See* Dilinoleate.

DIISOPROPYL OXALATE • Chelating ingredient. Toxic. Restricted to professional use only. E

DIISOPROPYL SEBACATE • Emollient and moisturizer. *See* Isopropyl Alcohol and Sebacic Acid.

DIISOPSTEARYL ADIPATE • Widely used fragrance and skin-conditioning ingredient in colognes, perfumes, bath products, moisturizers, and body and hand preparations. Made from stearic acid and adipic acid (*see both*).

DIKA • Made from the almondlike seeds of the *Irvingia barteri,* much used by natives of the west coast of Africa. *See* Irvingia Gabonensis.

DIKETENE • Colorless, non-water-absorbing liquid with a pungent odor. Obtained from acetone (*see*), it is used in the production of pigments, toners, pesticides, and food preservatives.

DILAURETH-7 CITRATE • Skin-conditioning ingredient and emulsifier. *See* Citric Acid.

DILAURETH-4 DIMONIUM CHLORIDE • *See* Quaternary Ammonium Compounds.

DILAURYL CITRATE • *See* Lauryl Alcohol and Citric Acid.

DILAURYL THIODIPROPIONATE • An antioxidant. White, crystalline flakes with a sweet odor. The CIR Expert Panel (*see*) concludes that based upon data available, this ingredient is safe for use in cosmetic products at concentrations not to exceed 0.05 percent.

DILAURYLDIMONIUM CHLORIDE • *See* Quaternary Ammonium Compounds.

DILINOLEAMIDOPROPYL DIMETHYLAMINE • An antistatic ingredient in hair preparations. *See* Linoleic Acid.

DILINOLEAMIDOPROPYL DIMETHYLAMINE DIMETHICONE PEG-7 PHOSPHATE • Used in hair conditioners. *See* Siloxanes and Silanes.

DILINOLEATE • Dimer Acid. Widely used emulsifier derived from linoleic acid (*see*).

DILINOLEIC ACID • Dilinoleic acid is an acid formed by a treatment of linoleic acid. It is used in hair coloring, bleaching, and conditioning. Also used in lipsticks. The CIR Expert Panel (*see*) says there were no adverse effects reported. The Panel did note that the concentration of use of diisopropyl dimer dilinoleate was reportedly as high as 53 percent in lipsticks, but that the highest concentration tested for irritation/sensitization was 27 percent. "Given the size of these molecules, their relative insolubility in water, their lipophilic nature, and the absence of any significant case reports of allergic reactions, a use concentration of 53% is not likely to be associated with any adverse effects," the CIR Expert Panel concluded. No toxicity tests were done.

DILINOLEIC ACID/ETHYLENEDIAMINE COPOLYMER • Made from dilinoleic acid and ethylenediamine (*see both*).

DILL • *Anethum graveolens.* A hardy herb native to southern Europe and western Asia as well as the Americas, it was said by the ancient Greek physician Galen that it "procureth sleep." The name dill is derived from a Saxon word meaning "to lull." It is used by herbalists to treat symptoms of colic in children and insomnia in adults caused by indigestion. Used in "organic" cosmetics. Chewing dill seeds supposedly cures bad breath, and drinking dill tea calms upset stomachs and hiccups. It contains a volatile oil that includes carvone, used by herbalists to break up intestinal gas, and limonene, used in foods as a flavoring. Dill in hot milk is recommended by herbalists as a drink that calms the nerves. Herbalists say that it increases milk production when taken by nursing mothers. Limonene can be a skin irritant and sensitizer.

DILUENT • Any component of a color additive mixture that is not of itself a color additive and has been intentionally mixed therein to facilitate the uses of the mixture in coloring cosmetics or in coloring the human body, food, and drugs. The diluent may service another functional purpose in cosmetics, as, for example, emulsifying or stabilizing. Ethylcellulose is an example.

DIMER ACID • *See* Dilinoleate.

DIMETHICONE • Dimethicone Copolyol. A silicone (*see*) oil, white, viscous, used as an ointment base ingredient, as a topical drug vehicle, and as a skin protectant. Very low toxicity.

DIMETHICONE AMINO ETHYL PROPANOL • Used as a wetting and lubricating ingredient in hair sprays. *See* Silicones.

DIMETHICONE PEG-8 MEADOWFOAMATE • Fatty acid derived from meadowfoam seed oil used as a hair conditioner and emollient for the skin. *See* Dimethicone.

DIMETHICONE PEG-7 PHOSPHATE • Made from dimethicone (*see*) and ethylene oxide (*see*), it is an emulsifier and cleansing ingredient used in hair-coloring and hair-conditioning ingredients. *See* Dimethicone.

DIMETHICONE PEG-8 PHTHALATE • A hair-conditioning ingredient. *See* Dimethicone and Phthalates.

DIMETHICONOL • Antifoaming and skin-conditioning ingredient used in moisturizers and blushers and other makeup. *See* Dimethicone.

DIMETHOXY BENZENE • Veratrole. Colorless crystals or liquid derived from methanol. It is used as an antiseptic.

p-DIMETHOXY BENZENE • A synthetic raspberry, fruit, nut, hazelnut, root beer, and vanilla flavoring ingredient for beverages, ice cream, ices, candy, and baked goods.

DIMETHOXY METHANE • Methylal. Solvent for cosmetic aerosols and pump formulations and perfumes. Has a formaldehydelike odor and is toxic by ingestion and inhalation.

***m*-DIMETHOXYBENZENE** • Resorcinol. A synthetic fruit, nut, and vanilla flavoring. Used on the skin as a bactericidal and fungicidal ointment. Has the same toxicity as phenol (extremely toxic), but causes more severe convulsions.

DIMETHOXYDICGLYCOL • A solvent. *See* Glycols.

2,6-DIMETHOXY-3,5-PYRIDINEDIAMINE • A hair coloring. *See* Coal Tar.

DIMETHYL • Ethane. A gaseous hydrocarbon (*see*) forming a constituent of ordinary illuminating gas. It is the second member of the paraffin series, and its most important derivatives are common alcohol, aldehyde, ether, and acetic acid.

DIMETHYL ANTHRANILATE • Colorless, pale yellow liquid with a grapelike odor. Used in perfumes and flavorings. *See* Benzoic Acid.

DIMETHYL ASPARTIC ACID • *See* Aspartic Acid.

DIMETHYL BEHENAMINE • *See* Behenic Acid.

DIMETHYL BENZYL CARBINOL • A flavoring ingredient. *See* Diphenolic Acid.

DIMETHYL BENZYL CARBINYL ACETATE • *See* Dimethyl Benzyl Carbinol and Acetic Acid.

DIMETHYL BRASSYLATE • Used in polyethylene films and water-resistant products.

DIMETHYL CITRACONATE • Fragrance that causes an allergic reaction. Banned in fragrances by the UK and the EU.

DIMETHYL COCAMINE • *See* Coconut Oil.

DIMETHYL ETHER • Methyl Ether. Colorless gas with an ethereal odor. Used as a propellant.

DIMETHYL ETHER RESORCINOL • A benzene derivative originally obtained from certain resins but now usually synthesized. *See* Dimethoxy Benzene.

DIMETHYL GLUTAMIC ACID • *See* Glutamic Acid.

DIMETHYL GLUTARATE • Nail polish remover ingredient. *See* Glutamic Acid.

DIMETHYL HEXAHYDRONAPHTHYL DIHYDROXYMETHYL ACETAL • Used as a fragrance ingredient.

DIMETHYL HYDANTOIN • *See* Hydantoin.

DIMETHYL HYDROGENATED TALLOWAMINE • *See* Tallow.

DIMETHYL HYDROQUINONE • *See* Hydroquinone.

N,N,DIMETHYL-N-HYDROXYETHYL-3-NITRO-*p*-PHENYLENE DIAMINE • *See* *p*-Phenylenediamine.

DIMETHYL IMIDAZOLIDINONE • A skin-conditioning ingredient. *See* Imidazolidinone.

DIMETHYL LAURAMINE • An antistatic ingredient. It has antifungal and antimicrobial properties. The CIR Expert Panel (*see*) concludes that there is insufficient data available to support the safety of this.

DIMETHYL LAURAMINE OLEATE • Hair-conditioning ingredient. *See* Lauric Acid and Oleic Acid.

DIMETHYL LAUROYL LYSINE • Amino acid used in skin conditioners. *See* Amino Acids.

DIMETHYL MALEATE • A solvent. *See* Maleic Acid and Methyl Alcohol.

DIMETHYL MYRISTAMINE • *See* Myristic Acid.

DIMETHYL OCTANOL • Synthetic flavoring, colorless, with a sweet, roselike odor.

DIMETHYL OCTANYL ACETATE • Synthetic roselike scent.

3,7-DIMETHYL-2-OCTEN-1-OL • Banned in fragrances by the UK. *See* Octanoic Acid.

DIMETHYL OCTYNEDIOL • *See* Citronellol.

DIMETHYL OXAZOLIDINE • A fragrance ingredient. *See* Oxazoline and Oxazolidine.

DIMETHYL PABA ETHYL CETEARYLDIMONIUM TOSYLATE • *See* Quaternary Ammonium Compounds.

DIMETHYL PALMITAMINE • *See* Palmitic Acid.

N,N-DIMETHYL-*p*-PHENYLENE DIAMINE SULFATE • *See* *p*-Phenylenediamine.

DIMETHYL PHTHALATE • Phthalic Esters. A colorless, aromatic oil insoluble in water. A solvent, especially for musk (*see*). Used to compound calamine lotion and as an insect repellent. Absorbed through the skin. Irritating to the eyes and mucous membranes. On the basis of the available information, the CIR Expert Panel (*see*) found it safe in the early 1980s but is considering new information to determine if the final safety assessment should be reaffirmed, amended, or have an addendum. *See* Phthalates.

N,N-DIMETHYL 2,6-PYRIDINEDIAMINE HCL • Used in hair coloring. *See* Pyridine.

DIMETHYL SOYAMINE • *See* Soy Acid.

DIMETHYL STEARAMINE • An antistatic ingredient in hair products. The CIR Expert Panel (*see*) concludes that there is insufficient data available to support the safety of this ingredient in cosmetics. *See* Stearic Acid.

DIMETHYL SULFATE • Sulfuric Acid. Dimethyl Ester. Colorless, oily liquid used as a methylating ingredient (to add methyl) in the manufacture of cosmetic dyes, perfumes, and flavorings. Methyl salicylate (*see*) is an example. Extremely hazardous, dimethyl sulfate has delayed lethal qualities. Liquid produces severe blistering, necrosis of the skin. Sufficient skin absorption can result in serious poisoning. Vapors hurt the eyes. Ingestion can cause paralysis, coma, prostration, kidney damage, and death.

DIMETHYL SULFONE • Organic compound used as an emulsifier. *See* Sulfonated Oils.

DIMETHYL SULFOXIDE • Water-absorbing liquid used as a solvent. It readily penetrates the skin and other tissues. It is approved by the FDA for humans but must comply with FDA regulations. It is used to help anti-inflammatory medicines to penetrate the skin. On the Canadian Hotlist (*see*). Banned by the EU in cosmetics.

DIMETHYL TALLOWAMINE • *See* Tallow.

DIMETHYLAMINE • Prepared from methanol (*see*) and ammonia (*see*), it is used in the manufacture of soaps and detergents. It also promotes hardening of plastic nails. Irritating to the skin and mucous membranes.

DIMETHYLHYDROXYMETHYLPYRAZOLE • A broad spectrum bactericide and fungicide compatible with proteins. *See* Pyrazole.

DIMETHYLADIPATE • A solvent that is used as a nail polish remover ingredient. *See* Adipic Acid.

DIMETHYLAMINOETHYL METHACRYLATE • *See* Acrylates.

1-DIMETHYLAMINOMETHYL-1-METHYLPROPYL BENZOATE (AMYLO-CAINE) AND ITS SALTS • An early local anesthetic once widely used but eventually abandoned because of side effects. The EU and ASEAN (*see*) banned it in cosmetics.

DIMETHYLAMINOPROPYL OLEAMIDE • *See* Oleic Acid.

DIMETHYLAMINOPROPYL STEARAMIDE • *See* Stearic Acid.

DIMETHYLOCTAHYDRO-2-NAPHTHALDEHYDE • A fragrance ingredient.

DIMETHYLOL ETHYLENE THIOUREA • A preservative.

DIMETHYLOL UREA • A preservative. May release formaldehyde (*see*).

DIMETHYL OXAZOLIDINE • A preservative. *See* Oxazolidine.

1,3-DIMETHYLPENTYLAMINE AND ITS SALTS • Used for organic synthesis and Chinese medicine, health products synthesis. This amine is an adrenergic compound used to provide temporary relief of nasal congestion, as well as treatment for hypertrophied or hyperplasic oral tissues. Banned in cosmetics by the EU and ASEAN (*see*).

DIMETHYLSILANOL HYALURONATE • *See* Hyaluronic Acid.

DIMYRISTYL THIODIPROPIONATE • Diester of myristyl alcohol and thiodipropionic acid (*see both*).

DINKUM OIL • *See* Eucalyptus Oil.

DINONOXYNOL-9-CITRATE • Diester of citric acid and nonoxynol-9. *See* Citric Acid and Nonoxynol-2.

DINONYL PHENOL • *See* Phenols.

DINOXYNOL-4 PHOSPHATE • *See* Nonoxynol and Surfactants.

DIOCTANOATE/DIISONONANOATE • A complex mixture of acids used as a texturizer (*see*).

DIOCTYL- • Containing two octyl groups. Octyl is obtained from octane, a liquid paraffin found in petroleum.

DIOCTYL ADIPATE • An emollient made from octyl alcohol and adipic acid. On the basis of available data, the CIR Expert Panel concludes that it is safe as presently used in cosmetics. *See* Adipic Acid.

DIOCTYL DIMER DILINOLEATE • A skin-conditioning ingredient. The CIR Expert Panel (*see*) concludes that there is insufficient data available to support the safety of this ingredient in cosmetics. *See* Dilinoleic Acid.

DIOCTYL MALEATE • *See* Malic Acid.

DIOCTYL PHTHALATE • An oily ester (*see*) used chiefly as a plasticizer, solvent, and fixative in perfumes and nail enamels. Because of its bitter taste, also used as a denaturant for alcohol (*see*). Irritating to mucous membranes, and a central nervous system depressant if absorbed through the skin. Linked to testicular cancer and cell mutation.

DIOCTYL SODIUM SULFOSUCCINATE • Docustae Sodium. A waxlike solid that is very soluble in water. It is used as a dispersing and solubilizing ingredient in foods and cosmetics. On the basis of available data, the CIR Expert Panel concludes that this ingredient is safe as presently used in cosmetics.

DIOCTYL SUCCINATE • A white wax, soluble in water, it is a wetting ingredient used in compounding calamine lotion. No known skin toxicity.

DIOCTYLAMINE • Di-2-Ethylhexyl-Amine. *See* Amines.

DIOCTYLDODECYL FLUOROHEPTYL CITRATE • Skin conditioner. *See* Citric Acid.

DIOCTYLDODECYL LAUROYL GLUTAMATE • A hair- and skin-conditioning ingredient. *See* Lauric Acid and Glutamic Acid.

DIOLEOYL EDETOLMONIUM METHOSULFATE • A pH (*see*) adjuster and emulsifier.

DIOLEOYLISOPROPYL DIMONIUM METHOSULFATE • *See* Quaternary Ammonium Compounds.

DIOLETH-8-PHOSPHATE • Direct Black 51. Synthetic compound from fatty acids. Used in hair coloring. The EU asked for an urgent review since it has been linked to bladder cancer. Proposed for a ban.

DIOLEYL TOCOPHERYL METHYLSILANOL • A fatty compound used in creams. *See* Tocopherol.

DIOSCOREA VILLOSA • *Dioscorea mexicana. D. paniculata.* Wild Yam. Colicroot. Rheumatism Root. Chinese Yam. Japanese researchers in 1936 discovered glycoside saponins of several Mexican yam species from which steroid saponin (*see*), primarily diosgenin, could be derived. These derivatives were then converted to progesterone, an intermediate in cortisone production. Steroid drugs derived from diosgenin include corticosteroids, oral contraceptives, androgens, and estrogens. For more than two centuries, American herbalists used wild yam roots to treat painful menstruation, ovarian pain, cramps, and problems of childbirth. Wild yam root also has been used to treat gallbladder pain, and ease the passage of gallstones. Wild yam root also reputedly can lower blood cholesterol and blood pressure. The most widely prescribed birth control pill in the world, Desogen, is made from the wild yam, confirming what the ancient Mexican women knew all along. They used wild yam as a contraceptive. Long-term use may cool libido. Contraindicated in pregnancy and kidney impairment. Used in anti-aging cosmetics. Any compound with an androgenic effect is banned by ASEAN (see).

DIOSMINE • An antioxidant. See Phenols.

DIOSPYROS KAKI • Persimmon. American Indians used the fruit from this tree grown in the southern and eastern United States. Used as a wax in cosmetics.

DIOXANE • 1,4-Dioxane. A colorless liquid used as a solvent for cellulose esters, a major component of plant cell walls, and used as a solvent for fats, greases, and resins and in various products including paints, lacquers, glues, cosmetics, and fumigants. In animals it affected the liver. Dioxane is primarily used in solvent applications for the manufacturing sector; however, it is also found in fumigants and automotive coolant. Additionally, the chemical is also used as a foaming agent. It is a suspected toxicant. Also an eye and respiratory tract irritant. It is suspected of causing damage to the central nervous system, liver, and kidneys. Accidental worker exposure to 1,4-dioxane has resulted in several deaths. Dioxane is classified by the International Agency for Research on Cancer (IARC) as possibly carcinogenic to humans due to the fact that it is a known carcinogen in animals. It also forms contamination plumes in groundwater when released to the environment. Groundwater supplies have been adversely impacted in several areas. It should not be confused with dioxin (see) but neither should it be in so many flavorings.

DIOXIN • The commonly used name for TCDD. 2,3,7,8-Tetrachlorodibenzo-*p*-Dioxin. It is a halogenated aromatic hydrocarbon, and it causes mutagenic and carcinogenic changes in animals. It is a by-product of additive orange (2,4-D and 2,4,5-T). It is the most toxic of chlorine-containing dioxin compounds. The long-term human consequences of exposure to this compound are controversial, but it certainly would be wise to avoid exposure to it. It is a suspected cancer-causing additive.

DIOXYBENZONE • Used in sunscreens in Austria and the United States. Has not been tested by their agencies. Is an organic compound used in sunscreen to block UVB. It is a derivative of benzophenone. A yellow powder with a melting point of 68°C, it is insoluble in water, but moderately soluble in ethanol and isopropanol.

DIPA • The abbreviation for diisopropanolamine.

DIPALMETHYL HYDROXYETHYLMONIUM METHOSULFATE • See Quaternary Ammonium Compounds.

DIPALMITAMINE • An antistatic ingredient in hair products. See Palmitic Acid.

DIPALMITOYL CYSTINE • A fatty compound with cystine (see) and used in creams.

DIPALMITOYL HYDROXYPROLINE • Fatty compound made with amino acids and used in creams.

DI-C12-15-PARETH-2-PHOSPHATE • A surfactant and emulsifying ingredient. See Phosphoric Acid.

DIPENTAERYTHRITYL HEXACAPRYLATE/HEXACAPRATE • Mixture of caprylic and capric acids and pentaerythritol (see all). Used in cosmetic creams and oils.

DIPENTAERYTHRITYL HEXAHYDROXYSTEARATE/STEARATE/ROSINATE • Mixture of an extract of algae and rosin used as a skin-conditioning ingredient.

DIPENTAERYTHRITYL PENTAHYDROXYSTERATE/PENTALISOSTER-ATE • Skin conditioner. *See* Pentanoic Acid and Stearic Acid.

DIPENTENE • *See* Limonene.

DIPERODON HYDROCHLORIDE • Obtained by condensing a piperdine and glycerol chlorohydrin with an alkali. Bitter taste. Soluble in alcohol. Used as an anesthetic solution.

DIPHENOLIC ACID • Prepared by condensing phenol (*see*) with another acid. Soluble in hot water. It is an intermediate for lubricating oil additives. Used in cosmetics as a surfactant and plasticizer. *See* Phenols for toxicity.

DIPHENYL ACETONITRILE • Diphenatrile. Yellow crystalline powder used in the preparation of antispasmodics and herbicides. Acetonitrile is on the Canadian Hotlist (*see*).

DIPHENYL DIMETHICONE • *See* Dimethicone.

DIPHENYL METHANE • Benzyl Benzene. Used chiefly as a perfume in soaps. Prepared from methylene chloride and benzene, with aluminum chloride as a catalyst. Smells like oranges and geraniums. A petroleum distillate and like all such substances can, when imposed, produce local skin irritation and more rarely a skin reaction to sunlight, which includes prickling, swelling, and sometimes pigmentation. Methylene chloride is no longer permitted in cosmetics.

DIPHENYL OXIDE • Colorless crystals or liquid with a geraniumlike odor. Derived from benzene, it is used in perfumery, particularly soaps. Toxic by inhalation of vapor.

DIPHENYLAMINE • Not permitted in fragrances by the UK or the EU.

DIPHENYLENE SULFIDE • *See* Dibenzothiophene.

DIPOTASSIUM AZELATE • The salt of azelic acid. Used as a plasticizer.

DIPOTASSIUM EDTA • *See* Ethylenediamine Tetraacetic Acid.

DIPOTASSIUM GLYCYRRHIZATE • The dipotassium salt of glycyrrhizic acid (*see*).

DIPOTASSIUM PHOSPHATE • A sequestrant. A white grain used as a buffering ingredient to control the degree of acidity in solutions. It is used medicinally as a saline cathartic.

DIPROPYLENE GLYCOL • Widely used fragrance and solvent ingredient in shampoos, powders, makeup, moisturizers, cleansers, suntan products, and deodorants. *See* Propylene Glycol.

DIPROPYLENE GLYCOL DIBENZOATE • Light colored liquid that is used as a plasticizer. *See* Propylene Glycol and Benzoic Acid.

DIPROPYLENE GLYCOL SALICYLATE • Insoluble in water, it is used as a plasticizer and in sunscreen lotions and fixative in hair sprays. *See* Propylene Glycol and Salicylates.

DIPSACUS SYLVESTRIS EXTRACT • Rusty Foxglove. Contains the heart stimulant digitalis. Used as a skin conditioner.

DIPTERYX ODORATA • The tree bears the tonka bean (*see*). Used as a fragrance ingredient. Contains coumarin (*see*).

DIRECT BLACK 51 • Classed as a diazo dye (*see*).

DIRECT BLUE 86 • A phthalocyanine color. *see* Phthalic Acid. *See also* Direct Dyes.

DIRECT DYES • These compounds need salts to be effective. When combined with aniline, they improve in fastness. Used in hair dyes and in some pigments. *See* Aniline Dyes.

DIRECT RED 23 • Fast Scarlet 4BSA • Classed chemically as a diazo color. *See* Colors.

DIRECT RED 80 • Classed chemically as a diazo color, it is a brilliant red. *See* Coal Tar.

DIRECT RED 81 • Benzo Fast. Red 8 BL. A diazo dye. *See* Azo Dyes and Direct Dyes.

DIRECT VIOLET 48 • A diazo dye. *See* Azo Dyes and Direct Dyes.

DIRECT YELLOW 12 • Chrysophenine G. A diazo dye. *See* Azo Dyes and Direct Dyes.

DISELENIUM SULFIDE • An antidandruff ingredient used in prescription items and OTC brands. *See* Selenium Sulfide.

DISILOXANE • An antifoaming ingredient and skin conditioner used in aerosol hair sprays.

DISODIUM ADENOSINE TRIPHOSPHATE • A preservative and skin conditioner derived from adenylic acid. *See* Adenosine Triphosphate.

DISODIUM ASCORBYL SULFATE • Used in skin care products. *See* Ascorbic Acid.

DISODIUM CAPROAMPHODIACETATE • Used as a hair conditioner and cleansing ingredient. *See* Quaternary Ammonium Compounds and Surfactants.

DISODIUM CAPROAMPHODIPROPIONATE • *See* Surfactants.

DISODIUM CAPRYLOAMPHODIACETATE • *See* Surfactants.

DISODIUM CAPRYLOAMPHODIPROPIONATE • *See* Surfactants.

DISODIUM CETEARYL SULFOSUCCINATE • The disodium salt of cetearyl alcohol and sulfosuccinic acid (*see both*).

DISODIUM COCAMIDO MIPA-SULFOSUCCINATE • *See* Coconut Oil and Surfactants.

DISODIUM COCAMPHODIACETATE • *See* Coconut Oil and Surfactants.

DISODIUM COCOAMPHOCARBOXYMETHYLHYDROXYPROPYL-SULFONATE • *See* Coconut Oil and Surfactants.

DISODIUM DECETH-6 SULFOSUCCINATE • *See* Sulfonated Oils.

DISODIUM DIMETHICONE COPOLYOL SULFOSUCCINATE • *See* Dimethicone and Succinic Acid.

DISODIUM DISTRYLBIPHENYL DISULFONATE • Use of this colorant in cosmetic products is prohibited in the United States and may be restricted in other countries.

DISODIUM EDTA-COPPER • Copper Versenate. Used as a sequestering ingredient. Permanently listed as a coloring for shampoos in 1974. *See* Ethylenediamine Tetraacetic Acid for toxicity.

DISODIUM HYDROGENATED COTTONSEED GLYCERIDE SULFO-SUCCINATE • *See* Sulfonated Oils.

DISODIUM HYDROGENATED TALLOW GLUTAMATE • *See* Hydrogenated Tallow.

DISODIUM ISODECYL SULFOSUCCINATE • *See* Sulfonated Oils.

DISODIUM ISOSTEARAMINO MEA-SULFOSUCCINATE • *See* Surfactants.

DISODIUM ISOSTEAROAMPHODIPROPIONATE • *See* Surfactants.

DISODIUM LANETH-5-SULFOSUCCINATE • *See* Sulfonated Oils.

DISODIUM LAURAMIDE PEG-2 SULFOSUCCINATE • *See* Surfactants.

DISODIUM LAURAMIDO MEA-SULFOSUCCINATE • *See* Surfactants.

DISODIUM LAURETH SULFOSUCCINATE • *See* Surfactants.

DISODIUM LAURIMINIDIPROPIONATE • *See* Surfactants.

DISODIUM LAUROAMPHODIPROPIONATE • An ingredient used in hair products as a conditioner and foam booster.

DISODIUM LAURYL SULFOSUCCINATE • *See* Surfactants.

DISODIUM MONOCOCAMIDOSULFOSUCCINATE • *See* Dioctyl Sodium Sulfosuccinate.

DISODIUM MONOLAURETHSULFOSUCCINATE • *See* Dioctyl Sodium Sulfosuccinate.

DISODIUM MONOLAURYLAMIDOSULFOSUCCINATE • *See* Dioctyl Sodium Sulfosuccinate.

DISODIUM MONOLAURYLSULFOSUCCINATE • *See* Dioctyl Sodium Sulfosuccinate.

DISODIUM MONOMYRISTAMIDOSULFOSUCCINATE • *See* Dioctyl Sodium Sulfosuccinate.

DISODIUM MONOOLEAMIDOSULFOSUCCINATE • *See* Dioctyl Sodium Sulfosuccinate.

DISODIUM MONORICINOLEAMIDO MEA-SULFOSUCCINATE • *See* Sulfonated Oils.

DISODIUM MYRISTAMIDO MEA-SULFOSUCCINATE • *See* Dioctyl Sodium Sulfosuccinate.

DISODIUM NONOXYNOL-10 SULFOSUCCINATE • *See* Surfactants.

DISODIUM OLEOAMPHODIPROPIONATE • An ingredient used in hair products as a conditioner and foam booster. *See* Oleic Acid.

DISODIUM OLEYL SULFOSUCCINATE • *See* Surfactants.

DISODIUM PALMITOLEAMIDO PEG-2 SULFOSUCCINATE • *See* Succinic Acid and Surfactants.

DISODIUM C12-15 PARETH SULFOSUCCINATE • The sodium salt of sulfosuccinic acid (*see*). *See* Surfactants.

DISODIUM PARETH-25 SULFOSUCCINATE • *See* Surfactants.

DISODIUM PEG-4-COCAMIDO MIPA-SULFOSUCCINATE • *See* Surfactants.

DISODIUM PHOSPHATE • *See* Sodium Phosphate.

DISODIUM PPG-2-ISODECETH-7 CARBOXYAMOPHODIACETATE • An organic salt that is used in hair products as a conditioning and foam booster.

DISODIUM PYROPHOSPHATE • Sodium Pyrophosphate. An emulsifier and texturizer used to decrease the loss of fluid from a compound. It is GRAS for use in foods as a sequestrant. *See* Sodium Pyrophosphate Peroxide.

DISODIUM RICINOLEAMIDO MEA-SULFOSUCCINATE • Widely used as a surfactant, it is the disodium salt of ethanolamide and sulfosuccinic acid (*see*).

DISODIUM SOYAMHOOLEATE • Used in hair products. *See* Soy and Oleic Acid.

DISODIUM STEARMIDO MEA-SULFOSUCCINATE • *See* Surfactants.

DISODIUM STEARMINODIPROPIONATE • *See* Steareth-2.

DISODIUM STEARYL SULFOSUCCINATE • *See* Sulfonated Oils.

DISODIUM SUCCINATE • *See* Succinic Acid.

DISODIUM SUCCINOYL GLYCYRRHETINATE • A flavoring ingredient. *See* Licorice.

DISODIUM TALLOW SULFOSUCCINAMATE • *See* Succinic Acid and Tallow.

DISODIUM TALLOWAMIDO MEA-SULFOSUCCINATE • *See* Surfactants.

DISODIUM TALLOWAMINODIPROPIONATE • *See* Surfactants.

DISODIUM TRIDECYLSULFOSUCCINATE • *See* Succinic Acid.

DISODIUM UNDECYLENAMIDO MEA-SULFOSUCCINATE • *See* Surfactants.

DISODIUM WHEAT GERMAMIDO MEA-SULFOSUCCINATE • *See* Surfactants.

DISODIUM WHEAT GERMAMIDO PEG-2-SULFOSUCCINATE • *See* Wheat Germ Oil and Surfactants.

DISOYADIMONIUM CHLORIDE • *See* Quaternary Ammonium Compounds.

DISOYAMINE • Antistatic ingredient. *See* Soybean Oil.

DISOYDIMONIUM CHLORIDE • Antistatic ingredient in hair products. *See* Soybean Oil.

DISPERSANT • A dispersing ingredient, such as polyphosphate, for promoting the formation and stabilization of a dispersion of one substance in another. An emulsion, for instance, would consist of a dispersed substance and the medium in which it is dispersed.

DISPERSE BLACK 9 • Nacelan Diazine Black JS. Classed chemically as an azo dye (*see*). This was not found to be carcinogenic or tetratogenic in rats or rabbits and was not cancer causing when applied to the skin of mice. At 3 percent suspension it did not irritate or sensitize the skin of human subjects. On the basis of available data, the CIR Expert Panel concludes that this ingredient is safe as presently used in cosmetics.

DISPERSE BLUE 1 • 1, 4, 5, 8-CI 64500. Tetraaminoanthraquinone. Classed chemically as an anthraquinone (*see*) color. A skin cancer study in mice was negative. There were questionable urinary bladder tumors in mice but due to calculi rather than arising from toxicity to the genes. Such bladder calculi, it is reported, do not form in humans. The ingredient is also poorly absorbed so that exposure to hair dyes is brief. On the basis of available data, the CIR Expert Panel concludes that this ingredient is safe as presently used in cosmetics.

DISPERSE BLUE 3 • CI 61505. Disperse Fast Blue. An anthraquinone (*see*) dye. *See also* Disperse Dyes.

DISPERSE BLUE 3:1 • Nacelan Brilliant Blue NR. Classed chemically as an anthraquinone (*see*).

DISPERSE BLUE 7 • An anthraquinone (*see*) color. The CIR Expert Panel (*see*) has listed this as top priority for review.

DISPERSE BROWN • 1 CI 11152. A monoazo color (*see*).

DISPERSE DYES • These compounds are only slightly soluble in water but are readily dispersed with the aid of sulfated oils. Used on nylon knit goods, sheepskins, and furs, they are in human hair dyes as well as resins, oils, fats, and waxes. Not permanently listed as safe.

DISPERSE ORANGE 3 • CI 11005. A monoazo color (*see*).

DISPERSE RED 11 • CI 62015. An anthraquinone (*see*) color.

DISPERSE RED 15 • CI 60710. An anthraquinone (see) color.

DISPERSE RED 17 • CI 11210. A monoazo color (*see*).

DISPERSE VIOLET 1 • Classed as an anthraquinone (*see*) color. Although there are limited human studies, on the basis of available data, the CIR Expert Panel concludes that this ingredient is safe as presently used in cosmetics.

DISPERSE ORANGE 3 • A monoazo color (*see*).

DISPERSE VIOLET 4 • CI 61105. Solvent Violet 12. Classed chemically as an anthraquinone color. *See* Colors.

DISPERSE VIOLET 15 • A hair coloring. *See* Coal Tar.

DISTARCH GLYCERYL ETHER • An anticaking ingredient. *See* Starch and Glycerin.

DISTARCH PHOSPHATE • A combination of starch and sodium metaphosphate. It is a water softener, sequestering ingredient, and texturizer. It is used in dandruff shampoos.

DISTEARDIONIUM HECTORITE • *See* Quaternary Ammonium Compounds.
DISTEARETH-6 DIMONIUM CHLORIDE • *See* Quaternary Ammonium Compounds.
DISTEARETH-2-LAUROYL GLUTAMATE • *See* Surfactants.
DISTEARETH-5 LAUROYL GLUTAMATE • *See* Surfactants.
DISTEARYL ETHER • A skin-conditioning ingredient. *See* Stearic Acid.
DISTEARYL EXPOXYPROPYLMONIUM CHLORIDE • *See* Quaternary Ammonium Compounds.
DISTEARYL PHTHALIC ACID AMIDE • Emollient. *See* Stearic Acid and Phthalic Acid.
DISTEARYL THIODIPROPIONATE • The diester of stearyl alcohol and thiodipropionic acid used as a stabilizer (*see all*).
DISTEARYLDIMETHYLAMINE DILINOLEATE • Used as a hair-conditioning ingredient. *See* Dilinoleic Acid and Dimer Acid.
DISTEARYLDIMETHYLAMINE DIMERATE • *See* Dimer Acid.
DISTEARYLDIMONIUM CHLORIDE • *See* Quaternary Ammonium Compounds.
DISTILLATE • The volatile material recovered by condensing the vapors of an extract, or material from fruit that is heated to its boiling point in a still.
DISTILLATION • The physical process of heating a product to the boiling point in a still and collecting the vapors by condensing them through cooling.
DISTILLED • The result of evaporation and subsequent condensation of a liquid, as when water is boiled and steam is condensed.
DISTILLED OIL • An essential oil obtained by the distillation of the portion of a botanical material, such as peel, leaves, and stem, containing the essential oil.
DITALLOWAMIDOETHYL HYDROXYPROPYLAMINE • Hair-conditioning ingredient. *See* Tallow.
DITALLOW AMMONIUM CHLORIDE • Used in hair products. *See* Tallow.
DITALLOWDIMONIUM CHLORIDE • *See* Quaternary Ammonium Compounds and Tallow.
DI-TEA-OLEAMIDO PEG-2-SULFOSUCCINATE • *See* Quaternary Ammonium Compounds.
DI-TEA-PALMITOYL ASPARTATE • A cleanser. *See* Aspartic Acid.
DITHIOMETHYLBENZYLAMIDE • A preservative. *See* Benzoic Acid.
DITHIOTHREITOL • Hair-waving and -straightening ingredient. *See* Thiogylcolic Acid Compounds.
DITHIODIGLYCOLIC ACID • *See* Thioglycolic Acid Compounds.
DITHIOMETHYLBENZYLAMIDE • A preservative. *See* Benzoic Acid.
DITHIOTHREITOL • Hair-waving and -straightening ingredient. *See* Thiogylcolic Acid Compounds.
DITRIDECYL ADIPATE • Emollient. Diester of tridecyl alcohol and adipic acid (*see both*).
DITRIDECYL DILINOLEATE • The diester of tridecyl alcohol and dilinoleic acid. *See* Dimer Acid.
DITRIDECYL DIMER DILINOLEATE • A skin-conditioning ingredient. The CIR Expert Panel (*see*) concludes that there is insufficient data available to support the safety of this ingredient in cosmetics. *See* Tridecyl Alcohol and Dilinoleic Acid.
DITRIDECYL SODIUM SULFOSUCCINATE • *See* Sulfonated Oils.
DITRIDECYL THIODIPROPIONATE • The diester of tridecyl alcohol and thiodipropionic acid (*see both*).

DISULFIRAM • Antabuse. Produces a sensitivity to alcohol that results in a highly unpleasant reaction when the patient under treatment ingests even small amounts of alcohol.

DIVINYLDIMETHICONE/DIMETHICONE CROSSPOLYMER • Film former and skin-conditioning ingredient. *See* Siloxane and Silanes.

DMAE • Abbreviation for dimethylaminoethanol.

DMAPAP ACRYLATES/ACRYLIC ACID/ACRYLONITROGENS CO-POLYMER • Synthetic polymer (*see*) used as a film former and thickener. *See* Acrylates.

DM HYDANTOIN • Preservative in many cosmetics including hair products, bath products, makeup, and baby products. *See* Hydantoin.

DMDM • The abbreviation for dimethylol dimethyl. *See* Methyl Alcohol and Imidazolidinone.

DMDM HYDANTOIN • A preservative. May release formaldehyde (*see*). Can be a skin irritant. On the basis of available data, the CIR Expert Panel concludes that this ingredient is safe as presently used in cosmetics. *See also* Hydantoin.

DMHF • The abbreviation for the resin formed by heating hydantoin and formaldehyde (*see both*).

DNA • Desoxyribonucleic acid. The complex substance that makes up genes; it contains the genetic information for all organisms.

DOCOSAHEXAENOIC ACID • *See* Behenic Acid.

DODECANEDIOIC ACID/CETEARYL ALCOHOL/GLYCOL COPOLYMER • The coconut oil, cetearyl alcohol, and ethylene glycol monomers, used to form a wax (*see all*).

DODECANOIC ACID • Lauric Acid. A common constituent of vegetable fats, especially coconut oil and laurel oil. Used in the manufacture of miscellaneous flavors. Its derivatives are widely used as a base in the manufacture of soaps, detergents, and lauryl alcohol (*see* Fatty Alcohols) because of their foaming properties. Has a slight odor of bay. A mild irritant but not a sensitizer. ASP

DODECYL GALLATE • The ester of gallic acid derived from tannin and used in ink.

DODECYLBENZENE SULFONIC ACID • A sulfonic acid anionic (*see*) detergent. Made from petroleum. May cause skin irritation. If swallowed, will cause vomiting.

DODECYLBENZYLTRIMONIUM CHLORIDE • *See* Quaternary Ammonium Compounds.

DODECYLHEXADECANOL • Alcohol used as emollient and emulsion stabilizer. *See* Hexanol.

DODECYLHEXADECYLTRIMONIUM CHLORIDE • An antistatic ingredient in hair conditioners and an emulsifier. *See* Quaternary Ammonium Compounds.

DODECYLTETRADECANOL • *See* Myristic Acid.

DODECYLXYLDITRIMONIUM CHLORIDE • *See* Quaternary Ammonium Compounds.

DODOXYNOL-5, -6, -7, -9, -12, -13 • Emulsifiers. *See* Phenols.

DOG ROSE EXTRACT • Extract of the fruit of *Rosa canina,* a wild rose. Used as a skin conditioner.

DOLOMITE • A common mineral, colorless to white or yellowish gray, containing calcium, phosphorous, and magnesium. It is one of the most important raw materials for magnesium and its salts. It is used in toothpaste as a whitener.

DOLLOF • *See* Filipendula Rubra.

DOMIPHEN BROMIDE • Clear, colorless, odorless crystalline powder with a slightly bitter taste. Soluble in water, but incompatible with soap, it is used as an antiseptic and detergent in cosmetics.

DONG QUAI • *Angelica sinensis.* Tang Kwei. The root of the herb is used for the treatment of female gynecological ailments, particularly menstrual cramps, irregularity, and malaise during the menstrual period. It is also used to relieve the symptoms of menopause. It is reputedly useful in treating anemia and constipation. Used in "organic" cosmetics. *See also* Angelica.

DRAIZE TEST • An animal test used to determine the effects of different substances on the eye. Animal rights advocates oppose the use of animals—usually rabbits—for this purpose. Replacements include laboratory techniques that use freshly isolated tissues, tissue-cultured cells, or nonliving systems. The widely criticized Draize rabbit test is the only eye toxicity test officially accepted worldwide for regulatory purposes in the classification of slightly and moderately irritating chemicals. Today, there are no in vitro alternatives that could be used as a complete replacement for the Draize eye test, although many scientists are trying to develop substitutes.

DRIED BUTTERMILK • The dehydration of the liquid recovered from churning cow's milk. Used as an emollient.

DRIED EGG YOLK • Used for coloring and protein in cosmetics. Particularly associated with eczema in children. May also cause reactions ranging from hives to anaphylaxis. Egg yolk may also be found in root beer, soups, sausage, and coffee.

DROMETRIZOLE • A derivative of benzene used as a solvent in nail polish and as an ultraviolet light absorber to make cosmetics less susceptible to light. On the basis of available data, the CIR Expert Panel concludes that this ingredient is not safe for use in cosmetics until such time as appropriate safety data has been obtained. *See* Benzene.

DROMICEIUS • *See* Emu Oil.

DROSERA • Common Sundew. *Drosera rotundifolia* Powder. A dried flowering plant that grows in Europe, Asia, and in North America as far south as Florida. Formerly used to treat chest disorders. Used as a mild astringent in skin lotions and perfumes.

DRY SHAMPOOS • Usually consist of a water-absorbent powder such as talc (*see*) and a mild alkali. The product is placed in the hair and then brushed out, carrying with it any oil or dirt. Many women use baby powder or bath powder to "dry-wash" their hair. *See* Shampoos.

DRYING INGREDIENTS • *See* Rosin.

DRYOPTERIS FILIX-MAS • Shield fern. A fern that grows in Bermuda. Used as a skin-conditioning ingredient.

DRYOUT • Just as the top note (*see*) is the first impression of a perfume, this is the last impression. It may begin to become apparent after an hour or several hours or even the next day. The dryout notes show the fixative (*see*) effects of the components and will reveal the body note (*see*). The dryout depicts the tenacity of the composition and the fixative's ability to hold the scent. The better the perfume, usually the better the dryout.

DUBOISIA LEICHARDTII • Pituri. Pitchiri. Pitcheri Emu Plant. Poison Bush. A perennial shrub or small tree with brown to purplish bark on the young stems and corky older bark. The chief constituent of it is nicotine and nornicotine, with a content reportedly up to 25 percent of the dried weight of the plant material. An extract is used in cosmetics as a skin conditioner. The powder is a popular drug used by Aboriginals in Australia where the plant is grown. The EU bans nicotine and its salts in cosmetics.

DUKU EXTRACT • *Ransium domesticum* Extract. Occurs in at least four cultivated forms, namely, duku, langsat (lansones), duku langsat, and dokong. They differ in tree form, fruit, and in fruit arrangement. Duku langsat is native to Malaysia, the Philippines, and Java where it is widely distributed. Used in cosmetics as an emollient. The fresh fruit is eaten. The oil is used in emollients.

DULCAMARA EXTRACT • Bitter Sweet Nightshade. Extract of the dried stems of

Solanum dulcamara. Belonging to the nightshade family, it is used as a preservative. The ripe berries are used for pies and jams. The unripened berries are deadly. It is made into an ointment by herbalists to treat skin cancers and burns. It induces sweating. *See also* Horse Nettle.

DUNALIELLA BARDAWIL • Green Alga. Accumulates very large amounts of beta-carotene when exposed to high light intensity. The accumulated beta-carotene is concentrated in small, oily globules within the chloroplast and has been suggested to protect the alga against photodamage by high irradiation. Used as a humectant and in skin conditioners.

DURVILLEA ANTARCTICA EXTRACT • An algae (*see*) extract used in anti-aging products.

DUSTING POWDER • Body powders, powders such as talcum powder or cornstarch (*see both*), applied to the body to help absorb oils and moisture and to impart fragrance. Aim is to help to absorb moisture. According to the trade group Cosmeticsinfo.org, the following ingredients (*see all*) are commonly found in dusting power:

- Calcium Carbonate
- Colors
- Fragrance
- Glycerin
- Kaolin
- Magnesium Carbonate
- Mineral Oil
- Preservatives
- Sodium Acrylates Copolymer
- Talc
- Titanium Dioxide
- Zinc Oxide

E

EAR ALLERGY • The condition *Serous otitis,* which is fullness in the ears associated with the formation of thick mucus behind the eardrum, is sometimes an allergic phenomenon. The first symptom may be hearing loss, and allergies of the nose contribute to the problem. Allergic contact dermatitis in and around the ear is not uncommon. Nickel in earrings, eyeglasses, hair dye, cologne or perfume, and otic drops and ointments applied to the ear are among the most common offenders.

EAR LOBE • Frequently a site of allergic contact dermatitis from earrings containing nickel. May also be affected by hair products.

EARTH WAX • General name for ozocerite, ceresin, and montan waxes. *See* Waxes.

EASTERN PINE EXTRACT • An extract of *Pinus strobus.* Pine preparations are used for their scent and for "healing" properties.

ECBALLIUM ELATERIUM • Squirting Cucumber. *See* Cucumber.

ECHA • Abbreviation for European Chemicals Agency (*see*).

ECHINACEA • *Echinacea angustifolia.* Snakeroot. Stone Flower. Cone Flower. The roots and leaves of this herb served as a medicine for the Plains Indians. It is said by herbalists to be a natural antibiotic and immune enhancer. It contains a volatile oil that is antiseptic and glycosides (*see*) as well as phenol, which is an antiseptic. It was widely used by Dr. Wooster Beach, who in the mid-1800s founded Eclectic Medicine, a blending of homeopathic and North American herbalism. It has been found that it increases the ability of white blood cells to fight, digest, and destroy toxic organisms that invade the body. Echinacea is taken to combat colds, infections, and inflammations. The herb produces a numbing sensation when held in the mouth for a few minutes. May worsen liver damage. Do not use if you are allergic to its relatives such as ragweed, asters, and chrysanthemums.

ECHINACIN • *See* Echinacea.

ECHIUM PLANTAGINEUM • Viper's Bugloss. Wax and oil from a weed that grows on roadsides, fields, and sandy areas near the sea. Used as a skin-conditioning ingredient.

ECLIPTA PROSTRATA • False Daisy. Swamp Daisy. An extract of an annual herb used in emollients.

ECOFLATION • The growing cost of cosmetic ingredients that are environmentally sensitive, such as wood, botanicals, water, paper, petroleum, and meet the cosmetic regulations of various agencies.

ECTOIN • A skin conditioner. *See* Carboxylic Acid.

ECVAM • Abbreviation for European Centre for the Validation of Alternative Methods. New laboratory test to replace using animals. ECVAM was created by a Communication from the Commission to the European Council and Parliament October 1991 requirement for the protection of animals used for experimental and other scientific purposes, which requires that the Commission and the member states should actively support the development, validation, and acceptance of methods which could reduce, refine, or replace the use of laboratory animals.

ECZEMA • Inflammation of the skin causing itching, scaling, and sometimes blisters.

EDATHAMIL DISODIUM • EDTA. Sodium edetate. A chelating ingredient (*see*) used to reduce minerals in compounds in many products, including moisturizers, cleansers, suntan products, bleaches, body and face creams, and lotions.

EDC • *See* Ethylene Dichloride.

EDC • Abbreviation for endocrine disrupter chemical (*see*).

EDELWEISS • An alpine plant (*Leontopodium alpinum*), native to Europe and having leaves covered with whitish down and small flower heads. Used in anti-aging creams, nail polishes, and sun care products.

EDTA SALTS • Chelating ingredients widely used in cosmetic and skin care preparations. *See* Ethylenediamine Tetraacetic Acid.

EGG • Particularly associated with eczema in children. May also cause reactions ranging from hives to anaphylaxis. Eggs may also be found in root beer, soups, sausage, coffee, and cosmetics.

EGG OIL • A mixture of the fat-soluble emollients and emulsifiers extracted from the whole egg. Provides protection against dehydration and has lubricating and antifriction properties when rubbed on the skin.

EGG POWDER • Used in many cosmetics, including shampoos, ointments, creams, face masks, and bath preparations. Dehydrated egg powder is often incorporated into shampoos on the theory that protein is beneficial to damaged hair. There is little scientific evidence to substantiate this, but the egg coating does make the hair more cohesive and more manageable. The oil of egg yolk, which mixes easily with other oils, is used in ointment bases and cosmetic creams. Egg albumen is used in facial masks to give a tight feeling. For a homemade egg treatment, four beaten eggs are required, with a jigger of rum mixed in. Then the solution is massaged into the scalp, followed by a rinse with cold (never hot) water; the hot water would make the egg sticky. For persons not allergic to egg products, the ingredients are harmless.

EGG YOLK • The yellow matter of chicken eggs.

EGG YOLK EXTRACT • The extract of egg yolk. *See* Egg Oil.

EGGPLANT • Aubergine. A tender perennial plant, *Solanum melongena,* of the nightshade family, closely allied to the potato. The fruit is a large, egg-shaped berry, varying in color from dark purple to red, yellowish, or white. Used in "organic" cosmetics.

EICOSANE • A white, crystalline solid that is a mixture of hydrocarbons. It is used as a lubricant or plasticizer in cosmetic preparations.

EICOSAPENTAENOIC ACID • EPA. Found in fish oil (*see*), it is used in creams. In the human body, it reduces production of thromboxane, a clotting ingredient, in the blood, thus making the platelets less "sticky."

EIJITSU • *Rosa multiflora.* The fruit of *R. multiflora* or other species of Roisaceae. Used as an abrasive in skin products.

ELAEISIS GUINEENSIS • *See* Palm Kernel Oil.

ELASTASE • A term used for an enzyme that dissolves elastin.

ELASTIN • A protein in connective tissue used in hair and skin products as a moisturizer and conditioner. It is elastic and allows many tissues in the body to resume their shape after stretching or contracting. Elastin helps skin to return to its original position when it is poked or pinched. Elastin is also an important load-bearing tissue in the bodies of mammals and used in places where mechanical energy is required to be stored. The source for cosmetics may be oxen neck ligaments and other animal products, including pig ligaments and fish.

ELASTOMERS • Used for face masks. Rubberlike substances that can be stretched from twice to many times their length. Upon their release, they return rapidly to almost their original length. Synthetic elastomers have similar properties and are actually superior to the natural ones. They have been in use since 1930. Thiokol was the first commercial synthetic elastomer. It is a condensation polymer (*see*); for example, neoprene and silicone rubber.

ELDER FLOWERS • *Sambucus nigra. S. canadensis.* Sambucus. Black Elder Bourtree. Judas Tree. Extracted from the honey-scented flowers of the elder tree. Herbal additive to China tea, it contains essential oil, terpenes, glycosides (*see*), rutin, quercitrin (*see*), mucilage, and tannin (*see*). The fruits are high in vitamin C. Used in skin and eye lotions and bath preparations. Mildly astringent, it supposedly keeps the skin soft and clean. Old-time herb doctors used it. Elder flowers increase perspiration and therefore reduce body water. Used to scent perfumes and lotions. Elder flower is used to treat colds and flu; in salves to treat burns, rashes, and minor skin ailments; and to diminish wrinkles. It was used by herbalists to soothe the nerves. Hippocrates mentioned its use as a purgative. The inner bark and the young leaf buds, as well as the juice root, are all considered cathartics. The berries induce sweating and act as a diuretic. Only the black elder is safe to use internally. Red elder is toxic.

ELDERBERRY JUICE POWDER • Dried powder from the juice of the edible berry of a North American elder tree. Used for red coloring.

ELECAMPANE EXTRACT • An extract of *Enula helenium,* a large, coarse European herb now grown in the United States. Do not use or even handle if you are allergic. Can cause skin rash similar to poison ivy.

ELECTROLYSIS • Removal of unwanted body hair using a needle epilator. A small electric current is passed through the device to kill the hair root.

ELEMI • A soft, yellowish, fragrant plastic resin from several Asiatic and Philippine trees. Slightly soluble in water but readily soluble in alcohol. Used for gloss and adhesion in nail lacquer and to scent soaps and colognes.

ELEOCHARIS DULCIS • Water Chestnut. *See* Cyperus.

ELETTARIA CARDAMOMUM • *See* Cardamom Oil.

ELEUTHEROCOCCUS SENTICOSUS • *Acanthopanax senticosus.* Devil's Root. Touch-me-not Siberian Ginseng (although it is not really related to ginseng). The root, the rhizomes (underground stem), and the leaves are being used in cosmetics as an astringent. In Chinese medicine, it is being used for many things, including chronic inflammation of bronchi, neurasthenia, low sexual function, weakness, low white cell count after radiation therapy. It is alleged to help reduce stress, to improve the immune system, and to fight cancer and aging and many other conditions, including reducing the effects of radiation and insomnia.

ELEUTHRERO GINSENG • *See* Ginseng.

ELGUEA CLAY • Clay from Cuba used as an abrasive and absorbent.

ELLAGIC ACID • A polyphenol (*see*) of great scientific interest. It is in various fruits and nuts and has been found to inhibit tumors caused by mold and hydrocarbons such as cigarette smoke. Used as an antioxidant in skin products.

ELM BARK • Extract of *Ulmus campestris.* Elm derivatives have been widely used in herbal medicine. The inner bark contains a lot of mucilage and is used in cosmetics, in baby products, and in herbal products to soothe the skin.

EMBILICA POWDER • Used in brown spot fade cream. Ayurveda considers this to be one of the best herbs for eliminating intestinal worms and other parasites.

EMBRYO EXTRACT • An oil extracted from fetal calves, often promoted in "youth-restoring" creams and lotions.

EMERALD • Green Fuchsite. A mineral used as an abrasive.

EMETINE CHLORIDE • A preservative. Made from ipecac (*see*), it is used in medicine to treat amebic dysentery. Acute toxicity can occur at any dose. On the Canadian Hotlist (*see*).

EMILIANIA HUXLEYI • An extract of *Emiliania huxleyi,* one of five thousand or so different species of phytoplankton—freely drifting, photosynthesizing microscopic organisms that live in the upper, sunlit layers of the ocean. Used as a skin conditioner.

EMOLLIENTS • Creams, Lotions, Skin Softeners, and Moisturizers. An emollient by whatever designation—night cream, hand cream, eye cream, skin softener, moisturizer, and so on—remains an emollient. The selection of a cream, spray, or lotion is really a matter of taste and the influence of advertising and packaging. The AMA's Committee on Cutaneous Health finds little difference between liquid, cream, lotion, drop, or dew emollients, since they all perform the same function. These preparations do help to make the skin feel softer and smoother and to reduce the roughness, cracking, and irritation of the skin; they may possibly help retard the fine wrinkles of aging. However, in any application of oil to the skin, what happens is that the roughened, scaly surface is coated with a smooth film, cementing down the dry flakes. And although the oil retards the evaporation of water, as far as the oil penetrating the skin, dermatologists say this has been overemphasized. Any dryness would be in the layer known as the stratum corneum, and it is due to insufficient water in the skin. Exposure to low humidities in artificially heated or cooled rooms, aging, and heredity may all contribute to dry skin. The ancient Greek physician Galen is credited with making the first emollient of beeswax, spermaceti, almond oil, borax, and rose water (*see all*).

Most emollients today are still a mixture of oils. If the oils have a low melting point, the emollient will feel greasy; with a high melting point, it disappears from the skin. Because emollients are usually colorless, and seem to be absorbed rapidly, they are called vanishing creams. But, according to the AMA, it is the water in such creams, and not the oil, that benefits dry skin. Experiments with a specimen of callused skin placed in oils for three years could not make it flexible again. However, when a brittle piece of callus is placed in water, it soon becomes flexible. Most emollients are intended to remain on the skin for a significant period of time, including overnight. Petrolatum (Vaseline) is one of the least expensive and one of the most efficient emollients. It tends to keep the loss of natural moisture from the skin at a minimum. Next in efficiency and also inexpensive is zinc oxide (*see*). Mineral oil, vegetable oil, and shortening also work well. All may be found on your supermarket shelf. Vitamin A and hormone creams (*see both*) are added to keep the skin moist and supple. However effective they are in doing so is a matter of medical controversy. Glycerin (*see*) is widely used in emollients and has been found to work best in humid air because it draws moisture from the air. (When the humidity is high, most people do not need emollients.) A simple conditioner or emollient cream may contain lanolin, petrolatum, and oil of sweet almond. A moisturizing cream may contain mineral oil, stearic acid, lanolin, beeswax, sorbitol, and polysorbates (*see all*).

Among other ingredients in emollients and lotions are natural fatty oils such as olive, coconut, corn, peach kernel, peanut, and sesame oils in hydrogenated form; natural fats such as cocoa butter and lard; synthetic fatty oils such as paraffin; alcohols such as cetyl, stearyl, and oleyl; emulsifiers, preservatives, and antioxidants, including vitamin E and parabens (*see all*); and antibacterials and perfumes, especially menthol and camphor (*see both*). Among the problems with creams and lotions reported to the FDA were body and hand rashes, swelling of the eyes and face, blood vessels on the surface of the nose, red and painful eyes, burning of the face, and skin eruptions and irritations.

EMU OIL • The emu is a large, flightless bird. The cosmetic and moisturizing properties of its oil were studied at the University of Sydney, Australia. It was found to have anti-inflammatory and skin-penetrating properties. It reportedly has better moisturizing properties than mineral oil and lower incidence of pore clogging.

EMULSIFIERS • Ingredients used to assist in the production of an emulsion. Among common emulsifiers in cosmetics are stearic acid soaps such as potassium and sodium stearates; sulfated alcohols such as sodium lauryl sulfate, polysorbates, poloxamers, and pegs; and sterols such as cholesterol. (*See all* under separate listings.)

EMULSIFYING OIL • Soluble Oil. Jan oil, when mixed with water, produces a milky emulsion. Sodium sulfonate is an example.

EMULSIFYING WAX • Waxes that are treated so that they mix more easily.

EMULSION • What is formed when two or more nonmixable liquids are shaken so thoroughly together that the mixture continues to appear to be homogenized. Most oils form emulsions with water.

ENCAPSULATION • Scents can be encapsulated in gelatin and are released when a fragrance product is placed in hot water. Some microencapsulated products contain coated perfume granules that are so small they give the impression of free-flowing powder.

ENDOCRINE SYSTEM • Made up of glands and hormones that regulate many body functions, including growth, development, and maturation as well as the way various organs do their work. The endocrine glands—including the pituitary, thyroid, adrenal, thymus, pancreas, ovaries, and testes—release carefully measured amounts of hormones into the bloodstream that act as natural chemical messengers, traveling to different parts of the body in order to control and adjust many life functions.

ENDOCRINE DISRUPTER CHEMICAL • A synthetic chemical that either mimics or blocks hormones and disrupts the body's normal functions. This disruption can happen through affecting normal hormone levels, halting or stimulating the production of hormones, or changing the way hormones operate. Many chemicals, particularly pesticides and plasticizers, are suspected endocrine disrupters.

ENDOMYCES FERMENT FILTRATE • From yeast, used as a skin conditioner.

ENFLEURAGE • The technique of making perfumes from flowers that cannot be subjected to steam distillation, such as roses and orange blossoms. It includes the use of glass trays that are lined with lard, on which flowers picked early in the morning are scattered. The trays are stacked on one another. The next day the flowers are removed from the fat and replaced with fresh ones. The cycle is repeated for several weeks. The lard is then scraped from the trays and mixed with alcohol. The alcohol in turn is removed by distillation, leaving behind the flower-scented essential oil, or "absolute." The process usually takes thirty-six days and is therefore expensive and done only for fine perfumes.

ENGELHARDTIA CHRYSOLEPIS • Skin conditioner from bark. *See* Cinnamon.

ENGLISH OAK EXTRACT • Extract of the bark of *Quercus robur.* The wood is used for cabinetmaking. The extract is used in chestnut brown dye.

ENMEISOU EKISU • Enmeiso. An extract obtained from the Japanese plant *Isodonis japonicus,* also called *Isodon japonicus* or *Plectranthus japonicus.* Used as a skin conditioner and a fragrance.

ENSULIZOLE • PBSA. Phenylbenzimidazole Sulfonic Acid. Potassium sulfonate phenylbenzimidazole sulfonate, sodium phenylbenzimidazole sulfonate, and TEA-phenylbenzimidazole sulfonate are salts of phenylbenzimidazole. Controversial sunscreen. The Personal Care and Safety Council (formerly CTFA) describes it on its website Cosmeticsinfo.org as being a white to pale beige powder. In the United States,it is used in sun protection products and is called ensulizole. In addition to the acid, the European Union also permits the potassium, sodium and triethanolamine (TEA) salts of phenylbenzimidazole sulfonic acid to be used in sun protection products. The Food and Drug Administration (FDA) reviewed the safety of phenylbenzimidazole sulfonic acid and approved its use as an active ingredient in OTC sunscreen drug products at concentrations up to 4 percent. The European Commission's Scientific Committee on Consumer Products (SCCP) reviewed the safety of phenylbenzimidazole sulfonic acid and its potassium, sodium, and TEA salts and concluded that the use of these ingredients in cosmetic products at a maximum concentration of 8 percent would not pose a health hazard. The CIR Expert Panel (*see*) has deferred evaluation of this ingredient because the safety has been assessed by FDA. This deferral of review is according to the provisions of the CIR Procedures.

ENTADA PHASEOLOIDES • Extract of *Entada phaseoloides.* Matchbox Beans. Brown, heart-shaped seed found along the seacoast of eastern South America and Australia. The wood and bark of *E. phaseoloides* (family Leguminosae) contain high concentrations of saponins, and they are used traditionally, occasionally by some rural communities, to prepare soapy solutions to wash their body parts and fabrics. The species is locally known as "Beluru" or "Sintok." In the preparation of herbal shampoos the saponins are used as the most important ingredient. Contraceptive and abortive uses have also been recorded. Toxic.

ENTERIC COATING • Coating on a compound allowing the slow release of the active ingredients.

ENTEROMORPHA COMPRESSA • The genus *Enteromorpha* is extremely common, consisting of very similar green seaweeds on all shore levels, found in bright green mats around the whole extent of the Irish coast, Europe, and North America. Used as a moisturizer in cosmetics. *See* Algae.

ENVIRONMENTAL WORKING GROUP • EWG. A nonprofit organization, the mission of which is to use the power of public information to protect public health and the environment.

ENZYME • Any of a unique class of proteins that catalyze a broad spectrum of biochemical reactions. Enzymes are formed in living cells. One enzyme can cause a chemical process that no other enzyme can. Among the enzymes used in cosmetics are amylase and chymotrypsin (*see both*).

EOSIN • Red crystalline powder soluble in alcohol and acetic acid. It is used as a coloring in cosmetic products. *See* Fluorescein.

EOSIN YELLOW • *See* Tetrabromofluorescein.

EPA GENETIC TOXICOLOGY PROGRAM • The U.S. Environmental Protection Agency has certain chemicals under study to determine their effects on genes, the parts of the cell that carry inherited characteristics. Damage to the mechanisms of genes can lead to birth defects and cancer, as well as other illnesses.

EPHEDRA • *Ephedra gerardiana. E. trifurca. E. sinica. E. equisetina. E. helvetica.* Ma Huang. Mormon Tea. There are about forty species of this herb mentioned in ancient scriptures of India and used by the Chinese for more than five thousand years. The stems contain alkaloids (*see*), including ephedrine (*see*). Herbalists use the herb to treat arthritis, asthma, emphysema, bronchitis, hay fever, and hives. It is a stimulant in cosmetics. *See also* Ephedrine. On the Canadian Hotlist (*see*).

EPHEDRINE • An alkaloid derived from the plant *Ephedra equisetina* and others of the forty species of ephedra produced synthetically. Ephedra has been used for more than five thousand years in Chinese medicine and has become more and more popular in Western medicine. Ephedrine acts like epinephrine (*see*) and is used as a bronchiodilator and nasal decongestant, to raise blood pressure, and topically to constrict blood vessels. On the Canadian Hotlist (*see*).

EPICHLOROHYDRIN • A colorless liquid with an odor resembling chloroform. It is soluble in water but mixes readily with alcohol and ether. Used as a solvent for cosmetic resins and nitrocellulose (*see*) and in the manufacture of varnishes, lacquers, and cements for celluloid articles; also a modifier for food starch. A strong skin irritant and sensitizer. Daily administration of 1 milligram per kilogram of body weight to skin killed all of a group of rats in four days, indicating a cumulative potential. Chronic exposure is known to cause kidney damage. A thirty-minute exposure to air concentrations of 8,300 parts per million was lethal to mice. Poisoned animals showed cyanosis, muscular relaxation or paralysis, convulsions, and death. Banned in cosmetics by Canada in 2009.

EPIDERMAL GROWTH FACTOR • Made up of human laboratory–made skin growth factor consisting of fifty-three amino acids (*see*) with fermentation of *E. coli.* Basically a protein product used in skin conditioners.

EPIDERMIS • Four to five layers of cells covering the skin (dermis).

EPIGAEA REPENS • *See* Arbutus Extract.

EPIGALLOCATECHIN • An oxidant. *See* Phenols.

EPILATORIES • Waxlike products that are softened by heat and applied when cool and then "yanked" off, taking embedded hair with them. (Some epilatories do not have to be heated.) They may be formulated from roses, paraffin, beeswax, ceresin, carnauba wax, mineral and linseed oils, and petrolatum. (See ingredients under separate listings.) Sometimes benzocaine is added in low concentrations for its local anesthetic effect. Benzocaine is on the Canadian Hotlist (*see*). *See* Depilatories.

EPILOBIUM ANGUSTIFOLIUM • Willow Herb. Fireweed. A widely grown herb used as a skin conditioner. May have anti-inflammatory properties.

EPIMEDIUM GRANDIFLORUM • Horny Goat Weed. Used as a tea, decoction, extract, tincture, dietary supplement, and soup vegetable. The Chinese consider it a premier libido lifter for men and women, and a top aid to erectile function in men. The plant has long been employed to restore sexual fire, boost erectile function, allay fatigue, and even alleviate menopausal discomfort. The Chinese Academy of Sciences recommends the regular use of it to slow the aging process.

EPINEPHRINE • Adrenalin. Adrenaline Chloride. The major hormone of the adrenal gland, epinephrine increases heart rate and contractions (vasoconstriction or vasodilation), relaxation of the muscles in the lungs and smooth muscles in the intestines, and the processing of sugar and fat. It is the hormone that readies us for "fight or flight" in stressful situations. In eye medications, it may cause redness, fluid retention, rash, severe stinging, burning, and tearing upon instillation, palpitations, and rapid heartbeat. Banned in cosmetics by the EU. Sulfonate permitted only in fragrances by the UK.

EPIPHYLLUM OXPETALUM • A cactus, an extract of which is used as a skin conditioner.

EPITHELIAL • Refers to those cells that form the outer layer of the skin, those that line all the portions of the body that have contact with external air, and those that are specialized for secretion.

EPITHELIUM • A thin layer of cells forming a tissue that covers surfaces and lines hollow organs.

EPOXY- • Chemical prefix describing an oxygen atom bound to two linked carbon atoms. Epoxies are used as chemical intermediates and are widely employed in thickening resins.

EPOXY RESINS • The versatile epoxy resins are used widely in manufacturing electrical equipment, in automobile plants, in paints for surface coating, and in aircraft and other industries for adhesive purposes. In cosmetics, they are used for adhesion, waterproofing, and emulsions.

EPOXY BUTANE • Banned in cosmetics by ASEAN. *See* Epoxy Resins and Butane.

EPSOM SALTS • *See* Magnesium Sulfate.

EQUISETUM ARVENSE • *See* Horsetail.

ERGOCALCIFEROL • Vitamin D$_2$. Used as a conditioner in skin and hair products. On the Canadian Hotlist (*see*). Banned in cosmetics by the EU.

ERGOSTEROL • Provitamin D$_2$. Derived from yeast or fungus ergot. It has vitamin D and estrogen activity. Used in skin conditioners.

ERGOT • *Claviceps purpurea.* A fungus most frequently growing on rye. The principal uses of ergot are as a uterine stimulant and a vasoconstrictor. Ergot was also used to check excessive menstrual bleeding. Ergot alkaloids are used widely today in the treatment of migraine and to stimulate the heart and other involuntary muscles. Ergot is known to contain a number of complex and potent alkaloids, some of which are very similar to lysergic acid (LSD). Long-term use may cause constriction of the blood vessels of the extremities, the end result of which may be gangrene. In the Middle Ages, epidemics of ergotism from eating contaminated rye flour produced both gangrene and convulsions. The FDA proposed a ban in 1992 on the use of ergot fluid extract to treat insect bites and stings because it has not been shown to be safe and effective for stated claims in OTC products. On the Canadian Hotlist (*see*).

ERICA CINEREA • Purple Heath. A shrub that yields a red coloring.

ERIGERON OIL • Horseweed. Fleabane Oil. Colt's-tail, Pride-weed, Scabious. Derived from the leaves and tops of a plant grown in the northern and central United States. An astringent that is sometimes used as a local application to hemorrhoids, bleeding from the anus, and small wounds. Used in fruit and spice flavorings for beverages, ice cream, ices, candy, baked goods, and sauces.

ERIOBOTRYA JAPONICA • Rosaceae family. Loquat. Japanese plum. Loquats contain amygdalin, which is also found in cherry bark and apricot kernel, both of which are used to treat coughs. In the 1950s, the flowers attracted the interest of the perfume industry in France and Spain, and some experimental work was done in extraction of the essential oil from the flowers or leaves. The product was appealing, but the yield was very small. The leaves possess a mixture of triterpenes and also tannin, vitamin B, and ascorbic acid; in addition, there are traces of arsenic. Young leaves contain saponin. Some individuals suffer headache when too close to a loquat tree in bloom. The emanation from the flowers is sweet and penetrating.

ERIODICTYON CALIFORNICUM • *See* Yerba Santa Fluid Extract.

ERUCA SATIVA • Garden Rocket Extract. From a small shrub that is related to broccoli. *See* Erucic Acid.

ERUCALKONIUM CHLORIDE • *See* Quaternary Ammonium Compounds.

ERUCAMIDE • Erucylamide. An aliphatic amide slightly soluble in alcohol and acetone. Used as a foam stabilizer; a solvent for waxes, resins, and emulsions; and an antiblock ingredient for polyethylene.

ERUCAMIDOPROPYL HYDROXYSULTAINE • An antistatic ingredient for hair products. *See* Erucic Acid and Betaines.

ERUCIC ACID • Cis-13-Docosenoic Acid. A fatty acid derived from mustard seed, rapeseed, and carambe seed. Used in polyethylene film, lipsticks, and water-resistant nylon.

ERUCYL ARACHIDATE • Ester of erucyl alcohol and arachidic acid. *See* Arachidic Acid.

ERYCYL ERUCATE • The ester of erucyl alcohol and erucic acid. A fatty alcohol derived from erucic acid that is used as a lubricant and surfactant, and in plastics and textiles.

ERYNGIUM MARITIMUM • Sea Holly. This European plant is found on sandy shores and is used by herbalists to treat many urinary ailments. A diuretic, it is often used to treat kidney stones and gravel, especially if there is urinary retention.

ERYTHORBIC ACID • Isoascorbic Acid. Antioxidant. White, slightly yellow crystals, which darken on exposure to light. Isoascorbic acid contains one-twentieth the vitamin capacity of ascorbic acid (*see*). The final report to the FDA of the Select Committee on GRAS Substances stated in 1980 that it should continue its GRAS status, with no limitations other than good manufacturing practices.

ERYTHRITOL • Isolated from algae, lichens, and grasses, it is about twice as sweet as sugar. It is used as a humectant (*see*) and a conditioning ingredient in moisturizing creams and lotions.

ERYTHROSINE • Sodium or potassium salt of tetraiodofluorescein, a coal tar derivative. A brown powder that becomes red in solution. FD & C Red No. 3 is an example. It is used in rouge. *See* Coal Tar for toxicity.

ERYTHULOSE • Erythulose is a specific sugar that is obtained by biotransformation from a sugar alcohol derived from algae or lichen. It reacts with substances of the epidermis leading to various brown polymers. These combine with proteins of the horny layer and can therefore not be washed off. It provides an even and uniform tan but this does not provide UV protection.

ESCHSCHOLTZIA • California Poppy. A perennial growing to a height of two feet. It has thin leaves, tapering to a fine tip and bright orange, yellow, pink, or red flowers. The fruit is oblong with small, globular seeds. It is found in western North America, central Europe, and southern France. The plant possesses analgesic, antispasmodic, febrifuge, nervine, and sedative properties. Although California poppy is closely related to the opium poppy, it has a very different effect on the central nervous system. California poppy is not a narcotic. In fact, rather than disorienting the user, it tends to normalize psychological function. Native American tribes used the sap for its painkilling properties, particularly for toothaches. The plant was also used to obtain a high because of its sedative effects. In cosmetics, it is used as a skin conditioner.

ESCIN • A saponin occurring in the seeds of the horse chestnut tree, *Aesculus hippocastanum*. Practically insoluble in water, it is used as a sunburn protective.

ESCULIN • Occurs in the bark and leaves of the horse chestnut tree. It has been used as a skin protectant in ointments and creams.

ESERINE ALKALOID AND SALTS • On the Canadian Hotlist (*see*). *See* Physostigmine.

ESSENCE • An extract of a substance that retains its fundamental or most desirable properties in concentrated form, such as a fragrance or flavoring.

ESSENCE OF MIRBANE • Used to scent cheap soap. *See* Nitrobenzene.

ESSENTIAL OIL • The oily liquid obtained from plants through a variety of processes. The essential oil usually has the taste and smell of the original plant. Essential oils are called volatile because most of them are easily vaporized. The only theories for calling such oils essential are (1) the oils were believed essential to life and (2) they were the "essence" of the plant. The use of essential oils as preservatives is ancient. A large number of oils have antiseptic, germicidal, and preservative action; however, they are used primarily for fragrances and flavorings. A teaspoon may cause illness in an adult, and less than an ounce may kill.

ESTER • A compound formed from an alcohol and an acid by elimination of water, as ethyl acetate (*see*). Usually, fragrant liquids used for artificial fruit perfumes and flavors. Esterification of rosin, for example, reduces its allergy-causing properties. Toxicity depends on the ester.

ESTERIFICATION • The process of forming an ester (*see*), as in the reaction of ethyl alcohol and acetic acid to form ethyl acetate.

ESTRADIOL • Most potent of the natural estrogenic female hormones. *See* Hormone Creams and Lotion. Also used in perfumes. It is on the Canadian Hotlist (*see*) and banned in Canada. May be found in products from Japan where it is permitted at 200 IU/g total estrogens.

ESTRADIOL BENZOATE • *See* Estradiol.

ESTRAGON OIL • Tarragon. A flavoring ingredient from the oil of leaves of a plant native to Eurasia, used in fruit, licorice, liquor, root beer, and spice flavorings for beverages, ice cream, ices, candy, baked goods, meats, liquor, and condiments. GRAS

ESTROGEN • A female hormone. *See* Hormone Creams and Lotion.

ESTRONE • A follicular hormone that occurs in the urine of pregnant women and mares, in human placenta, and in palm kernel oil (*see*). Used in creams and lotions as a "hormone" to improve the skin. Usually, there is not enough in the creams to have an effect. It can have harmful systemic effects if used by children. On the Canadian Hotlist (*see*) and banned in that country. May be found in products from Japan where it is permitted at 200 IU/g total estrogens.

ETHANE • Colorless, odorless gas used in propellants. *See* Ethylene.

ETHANOL • Ethyl Alcohol. Rubbing Alcohol. Ordinary Alcohol. An antibacterial used in mouthwashes, nail enamel, astringents, liquid lip rouge, and many other cosmetic products. Clear, colorless, and very flammable, it is made by the fermentation of starch, sugar, and other carbohydrates. When it is deliberately denatured (*see*), it is poisonous. Used medicinally as a topical antiseptic, sedative, and blood vessel dilator. Ingestion of large amounts may cause nausea, vomiting, impaired perception, stupor, coma, and death.

ETHANOLAMINE DITHIODIGLYCOATE • *See* Ethanolamines.

ETHANOLAMINE THIOGLYCOLATE • The CIR Expert Panel (*see*) has listed this as a high priority for review. *See* Ethanolamines.

ETHANOLAMINES • Three compounds—monoethanolamine, diethanolamine, and triethanolamine—with low melting points, colorless, and solid, which readily absorb water and form viscous liquids; soluble in both water and alcohol. They have an ammonia smell and are strong bases. Used in cold permanent-wave lotions as a preservative. Also form soaps with fatty acids (*see*), and are widely used as detergents and emulsifying ingredients. Very large quantities are required for a lethal oral dose in mice (2,140 milligrams per kilogram of body weight). They have been used medicinally as sclerosal ingredients for varicose veins. Can be irritating to skin if very alkaline. *See* Diethanolamine.

ETHER • An organic compound. Acetic ether (*see* Ethyl Acetate) is used in nail polishes as a solvent. Water-insoluble, fat-insoluble liquid with a characteristic odor. It is obtained chiefly by the distillation of alcohol with sulfuric acid and is used chiefly as a solvent. A mild skin irritant. Inhalation or ingestion causes central nervous system depression

ETHINYLESTRADIOL • Female hormone. On the Canadian Hotlist (*see*) and banned in that country. May be found in products from Japan where it is permitted at 200 IU/g total estrogens.

ETHIODIZED OIL • The ethyl ester of the fatty acids derived from poppy seeds with iodine. It is used as an antiseptic and skin conditioner. *See* Iodine.

ETHOXYDIGLYCOL • An alcohol compound widely used as a solvent or fragrance ingredient in indoor tanning products, cleansing creams, and hair bleaches as well as moisturizers. *See* Ethoxylate. Also forms soaps with fatty acids (*see*), and are widely used as detergents and emulsifying ingredients. Very large quantities are required for a lethal oral dose in mice. They have been used medicinally as sclerosal ingredients for varicose veins. Can be irritating to skin if very alkaline. *See* Diethanolamine.

ETHOXYDIGLYCOL ACETATE • Carbitol Acetate. Used as a solvent and plasticizer for nail enamels and resins and gums. Less toxic than ethoxydiglycol alone by ingestion but is more toxic when applied to the skin. *See* Butylene Glycol.

ETHOXYETHANOL • Cellosolve. Ethylene Glycol Monoethyl Ether. A solvent for nail enamels and a stabilizer in cosmetic emulsions, including shampoos. Obtained by heating ethylene chloride with alcohol and sodium acetate. Colorless and practically odorless. Acute toxicity is several times greater than polyethylene glycol (*see*) in animals. Produces central nervous system depression and kidney damage. Can penetrate the intact skin. The CIR Expert Panel (*see*) found this ingredient unsafe in 1999 for use because of its adverse effects on reproductive and developmental toxicity. On the Canadian Hotlist (*see*).

ETHOXYETHANOL ACETATE • Cellosolve Acetate. Used to give high gloss to nail polish and to retard evaporation. A colorless liquid with a pleasant odor. Somewhat less toxic than ethoxyethanol alone, it is a central nervous system depressant but does not cause as much kidney damage. It can be readily absorbed through the skin. The CIR Expert Panel (*see*) found this ingredient unsafe in 1999 for use because of its adverse effects on reproductive and developmental toxicity. On the Canadian Hotlist (*see*).

2-ETHOXYETHYL-*p*-METHOXYCINNAMATE • Slightly yellow, viscous liquid, practically odorless, almost insoluble in water. UV absorber in suntan preparations.

ETHOXYHEPTYL BICYCLOOCTANONE • Ethocyn. A skin-conditioning ingredient.

ETHOXYLATE • Ethyl (from the gas ethane) and oxygen are mixed and added to an additive to make it less or more soluble in water, depending upon the mixture. Ethoxylate acts as an emulsifier.

ETHOXYLATED FATTY ACIDS • *See* Ethoxylate and Fatty Acids.

ETHOXYLATED FATTY ALCOHOLS • *See* Ethoxylate and Fatty Alcohols.

ETHOXYLATED SURFACTANTS • Detergents, wetting ingredients, and emulsifiers that have been treated with ethane gas and oxygen to make them more or less soluble, depending upon the mixture. The FDA is studying these ingredients to determine their safety in cosmetics.

4-ETHOXY-*m*-PHENYLDIAMINE • *See* Phenylenediamine.

4-ETHOXY-SULFATE • On the Canadian Hotlist (*see*). *See* Phenylenediamine.

ETHYL ACETATE • A colorless liquid with a pleasant fruity odor that occurs naturally in apples, bananas, grape juice, pineapple, raspberries, and strawberries. A very useful solvent in nail enamels and nail polish removers. Also an artificial fruit essence for perfumes. It is a mild local irritant and central nervous system depressant. The vapors are irritating, and prolonged inhalation may cause kidney and liver damage. Irritating to the skin. Its fat solvent action produces drying and cracking and sets the stage for secondary infections. On the basis of available data, the CIR Expert Panel concludes that this ingredient is safe as presently used in cosmetics.

ETHYL ACETOACETATE • Acetoacetic Ester. A synthetic flavoring that occurs naturally in strawberries. Pleasant odor. Used in loganberry, strawberry, apple, apricot, cherry, peach, liquor, and muscatel flavorings for beverages, ice cream, ices, candy, baked goods, chewing gum, and gelatin desserts. Moderately irritating to skin and mucous membranes.

ETHYL ACRYLATE • Used for testing for acrylate allergy, which is common. *See* Acrylates. According to Dr. Frances Storrs, professor of dermatology at Oregon Health Sciences University, in 1997, more than 90 percent of patients who are allergic to acrylates found in artificial nails will test positive for ethyl acrylate, making it a good screener. Banned in fragrances by the UK and the EU.

ETHYL ALCOHOL • *See* Ethanol.

ETHYL ALMONDATE • An ester of fatty acids derived from sweet almond oil, it is used in hair and skin conditioners.

ETHYL AMINOBENZOATE • *See* Ethyl Anthranilate.

3-ETHYLAMINO-*p*-CREOSOL SULFATE • A coal tar (*see*) hair coloring.

ETHYL ANTHRANILATE • Colorless liquid, fruity odor, soluble in alcohol and propylene glycol. A synthetic flavoring ingredient, clear, colorless to amber liquid with an odor of orange blossoms. Used in berry, mandarin orange, floral, jasmine, neroli, fruit, grape, peach, and raisin flavorings for beverages, ice cream, ices, candy, baked goods, gelatin desserts, and chewing gum. Used in perfumery.

ETHYL APRICOT KERNELATE • An emollient derived from apricot kernel oil (*see*).

ETHYL ARACHIDONATE • The ester of ethyl alcohol and arachidonic acid (*see both*).

ETHYL ASCORBIC ACID • Antioxidant used in skin conditioners.

ETHYL ASPARTATE • The ester of ethyl alcohol and aspartic acid (*see both*).

ETHYL AVOCADATE • *See* Avocado.

ETHYL BENZOATE • Essence de Niobe. An artificial fruit essence used in perfumes. Almost insoluble in water. Also used in strawberry and raspberry flavorings. Used as a preservative. *See* Benzoates.

7-ETHYLBICYCLOOXAZOLIDINE • A preservative. *See* Oxazolidine.

ETHYL BIOTINATE • Used in hair and skin conditioners. *See* Biotin.

ETHYL BROMIDE • Colorless liquid from ethanol or ethylene and hydrobromic acid. Used as a solvent, anesthetic, and fumigant. Toxic by ingestion, inhalation, and skin absorption. It is a strong irritant.

ETHYL BUTYL VALEROLACTONE • A fragrance ingredient. *See* Valeric Acid.

ETHYL BUTYLACETYLAMINO PROPIONATE • An insect repellent.

ETHYL BUTYRATE • Pineapple Oil. An ingredient in perfumes; colorless, with a pineapple odor. It occurs naturally in apples and strawberries. Also used in synthetic flavorings such as blueberry and raspberry.

ETHYL CAPRATE • Colorless liquid with a fragrant odor used as a flavoring ingredient. *See* Capric Acid.

ETHYL CAPROATE • Colorless to yellowish liquid, pleasant odor, soluble in alcohol and ether. Used in artificial fruit essences.

ETHYL CARBONATE • Carbonic Acid Diethyl Ester. Pleasant odor, practically insoluble in water. Used as a solvent for nail enamels.

ETHYL CELLULOSE • Cellulose Ether. Binding, dispersing, and emulsifying ingredient used in cosmetics, particularly nail polishes and liquid lip rouge. Prepared from wood pulp or chemical cotton by treatment with an alkali. Also used as a diluent (*see*). Not susceptible to bacterial or fungal decomposition.

ETHYL CHLORIDE • Chloroethane. Prepared by the action of chlorine on ethylene in the presence of hydrochloric acid and light. Used as a topical anesthetic in minor operative procedures and to relieve pain caused by insect stings, burns, and irritation. Mildly irritating to mucous membranes. High concentrations of vapors cause unconsciousness. On the Canadian Hotlist (*see*).

ETHYL CINNAMATE • An almost colorless, oily liquid with a faint cinnamon odor. Used as a fixative for perfumes; also to scent heavy oriental and floral perfumes in soaps, toilet waters, face powders, and perfumes. Insoluble in water. Also used as a synthetic food flavoring. Has been reported to cause eye, skin, and respiratory irritation.

ETHYL CYANOACRYLATE • *See* Acrylates.

ETHYL CYCLOHEXYL PROPIONATE • A fragrance ingredient.

ETHYL DIHYDROXYPROPYL PABA • The ester of ethyl alcohol and *p*-dihydroxypropyl aminobenzoic acid. *See* Ethyl Alcohol and PABA.

ETHYL DIISOPROPYLCINNAMATE • *See* Cinnamic Acid.

ETHYL 2,2-DIMETHYLHYDROCINNAMAL • A fragrance ingredient. *See* Cinnamal.

5-ETHYL-3,7-DIOX-1-AZABICYCLO[3.3.0]OCTANE[7-ETHYLBICYCLO-OXAZOLADINE]. Prohibited by the UK in oral hygiene products and in products intended to come into contact with mucous membranes. *See* Octane.

ETHYL ESTER OF HYDROLYZED ANIMAL PROTEIN • The ester of ethyl alcohol and the hydrolysate of collagen (*see*).

ETHYL ESTER OF PVM/MA COPOLYMER • Used for its setting properties, it yields a nontacky film and is water resistant. It is used in hair-setting and -bodying preparations. On the basis of available data, the CIR Expert Panel concludes that this ingredient is safe as presently used in cosmetics. *See* Vinyl Polymers.

ETHYL FORMATE • Formic Acid. A colorless, flammable liquid with a distinct odor occurring naturally in apples and coffee extract. Used as a yeast and mold inhibitor. Also used as a synthetic flavoring ingredient. Irritating to the skin and mucous membranes, and narcotic in high concentrations. The final report to the FDA of the Select Committee on GRAS Substances stated in 1980 that it should continue its GRAS status with no limitations other than good manufacturing practices. *See* Formic Acid for further toxicity.

ETHYL FERULATE • Preservative. *See* Ferulic Acid.

ETHYL GLUCOSIDE • Skin conditioner. *See* Glucose.

ETHYL GLUTAMATE • The ester of ethyl alcohol and glutamic acid. *See* Glutamate.

ETHYL GUAIAZULENE SULFONATE • An astringent. *See* Sulfonic Acid.

ETHYL HEPTANOATE • A synthetic flavoring ingredient, colorless, with a fruity, winelike odor and taste, and a burning aftertaste. Used in blueberry, strawberry, butter, butterscotch, coconut, apple, cherry, grape, melon, peach, pineapple, plum, vanilla, cheese, nut, rum, brandy, and cognac flavorings for beverages.

ETHYL HEXANEDIOL • A solvent. It is absorbed through the skin and is metabolized and eliminated in the urine. It affected the growth and liver of test animals. Skin application also affected birth defects in female rats. In human studies, it was a weak sensitizer. On the basis of available data, the CIR Expert Panel concludes that this ingredient is safe as presently used in cosmetics. The panel, however, did express concern about the birth defects caused in some rats following skin exposure to undiluted ethyl hexanediol.

ETHYLHEXYLGLYCERIN • This is a natural preservative, used as an alternative to parabens products. It is derived from natural glycerin. Also used as a deodorizer and skin conditioner.

ETHYL HEXYLMETHOXYCINNAMATE • Used as a sunscreen in hypoallergenic cosmetics. *See* Cinnamic Acid.

ETHYL-*p*-HYDROXYBENZOATE • *See* Benzoic Acid.

ETHYL HYDROXYMETHYL OLEYL OXAZOLINE • A synthetic wax.

ETHYL ISOVALERATE • Colorless, oily liquid with a fruity odor derived from ethanol and valerate. Used in essential oils, perfumery, artificial fruit essences, and flavoring. *See* Valeric Acid.

ETHYL LACTATE • Colorless liquid with a mild odor. Derived from lactic acid with ethanol. Used as a solvent for nitrocellulose, lacquers, resins, enamels, and flavorings. *See* Lactic Acid.

ETHYL LAURATE • The ester of ethyl alcohol and lauric acid used as a synthetic flavoring. It is a colorless oil with a light, fruity odor. It is also used as a solvent.

ETHYL LAUROYL ARGINATE HCL • Hair and skin conditioner. *See* Lauric Acid.

ETHYL LEVULINATE • Colorless liquid soluble in water. Used as a solvent for cellulose acetate and starch and flavorings. *See* Levulinic Acid.

ETHYL LINALOOL • *See* Linalool.

ETHYL LINOLEATE • Used as a fragrance ingredient and emollient. The ester of ethyl alcohol and linoleic acid. Vitamin F. *See* Fatty Acids and Linoleic Acid.

ETHYL MALONATE • Colorless liquid, sweet ester odor. Insoluble in water. Used in certain pigments and flavorings.

ETHYL MALTOL • *See* Maltose.

ETHYL METHACRYLATE • The ester of ethyl alcohol and methacrylic acid. Birth defects were seen in rats injected with this ingredient. Positive evidence of mutagenicity were also observed in mouse cancers. Reports of human sensitivity to this ingredient have been made. On the basis of available data, the CIR Expert Panel concludes that this ingredient is safe as presently used in cosmetics but that skin contact should be avoided. *See* Acrylates.

ETHYL METHOXYCINNAMATE • Used as a sunscreen in hypoallergenic cosmetics. *See* Cinnamic Acid.

ETHYL METHYLPHENYLGLYCIDATE • Strawberry Aldehyde. Colorless to yellowish liquid having a strong odor suggestive of strawberry. Used in perfumery and flavors. *See* Phenols.

ETHYL MINKATE • Fatty acids from mink oil (*see*).

ETHYL MORRHUATE • Lipinate. Salt of morrhuic acid, a fatty acid obtained from cod liver oil. Used in creams and lotions.

ETHYL MYRISTATE • The ester of ethyl alcohol and myristic acid (*see both*).

ETHYL NICOTINATE • Used as a skin-conditioning ingredient. *See* Ethyl Alcohol and Nicotinic Acid.

N-ETHYL-3-NITRO PABA • Hair coloring. *See* Parabens.

ETHYL OLEATE • An ingredient in nail polish remover; yellowish, oily, insoluble in water. It is made from carbon, hydrogen, oxygen, and oleic acid (*see*) and used as a synthetic butter and fruit flavoring. Emollient. *See* Octadecenoic Acid.

ETHYL OLIVATE • Fatty acids derived from olive oil. Emollient and hair conditioner. *See* Olive Oil.

ETHYL PABA • An ultraviolet light absorber. *See* Parabens.

ETHYL PALMITATE • The ester of ethyl alcohol and palmitic acid (*see both*).

ETHYL PEG-15 COCAMINE SULFATE • *See* Coconut Oil.

ETHYL PELARGONATE • The ester of ethyl alcohol and pelargonic acid (*see both*) used in the manufacture of lacquers and plastics, derived from rice bran. Pelargonic acid is a strong irritant.

ETHYL PERSATE • Persic Oil Acid. Ethyl Ester. The ethyl ester of the fatty acids derived from either apricot kernel oil or peach kernel oil. *See* Apricot Kernel Oil and Peach Kernel Oil.

ETHYL PHENETHYL ACETAL • Used in fragrances. *See* Benzene.

ETHYL PHENYLACETATE • A fixative for perfumes, colorless or nearly colorless liquid, with a sweet honey rose odor. Also a synthetic flavoring ingredient in various foods.

ETHYL RICINOLEATE • Fragrance ingredient and emollient used in cleansing products. *See* Octanoic Acid.

ETHYL SALICYLATE • Used in the manufacture of artificial perfumes. Occurs naturally in strawberries and has a pleasant odor. Also used as a synthetic flavoring ingredient in fruit drinks, baked goods, and so on. At one time it was used to treat rheumatics. It may cause allergic reactions, especially in people who are allergic to other salicylates, including salicylates used in sunscreen lotions.

ETHYL SERINATE • The ester of ethyl alcohol and serine (*see both*).

ETHYL STEARATE • The ester of ethyl alcohol and stearic acid (*see both*).

ETHYL TOLUENESULFONAMIDE • Plasticizer for cellulose acetate and for ethylating. *See* Toluene.

ETHYL UNDECYLENATE • The ester of ethyl alcohol and undecylenic acid.

ETHYL UROCANATE • The ester of ethyl alcohol and urocanic acid. *See* Imidazoline.

ETHYL VALERATE • The ester of ethyl alcohol and valeric acid (*see both*).

ETHYL VANILLIN • An ingredient in perfumes. Colorless flakes, with an odor and flavor stronger than vanilla. Also a synthetic food flavoring.

ETHYL WHEAT GERMATE • Hair- and skin-conditioning ingredient. *See* Wheat Germ.

ETHYL XIMENYNATE • Emollient. *See* Octanoic Acid.

ETHYLENE • The sixth-highest-volume chemical produced in the United States, it is a colorless gas with a sweet odor and taste. It is derived from heat cracking hydrocarbon gases or from fluid removal from ethanol. It is used to make chemical compounds including those used to make plastics, refrigerants, anesthetics, and orchard sprays to accelerate fruit ripening.

ETHYLENE/ACRYLATE COPOLYMER • *See* Acrylates and Copolymers.

ETHYLENE BRASSYLATE • *See* Behenic Acid.

ETHYLENE/CALCIUM ACRYLATE COPOLYMER • *See* Acrylates.

ETHYLENE CARBONATE • A solvent. Highly flammable and potentially explosive. It can asphyxiate. *See* Carboxylic Acid.

ETHYLENE CHLORIDES • Solvents. No longer permitted in cosmetics.

ETHYLENE DEHYDROGENATED TALLOW AMIDE • *See* Tallow.

ETHYLENEDIAMINE • Solvent manufactured from ethylene dichloride and ammonia. It is strongly alkaline and may be irritating to the nose and respiratory system if inhaled. It can also cause kidney and liver damage. Colorless, clear, thick, and strongly alkaline. A bacteria-killing component in processing sugarcane. Also used as a solvent for casein, albumen, and shellac. Has been used as a urinary acidifier. It can cause sensitization leading to asthma and allergic skin rashes. On the Canadian Hotlist (*see*).

ETHYLENEDIAMINE TETRAACETIC ACID • EDTA. An important compound in cosmetics used primarily as a sequestering ingredient (*see*), particularly in shampoos. It may be irritating to the skin and mucous membranes and cause allergies such as asthma and skin rashes. Also used as a sequestrant in carbonated beverages. When ingested, it may cause errors in a number of laboratory tests, including those for calcium, carbon dioxide, nitrogen, and muscular activity. It is on the FDA list of food additives to be studied for toxicity. It can cause kidney damage. The trisodium salt of EDTA was fed to rats and mice for nearly two years. According to a summary of the report: "Although a variety of tumors occurred among test and control animals of both species, the test did not indicate that any of the tumors observed in the test animals were attributed to EDTA. The tests were part of the National Cancer Institute's Carcinogenesis Bioassay Program."

ETHYLENEDIAMINES/STEARYL DIMER DILIONOLEATE COPOLYMER • Used in oral care preparations and skin conditioners. *See* Ethylenediamine Tetraacetic Acid (EDTA) and Stearic Acid.

ETHYLENE DICHLORIDE • EDC. The halogenated aliphatic hydrocarbon derived from the action of chlorine on ethylene. It is used in the manufacture of vinyl chloride (*see*); as a solvent for fats, waxes, and resins; as a lead scavenger in antiknock gasolines; in paint, varnish, and finish removers; as a wetting ingredient; as a penetrating ingredient; in organic synthesis; and in the making of polyvinyl chloride (PVC) (*see*). EDC is also used as an ingredient in cosmetics and as a food additive. It is one of the highest-volume chemicals produced. It can be highly toxic whether taken into the body by ingestion, inhalation, or skin absorption. It is irritating to the mucous membranes. In cancer testing, the National Cancer Institute found this compound caused stomach cancer, vascularized cancers of multiple organs, and cancers beneath the skin in male rats. Female rats exposed to EDC developed mammary cancers—in some high-dose animals as early as the twentieth week of the study. The chemical also caused breast cancers as well as uterine cancers in female mice and respiratory tract cancers in both sexes.

ETHYLENE DIOLEAMIDE • *See* Fatty Acids.

ETHYLENE DISTEARAMIDE • *See* Fatty Acids.

ETHYLENE DODECANEDIOATE • A fragrance ingredient.

ETHYLENE GLYCOL • A slightly viscous liquid with a sweet taste. Absorbs twice its weight in water. Used as an antifreeze and humectant (*see*), also as a solvent. Toxic when ingested, causing central nervous system depression, vomiting, drowsiness, coma, respiratory failure, kidney damage, and possibly death. Polymers (*see*) of ethylene glycol are linked either with alcohols or fatty acids in many cosmetic ingredients. Some metabolites of ethylene glycol are reproductive and developmental toxins, according to the CIR Expert Panel (*see*). For example, 2-butoxyethanol caused adverse reproductive and developmental effects in oral administration but not when applied to the skin. In general, the panel concludes, these metabolites of concern are not expected to be included in cosmetic formulations that contain polymers of ethylene glycol.

ETHYLENE/MA COPOLYMER • A film former. *See* Maleic Acid.

ETHYLENE/MALEIC ANHYDRIDE COPOLYMER • Plastic material made from ethylene and maleic anhydride. Maleic anhydride is a powerful irritant causing burns. Contact with skin should be avoided. Ethylene is used in the manufacture of plastics and alcohols. High concentrations can cause unconsciousness.

ETHYLENE METHACRYLATE • Used in foundations, sunscreens, eye shadows, concealer, eye liner, face powder, bronzer/highlighter, blush, and brow liners. Considered safe based on assumption of low absorption. The CIR Expert Panel (*see*) determined it safe for use when formulated to avoid irritation, but it may contain harmful impurities. On the Canadian Hotlist (*see*). *See* Acrylates.

ETHYLENE/METHACRYLATE COPOLYMER • A film former. *See* Ethylene Methacrylate.

ETHYLENE OXIDE • Derived from petroleum. Used to make ethyoxylated ingredients such as PEG (*see*) derivatives. Suspected of causing cancer. On the Canadian Hotlist (*see*). Banned in cosmetics by the EU.

ETHYLENE UREA • *See* Urea.

ETHYLENE/VA COPOLYMER • Provides a continuous film for nail enamels or to control film in hair sprays.

2-ETHYLHEXOIC ACID • A mild-scented liquid, slightly soluble in water, it is used in paint and varnish driers and to convert some mineral oils to greases. Its esters (*see*) are used as plasticizers.

ETHYLHEXYL HYDROXYSTEARATE • Emollient. *See* Stearic Acid.

ETHYLHEXYL ISOPALMITATE • Widely used emollient in body and hand products, makeup, and tanning products. Also used as a fragrance. *See* Palmitic Acid.

ETHYLHEXYL PALMITATE • An emollient used in cosmetic creams. *See* Palmitic Acid.

ETHYLHEXYL PELARGONATE • An emollient used in makeup. *See* Ethyl Pelargonate.

ETHYLPARABEN • Widely used preservative. *See* Propylparaben.

ETIDRONIC ACIDS AND THEIR SALTS. Used in hair care and soap. In hair care, the EU limits it to 1.5 percent and for soap, 0.2 percent. *See* Benzyl Alcohol.

ETOCRYLENE • The organic ester derived from acrylic acid widely used in nail polish. *See* Acrylates.

EU • Abbreviation for European Union.

EUCALYPTOL • A chief constituent of eucalyptus and cajeput oils. Occurs naturally in allspice, star anise, bay, calamus, and peppermint oil. An antiseptic, antispasmodic, and expectorant. Used to flavor toothpaste and mouthwash and to cover up malodors in depilatories. It is not used in hypoallergenic cosmetics. Fatalities followed ingestion of doses as small as 3 to 5 milliliters (about a teaspoon), and recovery has occurred after doses as large as 20 to 30 milliliters (about 4 to 5 teaspoons).

EUCALYPTUS CITRIODORA • *See* Eucalyptus Oil.

EUCALYPTUS EXTRACT • *See* Eucalyptus Oil.

EUCALYPTUS OIL • Dinkum Oil. Yukari Ekisu. *Eucalyptus globulus.* Used in skin fresheners. The colorless to pale yellow, volatile liquid from the fresh leaves of the eucalyptus tree. It is 70 to 80 percent eucalyptol and has a spicy, cool taste and a characteristic aromatic, somewhat camphorlike odor. Used as a local antiseptic. Eucalyptus is used by practitioners to "refresh the nervous system and to treat tiredness, poor concentration & headaches." It does have antibiotic properties, which may make it helpful in the treatment of skin infections, wounds, herpes, and ulcers. Eucalyptus is also an insect repellant. It can cause allergic reactions, and fatalities have followed ingestion of doses as small as 3 to 5 milliliters (about equal to a teaspoon); about 1 milliliter has caused coma.

EUCHEUMA SPINOSUM • Extract of *Eucheuma spinosum,* a seaweed (*see*) used as a skin conditioner.

EUCOMMIA ULMOIDES • Kommi Gum. A Chinese tree that yields rubber.

EUGENIA CARYOPHYLLUS • *See* Clove Oil.

EUGENIA CUMINI • Jambul Extract. Used as a flavoring.

EUGENIA JAMBOS • Rose Apple. Native to the East Indies, it is an evergreen tree. Hair conditioner and used for skin, outbreaks on skin, acne, and chronic acne, especially on the nose and cheeks.

EUGENOL • An ingredient in perfumes and dentifrices obtained from clove oil. Occurs naturally in allspice, basil, bay leaves, calamus, pimento, and laurel leaves. It has a spicy, pungent taste. Used as a fixative in perfumes and flavorings. Eugenol also acts as a local antiseptic. When ingested, it may cause vomiting and gastric irritation. Because of its potential as an allergen, it is left out of hypoallergenic cosmetics. Methyleugenol, a flavoring, has also been found to cause tumors in rats. FEMA (*see*) says that at current use, it probably offers no danger to humans but nevertheless it requires further study. The UK has banned methyleugenol in cosmetics. Toxicity is similar to phenol, which is highly toxic. Death in laboratory animals given eugenol was due to vascular collapse. GRAS. ASP

EUGENYL ACETATE • Fragrance ingredient. *See* Eugenol.

EUGENYL GLUCOSIDE • Skin conditioner. *See* Eugenol and Glucose.

EUONYMUS JAPONICUS • Green Spire. Evergreen. Extract of *Euonymus japonicus* used as hair and skin conditioners. Poisonous if swallowed.

EUPATORIUM PURPUREUM • A perennial common to Europe, the eastern United States, and Canada, it grows in meadows. It was used to treat diarrhea and stomach upsets. Was also given for gout, arthritis, and flu. It is rich in vitamin C and contains salicylic acid and citric acid (*see both*).

EUPHORBIA CERIFERA • EU label name for Candelilla wax.

EUPHORBIA EXTRACT • Asthma Weed. Spurge Extract. Snake Weed Extract. An extract of the herb *Euphorbia pilulifera.* A large genus of plants of greatly diverse appearance, some being fleshy and cactuslike, and others being leafy and herbaceous or shrubby, but all having milky juice and flowers. The plant yielding castor oil belongs to this family.

EUROPEAN ASH • A tall Eurasian tree, *Fraxinus excelsior,* with leaves that are dark green with prominent veins.

EUROPEAN CHEMICALS AGENCY • ECHA. The agency, upon request of the European Commission, identifies substances of very high concern. The chemicals may be

- carcinogenic, mutagenic, or toxic to reproduction.
- persistent, bioaccumulative, and toxic or very persistent and very bioaccumulative.
- identified, on a case-by-case basis, from scientific evidence as causing probably serious effects to human health or the environment of an equivalent level of concern as those above.

The findings are made available to the public.

EUROPEAN HOLLY EXTRACT • The extract of *Lex aquifolium.*

EUROPEAN UNION • EU. Founded in 1967, a commission made up of elected representatives. Initiates EU policy on the economy in particular but, increasingly, also on environmental and foreign and security affairs. Among its interests are cosmetic safety and commerce.

EURPHRASIA • Eyebright Herbs. A derivative from any of several herbs, regarded as a remedy for eye ailments. It is used to soothe the eye in a rinse.

EUTERPE EDULIS • Assai. South American Palm. The juice extract form is used as a skin conditioner.

EUXYL K 400 • A newer preservative for cosmetics and toiletries rapidly increasing in use. It contains 1,2-dibromo-2,4-dicyanobutane and 2-phenoxyethanol. There are increasing reports of patients who are sensitive to it, and physicians are being encouraged to test for it in patients with allergic contact dermatitis (*see*).

EVENING PRIMROSE • *Oenothera biennis.* Sundrops. The leaves and oil from the seed are used by herbalists to treat liver and kidney dysfunctions. The oil has a high content of linoleic acid (GLA), an essential polyunsaturated fatty acid that is converted into prostaglandins (*see*) and hormones. It is used as a tonic for inflammatory conditions. It is used in "organic" cosmetics. It is said to relieve premenstrual tension, high blood pressure, and anxiety associated with inflammatory conditions. It has been recommended for infantile eczema, painful breasts, arthritis, and neurosis. It reputedly lowers cholesterol.

EVERLASTING EXTRACT • An extract derived from the flowering plant *Helichrysum italicum* and related species. Used in facial moisturizer/treatments, anti-aging products, sunscreens, body firming lotion, redness/rosacea treatment, hand cream, facial cleanser, around-eye cream, and skin fading/lighteners. May scavenge free radicals (*see*).

EVERNIA PRUNASTRI • A lichen, *Evemia* species, that grows on oak trees and yields a resin for use as a fixative (*see*) in perfumery. Stable, green liquid with a long-lasting characteristic odor. Soluble in alcohol. Used in fruit, honey, and spice flavorings for beverages, ice cream, ices, candy, baked goods, gelatin desserts, condiments, and soups. A common allergen in after-shave lotions.

EVODIA RUTAECARPA • Strongly fragrant small fruits that smell like concentrated black pepper. They have been used in traditional Chinese medicine for two thousand years against stomach troubles and pain. They kill *Helicobacter pylori,* the germ that causes stomach ulcers, and are often used against headaches. They decrease the clotting ability of the blood and thus are being studied for use in Alzheimer's treatment. They also contain Cox-2 inhibitors and so are helpful in arthritis pain. Large doses can stimulate the central nervous system and lead to visual disturbances and hallucinations, because they contain 5-MeO-DMT as well as other tryptamines. Herbalists consider evodia slightly toxic. They caution against long-term use and overdosage, but generally consider short-term use safe.

EXALTING FIXATIVES • A material that acts as an odor carrier, improving and fortifying transportation of the vapors of other perfume materials. Musk and civet are examples. *See* Fixative.

EXCIPIENT • A more or less inert substance added to a prescription as a diluent or vehicle or to give form or consistency when the medication is in pill form. Not infrequently, excipients may be "hidden" allergens.

EXFOLIANT • Ingredient that causes skin to shed. Ingredients such as the alpha-hydroxy acids (*see*) and salicylic acid are included in this category. *See* Exfoliation.

EXFOLIATION • Shedding of superficial cells of the skin. Many compounds containing acids are being used in products aimed at the older market as a means of peeling the skin to make it look younger. In the youth market, such products are sold to get rid of oily, blackhead-dotted top layers of skin. There is a question of whether such products are over-the-counter drugs or cosmetics. The cosmetic producers say they do not change the structure of the skin—just peel off the dead layers—and therefore, the products are cosmetics. Some early versions of the exfoliants were too strong and irritated the skin. The most recent versions are more gentle at peeling.

EXPOXIDIZED SOYBEAN OIL • A modified oil obtained from soybeans. *See* Epoxy- and Soybean Oil.

EXT. D&C • Colors that are certified by the FDA only for external use.

EXT. D & C VIOLET NO. 2 • CI 60730. Classed chemically as an anthraquinone color. Bluish scarlet. Permitted only for use in preformed hair colors, but textbooks list use in bath salts, soaps, and hair-waving fluids as well. The cosmetics industry has petitioned the FDA to allow wider use. Permanently listed for external use in 1982. However, in 2003, the FDA put a petition for the safe use of this coloring in externally applied drug products in abeyance (*see*). *See also* Colors.

EXT. D & C YELLOW NO. 7 • CI 10316. Formerly FD & C Yellow No. 1. Greenish yellow. A coal tar color. Classed chemically as a nitro color. It is the disodium salt of 2,4-dinitro-l-naphthol-7-sulfonic acid. Used in hair rinses and shampoos. *See* Colors.

EXT. D & C YELLOW NO. 7 ALUMINUM LAKE • CI 10316. Naphthol Yellow Lake. A coal tar color. Light yellow or orange-yellow powder. An insoluble pigment prepared from Ext. D & C Yellow No. 7 (*see*). *See* Colors.

EXTENDER • A substance added to a product, especially a diluent or modifier (*see both*). Petroleum jelly would be an example.

EXTENSIN • A protein that is a component of plant cell walls.

EXTRACT • The solution that results from passing alcohol or an alcohol-water mixture through a substance. Examples of extracts would be the alcohol-water mixture of vanillin, orange, or lemon extract found among the spices and flavorings on the supermarket shelf. Extracts are not as strong as essential oils (*see*).

EYE ALLERGY • There are many forms of allergy of the eye. The mucous membranes of the eye may be involved in allergic rhinitis. Such allergic conjunctivitis may also occur by itself without irritation of the nose. Another form, "spring pinkeye," is probably due to allergens in the air. Dust, mold spores, foods, and eye medications may all cause conjunctivitis. There is also a less severe, chronic form of allergic conjunctivitis. Symptoms include prolonged photophobia, itching, burning, and a feeling of dryness. There may be a watery discharge, and finding the source of allergy is often difficult.

EYE BRIGHT • *Euphrasia officinalis.* Euphrasy. An annual herb native to Europe and western Asia and grown in the United States, it belongs to the foxglove family. It contains tannins, iridoid glycosides, phenolic acids, and volatile oil. It has been mentioned in medical literature since the early 1300s. It had the reputation of being able to restore eyesight in very old people and is still used today as an eyewash for inflamed and tired eyes and to treat sinus congestion. Used in "organic" cosmetics. Astringent infusions are made by herbalists for coughs, colds, and sore throats. It is also occasionally used to treat jaundice, loss of memory, and dizziness.

EYE CREAMS • Eye Wrinkle Creams. So-called eye creams are slightly modified emollient creams (*see*), usually with the perfume omitted. There is less subcutaneous fat in the skin around the eyes, and it is likely for this reason that wrinkles first begin to develop there. According to the American Medical Association, eye creams will not prevent wrinkles but may make them less noticeable. Most eye creams contain essentially the same ingredients: lecithin, cholesterol, beeswax, lanolin, sodium benzoate, boric acid, mineral oil, ascorbyl palmitate, and almond oil (*see all*).

EYE MAKEUP REMOVER • Pads saturated with ingredients to remove eye makeup. They may contain a solvent such as acetone (*see*), an oil and/or lanolin (*see*), and perfume. Hypoallergenic (*see*) cosmetics manufacturers use cotton pads saturated with pure mineral oil. Eye irritations from eye makeup removers have been reported to the FDA within the past several years.

EYE MASCARA • Mascara is used to color and thicken eyelashes. Early mascara was composed of a pigment and soap. Today it still contains a salt of stearic acid (*see*) with pigments and/or lanolin, paraffin, and carnauba wax (*see all*). Within the past few years there have been a number of complaints of itching, burning, and swelling of eyes and eye irritation due to mascara.

EYE SHADOW • Shades of blue, green, brown, red, yellow, and white are used to color the lid and area under the eyebrow to highlight the eyes. The waterless type of eye shadow uses colors mixed with a lightening ingredient such as titanium dioxide (*see*) and are then mixed with petrolatum (*see*) on a roller mill. Eye shadows may also contain lanolin, beeswax, ceresin, calcium carbonate, mineral oil, sorbitan oleate, and talc (*see all*). The iridescent effect is achieved by adding very pure aluminum. There have been reports in recent years of eye irritation from eye shadow and one complaint of a package shattering in the eye and another of a sharp foreign article in the product applicator. Surfactants (*see*) are used to aid spreading; film formers to give an even, unbroken coat; and pH controllers to prevent skin oils or tears from altering the colors. Preservatives and antioxidants are added to increase shelf life. In 2004, it was reported that those allergic to rubber may have a problem with applicators used to apply eye shadow and sponges to remove it. Experts advise that you do not put your eye shadow on while driving and do not lend to others or use their eye shadows.

EYEBRIGHT HERBS • *See* Euphrasia.

EYEBROW DYES • No permanent dyes are approved for use around the eyes.

EYEBROW PENCILS • Usually contain lampblack, petrolatum, and paraffin (*see all*) and sometimes aluminum silicate and stearic acid (*see both*). The use of eyeliner pencils applied to the upper and lower border of the eyelids inside the lashes rather than to the eyelid behind the lashes is not recommended by physicians. According to a report by an eye specialist quoted by the American Medical Association, this may lead to various problems, including permanent pigmentation of the mucous membrane lining of the inside of the eye, moderate redness and itching, tearing, and blurring of vision.

EYEBROW PLUCKING CREAM • Used to soften the skin to allow the hairs to be pulled more easily and to alleviate the discomfort. Most eyebrow plucking creams contain benzocaine, a painkiller, and cold cream (*see both*). Benzocaine is on the Canadian Hotlist (*see*).

EYEDROPS, LOTIONS, AND WASHES • Soothe and clear eyes of redness. Work by constricting the blood vessels in the eyes, and by anesthetizing and soothing the eyes with anesthetics and emollients. Mild astringents such as boric acid or sodium chloride are used. Mild anesthetics used are antipyrine hydrastine hydrochloride and berberine hydrochloride. To contract the blood vessels, tetrahydrozoline hydrochloride is used. Included for their pleasant smell are camphor, peppermint, or witch hazel. Among the preservatives used are phenols, cresol, and formaldehyde. A wetting ingredient such as benzalkonium is also usually included. Reports of eye irritations are infrequent from eye treatment products, but the largest danger is from contamination because eye solutions are good mediums for the growth of bacteria and molds; therefore, they must be kept sterile. Tetrahydrozoline is banned in cosmetics by ASEAN.

EYELASH CREAMS • Used to make the lashes soft and shiny. Such creams usually contain lanolin, cocoa butter, paraffin, cetyl alcohol, and peach kernel oil (*see all*). However, ingredients may cause reactions in persons who are allergic to specific ingredients.

EYELASH DYES • Include eyebrow dyes. Brown, black, and blue certified oil-soluble dyes are used. Because of possible damage to the eyes, only certain ingredients and colors may be used in these preparations (*see* Colors). The U.S. Food and Drug Administration forbids the use of coal tar (*see*) dyes in the area of the eye. Highly purified inorganic pigments must be used, among them carbon black, charcoal black, black iron oxide, and ultramarine blue for black and blue shades. Iron oxides are used also for yellow and brown shades, carmine for red, chromic oxides for green, and titanium dioxide or zinc oxide for white. *See* Colors for toxicity.

EYELASH ENHANCER • Reportedly delivers statistically significant increases in eyelash length, thickness, and darkness. Allergan, its maker, said it would minimize risk by telling doctors and patients about potential drug side effects and instructing users not to use Latisse on lower eyelashes. The drug itself is based on bimatoprost, which is a synthetic prostaglandin analogue that is currently used to treat glaucoma. It was during clinical studies of the drug for glaucoma that Allergan discovered that some patients developed longer, darker, and thicker eyelashes. Approved by the FDA for lash enhancement in 2008.

EYELASH OILS • Used to make the lashes soft and shiny. Such oils usually contain lanolin, cocoa butter, cetyl alcohol, alcohol water, and olive oil. However, reactions may occur in persons allergic to specific ingredients.

EYELIDS • The skin of the eyelids is a common site of allergic contact dermatitis. The lesions, at first, may be swollen, red, and scaly, but as the victim tries to control the condition, the situation may become chronic and the skin of the lids thicken and roughen. Nail polish and perfume are among the most common allergens, but artificial eyelashes are also a source of trouble.

EYELINERS • Used to outline and accentuate the eyes, eyeliners may come in pencil or liquid form or in the newer pencil-brush container. Eyeliners usually contain an alkanolamine, a fatty alcohol, polyvinylpyrrolidone, cellulose ether, methyl paraben, antioxidants, perfumes, and titanium dioxide (*see all*). Waterproof eyeliners resist tears, moisture in the air, and perspiration. Some also resist ordinary soap and water. Most of the waterproof eyeliners are made of a pigment suspended in a gum or resin solution or a pigmented waxy base dissolved in a volatile solvent. Waterproof eyeliners must be removed with a solvent such as mineral oil or similar oils. Most facial cleansing lotions and creams contain such solvents. The FDA has found a persistent problem of bacterial contamination in some liquid eyeliners. Since bacterial infections around the eyes can lead to serious problems, it is probably better to purchase nonliquid eyeliners. There are also a significant number of persons allergic to eyeliners and other such products. The American Medical Association recommends that women stop using an eyeliner or eye makeup product if their skin becomes red, itchy, or swollen whenever an eye cosmetic is applied. The AMA also points out that because the eyelids are easily irritated, eye makeup, particularly eyeliner, should be removed with care. It also cautions against repeatedly applying eye makeup at one session because of the possibility of irritation. There have been a number of reports of swollen eyelids and eye irritation from well-known products.

EYEWASHES • *See* Eyedrops, Lotions, and Washes.

F

FABA BEAN EXTRACT • *Vicia faba.* Fava Bean. Common Bean. The extract of the seeds of *Vicia faba,* a member of the legume family. High-quality cosmetic oil. Inhalation or ingestion of the pollen of its flower can cause fever and headache in certain sensitized individuals.

FABIANA IMBRICATA • Pichi extract. A Peruvian shrub that yields a tonic, diuretic, and essential oil.

FACE MASKS AND PACKS • Claims are made for face masks and for the thicker face packs that they shrink pores, remove wrinkles, and relieve tension. Only the last may be true. According to the American Medical Association, there is no evidence that any cosmetic can safely shrink pores, and only surgery removes wrinkles. However, the apparent cooling or tight feeling derived from their use may induce a clean feeling. Clay face masks usually contain purified siliceous earth, kaolin, glycerin, and water. Face packs usually contain zinc stearate, zinc oxide, tragacanth, alcohol, glycerin, and lime-water. Both masks and packs may also contain acacia, balsam Peru, glyceryl mono-stearate, magnesium carbonate, wax, salicylic acid, spermaceti, Turkey-red oil, talc, titanium oxide, and/or zinc sulfate. (*See* ingredients above under separate listings.) Complaints to the FDA about face masks and packs include burning sensation, swelling, blisters and lumps, eye ailments, skin irritation, and corneal ulcers.

FACIAL FOUNDATIONS • Designed to add color, to cover blemishes, and to blend uneven facial color in women of all skin colors. Facial foundations available for white or light skin must be formulated in at least seven or eight shades; however, facial foundations for black or dark skin must be formulated in at least ten to twelve or more shades to cover the tremendous variation in skin pigmentation. In basic terms, a facial foundation is a pigmented moisturizer that can be customized to meet the needs of a variety of skin types. Dr. Zoe Draelos, a clinical associate professor at Wake Forest University School of Medicine and a private practitioner, says that this cosmetic type is applied to the entire face, used on a daily basis, and worn for an extended period of time. For this reason, facial foundation plays an important role in skin treatment, but it is also the facial cosmetic most likely to be problematic. She notes four basic facial foundation formulations are available: oil-based, water-based, oil-free, and water-free or anhydrous forms.

Oil-based products are designed for dry skin, while water-based products can be adapted for all skin types. Oil-free formulations are used for oily skin, while anhydrous forms are extremely long wearing and are used for camouflage or theatrical purposes. Oil-based foundations are water-in-oil emulsions containing pigments suspended in oil, such as mineral oil or lanolin alcohol. Vegetable oils (e.g., coconut, sesame, safflower) and synthetic esters (e.g., isopropyl myristate, octyl palmitate, isopropyl palmitate) also may be incorporated. The water evaporates from the foundation following application, leaving the pigment in oil on the face. This creates a moist skin feeling, which is especially desirable in patients with a dry complexion. Oil-based foundations do not shift color as they mix with sebum because the color is fully developed in the oily phase of the formulation. These foundations are easy to apply because the pigment can be spread over the face for up to five minutes prior to setting.

Water-based facial foundations are oil-in-water emulsions containing a small amount of oil in which the pigment is emulsified with a relatively large quantity of water. The primary emulsifier is usually soap (e.g., triethanolamine, nonionic surfactant). The secondary emulsifier, present in smaller quantity, is usually glyceryl stearate or propylene glycol stearate. These popular foundations are appropriate for minimally dry to normal skin. Because the pigment is already developed in oil, this foundation type also is not subject to color drift. The application time is shorter than with oil-based foundations because of the lower oil content. These products usually are packaged in a bottle.

Oil-free facial foundations contain no animal, vegetable, or mineral oils. They contain other oily substances, such as the silicones dimethicone or cyclomethicone. These foundations usually are designed for individuals with oily complexions because they leave the skin with a dry feeling. Silicone is noncomedogenic, nonacnegenic, and hypoallergenic, accounting for the tremendous popularity of this type of facial foundation formulation. These products usually are liquids packaged in a bottle. Oil-control facial foundations should not be confused with oil-free facial foundations. All facial foundations contain a blotter designed to absorb sebum. Oil-control facial foundations simply contain additional blotters, such as talc, kaolin, starch, or other polymers, designed to absorb sebum in higher concentration. Usually, these products are formulated with dimethicone; however, mineral oil may be added to some formulations. Thus, oil-control foundations are not necessarily oil-free.

Water-free or anhydrous foundations are waterproof. Vegetable oil, mineral oil, lanolin alcohol, and synthetic esters form the oil phase, which may be mixed with waxes to form a cream. High concentrations of pigment can be incorporated into the formulation, yielding an opaque facial foundation. The coloring agents are based on titanium dioxide with iron oxides, occasionally in combination with ultramarine blue. Titanium dioxide acts as a facial-concealing or covering agent. These products can be dipped from a jar, squeezed from a tube, wiped from a compact, or stroked from a stick. Dr. Draelos says these foundations are well suited for use in patients with facial scarring who desire camouflaging.

Facial foundations are manufactured in a variety of finishes, including the following: matte, semimatte, moist semimatte, and shiny. The finish is the surface characteristic of a cosmetic. Matte finish foundations yield a flat look with no shine and generally are oil-free. They are good for people with oily skin who tend to develop some shine after a foundation has been applied. A semimatte finish has minimal shine and is generally an oil-free foundation or water-based foundation with minimal oil content. This finish works well on slightly oily to normal skin. A foundation with more shine is known as a moist semimatte foundation and generally is water based with moderate oil content. This finish works well on normal-to-dry skin. Shiny finishes are found in oil-based foundations and are only appropriate for persons with dry skin. The shinier foundations with increased oil content also have increased moisturizing ability.

FACIAL POWDERS •
Provide coverage of complexion imperfections, oil control, a matte finish, and tactile smoothness to the skin, according to a dermatologist, Dr. Zoe Draelos, who is an expert in cosmetics, their benefits, and adverse reactions. She says that originally, facial powder was applied over a moisturizer to function as a type of powdered foundation. Liquid foundations have largely replaced the powdered foundation; however, for patients who wish sheer coverage with good oil control, a powdered foundation performs excellently. An appropriate moisturizer for the patient's skin type is first applied and allowed to set or dry, followed by application of a full coverage translucent powder. Dr. Draelos added: "Full-coverage powders contain predominantly talc (hydrated magnesium silicate) and increased amounts of covering pigments." The covering pigments used in face powder can be listed in order of increasing opaqueness, as follows: titanium dioxide, kaolin, magnesium carbonate, magnesium stearate, zinc stearate, prepared chalk, zinc oxide, rice starch, precipitated chalk, and talc. It generally is accepted that the optimum opacity is achieved with a particle size of 0.25 microns. Magnesium carbonate also can be used to improve oil blotting, to keep the powder fluffy, and to absorb any added perfume. Kaolin (hydrated aluminium silicate) also may function to absorb oil and perspiration. Full-coverage face powders usually are packaged in a compact and applied to the face with a puff. Transparent facial powders are more popular today to add coverage and to improve oil-blotting abilities of a previously applied liquid foundation. Transparent powders have the same formulation as full-coverage powders except they contain less talc, titanium dioxide, or zinc oxide because coverage is not a priority. Transparent facial powders commonly have a light shine, produced by nacre-

ous pigments, such as bismuth oxychloride, mica, titanium dioxide–coated mica, or crystalline calcium carbonate (*see all*). Facial powder usually includes iron oxides as the main pigment, but other inorganic pigments, such as ultramarine, chrome oxide, and chrome hydrate (*see all*), also may be used. These powders are designed to augment the underlying skin and foundation tones; therefore, transparent powders can be used by people who have difficulty finding an appropriately tinted facial foundation.

FACTOR • *See* SPF.

FAEX • EU name for compressed yeast. *See* Yeast.

FAGUS SYLVATICA • A member of the beech family. Used as a coloring.

FAKE NAILS • *See* Artificial Nails.

FALSE EYELASHES • Can be made of real or synthetic hair on a thin stringlike base that is pasted over the natural eyelashes on the eyelid. There have been cases of eye irritation and one case of blindness reported to the FDA. Whether the problems were the result of the adhesive used, the dye on the eyelashes, or other materials is not clear.

FAO/WHO • The Joint Expert Committee on Food Additives (JECFA) is an international expert scientific committee that is administered jointly by the Food and Agriculture Organization of the United Nations (FAO) and the World Health Organization (WHO).

FARNESENE • A hydrocarbon (*see*) used as a fragrance ingredient.

FARNESOL • Used in perfumery to emphasize the odor of sweet floral perfumes such as lilac. Occurs naturally in ambrette seed, star anise, cassia, linden flowers, seed oils, citronella, rose, and balsam. Also a food flavoring.

FARNESYL • The ester of farnesol and acetic acid (*see both*). Used as a fragrance ingredient, humectant, and moisturizer.

FAST GREEN FCF • A name applied to uncertified green coloring.

FATIGUE • Everyone's nose becomes "fatigued" when smelling a certain odor. No matter how much you like a fragrance, you can only smell it for a short interval. It is nature's way of protecting humans from overstimulation of the olfactory sense.

FATTY ACID ESTERS • The fatty acid esters of low-molecular-weight alcohols are widely used in hand products because they are oily but nongreasy when applied to the skin. They are emollients and emulsifiers. *See* Fatty Acids and Ester.

FATTY ACIDS • Fatty acids are used in bubble baths and lipsticks, but chiefly for making soap and detergents. One or any mixture of liquid and solid acidscapric, caprylic, lauric, myristic, oleic, palmitic, and stearic. In combination with glycerin, they form fat. Necessary for normal growth and healthy skin. In foods they are used as emulsifiers, binders, and lubricants. *See* Stearic Acid.

FATTY ALCOHOLS • Cetyl, Stearyl, Lauryl, Myristyl. Solid alcohols made from acids and widely used in hand creams and lotions. Cetyl and stearyl alcohols form an occlusive film to keep skin moisture from evaporating, and they impart a velvety feel to the skin. Lauryl and myristyl are used in detergents and creams. Very low toxicity.

FATTY ACID DIALKANOLAMIDES • Dialkanolamines, being strong bases (pK = 11–12), occur in cosmetic products almost exclusively in the form of the salts with organic or inorganic acids, functioning as buffering agents, emulsifiers, or surfactants; that is, functions due just to the properties of their salts. The EU attempted to ban this compound in 1999 because of the toxicological effects of the dialkanolamine salts and, in particular, their readiness to form nitrosamines (*see*). Therefore, there is no doubt that all the reports previously evaluated by the Scientific Committee on Cosmetology (SCC), concerning either nitrosamine contents of commercial cosmetic products or basic research on the mechanism(s) of nitrosamine formation, apply directly to dialkanolamine salts rather than to free dialkanolamines. The EU says fatty acid dialkanolamides' content must not exceed 0.5 percent dialkanolamines and it should not be used with nitrosating systems and kept in nitrate-free containers.

FD & C • Abbreviation for Food, Drug, and Cosmetic.

FD & C COLORS • Food, Drug, and Cosmetic Colors. A color additive is a term to describe any dye, pigment, or other substance capable of coloring a food, drug, or cosmetic, on any part of the human body. In 1900, there were more than eighty dyes used to color food. There were no regulations and the same dye used to color clothes could also be used to color candy. In 1906, the first comprehensive legislation for food colors was passed. There were only seven colors, which, when tested, were shown to be composed of known ingredients that demonstrated no harmful effects. Those colors were orange, erythrosine, ponceau 3R, amaranth, indigotin, naphthol yellow, and light green. A voluntary system of certification for batches of color dyes was set up. In 1938, new legislation was passed, superseding the 1906 act. The colors were given numbers instead of chemical names and every batch had to be certified. There were fifteen food colors in use at the time. In 1950, children were made ill by certain coloring used in candy and popcorn. These incidents led to the delisting of FD & C Orange No. 1, Orange No. 2, and FD & C Red No. 32. Since that time, because of experimental evidence of possible harm, Red 1 and Yellow 1, 2, 3, and 4 have also been delisted. Violet 1 was removed in 1973. In 1976, one of the most widely used of all colors, FD & C Red No. 2, was removed because it was found to cause tumors in rats. In 1976, Red No. 4 was banned for coloring maraschino cherries (its last use), and carbon black was also banned, because both contain cancer-causing additives. Earlier, in 1960, scientific investigations were required by law to determine the suitability of all colors in use for permanent listing. Citrus Red No. 2 (limited to 2 ppm) for coloring orange skins has been permanently listed; Blue No. 1, Red No. 3, Yellow No. 5, and Red No. 40 are permanently listed but without any restrictions.

In 1959, the Food and Drug Administration approved the use of "lakes," in which the dyes are mixed with alumina hydrate to make them insoluble. *See* FD & C Lakes. The other food coloring additives remained on the "temporary list." The provisional list permitted colors then in use to continue on a provisional, or interim, basis pending completion of studies to determine whether the colors should be permanently approved or terminated. FD & C Red No. 3 (erythrosin) is permanently listed for use in food and ingested drugs and provisionally listed for cosmetics and externally applied drugs. It is used in foods such as gelatins, cake mixes, ice cream, fruit cocktail cherries, bakery goods, and sausage casings. The FDA postoned the closing date for the provisionally listed color additives—FD & C Red No. 3, D and C Red No. 33, and D & C Red No. 36—to May 2, 1988, to allow additional time to study "complex scientific and legal questions about the colors before deciding to approve or terminate their use in food, drugs, and cosmetics." The agency asked for sixty days to consider the impact of the October 1987 U.S. Court of Appeals ruling that there is no exception to the Delaney Amendment (*see*), which says that cancer-causing additives may not be added to food.

On July 13, 1988, the Public Citizens Health Research Group announced that the FDA agreed to revoke by July 15, 1988, the permanent listing of four color additives used in drugs and cosmetics—D & C Red No. 8, D & C Red No. 9, D & C Red No. 19, and D & C Orange No. 17. In a unanimous decision in October 1987, the U.S. Court of Appeals for the District of Columbia said the FDA lacked legal authority to approve two of the colors, D & C Orange No. 17 and D & C Red No. 19, since they had been found to induce cancer in laboratory animals. The Supreme Court ruled against an appeal on April 18, 1988. Meanwhile, Public Citizen also brought a similar suit, challenging the use of D & C Red No. 8 and D & C Red No. 9, which was before the U.S. Circuit Court of Appeals in Philadelphia. Under an agreement between the FDA and Public Citizen, the case was sent back to the FDA, and the agency delisted these colors as well as D & C Orange No. 17 and D & C Red No. 19.

Other countries, as well as the World Health Organization, maintain there are inconsistencies in safety data and in the banning of some colors, which in turn affects international commerce. As of this writing, there is still a great deal of confusion about the colors, with the FDA maintaining that the cancer risk is minimal—as low as one in a billion—while groups such as Ralph Nader's Public Citizen maintain that any cancer risk for a food additive is unacceptable. In 1990, the lakes of Red. No. 3 were removed for all uses from the approved list. The color itself was also removed in 1990 for cosmetic and external drug use. It is still, as of this writing, approved for food and ingested drugs.

FD & C BLUE NO. 1 • Brilliant Blue FD & C. A coal tar derivative, triphenyl-methane, used for hair colorings, face powders, and other cosmetics. Also used as a coloring in bottled soft drinks, gelatin, desserts, cereals, and other foods. May cause allergic reactions. On the FDA permanent list of color additives. Rated 1A, that is, completely acceptable for nonfood use, by the World Health Organization. However, it produced malignant tumors at the site of injection and by ingestion in rats. *See* Colors.

FD & C BLUE NO. 2 • Moderate bright green. A coal tar derivative, triphenyl-methane, used in hair rinses and in mint-flavored jelly, frozen desserts, candy, confections, and cereals. It is a sensitizer in the allergic. Permanently listed for surgical sutures in 1971 and for food and ingested drug use in 1987. Produces malignant tumors at the site of injection when introduced under the skin of rats. *See* Colors.

FD & C BRILLIANT BLUE NO. 1 ALUMINUM LAKE • Aluminum salt of certified Brilliant Blue No. 1. *See* Colors and Lakes, Color.

FD & C GREEN NO. 3 • Permanently listed by the FDA for use in food, drugs, and cosmetics in 1982, except in the area of the eye.

FD & C LAKES • Aluminum or Calcium Lakes. Lakes are pigments prepared by combining FD & C colors with a form of aluminum or calcium, which makes the colors insoluble. Aluminum and calcium lakes are used in confection and candy products and for dyeing eggshells and other products that are adversely affected by water.

FD & C RED NO. 2 • Amaranth. Formerly one of the most widely used cosmetic and food colorings. A dark, reddish brown powder that turns bright red when mixed with fluid. A monoazo color, it was used in lipsticks, rouges, and other cosmetics as well as in cereals, maraschino cherries, and desserts. The safety of this dye was questioned by American scientists for more than twenty years. Two Russian scientists found that FD & C Red No. 2 prevented some pregnancies and caused some stillbirths in rats. The FDA ordered manufacturers using the color to submit data on all food, drug, and cosmetic products containing it. Controversial tests at the FDA's National Center for Toxicological Research in Arkansas showed that in high doses FD & C Red No. 2 caused a statistically significant increase in a variety of cancers in female rats. The dye was banned by the FDA in January 1976.

FD & C RED NO. 3 • Erythrosine. Bluish pink. A coal tar derivative, a xanthene color, used in toothpaste and in canned fruit cocktail, fruit salad, and cherry pie mixes as well as maraschino cherries. Has been determined a carcinogen. FD & C Red No. 3 was permanently listed for use in food and ingested drugs, but only provisionally listed for cosmetics and externally applied drugs. In 1990, the lakes (*see*) of FD & C Red No. 3 were removed for all uses from the approved list. The color itself was also removed in 1990 for cosmetic and external drug use. It is still, as of this writing, approved for food and ingested drugs!

FD & C RED NO. 4 • A monoazo color and coal tar dye. Used in mouthwashes, bath salts, and hair rinses. It was banned in food by the FDA in 1964, when it was shown to damage the adrenal glands and bladders of dogs. The agency relented and gave it provisional license for use in maraschino cherries. It was banned in all food in 1976 because it was shown to cause urinary bladder polyps and atrophy of the adrenal glands in animals. It was also banned in orally taken drugs but is still permitted in cosmetics for external use only. The uncertified version is called Ponceau SX. *See also* Colors.

FD & C RED NO. 20 • Permanently listed by the FDA in 1983 for general use in drugs and cosmetics (except in areas around the eyes).

FD & C RED NO. 22 • Permanently listed by the FDA in 1983 for general use in drugs and cosmetics (except in areas around the eyes).

FD & C RED NO. 40 • Allura Red AC. Newest color. Used widely in the cosmetics industry. Approved in 1971, Allied Chemical has an exclusive patent on it. It is substituted for FD & C Red No. 4 in many cosmetics, food, and drug products. Permanently listed in 1971 because, unlike the producers of "temporary" colors, this producer supplied reproductive data. However, many American scientists feel that the safety of FD & C Red No. 40 is far from established, particularly because all the tests were conducted by the manufacturer. Therefore, the dye should not have received a permanent safety rating. The National Cancer Institute reported that *p*-credine, a chemical used in the preparation of FD & C Red No. 40, was carcinogenic in animals. In rats, a high (3,800–8,350 mg/kg) oral dose of the coloring caused adverse reproductive effects. The FDA permanently listed Red No. 40 for use in foods and ingested drugs and cosmetics, including use around the eye area. Its lake (*see*) is permitted only for drug and cosmetic use.The British and European Parliaments, at this writing, are seeking to ban it because of its adverse affect on hyperactivity in children. The UK made a move in 2009 to phase out this color because of reports that it may contribute to hyperactivity in children. *See also* Azo Dyes and FD & C Colors. ASP. E

FD & C YELLOW NO. 5 • Tartrazine. A coal tar derivative, it is used as a coloring in hair rinses, hair-waving fluids, and bath salts. A pyrazole color, it is also found in prepared breakfast cereals, imitation strawberry jelly, bottled soft drinks, gelatin desserts, ice cream, sherbets, dry drink powders, candy, confections, bakery products, spaghetti, and puddings. Causes allergic reactions in persons sensitive to aspirin. The certified color industry petitioned for permanent listing of this color in February 1966, with no limitations other than good manufacturing practice. However, in February 1966, the FDA proposed the listing of this color with a maximum rate of use of 300 parts per million in food. The color industry had objected to the limitations. Yellow No. 5 was thereafter permanently listed as a color additive without restrictions. Rated 1A by the World Health Organization—acceptable in foods. It is estimated that half the aspirin-sensitive people plus 47,000 to 94,000 others in the nation are sensitive to this dye. It is used in about 60 percent of both over-the-counter and prescription drugs. Efforts were made to ban this color in OTC pain relievers, antihistamines, oral decongestants, and prescription anti-inflammatory drugs. Aspirin-sensitive patients have been reported to develop life-threatening asthmatic symptoms with ingestion of this yellow. Since 1981 it is supposed to be listed on the label if it is used. The uncertified version is Acid Yellow 23.

FD & C YELLOW NO. 5 ALUMINUM LAKE • The uncertified version is Pigment Yellow 100. *See* FD & C Yellow No. 5, Colors, and Lakes, Colors.

FD & C YELLOW NO. 6 • Sunset Yellow FCF. A coal tar, monoazo color, used in carbonated beverages, bakery products, candy, confectionery products, gelatin desserts, and dry drink powders. It is also used in hair rinses as well as other cosmetics. It is not used in products that contain fats and oils. Since there is evidence that this color causes allergic reactions, alcoholic beverages that contain it must list it on the label according to the Bureau of Alcohol. Rated 1A by the World Health Organization—acceptable in foods. Permanently listed December 22, 1986. In 1989, a ruling went into effect that it had to be listed on the labels because of its ability to induce allergic reactions. The British and the European Parliaments, at this writing, are seeking to ban it because of its reported effects on hyperactive behavior in young children. On the U.S. Codex Committee on Food Additives and Contaminants high-priority list for toxicology studies. *See* FD & C Colors. ASP. E

FD & C YELLOW NO. 6 ALUMINUM LAKE • The uncertified version is Pigment Yellow 104. *See* FD & C Yellow No. 6, Colors, and Lakes, Colors.

FEMA • Abbreviation for the Flavor and Extract Manufacturers Association.

FEMININE VAGINAL DEODORANTS. • *See* Vaginal Deodorants.

FENNEL OIL AND EXTRACT • *Foeniculum vulgare.* One of the earliest known herbs from the tall, beautiful shrub. Used in astringents and perfumes. The fennel flowers appear in June and are bright yellow. Compresses of fennel tea are used by organic cosmeticians to soothe inflamed eyelids and watery eyes. May cause allergic reactions.

FENUGREEK SEED • *Trigonella foenum-graecum.* Greek Hay. An annual herb grown in southern Europe, North Africa, and India, and used in hair tonics, supposedly to prevent baldness; also added to powders, poultices, and ointments. The seeds are used in making curry.

FERMENTED VEGETABLE • A mixture of cane sugar, molasses, and vegetable proteins. Used in "natural" cosmetics.

FERRIC AMMONIUM CHLORIDE • Brownish yellow, or orange, iron compound. Absorbs water readily. Used as a styptic and astringent. Irritating to the skin and not suitable for wide use.

FERRIC AMMONIUM FERROCYANIDE • Iron Blue. An inorganic salt used as a dark blue coloring for cosmetics. Permanently listed in 1977. *See* Iron Salts.

FERRIC FERROCYANIDE • Iron Blue. A coloring for externally applied cosmetics, including the eye area. Permanently listed in 1978. *See* Colors.

FERRIC GLYCEROPHOSPHATE • Used in oral care products. *See* Phosphorous and Glycerin.

FERRIC NITRATE • Derived from the action of concentrated nitric acid on scrap iron or iron oxide. Used for dyeing and for tanning.

FERRIC PYROPHOSPHATE • Used as a nutrient source of iron.

FERROUS AMMONIUM SULFATE • *See* Ammonia and Ferrous Sulfate.

FERROUS CHLORIDE • Iron Chloride. Greenish white crystals made from the action of hydrochloric acid on iron. Used in dyeing and in cosmetic and pharmaceutical preparations.

FERROUS FUMARATE • A salt of ferrous iron combined with fumaric acid. Odorless and tasteless, the reddish brown compound is used as a dietary supplement.

FERROUS GLUCOHEPTONATE • Skin conditioner. *See* Carboxylic Acid.

FERROUS SULFATE • Green or Iron Vitriol. Pale bluish green, odorless crystals, effluorescent in dry air. An astringent and deodorant. Used in hair dyes. A source of iron used medicinally.

FERULA ASSA-FOETIDA • Asafetida. *See* Asafoetida Extract.

FOETIDA • *See* Asafoetida Extract.

FERULA GALBANIFLUA • *See* Galbanum Oil.

FERULIC ACID • An antioxidant, preservative, and ultraviolet absorber. *See* Phenols.

FEVERFEW • *Chrysanthemum parthenium. Pyrethrum parthenium. Tanacetum parthenium.* Flirtwort. Bachelor's Buttons. Maydes' Weed. Wild Quinine. A small, hardy perennial herb, a member of the chamomile (*see*) family, it was introduced into Britain from Southeast Asia. Since ancient times it has been used by physicians for its action on the uterus. It was thought to promote menstrual evacuation and to aid in the expulsion of the placenta after childbirth. It was prescribed as an antidote against narcotic poisoning and was also considered a poultice herb with cooling and analgesic properties. Herbalists today use it as a laxative and to treat stings and bites. The name feverfew is derived from the word *febrifuge,* which means "to lower fever," the most common use for the herb by Greek physicians. It is now being investigated as a preventative for migraines. Used in "organic" cosmetics.

FIBROIN • Produced by silkworms. Used as a thickener.

FIBROIN/PEG-40/SODIUM ACRYLATE COPOLYMER • Film former used as a skin protectant. *See* Fibroin.

FIBRONECTIN • A fibrous protein widely distributed in connective tissue and membranes and present on cell surfaces. Acts as an adhesive and as a defense mechanism.

FICIN • An enzyme occurring in the latex of tropical trees and usually isolated from figs. Absorbs water. Used in cosmetics as a protein digestant. Used as a meat tenderizer. Ten to twenty times more powerful than papain tenderizers. Can cause irritation to the skin, eyes, and mucous membranes and in large doses can cause purging.

FICUS CARICA • *See* Fig Extract.

FIELD POPPY EXTRACT • Extract of the petals of *Papaver rhoeas* used in coloring and as an odorant.

FIG EXTRACT • From *Opuntia ficus.* Any of several woody plants with oblong fruit.

FIG LEAF ABSOLUTE • *Ficus carica.* Banned in fragrances based on its sensitizing and extreme phototoxic potential by the EU and the UK.

FIGWORT • *Scrophularia nodosa.* A perennial plant native to Britain and the United States, it used to be hung in houses and barns to ward off witches. Herbalists used it as an ointment to treat eczema, rashes, bruises, scratches, and small wounds, and for removing freckles.

FILIPENDULA RUBRA • Queen of the Prairie. Dollof. Bridewort. Used by American Indians to treat burns and abrasions. It contains salicylides (*see*).

FILM FORMER • Used to hold the hair in place. Used in small amounts in skin care products to leave a smooth feel to the skin. Used in nail enamels to produce a continuous film. Can be skin sensitizers for some.

FINGERNAIL POLISH • *See* Nail Polish.

FINGERNAIL POLISH REMOVER • *See* Nail Polish Remover.

FINISHING RINSE • A product that coats only the surface fibers of the hair and is used to add sheen and to remove tangles.

FIR NEEDLE OIL • Fir Oil. An essential oil obtained by the steam distillation of needles and twigs of several varieties of pine trees native to both Canada and Siberia. Used as a scent in perfumes and as a flavoring ingredient.

FIRST-AID PLANT • *See* Aloe Vera.

FISH CARTILAGE EXTRACT • Used in anti-aging products and moisturizers.

FISH GLYCERIDES • *See* Fish Oil and Glycerin.

FISH LIVER OIL • *See* Fish Oil.

FISH OIL • A fatty oil in soap manufacturing derived from fish or marine animals.

FIXATIVE • A chemical that reduces the tendency of an odor or flavor to vaporize by making the odor or flavor last longer. An example is musk (*see*), which is used in perfume.

FLAVONES • One of a group of plant pigments that produces ivory and yellow colors. They are reputed to have a wide range of activities, including reducing excess fluid and stimulating the heart. Some, such as rutin and hesperidin, are said to increase the strength of the capillaries and to lower blood pressure.

FLAVONOIDS • Flavonoids are a large group of compounds widely distributed throughout nature. They include quercetin, present in onion skins, and anthocyanins (*see*), the major commercially used group.

FLAVOR • Used to identify a product that contains a material or combination added to cosmetics to mask a bad taste. The word *flavor* can be used in the United States instead of saying whether it is made by compounding synthetic chemicals or natural ones from botanicals. In the European Union, the taste maker is referred to as simply "aroma."

FLAVOR ENHANCERS • One of the newest and fastest-growing categories of additives; potentiators, which enhance the total seasoning effect generally without contributing any taste or odor of their own.

FLAXSEED • The seed of the flax plant may be "hidden" in cereals and in the milk of cows fed flaxseed. It is also in flaxseed tea and the laxative flaxolyn. It is a frequent allergen when ingested, inhaled, or in direct contact. Flaxseeds are the source of linseed oil (*see*). Among other hidden sources are wave-setting preparations, shampoos, hair tonics, depilatories, patent leather, insulating materials, rugs, and some cloths.

FLEXIBLE COLLODION • A mixture of collodion (*see*) with camphor and castor oil to make collodion more malleable.

FLORAL BOUQUET • One of the basic perfume types, it is a blending of flower notes with no particular standouts. For balance and body, it may contain a medley of basic notes such as amber, musk, and vetiver, as well as a touch of the aromatic, but there is definitely the scent of a bouquet of flowers.

FLUORESCEIN • A yellow, granular or red, crystalline dye giving a brilliant yellow-green fluorescence in an alkaline solution. Very visible. *See* Tetrabromofluorescein for toxicity.

FLUORESCENT BRIGHTENERS • (46, 47, 52). Colorless, water- or solvent-soluble aromatic compounds with an affinity for fibers. They are usually violet, blue, or blue-green colors and are capable of increasing both the blueness and the brightness of a substrate, with a resulting marked whitening effect. They improve the brightness of tints and are included in detergents of all kinds to enhance cleansing action.

FLUORIDE • An acid salt used in toothpaste to prevent tooth decay and in nail products to strengthen nails. Fluorides cross the placental barrier and the effects on the fetus are unknown. Clinical evidence has shown kidney disturbance sometimes is due to the amount of fluoride in the blood. On the Canadian Hotlist (*see*). Not permitted in dentifrices, mouthwashes, or breath drops in Canada. *See* Sodium Fluoride and Stannous Fluoride.

FLUORINE COMPOUNDS • Addition of fluorine compounds to food is limited to that from fluoridation of public water supplies and to that resulting from the fluoridation of bottled water within limits set by the FDA. Fluorines are used in cosmetics in some hair and skin cleansers as well as in toothpastes.

FLUORO C2-8 ALKYL DIMETHICONE • An antifoaming ingredient. *See* Silicones.

4-FLUORO-6-METHYL SULFATE • Hair coloring. On the Canadian Hotlist (*see*). *See* Coal Tar.

FLUOROSALAN • A salicylide used as an antiseptic ingredient. *See* Salicylides.

FOAM STABILIZERS • Used in soft drinks and brewing. *See* Vegetable Gums.

FOAMING INGREDIENT • Associated psychologically with cleansing ability, foam or lather ingredients that bubble up when shaken with added water. They are used in shaving products, liquid bath detergents, and hair shampoos and mousses.

FOENICULUM VULGARE • *See* Fennel Oil and Extract.

FOLIC ACID • A yellowish orange compound and member of the vitamin B complex, used as a nutrient. Used in cosmetic emollients. Occurs naturally in liver, kidney, mushrooms, and green leaves. Aids in cell formation, especially red blood cells.

FOLLICLE • The tiny shaft in the skin through which a hair grows, and sebum (oil) is secreted from the sebaceous glands to the surface of the skin. *See* Hair.

FOMES OFFICINALIS • *See* Mushroom Extract.

FORESKIN • A British biomedical company, InterCytex, says it is aiming to bring its anti-aging and scar-repairing product Vavelta, consisting of human foreskins, to the U.S. market. The product is already available from accredited clinics in the UK through an injection process, but the company says, at this writing, it is now well under way with the process of getting it approved by the U.S. FDA. But besides the FDA, the company will also have to face the challenge of convincing potential consumers that injections containing a substance derived from collagen cells from babies' foreskins could prove a beneficial part of their beauty regime. The foreskins are evidently donated with the approval of mothers whose babies have just been circumcised, the basic idea being that the developing collagen derived from the skin samples can be used to encourage the growth of new collagen, rather than just replacing it. In fact, the company claims the strength of this is that instead of being a temporary treatment, the effects of the injections are permanent—an advantage that puts it well ahead of other injectable anti-aging treatments. It works because the formulation used in the injections relies on tiny skin cells known as fibroblasts that rejuvenate and revitalize damaged skin by repopulating areas where skin cells have been damaged. Those fibroblasts are formulated as a suspension— what the company terms human dermal fibroblasts (HDFs)—that are packaged in 1-ml cell storage mediums for the injection process. Like Botox, the treatment is targeted, as the injections are concentrated around the eyes, forehead, and mouth in the case of photoaging damage, and anywhere on the face or body in the case of scar or burn damage. It is approximately double the cost of a similar Botox injection treatment.

FOREST BLENDS • One of the basic perfume types, these blends are woody, mossy-leafy, or resinous. They either stand out alone with the aromatic notes of an individual nature, such as sandalwood, rosewood, the balsams, or cedar wood, or they have a combination of these notes. Quite often, the more pungent notes of geranium, lavender, fern, and herbs are used to give an earthy quality.

FORMALDEHYDE • A colorless gas obtained by the oxidation of methyl alcohol and generally used in watery solution. Vapors are intensely irritating to mucous membranes. It has been estimated that 4 to 8 percent of the general population may be sensitized to it. It is used in nail hardeners, nail polish, soap, and hair-growing products. It is widely used in cosmetics as a disinfectant, germicide, fungicide, defoamer, and preservative. Ingestion can cause severe abdominal pain, internal bleeding, loss of ability to urinate, vertigo, coma, and death. Skin reactions after exposure to it are very common because the chemical can be both irritating and allergy producing. Physicians have reported severe reactions to nail hardeners containing formaldehyde. Some surfactants, such as the widely used lauryl sulfate, may contain formaldehyde as a preservative, and other surfactants may have it without listing it on the label. Formaldehyde is an inexpensive and effective preservative, but there are serious questions about its safety. It is a highly reactive chemical that is damaging to the hereditary substances in the cells of several species. It causes lung cancer in rats and has a number of other harmful biological consequences. Researchers from the Division of Cancer Cause and Prevention of the National Cancer Institute recommended in April 1983 that, since formaldehyde is involved in DNA damage and inhibits its repair, since it potentiates the toxicity of X-rays

FOUNDATION MAKEUP   245

in human lung cells, and since it may act in concert with other chemical ingredients to produce mutagenic and carcinogenic effects, it should be "further investigated." Some shampoos contain formaldehyde. Among them at this writing are Breck Shampoo and L'Oréal Ultra Rich Gentle Shampoo.

The CIR Expert Panel (*see*) concludes that this ingredient is safe to the great majority of consumers. The panel believes, however, that "because of skin sensitivity of some individuals to this ingredient, the formulation and manufacture of a cosmetic product should be such as to ensure use at the minimal effective concentration of formaldehyde, not to exceed 0.2% measured as free formaldehyde. Formaldehyde is permitted in non-aerosol cosmetics, provided the concentration does not exceed 0.3% and is the minimum concentration to provide effective antimicrobial preservation. An exception is in nail hardeners where the concentration can be sold up to 5%. That product must be sold with nail shields, directions for use and caution regarding sensitization potential. It cannot be concluded that formaldehyde is safe in cosmetic products intended to be aerosolized." Formaldehyde is on the Canadian Hotlist (*see*). Banned in cosmetics in Sweden and Japan.

FORMIC ACID • Used as a rubefacient (*see*) in hair tonics; also a synthetic food flavoring. Colorless, pungent, highly corrosive, it occurs naturally in apples and other fruits. Also used as a decalcifier and for dehairing hides. Chronic absorption is known to cause albuminuria-protein in the urine. It caused cancer when administered orally in rats, mice, and hamsters in doses from 31 to 49 milligrams per kilogram of body weight. On the basis of available data, the CIR Expert Panel concludes that this ingredient is safe as presently used in cosmetics as a pH adjuster with a 64 ppm limit for the free acid.

FORSYTHIA SUSPENSA • Weeping forsythia is native to China. Extract of the fruit is used as an antioxidant and antibacterial.

FO-TI • *Polygonum multiforum.* Ho Shu Wu. One of the most popular herbs in China. Employed to treat skin ulcers and stomach ulcers as well as abscesses. The Chinese claim this herb has rejuvenating properties and can prevent gray hair and other premature signs of aging. It is also believed to increase fertility and maintain strength and vigor. Modern animal tests using fo-ti extracts have demonstrated antitumor activity. This herb also shows heart-protecting possibilities.

FOUNDATION MAKEUP • Aimed at covering blemishes, protecting the skin from drying out, and giving a glowing, healthy look. There is a cream-type foundation that vanishes from the skin but leaves a smooth, protective base for the application of pigmented makeup. Such creams are usually about 75 percent water, 15 percent stearic acid, and the remainder either sorbitan stearate or sorbitol. The pigmented foundation creams, which are designed to tint and cover the skin, usually contain about 50 percent water, mineral oil, stearic acid, lanolin, cetyl alcohol, propylene glycol, triethanolamine, borax, and insoluble pigments. They may also contain emulsifiers and detergents; humectants such as propylene glycol, glycerin, and sorbitol to absorb and retain water; lanolin derivatives; perfume; preservatives such as paraben; special barrier ingredients such as zinc stearate; cellulose derivatives and silicone; synthetic esters; thickeners such as sodium alginate, gum tragacanth, quince seed, and mucilage; and such waxes as beeswax and spermaceti. Stick-type makeup is made from isopropyl myristate, beeswax, carnauba wax, mineral oil, perfume, and dry pigment. Cake makeup, which is used by applying a wet sponge to the material and then applying the sponge to the face, is usually made of finely ground pigment, talc, kaolin, zinc, titanium oxide, precipitated calcium carbonate, and such inorganic pigments as iron oxides. To these may be added sorbitol, propylene glycol, lanolin, mineral oil, and perfume. If you check the above ingredients against those listed in the book, you will see that many—such as lanolin, perfume, beeswax, and paraben—are quite common allergens. However, by the very nature of the allergic response, you may not be allergic to a common allergen but to an uncommon one. The more ingredients to which you are exposed, of course, the greater the chances of developing an allergic response.

FRAGARIA CHILOENSIS AND F. VESCA • Flavoring. *See* Strawberry Juice.

FRAGILARIA PINNATA • Extract of algae used as an antioxidant and skin-conditioning ingredient.

FRAGRANCE • Any natural or synthetic substance or substances used solely to impart an odor to a cosmetic product. May be used without describing what is actually in the compound. Fragrances are widely used in topical formulations and can cause photoallergic or phototoxic reactions. To identify phototoxic effects, forty-three fragrances were evaluated in vitro with a photohaemolysis test using suspensions of human erythrocytes exposed to radiation sources rich in ultraviolet (UV) A or B in the presence of the test compounds. Haemolysis was measured by reading the absorbance values, and photo-haemolysis was calculated as a percentage of total haemolysis. Oakmoss caused photo-haemolysis of up to 100 percent with radiation rich in UVA and up to 26 percent with radiation rich in UVB. Moderate UVA-induced haemolysis (5–11%) was found with benzyl alcohol, bergamot oil, costus root oil, lime oil, orange oil, alpha-amyl cinnamic aldehyde, and laurel leaf oil. Moderate UVB-induced haemolysis was induced by hydroxy citronellal, cinnamic alcohol, cinnamic aldehyde, alpha-amyl cinnamic aldehyde, and laurel leaf oil. The phototoxic effects depended on the concentration of the compounds and the UV doses administered. Researchers conclude that some, but not all, fragrances exert phototoxic effects in vitro. Assessment of the correlation of the clinical effects of these findings could lead to improved protection of the skin from noxious compounds. Among the ingredients most likely to cause allergic responses in the sensitive are allyl alcohol, amyl cinnamal, amylcinnamyl alcohol, benzyl alcohol, benzyl salicylate, cinnamyl alcohol, cinnamal, citral, coumarin, eugenol, geraniol, hydroxycitronellal, hydroxymethylpentylcyclohexenecarboxaldehyde, isoeugenol, anisyl alcohol, enzyl benzoate, benzyl cinnamate, citronellol, farnesol, hexylcinnamaldehyde, lilial (2-(4-tert-butylbenzyl)propionaldehyde), *d*-Limonene, linalool, methyl heptine carbonate, and *g*-Methylionone (3-methyl-4-(2,6,6-trimethyl-2-cyclohexen-1-yl)-3-buten-2-one). Of course, there is no way to tell whether these are in your fragrances unless the law is changed. It now merely requires "fragrances" to be on the label. There is a consumer movement to get the fragrance ingredients identified but the manufacturers say they are protected under trade secrets. If you don't identify the problem by trial and error, you may call the cosmetic company and ask if certain ingredients are in the compound.

FRAGRANCE-FREE • Implies that a cosmetic so labeled has no perceptible odor. Products so labeled may still contain small amounts of fragrances to mask the fatty odor of soap or other unpleasant odors.

FRANGIPANI • *Plumeria alba.* A fragrance ingredient from the flowers of a small American shrub. *See* Jasmine.

FRANGULA ALNUS • *See* Buckthorn.

FRAXINUS EXCELSIOR • Common Ash. Tree native to England. *See* Fraxinus Ornus.

FRAXINUS ORNUS • Manna Ash. A member of the olive family, the seed extract is used as a skin-conditioning ingredient.

FREE RADICALS • Certain oxygen molecules that are underlying factors in aging and degenerative diseases because they damage DNA, the blueprint for life, within the cells. They also adversely affect enzymes, the workhorses of the cells, and damage cell membranes. Free radicals are formed during the course of normal metabolism, as well as from exposure to cigarette smoke and other environmental influences. Fat-soluble antioxidants, beta-carotene and other carotenoids, as well as vitamins C and E and pycnogenol (*see*), are believed to fight the damage from free radicals.

FREESIA REFRACTA • Sweet African herb used as an astringent ingredient.

FRENCH ROSE • An extract of *Rosa gallica* used in fragrances.

FRESHENER • *See* Skin Freshener.

FRUCTAN • *See* Fructose.

FRUCTOSE • A sugar occurring naturally in large numbers of fruits and honey. It is the sweetest of the foodstuffs. It is also used as a medicine and preservative. It caused tumors in mice when injected under the skin in 5,000-milligram doses per kilogram of body weight.

FRUITY BLENDS • One of the basic perfume types, fruity blends have other notes present but are noted for their clean, fresh citrus notes or a smooth, mellow, peachlike warmth.

FUCOCOUMARINS. In bronzing products. ASEAN has ruled it shall be below 1 mb/kg in a product. *See* Bergamot, Red and Coumarins.

FUCUS SERRATUS • Sea Oak. Sea Wrack. Toothed Wrack. An abundant seaweed, found in the Atlantic and Pacific oceans, with little bladders on its fronds that contain a gel. Used in bath gels, moisturizers, and lotions. Herbalists claim the gel strengthens weak limbs and relieves arthritis, sprains, and strains. They use it as a diuretic and as an aid in losing weight.

FUKITANPOPO EKISU • *See* Coltsfoot.

FULLER'S EARTH • Used in dry shampoos, hair colorings, beauty masks, and as a dusting powder; also used for lubricants and soaps. A white or brown, naturally occurring earthy substance. A nonplastic variety of kaolin (*see*) containing an aluminum magnesium silicate. Used as an absorbent and to decolorize fats and oils. No longer permitted as a color additive. *See* Magnesium Aluminum Silicate.

FUMARIA OFFICINALIS • Extract of a common weed thought to have antibacterial properties. Used as a skin-conditioning ingredient. *See* Fumitory Extract.

FUMARIC ACID • White, odorless, derived from many plants and essential to vegetable and animal tissue respiration; prepared industrially. An acidulant to adjust pH and used in apple, peach, and vanilla flavorings. Has been used to treat psoriasis but may cause skin irritation. GRAS

FUMITORY EXTRACT • *Fumaria officinalis.* Earth Smoke. Horned Poppy. Wax Dolls. An abundant weed in fields, the extract of the leaves, twigs, and flowers are used by herbalists in drinks for clearing obstructions from the liver or kidneys and to cure many diseases of the skin. It may also be used as an eyewash to ease conjunctivitis (*see*). Used as an odorant.

FUNGAL POLYSACCHARIDES • Many microorganisms such as bacteria and fungi possess so-called capsules made of polysaccharides (*see*), which protect these microorganisms from environmental insults and host immune defenses. Used in cosmetics to hold skin moisture. *See* Fungus and Polysaccharides.

FUNGICIDES • Any substances that kill or inhibit the growth of fungi. Older types include a mixture of lime and sulfur , copper oxychloride, and Bordeaux mixture. Copper naphthenate has been used to impregnate textile fabrics used for tenting and military clothing. Copper undecylenate with zinc undecylenate is used in foot powders and sprays.

FUNGUS • A plantlike organism that does not make chlorophyll. An organism of the kingdom Fungi, it feeds on organic matter; ranging from unicellular or multicellular organisms to spore-bearing syncytia. Mushrooms, yeasts, and molds are examples. The plural is fungi.

FURAN • A colorless, volatile liquid used in some chemical manufacturing industries. Furan has occasionally been reported to be found in foods. Scientists at FDA have discovered that furan forms in some foods more commonly than previously thought. The FDA says this discovery is likely a result of our ability to detect compounds at exceedingly low levels with the latest technology. The scientists think the furan forms in the food during traditional heat treatment techniques, such as cooking, jarring, and canning. The term "furans" is sometimes used interchangeably with "dioxins," but the FDA says furan is not a dioxin-like compound. The Dow Chemical Company, however, describes furans and dioxins as referring to a group of chemical compounds that share certain similar chemical structures and biological characteristics. Dioxins and furans are an unwanted by-product of combustion, both from natural sources such as forest fires and from man-made sources such as power plants, backyard burn barrels, and industrial processes. According to the EPA, dioxins and furans released into the air during combustion can be carried long distances before settling to the earth's surface. As a result, they are found almost everywhere at low levels. Dioxins and furans are produced by both natural and man-made processes and have therefore existed for centuries. The term "current background" is used to refer to the levels of dioxins and furans in the environment today. Dioxins and furans falling to land from air emissions tend to bind tightly to vegetation and soil. When dioxins and furans are released into water, they tend to settle into sediments where they can become trapped and stationary, or can be ingested by fish and other aquatic organisms. Dioxins and furans trapped in sediment can be further transported during activities that dislodge sediment, such as flooding or dredging. In the United States, the primary way people are exposed to dioxins and furans is through eating meat and dairy products. The animals we eat are exposed to background levels of dioxins and furans in the soil, on vegetation, and in some commercial animal feeds. Eating meat or dairy products exposes us to these low levels of dioxins and furans. Over time, we accumulate dioxins and furans in the fatty tissues of our own bodies. The term "furans" is sometimes used as shorthand for a group of environmental contaminants called the dibenzofurans, which have dioxin-like activity. In addition, the term "furans" refers to a large class of compounds of widely varying structures including, for example, nitrofurans. These chemicals have different effects than the furan that is now being studied. So far, FDA has focused on testing canned or jarred foods because these foods are heated in sealed containers. Furan has been found in such canned or jarred foods as soups, sauces, beans, pasta meals, and baby foods. Furan causes cancer in animals in studies where animals are exposed to furan at high doses. Because furan levels have been measured in only a few foods to date, it is difficult for FDA scientists to accurately calculate levels of furan exposure in food and to estimate a risk to consumers. The new data show furan in baby foods, but the FDA claims it is not of special concern. These data are exploratory and provide only a very limited and incomplete picture of the levels of furan in foods. These data alone do not indicate exposure or risk. FDA's preliminary estimate of consumer exposure is well below what FDA expects would cause harmful effects. FDA has no evidence that consumers should alter their infants' and children's diets and eating habits to avoid exposure to furan. In the course of investigations to confirm the accuracy of a report that furan may be formed in food under certain circumstances, however, FDA scientists discovered that a wider variety of heat-treated foods than previously thought contained varying levels of furan. The National Institutes of Health say furan is on the Department of Health and Human Services list of carcinogens, and is considered as possibly carcinogenic by the International Agency of Research on Cancer, based on studies in laboratory animals at high exposures. The concern is whether furan may also cause cancer in humans through long-term exposure to very low levels of furan in foods.

A number of the new flavorings, as you will read in this book, are derived from furan. The ECHA (*see*) says furan is an SIN, meaning something else should be substituted for now.

FURFURAL • Artificial Ant Oil. Used as a solvent, insecticide, fungicide, to decolor resins, and as a synthetic flavoring in food. A colorless liquid with a peculiar odor. Occurs naturally in angelica root, apples, coffee, peaches, and skim milk. Darkens when exposed to air. It irritates mucous membranes and acts on the central nervous system. Causes tearing and inflammation of the eyes and throat. Ingestion or absorption of .06 grams produces persistent headache. Used continually, it leads to nervous disturbances and eye disorders.

FURZE EXTRACT • Gorse. Extract of *Ulex europaeus,* a spiny evergreen shrub with yellow flowers. This common plant is often used for fuel and fodder.

FUSANUS SPICATUS • *Fusanus spicatus.* Wood Oil. Used as a fragrance ingredient in cleansing products. *See* Sandalwood.

FUSCOPORIA • Fungi used as a skin-conditioning ingredient and a humectant.

G

GADI LECUR • The name is used only on EU (*see*) products. *See* Cod Liver Oil.

GALACTARIC ACID • A chelating ingredient. *See* Carboxylic Acid.

GALACTOARABINAN • Larch Tree Extract. A polysaccharide extracted with water from larch wood used in the minimum quantity required to be effective as an emulsifier, stabilizer, binder, or bodying ingredient in essential oils. Used in hair products. Also used in artificial sweeteners.

GALACTOSE • White crystals occurring in milk sugar or lactose. Used as a diagnostic aid.

GALACTURONIC ACID • Obtained from plant pectins by hydrolysis, it is used in combination with allantoin (*see*) in creams and lotions.

GALANGAL • *Alpinia officinarum.* An herb cultivated in China, the rhizomes are unearthed in late summer and early autumn, cut into segments, and dried. It is used by some Chinese herbalists to break up intestinal gas and to treat heartburn and nausea.

GALBANUM GUM • *See* Galbanum Oil.

GALBANUM OIL • *Ferula galbaniflua.* A yellowish to green or brown, aromatic, bitter gum resin from an Asiatic plant used as incense. The oil is a fruit, nut, and spice flavoring for beverages, ice cream, ices, candy, baked goods, and condiments. Has been used medicinally to break up intestinal gas and as an expectorant.

GALEGA OFFICINALIS • Goat's Rue. Used as a skin conditioniner. *See* Galega Extract.

GALEGA EXTRACT • Goat's Rue. Extract of the herb *Galega officinalis.* This wildflower plant contains alkaloids, saponins, flavone, glycosides, tannin (*see all*), and bitters. In cosmetics it is used in an antidiabetic cream product that can penetrate human skin to deliver active antidiabetic elements. It is used to reduce blood sugar levels. It is also a powerful milk inducer in breast-feeding women. Used in cosmetics as a skin conditioner.

GALENICAL PREPARATION • Made up of herbal and/or vegetable matter.

GALLIC ACID • Obtained from tannins in nutgalls and also from broths of *Penicillin glaucum* or *Aspergillus niger.* Used as an astringent and antioxidant. *See* Propyl Gallate.

GALIUM APARINE EXTRACT • Goose Grass. Cleavers. From the herb *Gallium aparine. See* Cleavers.

GAMBIR EXTRACT • *Uncaria gambir.* A flavoring. *See* Catechu Extract.

GAMMA LINOLENIC ACID • *See* Linolenic Acid.

GAMMA-ORIZANOL • *See* Oryzanol.

GANODERMA LUCIDIUM and G. JAPONICUM • *See* Mushroom Extract.

GARCINIA CAMBOGIA EXTRACT • Kokum Butter. Extract from a large Asiatic tree used in creams and lotions.

GARDEN BALSAM EXTRACT • From the flowers of *Impatiens balsamina. See* Impatiens.

GARDENIA • The white or yellow flowers used in fragrances. Obtained from a large genus of Old World tropical trees and shrubs.

GARLIC EXTRACT • An extract from *Allium sativum,* a yellowish liquid with a strong odor used in fruit and garlic flavorings. It is being tested as an antibiotic and has been used to counteract intestinal worms.

GAULTHERIA PROCUMBENS • *See* Wintergreen Oil.

GAYLUSACCIA BACCATA • Huckleberry. Low shrub of the eastern United States bearing shiny black edible fruit; best known of the huckleberries. Used as flavoring.

GEL • A semisolid, apparently homogeneous substance that may be elastic and jellylike (gelatin) or more or less rigid (silica gel), and that is formed in various ways, such as by coagulation or evaporation. Gel compositions have been used in a variety of cosmetic and health and beauty applications. Some gel compositions have proven to be convenient and efficient vehicles or carriers for the application of various active ingredients to the skin. Such active ingredients include sunscreens, antiperspirants, deodorants, perfumes, cosmetics, emollients, insect repellants, medicaments, and the like. Cosmetic and health and beauty products incorporating a gel composition and those made entirely from a gel composition may be in the form of a liquid, soft gel, semisolid, or solid. Rubbing a liquid, soft gel, semi-solid, or solid containing an effective amount of an active ingredient dissolved or dispersed therein against the skin causes transfer of the gel composition to the skin surface in a layer form, leaving the active ingredient within the layer on the desired skin surface. For cosmetic and health and beauty applications, a gel composition preferably should have one or more of the following desired properties: transparency, compatibility with an active ingredient, controlled release of an active ingredient, minimization of skin irritation, and the ability to suspend organic and inorganic materials such as colored pigments, glitters, water, air, metal oxides, sunscreen active particulates, and fragrances. A gel composition used in cosmetic and health and beauty applications should moisturize the skin and exhibit water wash-off resistance.

GELATIN • Used in protein shampoos because it sticks to the hair and gives it "more body," peelable face masks, and as a fingernail strengthener. Gelatin is a protein obtained by boiling skin, tendons, ligaments, or bones with water. It is colorless or slightly yellow, tasteless, and absorbs five to ten times its weight of cold water. Also used as a food thickener and stabilizer and a base for fruit gelatins and puddings. Employed medicinally to treat malnutrition and brittle fingernails.

GELATIN/KERATIN AMINOACIDS/LYSINE HYDROXYPROPLYTRI-MONIUM CHLORIDE • A gelatin (*see*) made from a mixture of animal skins.

GELIDIUM CARTILAGINEUM • EU name for red algae (*see*).

GELLAN GUM • A gum produced by the fermentation of a carbohydrate with *Pseudomonas elodea.* Used as an emulsifier and thickener.

GELLIDIELA ACEROSA AND EXTRACT • Algae Extract. Seaweederm. An extract derived from *Gellidiela acerosa.* Widely used in skin, bath, and hair products as an emollient.

GENDER BENDER • *See* Endocrine Disrupter Chemical (EDC). The name is derived from the observation that these chemicals could mimic female hormones in both men and women.

GENE • The smallest genetic unit of a chromosome. It is a piece of DNA that contains the hereditary information for the production of a protein.

GENIPA AMERICANA • Huito. The ripened fruit is often eaten raw or made into jam. The genipap is native to wet or moist areas of Cuba, Hispaniola, Puerto Rico, the Virgin Islands, and from Guadeloupe to Trinidad; also from southern Mexico to Panama, and from Colombia and Venezuela to Peru, Bolivia, and Argentina. Its usefulness to the Indians was reported by several European writers in Brazil in the sixteenth century. Used as body paint among natives. Found to have antibacterial activity. The fruit is brewed into a tea and taken as a remedy for bronchitis.

GENISTEIN • A plant estrogen found in the urine of people with diets rich in soybeans and, to a lesser extent, in the cabbage family vegetables, this compound seems to block the growth of new blood vessels, essential for some tumors to grow and spread. Sheep grazing on some clovers are prone to reproductive failure because of genistein in the plants.

GENTIAN • *Gentiana campestris. G. lutea.* Baldimony. Felwort. Field Gentian. An annual plant that grows in dry, chalky soil in Great Britain, it is used in modern medicine. Herbalists make an infusion for heartburn or gas after eating. They also use it to stimulate the appetite. In 1992, the FDA proposed a ban on *G. lutea* in oral menstrual drug products because it has not been shown to be safe and effective for its stated claims. It is used in cosmetic creams and bath products to soothe the skin.

GENTIANA BUNGE • Tundra Gentian. Extract of the root contains a number of bioactive substances such as xanthones and flavonoids. It is being used to enhance skin coloring but also being tested against skin cancer and white skin patches known as vitaligo. *See* Gentian.

GERANIOL • Used in perfumery to compound artificial attar of roses and artificial orange blossom oil. Also used in depilatories to mask odors. Oily sweet, with a rose odor, it occurs naturally in apples, bay leaves, cherries, grapefruit, ginger, lavender, and a number of other essential oils. Geraniol is omitted from hypoallergenic cosmetics. Can cause allergic reactions. Whereas no specific toxicity information is available, deaths have been reported from ingestion of unknown amounts of citronella oil (*see*), which is 93 percent geraniol; gastric mucosa was found to be severely damaged. GRAS. ASP

GERANIUM • An essential oil used as flavoring. There are several types of geranium oil, the main ones being Reunion or Bourbon, Algerian, Moroccan, and French. The oils are composed chiefly of geraniol, citronellol, linalool, citronellyl formate, and several other compounds. Reunion oil is very rich in citronellol and has a heavy rose and minty odor. Algerian oil has a delicate odor. Moroccan oil is similar to Algerian oil. French oil is thought to possess the finest roselike odor. The concrete and absolute of geranium are also available commercially. The oil of geranium, widely used in perfumery and cosmetics, is stable and blends well with other fragrances. Dried leaves are used in sachets and potpourris. Leaves of geranium are also used in herbal teas and the oil is used in baked goods and fruit desserts. As a medicinal plant, geranium has traditionally been considered an astringent and used as a folk remedy in the treatment of ulcers. A terpine hydrate synthesized from geraniol is known to be an effective expectorant. Leaves are reported to have antifungal activity. Scented geranium and oil of geranium are reported to cause contact dermatitis. Geranium is reported to repel insects because of its citronellol content. *See* Geranium Rose Oil. GRAS

GERANIUM, EAST INDIAN, OIL • *Cymbopogon martini. See* Geranium. ASP

GERANIUM MACULATUM • The roots of this plant were used by herbalists to treat canker sores, sunburn, and inflammation. It is being used in "anti-aging" products.

GERANIUM OIL • Used in perfumery, dusting powder, tooth powder, and ointments. It is the light yellow to deep yellow oil of plants of the genus *Pelargonium* or of rose geranium leaves, with the characteristic odor of rose and geraniol. A teaspoon may cause illness in an adult, and less than an ounce may kill. May affect those allergic to geraniums.

GERANIUM ROSE OIL • *Pelargonium graveolens.* A synthetic flavoring additive that occurs naturally in geranium herbs and rose petals. Used in strawberry, lemon, cola, geranium, rose, violet, cherry, honey, rum, brandy, cognac, nut, vanilla, spice, and ginger ale flavorings for beverages, ice cream, ices, candy, baked goods, gelatin desserts, chewing gum, and jelly. A teaspoon may cause illness in an adult and less than an ounce may kill. May affect those allergic to geraniums. ASP

GERANYL ACETATE • Geraniol Acetate. Clear, colorless liquid with the odor of lavender, it is a constituent of several essential oils. Used in perfumery and flavoring. *See* Geraniol.

GERANYL ACETOACETATE • A synthetic fruit flavoring additive for beverages, ice cream, ices, candy, and baked goods. ASP

GERANYL BENZOATE • A synthetic flavoring additive, slightly yellowish liquid, with a floral odor. Used in floral and fruit flavorings for beverages, ice cream, ices, candy, baked goods, and candy. *See* Benzoate. ASP

GERANYL BUTYRATE • Geraniol Butyrate. Colorless liquid found in several essential oils, it is used in perfumes, soaps, and flavorings and as a synthetic attar of rose. *See* Geraniol.

GERANYL FORMATE • Geraniol Formate. Colorless liquid with a roselike odor, insoluble in alcohol, it occurs in several essential oils. Used in perfumes, soaps, and flavorings as a synthetic neroli bigarade oil (*see*). *See* Geraniol.

GERANYL PHENYLACETATE • Phenylacetic Acid. A synthetic flavoring, yellow liquid, with a honey-rose odor. Used in fruit flavorings for beverages, ice cream, ices, candy, baked goods, and chewing gum. *See* Geraniol for toxicity.

GERANYL PROPIONATE • Geraniol Propionate. Colorless liquid with a roselike odor, it is soluble in most oils and is used in perfumery and flavoring. *See* Geraniol.

GERANYL TIGLATE • *See* Geraniol.

GERIANAL • *See* Citral.

GERIANALDEHYDE • *See* Citral.

GERMANDER EXTRACT • An extract of the herb *Teucrium scorodonia* or *T. chamaedrys.* Wall Germander. A member of the mint family, it has long been used by herbalists as far back as Hippocrates and Pliny. The Greeks used it as a tonic. In the mid-eighteenth century, herbalists used it to treat gout. It is an astringent, antiseptic, diuretic, and stimulant and has been used in the treatment of jaundice, excess fluid due to heart failure, and ailments of the spleen. It continues to be used in folk medicine to heal ulcers and sores. Cases of its use in tea or capsules has been reported to the Centers for Disease Control as causing liver toxicity.

GERMANIUM • Suma. Occurs in the earth's crust, it is a naturally occurring isotope that is recovered from residues from refining of zinc and other sources. It is also present in some coals. It is used in infrared transmitting glass and electronic devices. It is used by Third World women as an eye makeup, a practice that is being discouraged because of its lead content. Also used as an intestinal astringent.

GERMANIUM SESQUIOXIDE • *See* Germanium.

GEROTINE • *See* Spermine.

GEUM RIVALE • *Avena geum* Rivale. *See* Avens and Clove Oil.

GEVUINA AVELLANA OIL • Natural Antioxidant Alpha Tocotrienol (vitamin E) present in Chilean hazelnut seed oil. Used in skin conditioners. *See* Hazelnut Oil.

GHATTI GUM • Indian Gum. The gummy exudate from the stems of a plant abundant in India and Ceylon. Used as an emulsifier and in butter, butterscotch, and fruit flavorings. Has caused an occasional allergy, but when ingested in large amounts, it has not caused obvious distress.

GIGARTINA STELLATA • Red algae mostly from the Pacific. *See* Algae.

GINGER • *Zingiber officinale.* Gan Jiang. Native to Asia but cultivated in many parts of the tropics, Hippocrates used ginger as a medicine. Widely used in many forms in cosmetics. Externally, ginger is a rubefacient (*see*). Modern studies have shown that ginger inhibits prostaglandins (*see*) and thus reduces inflammation. In 1992, the FDA issued a notice that ginger had not been shown to be safe and effective as claimed in OTC digestive aid products. Contraindicated in individuals suffering from a skin disease. An excessive dose can cause irritation of the mucous membrane lining of the stomach. It can also promote menstruation.

GINGER OIL • Obtained by steam distillation of dried ginger root. *See* Ginger.

GINKGO EXTRACT • Maidenhair. An extract of *Ginkgo biloba.* A sacred tree of the Chinese, the fruit has an offensive odor but is resistant to smoke, disease, and insects. Used in perfumes and as an insecticide and as a skin-conditioning ingredient in creams and in hair-grooming products. May be anti-inflammatory on the skin.

GINSENG • *Panax ginseng* (Asia). *P. quinquefolium* (North America). *Eleutherococcus senticosus* (Siberian Ginseng). Jen Shang. Chinese esteem ginseng as an herb of many uses. Panax comes from the Greek word *panakos,* meaning "panacea." Among ginseng's active ingredients are amino acids, essential oils, carbohydrates, peptides, vitamins, minerals, enzymes, and sterols. It has been found to normalize high or low blood sugar. In Asia, ginseng is esteemed for its abilities to preserve health, invigorate the system, and prolong life. It is taken in an herbal tea as a daily tonic. North American Indians used ginseng as a love potion. Russian scientists are studying ginseng for the treatment of insomnia and general debility. Japanese scientists recently reported isolating a number of compounds—rare in nature—from ginseng, some of which have anticancer properties. It is used in American cosmetics as a demulcent (*see*) and as a hair conditioner.

GLA • *See* Gamma Linolenic Acid.

GLANDULAR SUBSTANCES • Extracts of animal glands widely used in the cosmetic industry for various purposes.

GLASS AND GLASS BEADS • Suspending ingredients.

GLAUBER'S SALT • Crystalline sodium sulfate (*see*) used as an opacifier in shampoos and as a detergent in bath salts. Named for a German chemist, Johann R. Glauber, who died in 1668. Also used medicinally as a laxative. Skin irritations may occur.

GLECHOMA HEDERACEA • *See* Ground Ivy Extract.

GLEDITSIA AUSTRALIS • A thorny tree with green spikes of flowers. Sweet extract used as flavoring and as an emollient ingredient.

GLIADIN • A protein derived from wheat. *See* Wheat Germ Extract.

GLISODIN • A dietary supplement that reportedly has been shown to help protect the skin from the inside, complementing topical sunscreens and protective clothing. An antioxidant catalyst, meaning it works to increase the body's own production of its natural antioxidant defenses, including superoxide dismutase (SOD), helping the body to disarm the reactive oxygen species triggered by sun rays. This protective benefit is particularly beneficial for the sun sensitive.

GLOIOPELTIS • Skin conditioner. *See* Red Algae.

GLOSS WHITE • No longer permitted as a coloring in cosmetics. *See* Aluminum Hydrate.

GLUCAMINE • An organic compound prepared from glucose (*see*). Used in skin conditioners as a humectant.

GLUCAN • Alpha-Glucan Oligosaccharide. Beta-Glucan. Skin conditioners in lotions and cleansing products.

GLUCARIC ACID • A sugar acid derived from D-glucose. A conditioner used in hair products. *See* Saccharin.

GLUCAROLACTONE • *See* Saccharin and Lactic Acid.

GLUCOHEPTONIC ACID • A pH adjuster and skin-conditioning ingredient. *See* Glucose.

GLUCOHEPTONOLACTONE • Skin-conditioning ingredient. *See* Glucose.

GLUCONIC ACID AND SALTS • A light, amber liquid with the faint odor of vinegar, produced from corn. In cosmetics and personal care products, gluconic acid and its derivatives may be used in the formulation of mouthwashes, bath products, cleansing products, skin care products, and shampoo. It is water soluble and used as a dietary supplement and a sequestrant (*see*). The magnesium salt of gluconic acid has been used as an antispasmodic. *See* Sodium Gluconate. GRAS

GLUCONIC LACTONE • Derived from oxidation of glucose. *See* Gluconic Acid and Salts.

GLUCONOLACTONE • Made from milk sugar, it is a polyhydroxy acid (*see*) used in anti-aging creams to exfoliate the skin. Reportedly less irritating than earlier alphahydroxy acids (*see*). Also used as a fragrance ingredient in shampoos. *See* Glucose and Lactic Acid.

4-(2-b-GLUCOPYRANOSILOXY)PROPOXY-2-HYDROXYBENZOPHENONE • Sunscreen ingredient. *See* Benzophenones.

GLUCOSAMINE • Found in chitin (*see*). pH adjuster in cosmetics. It also is used in medicine to treat arthritis.

GLUCOSAMINE COMPLEX • An amino derivative of glucose that is found especially in polysaccharides such as chitin and in cell membranes. The main component of glucosamine complex is glucosamine itself. A natural mineral-like compound, glucosamine is naturally found in the body since birth. It is found in most living things, including some plants. Glucosamine helps the body to produce collagen. The therapeutic use of oral glucosamine has been shown to have some benefit against cartilage degeneration, and possibly in a case of spinal disc degeneration. The FDA was asked to cease evaluating a company's request for GRAS status for glucosamine as a food additive because of changes in the manufacture of glucosamine, with the understanding that the company may, in the future, submit another GRAS notification. Most of the glucosamine additives apparently are made in China. Glucosamine complex, when applied to the surface of skin, is claimed to exfoliate the surface of the skin. The producers of the complex claim it "tightens and firms the skin and keeps it soft and young-looking."

GLUCOSE • Used as a flavoring, to soothe the skin, and as a filler in cosmetics. Occurs naturally in blood and in grape and corn sugars. A source of energy for plants and animals. Sweeter than sucrose (*see*). Confectioners frequently suffer erosions and fissures around their nails, and the nails loosen and sometimes fall off.

GLUCOSE GLUTAMATE • Used as a humectant in hand creams and lotions, it occurs naturally in animal blood and in grape and corn sugars, and is a source of energy for plants and animals. It is sweeter than sucrose. The FDA has asked for further studies as to its potential mutagenic, teratogenic, subacute, and reproductive effects. The CIR

Expert Panel (*see*) concludes that there is insufficient data to support the safety of this ingredient when used in cosmetics.

GLUCOSE LACTO PEROXIDE • A natural preservative. *See* Lacto Peroxide.

GLUCOSE LACTOSE PEROXIDE • A natural preservative. *See* Lacto Peroxide.

GLUCOSIDES • Compounds with sugar and alcohol.

GLUCOSYL HESPERIDIN • Humectant and skin conditioner. *See* Glucose and Phenols.

GLUCOSYLRUTIN • Derived from rutin (*see*), it is an antioxidant. *See* Phenols.

GLUCOSYL STEVIOSIDE • A flavoring. *See* Glucose and Stevioside.

GLUCURONIC ACID • A carbohydrate widely distributed in the animal kingdom. Used as a pH adjuster, skin conditioner, and humectant.

GLUCURONOLACTONE • *See* Glucuronic Acid and Lactic Acid.

GLUTAMATE • Ammonium and monopotassium salt of glutamic acid (*see*). Used to enhance natural flavors and to improve the taste of tobacco. It is used as an antioxidant in cosmetics to prevent spoilage. It is being studied by the FDA for mutagenic, teratogenic, subacute, and reproductive effects. The final report to the FDA of the Select Committee on GRAS Substances stated in 1980 that there is no evidence in the available information that it is a hazard to the public when used as it is now and it should continue its GRAS status with limitations on the amount that can be added to food. The European Parliament stated in 2003 that this taste enhancer can provoke in certain cases nervous symptoms (decreased sensibility in neck, arms, and back) and irregular heartbeat. In animal testing, it provoked reproductive disorders in rats. It also is reported to cause problems for asthmatic persons.

GLUTAMIC ACID • A white, practically odorless, free-flowing crystalline powder, a nonessential amino acid (*see*) usually manufactured from vegetable protein. It is used to enhance food flavors, as an antioxidant and humectant in cosmetics, and as a softener in permanent wave solutions to help protect against hair damage. It is being studied by the FDA for mutagenic, teratogenic, subacute, and reproductive effects.

GLUTAMINE • A nonessential amino acid (*see*) used as a medicine and in cosmetics as a hair and skin conditioniner.

GLUTAMYL HISTAMINE • A hair-conditioning ingredient. *See* Glutamic Acid.

GLUTARAL • Glutaraldehyde. An amino acid (*see*) that occurs in green sugar beets. Used in a wide variety of cosmetics such as creams and emollients as a germicide and preservative. It has a faint, agreeable odor. In a two-year drinking test in rats, there was an increase in leukemia only in females. In humans, there is some evidence of skin irritation and sensitization. Occupational data and animal studies indicate that inhalation of this ingredient can cause respiratory irritation in addition to its skin effects. The CIR Expert Panel (*see*) is concerned about the carcinogenic potential of this ingredient when used in "leave-on" products. Based upon the animal and human data, the panel concluded that glutaral is safe for use at concentrations up to 0.5 percent in rinse-off products. There is insufficient data to determine the safety of it in leave-on products. The committee said it should not be used in aerosol products. *See* Glutaric Acid.

GLUTARALDEHYDE • A major allergen in the medical and dental workplace. It is used as a base in some waterless hand soaps. *See* Glutaral.

GLUTARIC ACID • Pentanedioic Acid. A crystalline fatty acid that is soluble in oil. Widely used in oriental medicine as an aromatic bitter. It is used in American cosmetics as a demulcent (*see*) and as a pH adjuster.

GLUTATHIONE • Cloves, caraway, dill weed, parsley, lemongrass oil, and celery have been found to have significant amounts of this protein. Acts to stimulate enzymes and is used in anti-aging products and as an emulsifier.

GLUTEN • A mixture of proteins from wheat flour.

GLY- • The abbreviation for glycine (*see*).

GLYCERETH-12-26 • Polyethylene glycols mixed with glycerin. The viscosity depends upon the number after glycereth. *See* Glycerin and Polyethylene Glycol.

GLYCERETH-7 TRIACETATE • A solvent used in emollients. *See* Polyethylene Glycol and Triacetin-26. Made from glycerin and polyethylene glycol (*see both*), it is widely used in cosmetics as a skin-conditioning ingredient and humectant.

GLYCERIDES • Any of a large class of compounds that are esters (*see*) of the sweet alcohol glycerin. They are also made synthetically. They are used in cosmetic creams as texturizers and emollients.

GLYCERIN • Glycerol. Any by-product of soap manufacture, it is a sweet, warm-tasting, oily fluid obtained by adding alkalis (*see*) to fats and fixed oils. A solvent, humectant, and emollient in many cosmetics, it absorbs moisture from the air and, therefore, helps keep moisture in creams and other products, even if the consumer leaves the cap off the container. Also helps the products to spread better. Among the many products containing glycerin are cream rouges, face packs and masks, freckle lotions, hand creams and lotions, hair lacquers, liquid face powder, mouthwashes, protective creams, skin fresheners, and toothpastes. In concentrated solutions it is irritating to the mucous membranes, but as used it is nonirritating and nonallergenic. Draws moisture from inside the skin and holds it on the surface for a better "feel." Dries skin from the inside out. The FDA issued a notice in 1992 that glycerin has not been shown to be safe and effective as claimed in OTC poison ivy, poison oak, and poison sumac products as well as in diaper-rash drug products.

GLYCEROL • *See* Glycerin.

GLYCERYL ADIPATE • Ester of glycerin and adipic acid (*see both*). Used as an emollient.

GLYCERYL ALGINATE • Used as an emollient. The ester of glycerin and alginic acid (*see both*). *See also* Ester.

GLYCERYL-*p*-AMINOBENZOATE • A semisolid, waxy mass or syrup with a faint aromatic odor, liquefying and congealing very slowly, used in cosmetic sunscreen preparations. *See* Benzoic Acid.

GLYCERYL ARACHIDONATE • Used as an emollient, emulsifier, and thickener. The ester of glycerin and arachidonic acid (*see both*). *See also* Ester.

GLYCERYL BEHENATE • Ester of glycerin and behenic acid (*see both*). Used as an emollient. *See also* Ester.

GLYCERYL CAPRATE • Emollient. *See* Glycerin and Caprylic Acid.

GLYCERYL CAPRYLATE • Emollient. *See* Glycerin and Caprylic Acid.

GLYCERYL CAPRYLATE/CAPRATE • Emollient. A mixture of caprylic acid and capric acid (*see both*).

GLYCERYL COCONATE • Emollient. *See* Glycerin and Coconut Oil.

GLYCERYL COLLAGENATE • Ester (*see*) of glycerin and collagen (*see both*). Used as a hair-conditioning ingredient and as an emollient in skin creams.

GLYCERYL DIBEHENATE • A mixture of glycerin and beheneic acid (*see both*) used as an emollient ingredient.

GLYCERYL DIERUCATE • Made from glycerin and erucic acid (*see both*). Emollient.

GLYCERYL DILAURATE • Widely used in cosmetics as an emollient in hand preparations, makeup, and cold creams. *See* Glycerin and Lauric Acid.

GLYCERYL DIMYRISTATE • *See* Glycerin and Myristic Acid.

GLYCERYL DIOLEATE • The diester of glycerin and oleic acid (*see both*).

GLYCERYL DIPALMITATE • *See* Glycerin and Palmitic Acid.

GLYCERYL DISTEARATE • Made from glycerin and stearic acid (*see both*) and widely used as an emollient in moisturizers, cuticle softeners, eye lotions, skin fresheners, mascara, and shampoos.

GLYCERYL ERUCATE • *See* Glycerin and Erucic Acid.

GLYCERYL HYDROGENATED ROSINATE • A mixture of glycerin and rosin (*see both*).

GLYCERYL HYDROSTEARATE • *See* Glyceryl Monostearate.

GLYCERYL HYDROXYSTEARATE • Made from glycerin and hydroxystearic acid (*see both*), widely used as an emollient and emulsifier in moisturizers, body and hand products, face and neck creams, cleansing lotions and pads, and other products.

GLYCERYL ISOSTEARATE • Widely used as an emollient and emulsifier in foundations, eye shadows, body and hand creams, cleansing lotions, bath products, and moisturizers. *See* Glyceryl Monostearate.

GLYCERYL LANOLATE • Used in hair and skin products as a conditioner. *See* Glycerin and Lanolin.

GLYCERYL LAURATE • Made from lauric acid and glycerin (*see both*), it is widely used as an emulsifier and emollient in permanent waves, shampoos, moisturizers, bath products, underarm deodorants, body and hand creams, and eye makeup.

GLYCERYL LINOLEATE • *See* Glycerin and Linoleic Acid.

GLYCERYL MONOSTEARATE • Emulsifying and dispersing ingredient used in baby creams, face masks, foundation cake makeup, liquid powders, hair conditioners, hand lotions, mascara, and nail whiteners. It is a mixture of two glyceryls, a white, wax-like solid, or beads. Lethal when injected in large doses into mice.

GLYCERYL MYRISTATE • *See* Glycerin and Myristic Acid.

GLYCERYL OLEATE • Used as an emulsifier in cosmetics up to 5 percent. Found to be nonirritating in humans. May cause allergies. Based on human and animal studies, the CIR Expert Panel (*see*) concludes that this additive is safe as a cosmetic ingredient in the present practices of use and concentration. Has reportedly caused allergic reactions. *See* Glycerin and Oleic Acid.

GLYCERYL PABA • Sunscreen ingredient. The ester of glycine and *p*-aminobenzoic acid (*see both*).

GLYCERYL PALMITATE LACTATE • Emollient. The lactic acid ester (*see*) of glyceryl palmitate.

GLYCERYL PALMITATE/STEARATE • An ester of glycerin and a blend of palmitic and stearic acids (*see all*).

GLYCERYL PHOSPHATES • *See* Glycerin and Phosphates.

GLYCERYL POLYMETHACRYLATE • Derived from glycerin and acrylic acid (*see both*), it is a film former widely used in moisturizers, body and hand products, fragrances, and eye makeup and lotions.

GLYCERYL RICINOLEATE • An emollient. The CIR Expert Panel (*see*) concludes that there is insufficient data to determine the safety of this ingredient in cosmetics. *See* Glycerin.

GLYCERYL SESQUIOLEATE • *See* Glycerin.

GLYCERYL STARCH • *See* Starch and Glycerol.

GLYCERYL STEARATE • Widely used as an emulsifier and skin-conditioning ingredient. It is in makeup, lotions, powders, and creams as well as foot powders and cuticle softeners. Based on available animal data and human experience, the CIR Expert Panel (*see*) concluded this ingredient is safe for use in applications to humans in the present practices of use and concentration. On the basis of the available information, the CIR

Expert Panel found it safe in the early 1980s but is considering new information to determine if the final safety assessment should be reaffirmed, amended, or have an addendum. May cause allergies. *See* Glycerin.

GLYCERYL STEARATE LACTATE • The lactic acid ester of glyceryl stearate. *See* Lactic Acid and Glycerin.

GLYCERYL STEARATE SE • A widely used emulsifier containing glyceryl stearate that contains some sodium and some potassium. Based on available animal data and human experience, the CIR Expert Panel (*see*) concluded this ingredient is safe for use in current concentrations. On the basis of the available information, the CIR Expert Panel found it safe in the early 1980s but is considering new information to determine if the final safety assessment should be reaffirmed, amended, or have an addendum. *See* Glycerin Monostearate.

GLYCERYL THIOGLYCOLATE • Found in permanent wave solutions, this is a common allergen among European hairstylists and is the second most common among U.S. beauticians. The CIR Expert Panel (*see*) concluded this ingredient is a potential sensitizer but can be safely used infrequently. Hairdressers who apply it to clients frequently are the most at risk for sensitization. *See* Glycerin and Thioglycolic Acid Compounds.

GLYCERYLTRIACETYL HYDROXYSTEARATE • *See* Glycerin and Octadecanoic Acid

GLYCERYL TRIMYRISTATE • *See* Glycerin and Myristic Acid.

GLYCERYL TRIOCTANOATE • *See* Glycerin.

GLYCERYL TRIOLEATE • *See* Glycerin and Oleic Acid.

GLYCERYL TRIUNDECANOATE • The triester of glycerin and undecanoic acid (*see both*).

GLYCERYL/SORBITOL OLEATE/HYDROXYSTEARATE • A mixed esterification product of glycerin and sorbitol with hydroxystearic acid and oleic acids (*see all*).

GLYCINE • Used as a texturizer in cosmetics. An amino acid (*see*) classified as nonessential. Made up of sweet-tasting crystals, it is used as a dietary supplement and as a gastric antacid.

GLYCINE SOJA • Soybean Flour and Oil. Flour used as an abrasive and thickener and oil as an emollient. *See* Soybean.

GLYCO- • Prefix from the Greek meaning "sweetness."

GLYCOFUROL • The ethoxylated ether of tetrahydrofurfuryl alcohol. *See* Furfural.

GLYCOGEN • Distributed throughout cell protoplasm, it is an animal starch found especially in liver and muscle. Used as a skin conditioner.

GLYCOL • The general name for alcohols that are very similar to glycerol (*see*). Used as fragrances, humectants, solvents, and thinners.

GLYCOL DILAURATE • *See* Ethylene Glycol and Lauric Acid.

GLYCOL DIOCTANOATE • *See* Ethylene Glycol.

GLYCOL DISTEARATE • Widely used surfactant made from glycerin and stearic acid. It is also used as an opacifier (*see*). On the basis of the available information, the CIR Expert Panel (*see*) found it safe in the early 1980s but is considering new information to determine if the final safety assessment should be reaffirmed, amended, or have an addendum.

GLYCOL DITALLOWATE • The diester of ethylene glycol and tallow acid (*see both*).

GLYCOL ESTERS • *See* Glycols and Ester.

GLYCOL ETHERS • Cellosolve. Carbitol. Dowanol. Ektasolve. EGME. Glycol ether is the name for a large group of chemicals. Most glycol ether compounds are clear, colorless liquids. Some have mild, pleasant odors or no smell at all; others (mainly the acetates) have strong odors. Cosmetics and toiletries benefit from the performance of glycol ethers, according to a manufacturer, because properties allow glycol ethers to prevent a component from separating out of the formulation, and to help maintain the clarity of a cosmetic formulation, even when the product is exposed to temperature extremes in shipping and storage. Glycol ether is an effective mutual solvent for ingredients of cosmetic preparations, the producers say, because it has similar emollient properties, it can also be used as a low-cost replacement for fatty acid isopropyl esters (*see*). Glycol ether is now in some personal care products as a preservative and may be used at levels up to 1.0 percent. The common belief that glycol ethers never evaporate fast enough to create harmful levels in the air is false, according to the Hazard Evaluation System and Information Service of California. Some evaporate quickly and can easily reach hazardous levels in the air; others evaporate very slowly and therefore are less hazardous by inhalation. The glycol ethers are widely used industrial solvents. Glycol ethers enter your body when they evaporate into the air you breathe, and they are rapidly absorbed into your body if the liquids contact your skin. Cases of poisoning have been reported where skin contact was the main route of exposure, even though there was no effect on the skin itself. The effects of overexposure can include anemia, mild intoxication, and irritation of the skin, eyes, nose, and throat. Some glycol ethers are hazardous to the male and female reproductive systems. Within the class of glycol ethers, toxicity varies. All propylene glycol ethers are currently believed to be relatively safe, according to California's Hazard Evaluation System and Information Service. Most ethylene glycol ethers with "methyl" in their names are relatively toxic.

GLYCOL HYDROXYSTEARATE • The ester of ethylene glycol and hydroxystearic acid. *See* Ethylene Glycol and Stearic Acid.

GLYCOL MONTANATE • The ester (*see*) of glycol and montan wax (*see both*). Used as emulsion stabilizers and opacifying ingredients in emollients.

GLYCOL RICINOLEATE • The ester of ethylene glycol and ricinoleic acid (*see both*).

GLYCOL SALICYLATE • The ester of polyethylene glycol and salicylic acid.

GLYCOL STEARATE • One of the most widely used bases for cosmetic creams at concentrations ranging from less than 0.1 to 10 percent. Low toxicity. On the basis of the available information, the CIR Expert Panel found it safe in the early 1980s but is considering new information to determine if the final safety assessment should be reaffirmed, amended, or have an addendum. *See* Glycols and Stearic Acid.

GLYCOL STEARATE SE • Widely used as an emollient, opacifying ingredient, and emulsifier in many cosmetic products including moisturizers, hair dyes, bath products, and shampoos. The self-emulsifying grade of glycol stearate that contains some sodium and/or potassium. On the basis of the available information, the CIR Expert Panel (*see*) found it safe in the early 1980s but is considering new information to determine if the final safety assessment should be reaffirmed, amended, or have an addendum. *See* Glycols and Stearates.

GLYCOLIC ACID • Contained in sugarcane juice and fruit, it is an odorless, slightly water-absorbing acid used to control the acid/alkali balance in cosmetics and whenever a cheap organic acid is needed. It is also used as an exfoliant (*see*). It is a mild irritant to the skin and mucous membranes. One of the more controversial services offered by skin care salons is the glycolic acid peel, a procedure that is also being performed by dermatologists. Glycolic acid is a compound related to alpha-hydroxy acids. As of this writing, glycolic acid is not considered a drug. Its marketers maintain it is a cosmetic because it does not change the structure of the skin. Has the potential of causing sun sensitivity and irritation. *See* Alpha-Hydroxy Acids.

GLYCOLIPIDS • A mixture of fats, oils, and carbohydrates used in emollients.

GLYCOLS • Propylene Glycol. Glycerin. Ethylene Glycol. Carbitol. Diethylene Glycol. Literally it means "glycerin" plus "alcohol." A group of syrupy alcohols derived from hydrocarbons (*see*) that are widely used in cosmetics as humectants. The FDA cautions manufacturers that glycols may cause adverse reactions in users. Propylene glycol and glycerin (*see both*) are considered safe. Other glycols in low concentrations may be harmless for external application, but ethylene glycol, carbitol, and diethylene glycol are hazardous in concentrations exceeding 5 percent even in preparations for use on small areas of the body. Therefore, in sunscreen lotions and protective creams where the area of application is extensive, they should not be used at all. Wetting ingredients (*see*) increase the absorption of glycols and therefore their toxicity. Glycols have also been associated with eczema (*see*).

GLYCOPROTEINS • Sweet proteins from milk sugar.

GLYCOSAMINOGLYCANS • An ingredient in wrinkle creams. Derived from various animal tissues. *See* Mucopolysaccharides.

GLYCOSIDES • Many flowering plants contain cardiac glycosides. The best known are foxglove, lily of the valley, and squill. Cardiac glycosides have the ability to increase the force and power of the heartbeat without increasing the amount of oxygen needed by the heart muscle. Among the glycosides in plants are cyanogens, goitrogens, estrogens, and saponins. They are found in lima beans, cassava, flax, legumes, broccoli and other brassicas, most legumes, and grasses.

GLYCOSPHINGOLIPIDS • GSL. Sugary, fatty acid compounds, one of which was said to be developed by Christiaan Barnard, the pioneer heart surgeon, in Switzerland, to counteract wrinkles. Some companies, charging a great deal of money, claim their product contains Dr. Barnard's GSL, which can "accelerate cell renewal." If that were proven, it would have to be a drug, not a cosmetic.

GLYCYL GLYCINE • A combination of amides and amino acids (*see both*) used in hair conditioners and skin conditioners.

GLYCYRRHETINIC ACID • Used as a flavoring, to soothe skin, and as a vehicle for other chemicals. Prepared from licorice root, it has been used medicinally to treat a disease of the adrenal gland.

GLYCYRRHETINYL STEARATE • The stearic acid ester of glycyrrhetinic acid (*see*).

GLYCYRRHIZA GLABRA • The EU name for licorice.

GLYCYRRHIZIC ACID • Used as a flavoring and coloring, and to soothe the skin in cosmetics. Extracted from licorice, the crystalline material is soluble in hot water and alcohol. *See* Glycyrrhetinic Acid.

GLYOXAL • Oxaldehyde. Prepared by the oxidation of acetaldehyde (*see*), it consists of yellow prisms or irregular pieces that turn white when cooled. Used in the manufacture of cosmetics and as germicides and glues. Moderately irritating to the skin. Also may be a sensitizer. Based on available animal data and human experience, the CIR Expert Panel (*see*) concludes this ingredient is safe. It is being used as a safer replacement for formaldehyde (*see*) in an increasing number of compounds.

GLYOXYLIC ACID • Used as a coloring. Syrup or crystals that occur in unripe fruit, young leaves, and baby sugar beets. Malodorous and a strong corrosive. Forms a thick syrup, very soluble in water, sparingly soluble in alcohol. It absorbs water from the air and condenses with urea to form allantoin (*see*) and gives a nice blue color with sulfuric acid. It is a skin irritant and corrosive.

GNAPHALIUM POLYCEPHALUM • *See* Cudweed Extract.

GOAT BUTTER • The fat from goat's milk used in emollients.

GOAT MILK • The whole milk obtained from goats used as a skin-conditioning ingredient.

GOAT'S RUE • *See* Galega Extract.

GOATWEED EXTRACT • *See* Saint John's Wort.

GOJI BERRIES • *Lycium barbarum.* Wolfberry. Gou Qi Zi. *Fructus lycii.* Snow Berry. Goji berries grow on an evergreen shrub found in temperate and subtropical regions in China, Mongolia, and in the Himalayas in Tibet. They are in the nightshade (Solonaceae) family. Increasingly used in skin creams. The berries have been used in Asia for thousands of years. Tibetan medicine includes these berries in the treatment of kidney and liver problems. They are also used in Tibet to lower cholesterol, lower blood pressure, and cleanse the blood and to increase longevity. The berries have a long history of use in the treatment of eye problems, skin rashes, psoriasis, allergies, insomnia, chronic liver disease, diabetes, and tuberculosis. They are reported to contain eighteen amino acids (six times higher than bee pollen), more beta-carotene than carrots, more iron than spinach, and twenty-one trace minerals. They have a sweetish tart aroma. The berries also contain vitamins B_1, B_2, B_6, and Vitamin E and are 13 percent protein.

GOLD • Used as a coloring and to give shine to cosmetics. The soft yellow metal is found in the earth's crust and used in jewelry, gold plating, and in medicine to treat arthritis. The pure metal is safe, but the gold salts can cause allergic skin reactions. On the Canadian Hotlist (*see*). The EU has banned it in cosmetics.

GOLD OF PLEASURE • *Camelina sativa.* A European false flax cultivated for its oil-rich seeds. Also grown in North America. Used as a skin-conditioning ingredient.

GOLDEN SEAL • *Hydrastis canadensis.* Puccoon Root. Yellow Root. American Indians were the first to use it for sore eyes. Early pioneers, along with many Indian tribes, used it as a general tonic. The rhizome and root are used by herbalists to treat heartburn and acid indigestion, colitis, duodenal ulcers, heavy menstrual periods, and as a general tonic for the female reproductive tract. It is also used for penile discharge, eczema, and skin disorders. Herbalists claim it dries and cleanses the mucous membranes and is good for liver dysfunction and for all inflammations. It reputedly has potent antibiotic and antiseptic properties. It does contain berberine (*see*). It is contraindicated during pregnancy and for persons suffering from high blood pressure and ischemia (insufficient blood flow). The FDA issued a notice in 1992 that *H. canadensis* and hydrastis fluid extract have not been shown to be safe and effective as claimed in OTC digestive aid products and in oral menstrual products.

GOLDENROD • *Solidago virgaurea* is a perennial that includes 125 species. It was valued for its medicinal properties by women in Elizabethan London. The name *solidago means* "makes whole" and herbalists say it helps to heal wounds and, in fact, at one time it was called "woundwort." During the Boston Tea Party, the colonists drank goldenrod tea, which was nicknamed the "Liberty Tea." In the past, the oil was used for treating digestive disorders, throat problems, and disorders of the nervous system. It is used in eye shadow. It is used by herbalists as an antiseptic. The pulped leaves, stalks, and flowers are good for stanching blood. American Indians used it to treat bee stings. It is best not to use goldenrod oil on damaged and sensitive skin. It is a popular massage oil, but its producers suggest you do not use the oil on children or during pregnancy. It is also suggested you put the oil on a patch of skin before applying it, to eliminate possibilities of skin irritations and allergies.

GOOSEBERRY • *See* Phyllanthus Emblica and Melanin.

GOSSYPIUM • The EU name for cotton.

GOTU KOLA • *Centella asiastica.* Thickleaved. Pennywort. An herb grown in Pakistan, India, Malaysia, and parts of eastern Europe, it is commonly used for diseases of the skin, blood, and nervous system. In homeopathy, it is used for psoriasis, cervicitis, pruritus vaginitis, blisters, and other skin conditions. Gotu kola is used in the Far East to treat leprosy and tuberculosis. It is also used as a sedative.

GOURD EXTRACT • The extract of various species of Cucurbitaceae.

GRAM • g. A metric unit of mass. One U.S. ounce equals 28.4 grams; one U.S. pound equals 454 grams. There are 1,000 milligrams (mg) in one gram.

GRAMICIDIN • Cortisporin Cream. Mycolog II Cream. Neosporin Ophthalmic Solution. Spectrocin Ointment. Introduced in 1949, it is a naturally occurring antibiotic produced by bacteria. Available only in combined preparations, it is used with other antibiotics to treat skin and eye infections. Some gramicidin medications contain corticosteroids (*see*) to relieve itching and inflammation. Gramicidin is also combined with antifungal drugs such as nystatin (*see*) to treat mixed fungal and bacterial infections. May cause rash and irritation in some people.

GRAPE EXTRACT • The extract of the pulp of *Vitis vinifera* used as a coloring.

GRAPE JUICE • The liquid expressed from fresh grapes used as a coloring.

GRAPE LEAF EXTRACT • The extract obtained from the leaves of *Vitis vinifera.*

GRAPEFRUIT EXTRACT • The extract of the seeds of the grapefruit, *Citrus paradisi.*

GRAPEFRUIT JUICE • The liquid expressed from the fresh pulp of *Citrus paradisi.*

GRAPEFRUIT OIL • *Citrus grandis.* An ingredient in fragrances obtained by expression from the fresh peel of the grapefruit. The yellow, sometimes reddish liquid is also used in fruit flavorings.

GRAPEFRUIT PEEL EXTRACT • The extract of *Citrus decumana* or *C. paradisi.* See Grapefruit Oil.

GRAPE-SEED OIL • A vegetable oil pressed from the seeds of *Vitis vinifera* grapes. It is used for massage oil, hair products, body hygiene creams, lip balm, and hand creams.

GRAPHITE • Black Lead. Obtained by mining, especially in Canada and Ceylon. Usually soft, black, lustrous scales. A pigment for cosmetics. Also used in lead pencils, stone polish, and as an explosive. The dust is mildly irritating to the lungs. No longer permitted in cosmetics.

GRAS • The Generally Recognized As Safe list was established in 1958 by Congress. Those substances that were being added to food over a long time, which under conditions of their intended use were generally recognized as safe by qualified scientists, would be exempt from premarket clearance. Congress had acted on a very marginal response—on the basis of returns from those scientists sent questionnaires. Approximately 355 out of 900 responded, and only about 100 of those responses had substantive comments. Three items were removed from the originally published list. Since then developments in the scientific fields and in consumer awareness have brought to light the inadequacies of the testing of food additives and, ironically, the complete lack of testing of the GRAS list. President Richard Nixon directed the FDA to reevaluate items on the GRAS list. The reevaluation was completed, and a number of items were removed from the list. A number were put on a priority list for further studies, but as of this writing, nothing new has been reported. The GRAS status is designated for substances considered safe in foods. No testing is required for other routes of entry into the body other than in foods. Substances that may be safe for ingestion may not be safe for inhalation. In many industries, GRAS status is considered a blanket statement of the safety of a substance even though there has been little testing in other routes of exposures. Toxicity of a substance varies greatly on the route of administration. The fragrance industry uses GRAS status as an indication that a substance may be safely used to fragrance products. Yet GRAS status requires no safety testing of a substance's effect on the skin, the respiratory system, or on the nervous system. Dermal, olfactory, and respiratory pathways are the primary routes of exposure to fragranced products. Science has come a long way since January 1, 1958. Substances considered safe then are no longer considered so. Yet many remain on the GRAS list. So they are still widely used in the food and fragrance industries. In the case of flavors and fragrances, individual chemicals are not listed on the label, just the word *flavors* or *fragrance.*

GRAVEOLENS SATIVA MEAL AND BRAN • *See* Oatmeal and Oat Bran.

GRAY HAIR RINSES • To cover yellowish tinge that often appears in gray hair. Usually compounded with acids such as adipic or citric (*see both*) and color rinses such as Acid Violet 9 and Acid Black 52 (*see both*).

GREAT BURNET • *Sanguisorba officinalis. Poterium officinale.* Used in medieval medicine as an astringent herb to stop hemorrhages. Also used in salves for ulcers and wounds.

GREAT PERIWINKLE • *Vinca major.* An ever-blooming perennial herb or small shrub, it is popular in gardens. The tropical periwinkle is an example of a folk medicine that made its way into modern medicine. In 1953, Dr. Faustino Garcia reported at the Pacific Science Congress that the plant, taken orally, is a folk medicine in the Philippines for the treatment of diabetes. Researchers at the Eli Lilly Company screened the plant and found that it showed good anticancer activity in test animals. The result was the discovery of two alkaloids that are useful in treating cancer. It has also been found useful in treating diabetes. Periwinkle has been found to stop external hemorrhages, apparently because it contains tannins (*see*). The effects of controlling menstrual hemorrhaging may be due to vincamine, which dilates blood vessels.

GREEN 3 • CI 42053. Fast Green. Used in shampoos, bath products, cleansers, shaving products, underarm deodorants, hair conditioners, colognes, and hair colorings. *See* FD & C Green No. 3.

GREEN 3 LAKE • The salt of Green 3 (*see*).

GREEN 5 • CI 61570. Japanese name Midori 201. An antraquinone color. Used in many products including shampoos, deodorants, after-shave lotions, hair conditioners, hand and body lotions, and bath products. A coal tar (*see*) color that must be certified in the United States. *See* D & C Green No. 5.

GREEN 6 • *See* D & C Green No. 6.

GREEN 8 • *See* D & C Green No. 8.

GREEN BEAN EXTRACT • Extract of unripe beans of domesticated species of *Phaseolus.*

GREEN MOVEMENT • Active through Green parties in many nations since the early 1980s. The political term *Green,* a translation of the German *Grün,* was coined by die Grünen, the first successful Green party, formed in the late 1970s. The term *political ecology* is sometimes used in Europe and in academic circles. Supporters of Green politics, called Greens, share many ideas with the ecology, conservation, environmental, feminist, and peace movements. In addition to democracy and ecological issues, Green politics is concerned with civil liberties, social justice, and nonviolence.

GREEN SOAP • A liquid soap made with potassium hydroxide and a vegetable oil other than coconut or palm kernel oil.

GREEN TEA EXTRACT • *Camellia sinensis* Leaf Extract. The catechins in green tea were found to inhibit *Staphylococci* and *Yersinia enterocolitica.* Green tea extracts may make strains of drug-resistant bacteria more sensitive to penicillin. In vitro studies on particular antibiotic resistant strains of *Staphylococcus aureus* revealed that addition of green tea extract induced reversal of penicillin resistance. It was found that epicatechin gallate markedly lowered the minimum inhibitory concentration of oxacillin and other beta-lactams. Extracts of green tea were found to strongly inhibit *Escherichia coli,* *Streptococcus salivarius,* and *Streptococcus mutans,* microorganisms found in the saliva and teeth of people suffering from dental caries.

GRINDELIA • A coarse, bumpy, or resinous herb grown in the western United States. It has flower heads with spreading tips. The dried leaves and stumps of these various gum weeds are used internally as a remedy in bronchitis and topically to soothe poison ivy rashes. Grindelia contains resin and an oil used in cosmetics.

GROUND IVY EXTRACT • *Glechoma hederacea.* Alehoof. Benth. Cat's Foot. Devil's Candlesticks. Hale House. Hay House. May House. Hay Maids. Hedge Maids. Thunder Vine. Tun-Hoof. Common plant in wastelands, it is used by herbalists for coughs, headaches, and backaches caused by sluggishness of the liver or obstruction of the kidneys. It contains tannin, volatile oil, bitter principle, and saponin (*see all*). Mixed with yarrow, the herb makes a poultice that has been used by folk doctors for "gathering tumors" and to clear the head and relieve aching backs. The astringency of the herb helps in the treatment of diarrhea and hemorrhoids.

GROUNDNUT • *See* Voandzeia Subterranea.

GROUNDSEL EXTRACT • Extract of *Senecio vulgaris.* Any plant of the very large genus *Senecio,* widely distributed herbs and (in the tropics) shrubs or trees of the family Asteraceae (aster family). Many grow as vines. Most North American species have small, yellow, daisylike flowers; they are especially abundant in the Plains region. Some species of the genus are better known as ragworts. Used in the treatment of the hair and skin in compounds that comprise at least 5 percent weight of pulverized particles of at least one plant. Ragwort (*see*) was used as a menstrual flow wound healer by Native Americans and settlers. A few have been found to be poisonous to livestock, although others are useful for grazing. Cornell Medical Center–Sloan Kettering researchers reported that groundsel contains a potent and often fatal liver toxin. The common groundsel (*S. vulgaris*), naturalized from Europe, is one of the species that is sometimes cultivated. Used as a skin conditioner probably for its hormonelike activity.

GROWTH FACTORS • Naturally occurring proteins that cause cells to grow and divide.

GROWTH HORMONE • GHRH. HGH. Protropin. Somatonorm. Somatrem. Somatropin. A hormone produced in the front of the pituitary gland that stimulates the production of bone-forming cells and growth. A child whose body produces insufficient HGH will not reach normal height as an adult. Beginning in the late 1950s, such children were treated with HGH extracted from cadaver pituitaries. This not only was extremely expensive, but exposed youngsters to the risk of infection from viral contamination of the hormone. Today, genetic engineering technology makes available pure supplies of HGH. Somatrem and somatropin are laboratory-created versions of growth hormone. Research is continuing to find other beneficial applications of this product. In rare instances, growth hormone may induce the onset of diabetes mellitus or thyroid dysfunction. Growth hormone (GH) is illegal for off-label anti-aging use, according to an article in the October 26, 2005, issue of *JAMA*. This article reviews the literature concerning the uses and adverse effects of GH as well as the legal ramifications of selling, using, or prescribing it. Although GH has been documented to improve some measures of body composition, including increased muscle mass, decreased total body fat, improved skin elasticity, and reduced rate of bone demineralization, these positive effects may be modest and short-lived. Benefits have not been demonstrated on strength, functional capacity, or metabolism. Significant adverse effects reported with GH include carpal tunnel syndrome, glucose intolerance, diabetes, arthralgia, myalgia, peripheral edema, and elevated triglyceride levels. Long-term GH treatment has raised concerns of an increased cancer risk and the potentiating effects of insulin-like growth factors on cancer. When sold through Web sites, GH may be expensive, and in some cases distributed without physician supervision. Formulations may include tablets, sprays, or injectables, ranging in cost from $200 to $1,000 monthly. The Federal Trade Commission estimated that one Internet site generated more than $70 million in sales of pills and sprays purported to contain GH or to stimulate its production. In 2004, U.S. sales of GH totaled $622 million for nearly 213,000 prescriptions, not including Web site sales. Worldwide annual sales of GH are estimated at $1.5 to $2 billion. Corticosteroids (*see*) may make growth hormone less effective. There are more than one hundred companies selling tablets, sprays, and creams claiming the products include human growth hormone but if the products do contain the hormone, they could have adverse effects; if they don't, they are fraudulent.

GSL • *See* Glycosphingolipids.

GUAIACOL • Obtained from hardwood tar or made synthetically. White, or yellow, crystalline mass with a characteristic odor. Darkens when exposed to light. Used as an antiseptic both externally and internally. Ingestion causes irritation of the intestinal tract and heart failure. Penetrates the skin. Produces pain and burning and then loss of sensitivity when applied to mucous membranes. Causes the nose to run and the mouth to salivate. Deep irritant on the skin. Also used as a flavoring.

GUAIACUM OFFICINALE • The EU name for extract from guaiac wood. *See* Guaiacwood Oil.

GUAIACWOOD OIL • Yellow to amber semisolid mass with a floral odor. Soluble in alcohol. Derived from steam distillation of guaiac wood. Used as a perfume fixative and modifier, soap odorant, and in fragrances.

GUAIAZULENE • A color additive also called azulene. Permanently listed in 1978 as a cosmetic for external use only. *See* Azulene.

GUANIDINE CARBONATE • Used to adjust pH (*see*) and to keep cosmetics moist. Colorless crystals, soluble in water, found in turnip juice, mushrooms, corn germ, rice hulls, mussels, and earthworms. Occurs as water-absorbing crystals, which are very alkaline. Used in hair straighteners and other hair products. It is a muscle poison if ingested.

GUANINE • Pearl Essence. Obtained from scales of certain fish, such as alewives and herring, by scraping. It is mixed with water and used in nail polish. However, it has been largely replaced with either synthetic pearl (bismuth oxychloride; *see* Bismuth Compounds) or aluminum and bronze particles. Lethal when injected into the abdomens of mice but not in humans. Permanently listed as a cosmetic coloring in 1977.

GUANOSINE • An organic compound that is found in the pancreas, clover, coffee plant, and pine pollen. Usually prepared from yeast. It is used as a skin conditioner in skin care products and cleansing lotions.

GUAR GUM • Used in emulsions, toothpastes, lotions, and creams. From the ground, nutritive seed tissue of plants cultivated in India, it has five to eight times the thickening power of starch. Employed also as a bulk laxative, appetite suppressant, and to treat peptic ulcers. A stabilizer in foods and beverages.

GUAR HYDROXYPROPYLTRIMONIUM CHLORIDE • *See* Quaternary Ammonium Compounds.

GUARANA EXTRACT • *Paullina cupana*. The dried paste consisting mainly of crushed seed from a plant grown in Brazil. Contains about 4 percent caffeine. Used in anti-aging products and in cola flavorings for beverages and candy. *See* Caffeine for toxicity.

GUAVA • *Psidium guajava*. A small, shrubby, tropical tree that is widely cultivated for its yellow fruit. It is used in "organic" cosmetics.

GUEVINA AVELLANA • Skin-conditioning ingredient. *See* Hazelnut Oil.

GUM • True plant gums are the dried exudates from various plants obtained when the bark is cut or other injury is suffered. Today, the term gum usually refers to water-soluble thickeners, either natural or synthetic; thickeners that are insoluble in water are called resins. They are soluble in hot or cold water and sticky. Gums are used in perfumes, dentifrices, emollient creams, face powders, hair-grooming aids, hair straighteners, hand creams, rouges, shampoos, skin bleach creams, and wave sets. Gums are also used as emulsifiers, stabilizers, and suspending agents in cosmetics.

GUM ARABIC • Acacia Gum. The exudate from acacia trees grown in the Sudan used in face masks, hair sprays, setting lotions, rouges, and powders for compacts. Serves as an emulsifier, stabilizer, and gelling ingredient. It may cause allergic reactions such as hay fever, dermatitis, gastrointestinal distress, and asthma.

GUM BENZOIN • Used as a preservative in creams and ointments and as a skin protective. It is the balsamic resin from benzoin grown in Thailand, Cambodia, Sumatra, and Cochin China. Also used to glaze and polish confections.

GUM DAMMAR • *See* Damar.

GUM GUAIAC • Resin from the wood of the guaiacum used widely as an antioxidant in cosmetic creams and lotions. Brown or greenish brown. Formerly used in treatment of rheumatism.

GUM KARAYA • Sterculia Gum. Used in hair sprays, beauty masks, setting lotions, depilatories, rouges, powder for compacts, shaving creams, denture adhesive powders, hand lotions, and toothpastes. It is the dried exudate of a tree native to India. Karaya came into wide use during World War I as a cheaper substitute for gum tragacanth (*see*). Karaya swells in water and alcohol but does not dissolve. It is used in finger-wave lotions, which dry quickly and are not sticky. Because of its high viscosity at low concentrations, its ability to produce highly stable emulsions, and its resistance to acids, it is widely used in frozen food products. In 1971, however, the FDA put this additive on the list of chemicals to be studied for teratogenic, mutagenic, subacute, and reproductive effects. It can cause allergic reactions such as hay fever, dermatitis, gastrointestinal diseases, and asthma. It is omitted from hypoallergenic cosmetics.

GUM ROSIN • *See* Rosin.

GUM SUMATRA • *See* Gum Benzoin.

GUM TRAGACANTH • An emulsifier used in brilliantines, shaving creams, toothpastes, face packs, foundation creams, hair sprays, mascaras, depilatories, compact powders, rouges, dentifrices, setting lotions, eye makeup, and hand lotions. It is the gummy exudate from a plant grown in Iran and Asia Minor. Its acid forms a gel. It may cause allergic reactions such as hay fever, dermatitis, gastrointestinal distress, and asthma.

GUTTA-PERCHA • Gummi Plasticum. The purified, coagulated, milky exudate of various trees grown in the Malay archipelago. Related to rubber; on exposure to air and sunlight, it becomes brittle. Used in cosmetics as a film former. Used in dental cement, in fracture splints for broken bones, and to cover golf balls.

GYMNEMA SYLVESTRIS • The Hindi name for this herb is *gurmar*, meaning "sugar destroyer." Said to be effective at blocking the taste of sugar from the system. The active ingredient in gymnema is gymnemic acid, which is composed of molecules with a similar atomic arrangement to glucose molecules. Cosmetic astringent.

GYNOSTEMMA PENTAPHYLLUM • Cylindrica Extract. The leaves of this plant help to regulate body fat metabolism and supposedly can help you lose weight. Skin conditioner.

GYPSOHILIA PANICULATA • *See* Saponaria Extract.

GYPSUM • A widespread colorless, white, or yellowish mineral, $CaSO_4 \cdot 2H_2O$, used in the manufacture of plaster of Paris, various plaaster products, and fertilizers.

H

HAEMATOCOCCUSPLUVIALIS • Antioxidant, coloring and skin protectant. It is a ubiquitous, unicellular green alga that produces the carotenoid pigment, astaxanthin (*see*).

HAEMATOXYLON CAMPECHIANUM • *See* Logwood.

HAIR • An outgrowth of skin, hair emanates from structures called follicles, of which the body has some 5 million—100,000 on the scalp alone, at least in youth. By the time a hair emerges into view from its follicle deep beneath the skin, it is dead; its cells are no longer capable of dividing to produce new hair. Hair texture depends on the diameter and shape of the hair's follicle and the proportion of hardshell cuticle in the hair's makeup. If the hair and its follicle are small in diameter, the hair will be fine. Whether it is straight or curly depends on how the cells in the follicle grow. An even growth pattern in the follicle produces straight hair, and an uneven pattern produces curly hair. *See also* Cellular Membrane Complex.

HAIR BLEACH • Among the most ancient of cosmetic preparations the Roman maidens used were various native minerals, such as quicklime mixed with lime, to produce reddish gold tresses. The most widely used bleach today is simply hydrogen peroxide. It has been employed to bleach hair since 1867. Reports of problems with hair bleach include nausea, burned scalp, severe life-threatening allergic reactions, and swelling of the face.

HAIR COLOR RINSE • This is a temporary hair color that covers the cuticle layer of the hair only and does not affect natural color pigment inside the hair shaft. Used after shampooing, it is usually washed out with the next shampooing. There are color shampoos formulated with a synthetic detergent and color, and there are powders, crayons, wave sets, and lacquers that are also used for temporary coloring. The most common color rinses today combine azo dyes (*see*). Acids used in hair color rinses are usually citric and tartaric. The rinses may also contain fatty acids, alcohols or amides, borax, glycols, thickening ingredients, and isopropyl alcohol. Recent complaints to the FDA about hair rinses include ear numbness, headaches, and hair turning the wrong color. One of the problems with hair rinses is that when customers are allergic to permanent dyes, they become allergic to rinses, although the chemicals are not the same.

HAIR COLORING • Permanent hair-coloring products change the color of the hair. They cannot be shampooed away but remain until the hair grows out or is cut off. The root hair must be "retouched" as it grows in. There are basically three types: natural organics, synthetics, and metallics. Natural organics such as henna and chamomile have been used for centuries to color hair. Such dyes are placed on the hair and removed when the desired shade has been obtained. They are more difficult to apply, less reliable than manufactured dyes, and less predictable as far as color is concerned. They can cause allergic reactions to specific ingredients but are harmless otherwise. Synthetic dyes such as para- or amino derivatives work by oxidation—that is, they are applied cold and depend on the development of the shade by the action of a compound such as hydrogen peroxide to liberate oxygen. They frequently cause skin rashes and allergic skin reactions, and the laws in most states require that patch testing be done before use. This means applying the dye to the skin twenty-four hours in advance to see if any irritation or reaction occurs. This precaution is rarely observed. Furthermore, there is evidence that *p*-phenylenediamine products may cause cancer. Semipermanent dyes, which also carry a warning to patch-test, require no mixing before use; there is a notice that they will last only for several shampoos. Metallic hair dyes offer no shade selection and directions indicate they develop gradually with each use.

Recent reports of injuries from hair coloring to the FDA include scalp irritation, hair breakage and loss, contact dermatitis, swelling of the face, and itching. In 1977, the National Cancer Institute reported that studies on laboratory animals showed those fed large amounts of hair dye developed thyroid and skin tumors. The agency warned that the studies indicated potential cancer danger to women who might absorb cancer-causing ingredients through their scalps. In 1978, a New York University Medical Center researcher reported that a study of 129 women with breast cancer and 193 without showed that the breast tumors were more likely to develop among hair-dye users who would otherwise be considered "at lower natural risks" for breast cancer. The cancers appeared about ten years after dyes were in use. The cosmetics manufacturers voluntarily removed 4MMPD, the dye ingredient known to be a cancer-causing ingredient. However, others in the phenylalanine group and other coal tar derivatives remain and women continue to dye their hair.

In 1979, the FDA attempted to force cosmetics manufacturers to include a cancer warning for coal tar hair dyes containing 4-methoxy-O-phenylenediamine, 2,4-diaminoanis. Japanese researchers showed that another hair dye intermediate, 2,4-diaminotoluene (2,4-DAT), caused cancer in animals. It was removed from most hair dyes in 1971 but was still a part of seven dyes in late 1977. The National Cancer Institute data shows that two other hair dye components cause cancer in laboratory animals: 2-nitro-*p*-phenylenediamine, contained in at least 354 hair dyes in 1979, and 4-amino-2-nitrophenol, contained in at least 90 hair dyes. Six other hair dye ingredients are positive on the AMES test, which shows 150 of 169 permanent hair dyes are mutagenic. The AMES test used genetic damage in bacteria as a signal that a chemical is potentially carcinogenic.

Available evidence indicates that chemicals related to hair dyes can be absorbed through the skin and distributed throughout the body in small but significant amounts. The scalp is a good route for absorption of hair dyes into the system because it is a large surface with a large number of sebaceous glands. In 1998, an eight-year retrospective survey of 4,108 persons by a University of San Francisco researcher under a grant from the NIC found that hair coloring wasn't linked to any cancers in women. There was a "slightly higher non-Hodgkin's lymphoma" rate in men who used semipermanent hair dye frequently. The NCI and the American Cancer Society continue to study the dark hair dyes, and their research results are expected soon. The FDA does not permit sale or distribution of a colorant that it has not approved. The exception to this ban concerns coal tar hair dyes whose labels display the following: "Caution: This product contains ingredients which may cause skin irritation on certain individuals and a preliminary test according to accompanying directions should first be made. This product must not be used for dyeing eyelashes or eyebrows; to do so may cause blindness." Semipermanent dyes penetrate into the hair shaft and do not rinse off with water, as do temporary colorings. They do wash out of the hair after several shampoos. Semipermanent dyes usually come in liquid, gel, or aerosol foam forms. Temporary hair colors are applied in the form of rinses, gels, mousses, and sprays. These products merely sit on the surface of the hair and are usually washed out with the next shampoo, although some may last two to three washings. If the hair gets wet during a rainstorm, for example, the color can run from the hair onto the face or clothing. Gradual or progressive dyes are in the form of a rinse. They slightly darken the hair by binding to compounds on the hair's surface. Gradual dyes are usually applied daily until the desired shade is achieved. Unlike temporary dyes, gradual dyes don't wash off readily or run when the hair gets wet. Compounds suspected of causing cancer are found in temporary, semipermanent, and permanent dyes.

HAIR CONDITIONERS • Hair conditioners try to undo the damage from other hair preparations, particularly bleaches and dyes, and from the drying effects of the sun as well as the aging process. They include humectants, finishing ingredients, and emulsions. Hair is softened by water. Consequently, humectants bring moisture into the hair and reduce brittleness. Glycerin, propylene glycol, sorbitol, and urea (*see all*) help retain moisture and keep water from evaporating and consequently keep hair softer. Finishing ingredients, which include cream rinses, are added to shampoos or applied after shampooing. They leave a film on the hair to make it feel soft and look shiny. Isopropyl myristate and balsam are examples (*see both*). Emulsions, including cream and protein conditioners, are applied before, during, or after shampooing and sometimes between shampoos. They should be nonsticking and, if rubbed between the hands, they should disappear. Such products usually contain lanolin, alcohols, sterols, glyceryl monostearate, spermaceti, glycerin, mineral oil, water, and perfume (*see all*). The aerosol type of hair conditioner is made by preparing a "concentrate" from lanolin, isopropyl palmitate (*see*), perfume oil, and some propellant. Protein conditioners contain a protein (*see*), such as beer or egg, aimed at replacing lost protein. However, according to the American Medical Association, there is little, if any, evidence to substantiate this activity. There is no proof that protein from hair conditioners can penetrate the hair shaft and reconstruct healthy hair. If there is any effect, it is merely a coating similar to those of cream rinses (*see*). Except for individual allergies, hair conditioners are considered nontoxic.

HAIR DYE BANS • In light of the hair dye strategy, the European Commission considered the banning of 49 substances used in hair dye products by amending Council Directive in July 2007. These substances were proposed to be included in the "List of substances which must not form part of the composition of cosmetic products" under Annex II of the Cosmetics Directive. In view of safety concerns expressed in relation to the use of some hair dyes, the Commission agreed in April 2003, together with member states and the stakeholders, on an overall detailed strategy to regulate hair dye substances within the framework of the Cosmetics Directive. The strategy was published as an "Information note on the use of ingredients in permanent and non-permanent hair dye formulations (dye precursors and direct dyes)" on the following website of the Commission: http://europa.eu.int/comm/enterprise/cosmetics/doc/hairdyestrategyinternet .pdf. The overall objective of this strategy is to regulate the use of hair dye substances on the basis of a scientific evaluation of safety data according to the most recent safety requirements of the SCCP. The main element of the strategy is a tiered, modulated approach, requiring industry to submit, by certain deadlines, safety files on hair dye substances to be assessed by the Scientific Committee on Consumer Products (SCCP).

HAIR EXTRACT • An extract obtained from mammal hair. Used as a protein ingredient in hair products and emollients.

HAIR KERATIN AMINO ACIDS • Obtained by the hydrolysis (*see*) of human hair. Used as a hair- and skin-conditioning ingredient.

HAIR LACQUERS AND SPRAYS • These products "hold the set" and keep the hair looking as if it were just done at the beauty parlor. Once this was strictly a woman's product, but men now freely spray their hair. Hair lacquers usually come in either a plastic squeeze bottle or an aerosol. The early products contained shellac, and some still do. The shellac type is made by dissolving perfume in alcohol and adding shellac (the excretion of certain insects), and then adding a mixture of triethanolamine (*see*) and water. PEGs, lanolin, alcohols, and castor oil may also be included in the mixture (*see all*). The early shellacs made hair shine but caused it to be brittle to the touch. The addition of lanolin, castor oil, and glycol counteract this effect. The newer hair lacquers contain a product used as a blood extender in medicine—polyvinylpyrrolidone (PVP). Related to plastics and similar to egg albumen in texture, it slightly stiffens the hair to keep it in place. PVP is dissolved in ether and then in glycerin, and perfume is added. The solution may also include polyethylene glycol, cetyl alcohol, and lanolin alcohols (*see all*). Pressurized hair sprays contain PVP, alcohol, sorbitol, and water. Additional ingredients may be lanolin, perfume, shellac, silicone, sodium alginate, or vegetable gums such as gum karaya, acacia, or gum tragacanth (*see all*). The propellant is usually Freon, the same one used as a coolant in air conditioners. Most sprays can cause eye and lung damage and should be used with caution. The pump sprays are a better choice than aerosols because they are not as fine and, thus, not as easily inhaled. Complaints to the FDA about hair sprays include headache, hair loss, rash, change in hair color, throat irritation, suspected lung lesions, and death. In one case, the hair ignited after a cigarette was lit. *See* Aerosols.

HAIR RELAXERS • *See* Hair Straighteners.

HAIR RINSES • Aimed at improving the feel and appearance of hair. Usually made of water-soluble material that can be dissolved and dispersed after application. When water has evaporated, a deposit is left behind, which forms a film. Among ingredients used are gums, certain protein derivatives, and synthetic polymers. A basic cream rinse contains glyceryl monostearate, 3 percent; benzalkonium chloride, 3 percent; water, about 94 percent; perfume; and coloring. The American Medical Association maintains that cream rinses cannot repair damaged hair as claimed in advertisements. *See* Hair Conditioners.

HAIR SPRAYS • A study reported in 2008, which adds to a growing body of research into the potential health risks posed by certain phthalates, linked hair-spray exposure to a genital birth defect. Exploring the factors influencing the risk of developing hypospadias, a birth defect affecting the urinary opening of the penis, scientists raised the alarm about hair sprays. Hair-spray exposure more than doubles defect risk.

In research published in *Environmental Health Perspectives,* researchers said women who came into contact with hair spray at work in the first three months of pregnancy were two to three times more likely to give birth to a son with hypospadias. Affecting an average of 1 in 250 boys in the United Kingdom and the United States, hypospadias is common enough for a two- to threefold increase in risk to be significant. Scientists concluded hair spray was the cause after conducting detailed telephone interviews in the UK with 471 mothers whose sons had been referred to surgeons for hypospadias, alongside 490 controls. They asked the women a range of questions about their health and lifestyle, including their occupation and other activities to establish exposure to different chemical substances. Picking out hair spray as a risk-inducing factor, the scientists suggested that the presence of phthalates was to blame. They said that significant excess risk of hypospadias was found for boys of mothers exposed to phthalates at work compared with those with no exposure. Previous studies indicating that phthalates may disrupt hormonal systems and reproductive development were cited in support of this position. However, the scientists were careful not to jump to any definitive conclusions. Professor Paul Elliot, head of epidemiology and public health at Imperial College London, said: "Further research is needed to understand better why women exposed to hairspray at work in the first 3 months of pregnancy may have increased risk of giving birth to a boy with hypospadias." In response to the study, the Cosmetic Toiletry and Perfumery Association (CTPA) defended hair spray and the safety of diethyl phthalate (DEP) (*see*), which is the only phthalate allowed for use in cosmetics in Europe. The UK trade association said DEP had most recently been reviewed by the European Commission's independent scientific expert committee SCCP in March 2007 and was approved for safe use in cosmetic products. If you wish to evaluate the study, at this writing you could check

G. Ormond et al., "Endocrine Disruptors in the Workplace, Hair Spray, Folate Supplementation, and Risk of Hypospadias: Case-control Study," *Environmental Health Perspectives,* November 20, 2008.

HAIR STRAIGHTENERS • Half the population wants curly hair, and the other half wants straight hair. There are three methods, none perfect, for straightening hair: pomades that coat the hair and glue it straight; the much-advertised hot combs and irons; and chemical straighteners. Pomades, of course, are the least effective but the least damaging. The hair relaxers do their work by breaking about one-third of the chemical bonds that twist strands into curls, usually by hydrolyzing them with a 2 to 2.4 percent emulsion of sodium hydroxide. The emulsion reportedly not only coats the hair but invades it, causing it to swell up to 50 percent more than its original size. A water rinse then makes it swell even more. Heating the hair, when done properly at 300° to 500°F, does straighten the strands when tension is applied. Burns of the scalp are not uncommon, and the hair is dried out and may become very brittle. Chemical straighteners are effective but can cause burns, irritations, and hair damage. They usually contain either thioglycolic acid compounds (*see*) or alkalies such as sodium hydroxide, as well as polyethylene glycol, cetyl alcohol, stearyl alcohol, a triethanolamine, propylene glycol (*see all*), perfume, and water. The glycols and alcohols may be caustic. The thioglycolate curl relaxers require the application of a neutralizer to the hair to stop the straightening process. Although there are home hair-straightening kits, there is a fine line between enough straightening and too much. If possible, the procedure should be done by a professional. The alkali curl relaxants, which are more effective for kinky hair, straighten the hair in about five to ten minutes while a comb is run through. The hair is then rinsed with water to stop the chemical action. The FDA has received complaints about scalp irritation and hair breakage related to both lye and "no lye" relaxers. Both types can be caustic. Again, there is a fine line between enough and too much, and the procedure should be done by a professional. Alkali straighteners contain strong burning ingredients, and first- to third-degree chemical burns can occur. They can also cause allergic reactions and swelling of the face and scalp. The greatest danger from these products is eye damage. Extreme caution must be used to avoid contact with the eyes. The hair will become fragile with any form of chemical or heat straightening. Bleached hair is particularly susceptible, and straightening of bleached hair is usually not recommended. Recent reports to the FDA of injuries include scalp irritation, loss of hair, and scalp burns.

HAIR THICKENERS • *See* Hair Tonics, Lotions, and Thickeners.

HAIR TONICS, LOTIONS, AND THICKENERS • Hair tonics and lotions are designed to keep the hair in place and looking healthy. There are three basic types: alcoholic, emulsion, and drug/tonic. Alcoholics may consist of an oil mixed with alcohol, glycerin (*see*), and perfume. Emulsions may be made by heating mineral oil and stearic acid (*see*), mixing it with hot water and triethanolamine (*see*), and adding perfume. The tonic or drug-type hairdressing usually contains antiseptics and may affect the function or structure of the human body or are designed to treat a diseased condition. They also contain low concentrations of rubefacients (these are products that cause a reddening and thus stimulation of the skin). Antiseptics employed may be creosols, phenols, chlorothymol, or resorcinol (*see all*). There is another type of hairdressing, used mostly by men, which is similar to a wave set common to women. It contains natural gums such as tragacanth, and karaya, or sodium alginate with alcohol, water, perfume, and glycerol. Among other chemicals in hair tonics and lotions are benzalkonium chloride, betanaphthol, camphor oil, cantharides tincture, chloral hydrate, phosphoric acid, pilocarpine, glycols, quinine, sorbitan derivatives, salicylic acid, and tars (*see all*). Hair thickeners contain oils and proteins that coat the hair with an invisible film, thus giving it body. The thickeners make the hair feel smoother, and it is more manageable. A common hair tonic formula contains resorcinol, 0.8 percent; chloral hydrate, 1.5 percent; ethanol, 80 percent; beta-naphthol, 0.8 percent; Turkey-red oil, 16.9 percent; perfume; and color (*see all*). Complaints to the FDA about hair conditioners and dressings include hair loss, eye irritation, pimples, inflamed scalp, hair shrunk into knots, face irritation, dryness, and rash. The EU bans pilocarpine (*see*) and its salts in cosmetics.

HAIRDRESSERS • You wouldn't believe hairdressers are at risk at their jobs except from dissatisfied customers. Actually, in all seriousness, they are at greater risk of developing bladder cancer because of the chemicals present in the hair dyes they use daily, according to research published in the *Lancet Oncology*. The conclusion was reached by a panel of scientists at the International Agency for Research on Cancer (IARC) in Lyon, who were brought together in 2007 to review the evidence on the cancer link that has built up over the preceding fifteen years. In the report published, Dr. Robert Baan, the lead author said, "A small but consistent risk of bladder cancer was reported in male hairdressers and barbers." While the panel was agreed that regular occupational exposure to hair dye increased cancer risk, they found data on personal use inconclusive. The evidence was judged to be insufficient to make a definitive conclusion on the carcinogenicity of hair dye when exposure is limited to personal use. The scientists also reviewed the data related to the cancer-causing potential of aromatic amines and organic dyes and added the following chemicals to its list of probable and definite carcinogens. Among the cancer-causing agents suspected: ortho-toluidine, 4-chloro-ortho-toluidine (probably carcinogenic), 4,4′-methylenebis, and benzidine-based dyes. The report was to be published again in Volume 99 of the monographs of the IARC, which is an arm of the World Health Organization (WHO). The publication of the *Lancet* findings adds to the mounting body of studies. One reason that the known carcinogenic hair dyes are still used is that there are said to be no acceptable alternatives. Another reason is that ingredient labeling is not required on professional hairdressers' products.

HAKKA YU • Essential oil obtained from *Mentha arvensis. See* Wild Mint Extract.

HALOGEN • Elements that include fluorine, chlorine, bromine, and iodine (*see all*). Fluorine is the most active.

HALOGENATED SALICYLANILIDES • Pertaining to a substance to which a halogen is added. An efficient fluke and worm killer. These halogenated salicylanilides are deleterious substances that render any cosmetic that contains them injurious to users. Therefore, any cosmetic product that contains such a halogenated salicylanilide as an ingredient at any level for any purpose is deemed to be adulterated. Banned by the FDA. Halogenated salicylanilides (tribromsalan [TBS,3,4′,5–tribromosalicylanilide]), dibromsalan (DBS,4′5–dibromosalicylanilide), metabromsalan (MBS,3,5–dibromosalicylanilide), and 3,3′,4,5′–tetrachlorosalicylanilide (TCSA) have been used as antimicrobial agents for a variety of purposes in cosmetic products. These halogenated salicylanilides are potent photosensitizers and cross-sensitizers and can cause disabling skin disorders. In some instances, the photosensitization may persist for prolonged periods as a severe reaction without further exposure to these chemicals. Safer alternative antimicrobial agents are available.

HALOGENATION • Incorporation of one of the halogen (*see*) elements, most often chlorine or bromine, into a chemical compound. Halogenation plays a frequent significant role in establishing the bioactivity of a compound. For example, benzene is treated with chlorine to form chlorobenzene, and ethylene is treated with bromine to form ethylene dibromine.

HALOPTERIS SCOPARIA • Brown algae from Africa has antibacterial properties. Used in cosmetics as a skin conditioner. *See* Algae.

HAM • Abbeviation for Hamamelis Water.

HAMAMELIS WATER • *See* Witch Hazel.

HAND CREAMS AND LOTIONS • These are emollients, which apply easily and without stickiness. Most contain stearic acid, lanolin, and water. They may also contain cetyl alcohol, mineral oil, glycerin, potassium hydroxide, perfume, and glyceryl mono-stearate (*see all*). The newer formulas may also contain healing ingredients such as allantoin (*see*) and water-repellent silicones (*see*) to protect the hands against further irritation from water, detergents, or wind. Most leading hand creams and lotions are uncolored, though surveys show that pink or blue hand creams are preferred; women over twenty-five prefer pink and teenagers blue. The pH (*see*) level of most hand creams and lotions is between 5 and 8. A typical formula for hand cream contains cetyl alcohol, 2 percent; lanolin, 1 percent; mineral oil, 2 percent; stearic acid, 13 percent; glycerin, 12 percent; methylparaben, 0.15 percent; potassium hydroxide, 1 percent; water, 68 percent; and perfume in sufficient amounts (*see all*). A typical hand lotion contains cetyl alcohol, 0.5 percent; lanolin, 1 percent; stearic acid, 3 percent; glycerin, 2 percent; methylparaben, 0.1 percent; triethanolamine, 0.75 percent; water, 85 percent; and perfume in sufficient amounts (*see all*). Among problems reported to the FDA concerning hand preparations were rash, blisters, and swollen feet. Lanolin derivatives, colors, and perfumes, of course, are possible allergens.

HANDKERCHIEF PERFUMES • A woman's perfume in a retail shop. The name was derived from the practice of dabbing scent on a handkerchief to allow the sniffer to distinguish among perfume compounds.

HARD WATER • Contains minerals. The EU regulates the minimum amount of calcium content in drinking water. After hair is washed with hard water, minerals may remain and affect its texture. Conditioners are used to counteract its effects.

HARPAGOPHYTUM EXTRACT • The extract of *Harpagophyton procumbens*. Devil's Claw. Grapple Plant. Devil's Craw Root. A perennial herb introduced into North America relatively recently, it has been used in South Africa for more than 250 years. It is used there by the natives as a tonic for arthritis. In cosmetics, it is used for hand and body lotions.

HARUNGANA MADAGASCARIENSIS • A tree or shrub, with orange-colored sap native to Madagascar. Skin-conditioning ingredient.

HASLEA OSTREARIA • Blue Algae. A rich source of vitamin E, zinc, iron, and copper. It reportedly has a soothing effect on the skin. It is used in anti-aging products.

HATOMUGI SHUSHI EKISU • Seeds of *Coix lacryma-jobima*. Used as a skin-conditioning ingredient. *See* Job's Tears.

HAWAIIAN WHITE GINGER • From the roots of *Hedychium coronarium*. Used in "organic" cosmetics. *See* Ginger.

HAW BARK • *See* Viburnum Extract.

HAWKWEED EXTRACT • *Pilosella officinarum*. Mouse Ear. An extract of the various species of *Hieracium*, its ingredients include coumarin, flavones, and flavonoids. Small plant with yellow flowers. Is slightly astringent and anti-inflammatory. It is used for respiratory problems where there is inflammation and a lot of mucus being formed. It has been used in poultices for wound healing. Used in skin-conditioning and facial masks.

HAWTHORN BERRY • *Crataegus oxycantha*. Mayblossom. A spring-flowering shrub or tree. A number of scientific studies in central Europe and the United States have found hawthorn berries can dilate the blood vessels and lower blood pressure. It has been used in Canada in poultices to reduce inflammation. They are used in "organic" cosmetics and in products to relieve acne. The berries reportedly can also increase the enzyme metabolism of the heart and make the heart's use of oxygen during exercise more efficient. Hawthorn extracts are also believed to have some diuretic properties. In the 1800s, the berries were used to treat digestive problems and insomnia. They do contain bioflavonoids, compounds that are necessary for vitamin C function and that also help strengthen blood vessels.

HAYFLOWER EXTRACT • An extract of hayflowers used in bath salts.

HAZEL EXTRACT • Extract of the leaves of the European nut *Corylus avellana* or *C. americana*. The hazelnut is in the family Betulaceae, which also contains birches, alders, and hornbeams. The hazelnut bears a certain resemblance to these other trees, particularly to the alder. The hazelnut had many uses as a magical tree: in Ireland, sticks of hazelnut protected the carrier against snakes, spirits and evil, and abduction by fairies. The Irish also believed a hazelnut in the pocket warded off rheumatism or lumbago, which is an elf-shot disease. A stalk of hazel with two nuts on it is supposed to cure toothache in England. Hazelnut was one of the magical, protective plants brought into the house on May Day, along with hawthorn and rowan. The hazelnut was regarded as the Tree of Knowledge in Ireland, and so it was the proper material for all rods of power. The hazelnut was a medieval symbol of fertility; perhaps this is related to the old symbolism of nuts as testicles. Used as a "brewed coffee" flavoring.

HAZELNUT OIL • The oil obtained from the various species of the hazelnut tree, genus *Corylus*. Used as a greaseless emollient.

HC • The abbreviation for hair color.

HC BLUE NO. 1 • Commercial hair coloring. Associated with fetal bone abnormalities in rats. In male rats, liver cancers occurred. Mice of both sexes also showed liver cancer in feeding studies. Based upon available data, the CIR Expert Panel (*see*) concludes that HC Blue No. 1 is not safe for use in cosmetics because of possible carcinogenicity. *See p*-Phenylenediamine and Colors.

HC BLUE NO. 2 • Commercial hair coloring. Found in hair dyes at around 1.7 percent and in human volunteers, less than one-tenth of 1 percent was absorbed over a period of thirty days. A National Toxicology Program oral-feeding study showed this to be nontoxic. It also was nonirritating in animals. On the basis of available data, the CIR Expert Panel (*see*) concluded this is safe for use in cosmetics. *See p*-Phenylenediamine and Colors.

HC BLUE NO. 4 • A reaction product of diaminoanthraquinone, epichlorohydrin, and diethanolamine. It contains benzenediamine. *See p*-Phenylenediamine.

HC BLUE NO. 5 • A reaction product of 2-nitro-*p*-phenylenediamine, epichlorohydrin, and diethanolamine. Contains benzenediamine. *See p*-Phenylenediamine.

HC BLUE NO. 6 • A commercial hair color. *See* Phenylenediamine.

HC BLUE NO. 7 • A commercial hair coloring. *See* Azo Dyes.

HC BLUE NO. 8 • A commercial hair coloring. *See* Anthraquinone.

HC BLUE NO. 9 • A commercial hair coloring. *See* Nitrophenol.

HC BLUE NO. 10 • A commercial hair coloring. *See* Nitrophenol.

HC BLUE NO. 11 • A commercial hair coloring. *See* Nitrophenol.

HC BLUE NO. 12 • A commercial hair coloring. *See* Nitrophenol.

HC BROWN NO. 1 • Capracyl Brown 2R. Commercial hair coloring. *See* Colors.

HC BROWN NO. 2 • A commercial hair coloring. *See* Azo Dyes.

HC GREEN NO. 1 • A commercial hair coloring. *See* Aniline Dyes.

HC ORANGE NO. 1 • 2-Nitro-4-Hydroxydiphenylamine. Commercial semipermanent hair coloring. While it may be a mild eye irritant, it has not been shown to be a skin irritant or sensitizer in animals. In humans, the concentrations of 3 percent tested produced no significant sensitization. The CIR Expert Panel (*see*) concluded that this is safe for use in hair dye formulations at concentrations up to 3 percent. *See* Nitrophenol.

HC ORANGE NO. 2 • A commercial semipermanent hair coloring.

HC ORANGE NO. 3 • 1-(2,3-Dihydroxypropyl)oxy-3-Nitro-4-(2-Hydroxyethyl)Aminobenzene. Used in hair dye. *See* Alkanes. May cause bladder cancer after long use.

HC RED NO. 1 • 4-Amino-2-Nitrodiphenylamine. Commercial semipermanent hair coloring. Nonirritating. Approximately 1.6 percent was absorbed through the skin in laboratory tests. On the basis of the animal and clinical data, the CIR Expert Panel (*see*) concluded that this is safe for use in hair-dye formulations at concentrations less than 0.5 percent. *See* p-Phenylenediamine and Colors.

HC RED NO. 3 • NI-(2-Hydroxyethyl)-2-Nitro-*p*-Phenylenediamine. Commercial semipermanent hair coloring. Was mutagenic in the Ames Test (*see*). In a two-year feeding study, there was no evidence of cancer in either male or female rats. There was equivocal evidence in male mice and inadequate evidence to make a judgment of cancer-causing in female mice. On the basis of the available data, the CIR Expert Panel concludes that this dye is safe as a "coal tar" dye ingredient at the current concentrations of use, with the condition that it should not be used in products containing nitrosating (*see*) ingredients. *See* p-Phenylenediamine and Colors.

HC RED NO. 7 • A commercial hair coloring. The CIR Expert Panel (*see*) has listed this as top priority for review. *See* Nitrophenol.

HC RED NO. 8 • A commercial hair coloring. *See* Anthraquinone.

HC RED NO. 9 • A commercial hair coloring. *See* Nitrophenol.

HC RED NO. 10 • A commercial hair coloring. *See* Nitrophenol.

HC RED NO. 11 • A commercial hair coloring. *See* p-Phenylenediamine.

HC RED NO. 12 • A commercial hair coloring. *See* Nitrophenol.

HC RED NO. 13 • A commercial hair coloring. *See* Nitrophenol.

HC RED NO. 14 • A commercial hair coloring. *See* Amines.

HC VIOLET NO. 1 • A commercial hair coloring. *See* Nitrobenzene.

HC VIOLET NO. 2 • A commercial hair coloring. *See* Benzene.

HC YELLOW NO. 2 • A commercial semipermanent hair coloring. Not a mutagen but can cause sensitivity. On the basis of the available data, the CIR Expert Panel (*see*) concludes that this dye is safe at concentrations up to 3 percent. The limitation on the concentration is based upon the available tests in humans. *See* Aniline Dyes.

HC YELLOW NO. 4 • Commercial hair coloring. Body weight decreases were found in animals given this ingredient by mouth. It did not produce irritation, sensitization, or photosensitization in animal tests. In some feeding studies, fetal toxicity was observed. It was mutagenic in several assays, but no evidence of cancer-causing was found in oral or skin studies. No sensitization was found in patch tests on two hundred human volunteers. Little HC Yellow No. 4 is absorbed through the scalp. On the basis of the available data, the CIR Expert Panel (*see*) concluded that this dye is safe. *See* p-Phenylenediamine and Colors.

HC YELLOW NO. 5 • N′-2-(Hydroxyethyl)-4-Nitro-*o*-Phenylenediamine. Commercial hair coloring. The CIR Expert Panel (*see*) has listed this as top priority for review. *See* p-Phenylenediamine.

HC YELLOW NO. 6 • Commercial hair coloring. *See* p-Phenylenediamine and Coal Tar.

HC YELLOW NO. 7 • A commercial hair coloring. *See* Coal Tar.

HC YELLOW NO. 8 • A commercial hair coloring. *See* Coal Tar.

HC YELLOW NO. 9 • A commercial hair coloring. *See* Nitrophenol.

HC YELLOW NO. 10 • A commercial hair coloring. *See* p-Phenylenediamine.

HC YELLOW NO. 11 • A commercial hair coloring. *See* p-Phenylenediamine.

HC YELLOW NO. 12 • A commercial hair coloring. *See* Nitrophenol. Proposed for a ban by the EU.

HC YELLOW NO. 13 • A commercial hair coloring. *See* Aniline.
HC YELLOW NO. 14 • A commercial hair coloring. *See* Nitrobenzene.
HC YELLOW NO. 15 • A commercial hair coloring. *See* Amines.
HCL • Abbreviation for hydrochloride.
HDI/TRIMETHYLOL HEXYLLACTONE CROSSPOLYMER • Used as an anticaking ingredient. *See* Isocyanate and Polymers.
HEALING INGREDIENTS • Medications added to hand creams and lotions (*see*) to treat chapped and irritated hands. Allantoin (*see*) is probably the most widely used healing ingredient in hand creams and lotions. Urea (*see*) has also been used.
HEART EXTRACT • The extract of animal heart tissue.
HEART HYDROLYSATE • The heart hydrolysate derived by acid, enzyme, or other method of hydrolysis.
HEATHER EXTRACT • An extract of *Calluna vulgaris,* also called ling extract. An evergreen shrub that grows in sandy, slightly acidic grasslands and woodlands, heather is a multifunctional plant. It serves as a food source for several mammals, reptiles, and insects; people have also used it in folk remedies. Heather contains anti-inflammatory, antioxidant, and antimicrobial materials. Traditionally, heather has been used to treat bronchitis, circulatory disorders, bile deficiency, open wounds, insomnia, hypotension, and many other ailments. The flowers and stems of heather are often dried and used in teas. The dried herb is also used in aromatherapies and hot baths for soaking sore feet or aching muscles. Scientific research has even demonstrated that components of the heather plant have antiproliferative effects on HL60 (human leukemia) cancer cells. It is also being promoted as an "anti-aging" compound in cosmetics.
HECTORITE • An emulsifier and extender. A clay consisting of silicate of magnesium and lithium, it is used in hair bleaches and in foundations and eyeliners. The dust can be irritating to the lungs.
HEDGE PARSLEY EXTRACT • Extract of the herb *Anthriscus sylvestris.*
HEDRA HELIX • Ivy Extract. Golden Ingot. Stimulant and toning agent primarily used in anti-aging creams. A mild irritant, it reportedly stimulates and tightens. Has been used by homeopathic physicians to treat cataracts, blood vessels, menstrual pain, and brain pressure as well as depression and skin irritation. May cause contact dermatitis (*see*).
HEDTA • Hydroxyethyl Ethylenediamine Triacetic Acid. A liquid with an ammonia odor, it is used as a chelating (*see*) ingredient in permanent waves. Low toxicity.
HEDYCHIUM SPICATUM EXTRACT • White Ginger. *See* Ginger.
HEILMOOR CLAY • Natural therapeutic mud containing high amounts of humic acids (humus) and extracted from deposits in lower Austria. It is used in cosmetics for beauty, face, and body treatments and as an additive for bath products. Nontoxic if sanitized.
HELICHRYSUM • *See* Everlasting Extract.
HELIOTROPE • Desert Heliotrope. Bluish purple flowers on a stem that coils in the shape of a fiddle neck. It grows throughout the southwestern United States and is a frequent cause of allergic contact dermatitis on the legs and ankles of persons walking through the desert.
HELIOTROPIN • Heliotropine. Piperonal. A purple diazo dye used in perfumery and soaps. Consists of colorless, lustrous crystals that have a heliotrope odor. Usually made from the oxidation of piperic acid. Ingestion of large amounts may cause central nervous system depression. Applications to the skin may cause allergic reactions and skin irritations. Not recommended for use in cosmetics or perfumes.
HELIX • Ivy. Duck Foot. Woody evergreen or vine that is poisonous by ingestion. Widely used as a skin conditioner in body, face, hair, and hand products and bathing

products. Application for insect bites. Can cause severe skin rashes including blisters and itching.

HELLEBORE • Perennial herbs of the lily family having thick toxic rhizomes. A genus of perennial herbs (*Helleborus*) of the crowfoot family, mostly having powerfully cathartic and even poisonous qualities. *H. niger* is the European black hellebore, or Christmas rose, blossoming in winter or earliest spring. *H. officinalis* was the hellebore of the ancients. *See* Veratum.

HEMA • *See* Methacrylates.

HEMATIN • The iron-containing portion of blood. Used as an anticaking ingredient.

HEMATITE • Used in skin creams to "strengthen the skin."

HEMEROCALLIS FULVA • *See* Water Lily.

HEMLOCK OIL • Spruce Oil. A natural flavoring extract from North American or Asian nonpoisonous hemlock. Used in fruit, root beer, and spice flavorings for beverages, ice cream, ices, candy, baked goods, gelatin desserts, puddings, and chewing gum.

HEMOGLOBIN • The red blood cells that carry oxygen from the lungs to the tissues where the oxygen is released.

HEMOLYMPH EXTRACT • An extract of crustacean blood.

HENNA • *Lawsonia inermia*. Henna Leaves. An ancient hair cosmetic obtained from the ground-up dried leaves and stems of a shrub found in North Africa and the Near East. A paste of henna and water is applied directly to the hair, and a reddish color is produced. Allergic skin rashes may occur. Those who are allergic to other dyes may be able to use henna without problems. Although it is rather messy and unpredictable to use, there is renewed interest in the dye because of the desire to return to "natural" products rather than using man-made cosmetics. The FDA ruled that henna is safe for coloring hair only. It may not be used for coloring eyelashes or eyebrows or in the area of the eyes. Permanently listed in 1965.

HEPARIN SALTS • An ingredient that prevents blood coagulation derived from beef, lung, or porcine intestinal mucosa. It is used to prevent lumping in cosmetics. In medicine, it is used to prevent and to treat deep vein blood clots, blood clots to the lung, and to treat heart attacks. It is used to flush and maintain in-dwelling catheters. Potential adverse reactions include hemorrhage, irritation, mild pain, and hypersensitivity reactions, including chills, fever, itching, runny nose, burning of feet, red eyes, tearing, joint pain, and hives.

HEPTADECADEINYL FURAN • A skin-conditioning ingredient. *See* Avocado.

N-HEPTADECANOL • Colorless liquid, slightly soluble in water. Used in perfume fixatives, soaps, and cosmetics, and in the manufacture of wetting ingredients and detergents. May be irritating to the skin.

HEPTANE • An aliphatic hydrocarbon. Volatile, colorless liquid derived from petroleum and used as an anesthetic and solvent. Highly flammable. Toxic by inhalation.

HEPTANOIC ACID • Enanthic Acid. Found in various fuel oils and in rancid oils, it has the faint odor of tallow. It is made from grapes and is a fatty acid used chiefly in making esters (*see*) for flavoring materials.

2-HEPTANONE • Used in perfumery as a constituent of artificial carnation oils. Found in oil of cloves and in cinnamon bark oil. It has a peppery, fruity odor that is very penetrating. Heptanone is responsible for the peppery odor of Roquefort cheese. Can be irritating to human mucous membranes and is narcotic in high doses.

HEPTAPEPTIDE-6 • Promotes the activity of sirtuins, enzymes that are claimed by cosmetic companies to help rejuvenate aging cells by strengthening their DNA repair processes and stimulating production of protective antioxidants. In an article in the journal *Nature,* Harvard Medical School lead researcher Dr. David Sinclair reported, "It's looking like these sirtuins [*see*] serve as guardians of the cell. These enzymes allow cells to survive damage and delay cell death. . . . What we think is that if a cell is at a point of deciding whether to live or die, these sirtuins push toward the survival mode and let the cell try a little harder and longer to fix itself."

2-HEPTENAL • Green-grassy, herbaceous, spicy, fruity esterlike synthetic flavoring. Suggested use in apple, fruit, cucumber, pear, grape flavorings; also used in fragrances for fruity top notes; also geranium and galbanum. Oily, colorless liquid with a penetrating fruit odor made from castor oil. Used in perfumery, pharmaceuticals, and flavoring. UK has banned trans-2-heptenal in fragrances. ASP

1-HEPTYL ACETATE • Liquid with fruit odor used in artificial fruit essences. *See* 2-Heptanone.

HEPTYL ALCOHOL • 1-Heptanol. Colorless, fragrant liquid miscible with alcohol. Used in perfumery. *See* 2-Heptanone.

HEPTYL FORMATE • Used in artificial fruit essences. *See* 2-Heptanone.

HEPTYL HEPTOATE • Colorless liquid with fruity odor used in artificial fruit essences. *See* 2-Heptanone.

HEPTYL PELARGONATE • Liquid with pleasant odor used in flavors and perfumes. *See* 2-Heptanone.

HEPTYLCYCLOPENTANONE • A fragrance ingredient. *See* Pentanoic Acid.

n-HEPTYLIC ACID • *See* Heptanoic Acid.

HEPTYLUNDECANOL • Synthetic substance secreted by the jaw glands of queen bees to keep other bees from becoming rivals. Used as an emollient. *See* 2-Heptanone.

HEPTYLUNDECYL HYDROXYSTEARATE • Emollient. *See* Stearic Acid.

HERB ROBERT EXTRACT • Extract of the entire plant *Geranium robertianum*. *See* Geranium Oil.

HERBAL SHAMPOOS • Many contain saponins, a class of substances found in many plants. They possess the common properties of foaming, or making suds when agitated in water. They also hold resins and fatty substances in suspension in water. These products clean the scalp and reduce scaliness. Here is the typical formula for herbal shampoos: quillaja extract, powdered, 5 percent; ammonium carbonate, 1 percent; borax, 1 percent; bay oil, 1 percent (*see all*); and water, 92 percent. Saponins can be irritating when applied to the skin, and when given internally can cause nausea. Toxicity of herbal shampoos depends on ingredients and amounts used. The allergic potential of the shampoos also depends on sensitivity and the herbs used, as well as the other ingredients, such as quillaja bark and ammonium carbonate.

HERNIARIA GALABRA EXTRACT • Rupture Wort. Green Carpet. A small herb with tiny green flowers related to carnations. Believed to be good for hernias and has also been found to have water-reducing properties. Herniaria, a native of Europe, was used in the past for hernias and skin cuts. Extractives and their physically modified derivatives such as tinctures, concretes, absolutes, essential oils, oleoresins, terpenes, terpene-free fractions, distillates, residues, etc., are used in cosmetics.

HESPERETIN LAURATE • An antioxidant and humectant used in skin conditioners. *See* Phenols and Lauric Acid.

HESPERIDIN • A natural bioflavonoid (*see*). Fine needles from citrus fruit peel. Used as a synthetic sweetener. One of the most expensive skin creams claims to have hesperidin Smart Crystals, which is a nanotechnology (*see*) "that transports anti-oxidants to the skin and guards DNA's natural repair mechanism."

HEVEA BRASILIENSIS • Rubber Plant.

HEXACHLOROPHENE • An antibacterial formerly used in baby oil, baby powder, brilliantine hairdressings, cold creams, emollients, deodorants, antiperspirants, face masks, hair tonics, shampoos, and medicated cosmetics products. In 1969, scientists reported microscopically visible brain damage in rats from small concentrations of the antibacterial. The company that had the patent on hexachlorophene, Swiss-based Givaudan Corporation, sold the chemical only to those companies that could demonstrate a safe and effective use for it. Givaudan refused to sell hexachlorophene for use in toothpastes and mouthwashes. However, when the patents expired in the mid-1960s, the FDA allowed hexachlorophene to be used in toothpastes and mouthwashes. In 1971, the chemical was an ingredient of nearly four hundred products ranging from fruit washes to baby lotion. Chloasma, a pigmenting of the face, was reported in 1961 in persons who had used hexachlorophene-containing products. Coma was reported in burn patients washed in hexachlorophene products in 1968.

On March 29, 1971, August Curley and Robert E. Hawk of the U.S. Environmental Protection Agency (EPA) presented a paper in Los Angeles at the American Chemical Society meeting stating that hexachlorophene has been found toxic to experimental animals, capable of penetrating the skin, and present in the blood of some human beings. Tests on thirteen human volunteers showed hexachlorophene levels of one part in a billion parts of blood to 89 ppb. Curley, chief research chemist at the EPA at the time, said that the agency thought the material was absorbed through the skin. He pointed out: "For over two decades, hexachlorophene has been widely used as a bactericide in the United States. However, relatively little quantitative data is available concerning its dermal absorption in either experimental animals or humans."

On May 17, 1971, the American Academy of Pediatrics warned that products containing hexachlorophene that are intended for oral use, such as certain toothpastes or throat lozenges, may be poisonous to children. In December 1971, the FDA curbed the use of hexachlorophene-containing detergents and soaps for total body bathing. Winthrop, the makers of pHisoHex, which contained 3 percent hexachlorophene, sent out further information to doctors saying that the product should not be used as a lotion, left on the skin after use, used as a wet soak or compress, or transferred to another container that would allow for misuse. It should always be rinsed thoroughly from the skin after any use, should be used in strict accordance with directions, and should always be kept out of the reach of children. The FDA has limited it up to 0.75 percent. Products containing up to 0.75 percent will be able to continue on the market with a warning: "Contains hexachlorophene. For external use only. Rinse thoroughly." Still used as a germicide and deodorant in some cosmetics. According to the summary of the report included in the *Federal Register,* the cancer-testing program showed that hexachlorophene did not cause tumors in rats under test conditions. However, NIOSH (the National Institute of Occupational Safety and Health) says that short-term exposure may cause effects on the central nervous system, resulting in convulsions and respiratory failure, and repeated or prolonged contact with skin may cause dermatitis. Repeated or prolonged contact may cause skin sensitization. Repeated or prolonged inhalation exposure may cause asthma. The substance may have effects on the nervous system, resulting in tissue lesions and blindness. Animal tests show that this substance possibly causes malformations in human babies. It is on the Canadian Hotlist (*see*). The EU has banned hexachlorophene in cosmetics. Following is the FDA statement concerning hexachlorophene at this writing:

Cosmetics. Hexachlorophene may be used as a preservative in cosmetic products other than those which in normal use may be applied to mucous membranes or which are intended to be used on mucous membranes, at a level that is no higher than necessary to achieve the intended preservative function, and in no event higher than 0.1 percent. Such use of hexachlorophene shall be limited to situations where an alternative preservative has not yet been shown to be as effective or where adequate integrity and stability data for the reformulated product are not yet available. The component of a preservative system, whether hexachlorophene or other antimicrobial agent, should be selected on the basis of the effect on the total microbial ecology of the product, not merely on gram-positive bacteria.

(1) Adequate safety data do not presently exist to justify wider use of hexachlorophene in cosmetics.

(2) Antibacterial ingredients used as substitutes for hexachlorophene in cosmetic products, and finished cosmetic products containing such ingredients, shall be adequately tested for safety prior to marketing. Any such ingredient or product whose safety is not adequately substantiated prior to marketing may be adulterated and will in any event be deemed misbranded unless it contains a conspicuous front panel statement that the product has not been adequately tested for safety and may be hazardous.

HEXACOSYL GLYCOL • An alcohol used in skin products as an emollient. *See* Glycol.
HEXADECANOIC ACID • *See* Palmitic Acid.
HEXADECANOLIDE • *See* Palmitic Acid.
HEXADECENE • Solvent.
HEXADECYL AMMONIUM FLUORIDE • Oral hygiene product the EU calculates at 0.15 percent when mixed with fluorine compounds. Fluorine concentration must not exceed 0.15 percent, and the EU label says, "Contains hexadecyl ammonium fluoride." *See* Fluoride.
HEXADECYL METHICONE • A silicone wax. *See* Silicones.
HEXADECYL STEARATE • *See* Stearic Acid.
2-4-HEXADIENAL • Hexa-2,4-Dienal; 2,4-Hexadienal; 2,4-Hexadien-1-ol; 2,4-Hx; 1,3-Pentadiene-1-Carboxaldehyde; 2-Propylene Acrolein; Sorbaldehyde; Sorbic Aldehyde 2,4-Hexadienal. A colorless to yellow liquid with a pungent "green" or citrus odor, is used as a food additive for flavor enhancement, as fragrance agent, as a starting material or intermediate in reactions in the chemical and pharmaceutical industries, as a fumigant, and as a corrosion inhibitor for steel. 2,4-hexadienal was selected for study by the National Cancer Institute because of the potential for carcinogenicity based on its structure and the potential link between exposure to lipid (*see*) peroxidation products in the diet and human malignancies. Male and female rats and mice received 2,4-hexadienal in corn oil by stomach tube for sixteen days, fourteen weeks, or two years. Under the conditions of these two-year stomach tube studies, there was clear evidence of cancer activity of 2,4-hexadienal in rats and mice based on increased incidences of squamous cell neoplasms of the forestomach. The occurrence of squamous cell carcinoma of the tongue in male mice may have been related to the administration of 2,4-hexadienal. The NTP (*see*) Board of Scientific Counselors Technical Reports Review Subcommittee, October 18, 2001, accepted the toxicology findings. This additive, of course, should be banned. ASP
HEXADIMETHRINE CHLORIDE • *See* Polymer.
HEXAMETHYLDISILOXANE • *See* Disiloxane.
HEXAMETHYLINDANOPYRAN • A fragrance ingredient. *See* Benzophenones.
HEXAMIDINE • A preservative. The CIR Expert Panel (*see*) has listed this as top priority for review. May cause contact dermatitis (*see*). *See* Benzoic Acid.

HEXAMIDINE DIISETHIONATE • Organic salt derived from petroleum distillate (*see*) used as a topical antiseptic. May cause contact dermatitis (*see*). The CIR Expert Panel (*see*) has listed this as top priority for review.

HEXANE • *See* Paraffin.

HEXANEDIOL DISTEARATE • The diester of hexanediol and stearic acid used as a wax and a plasticizer. It is derived from ethyl alcohol and stearic acid (*see both*).

1, 2, 6-HEXANETRIOL • An alcohol used as a solvent. No known skin toxicity.

HEXANOIC ACID • A synthetic flavoring additive that occurs naturally in apples, butter acids, cocoa, grapes, oil of lavender. Moderately toxic by ingestion and skin contact. Severe eye irritant. Has caused mutations in laboratory animals. ASP

HEXANOL • Hexyl Alcohol. Used as an antiseptic and preservative in cosmetics, it occurs as the acetate (*see*) in seeds and fruits of *Heracleum sphondylium* and Umbelliferae. A colorless liquid, slightly soluble in water, it is miscible with alcohol.

HEXAPEPTIDE-1, 2 • Amino acids (*see*) used as a skin-conditioning ingredient.

HEXENAL • (Z)-3-Hexenal. Leaf aldehyde. A colorless liquid and an aroma compound with an intense odor of freshly cut green grass and leaves. It is one of the major volatile compounds in ripe tomatoes. It is produced in small amounts by most plants and it acts as an attractant to many predatory insects. It is also a pheromone (*see*) in many insect species. Hexenal, at concentrations found in food, exerts genotoxic effects in cells from rat and human gastrointestinal tracts. The UK has banned several hexenal compounds in fragrances.

HEXENE • Solvent. *See* Hydrocarbons.

HEXENOL • Liquid with odor of green leaves. It occurs in grasses, leaves, herbs, and tea. Used in fragrances.

HEXETIDINE • An organic compound used as an antifungal ingredient.

HEXYL ALCOHOL • Used in antiseptics and in perfumery. *See* Hexanol.

HEXYL CINNAMAL • A fragrance ingredient. *See* Cinnamal.

HEXYLDECANOIC ACID • A cleansing ingredient. *See* Decanoic Acid.

HEXYLDECANOL • An alcohol of hexyldecanoic acid. Widely used as an exfoliant (*see*) and as an emollient.

HEXYLDECETH-2, 20 • Emulsifiers. *See* Hexyldecanol.

HEXYLDECYL ESTER OF HYDROLYZED COLLAGEN • A hair- and skin-conditioning ingredient. *See* Hydrolyzed Collagen.

HEXYLDECYL LAURATE • Skin-conditioning ingredient. *See* Lauric Acid.

HEXYLENE GLYCOL • Solvent. A widely used aliphatic alcohol. *See* Glycols.

HEXYL LAURATE • The ester of hexyl alcohol and lauric acid. Used as an emulsifier.

HEXYL NICOTINATE • The ester of hexyl alcohol and nicotinic acid (*see both*).

4-HEXYLRESORCINOL • Used in mouthwashes and sunburn creams. A pale yellow, heavy liquid that becomes solid upon standing at room temperature. It has a pungent odor and a sharp astringent taste and has been used medicinally as an antiworm medicine and antiseptic. It can cause severe gastrointestinal irritation; bowel, liver, and heart damage has been reported. Concentrated solutions can cause burns of the skin and mucous membranes.

HIBISCUS • A widely distributed genus of herbs, shrubs, or small trees of the family Malvaceae, with lobed leaves and large showy flowers. The petals were used in folk medicine to soothe inflammation. Used today in "organic" cosmetics.

HIERACIUM PILOSELLA • *See* Hawkweed Extract.

HIEROCHLOE ODORATA • *See* Sweet Grass Extract.

HIGHLIGHTS • Streaks of colored, bleached, or natural hair that are lighter than the rest of tresses. The color can be temporary or permanent.

HIMANTHALIA ELONGATA • Seaweed containing vitamins A, C, and E as well as amino acids. Used in "natural cosmetics."

HINOKITIOL • The organic compound distilled from the leaves of arborvitae, it is a pale yellow oil with a camphor smell and is used in perfumery and flavoring. Low toxicity.

HIPPOPHAE RHAMNOIDES • Sea Buckthorn. A seaweed containing high concentrations of vitamins C, E, and A as well as carotenes, flavonoids, and fatty acids. Used in "natural cosmetics" as an antioxidant and to soothe skin ulcers and as a fragrance ingredient.

HIRUDINEA EXTRACT • Obtained from leeches. Used in emollients.

HISTAMINE • A chemical released by mast cells and considered responsible for much of the swelling and itching characteristics of hay fever and other allergies.

HISTIDINE • A basic essential amino acid (*see*) used as a nutrient. It is a building block of protein and used in cosmetic creams and permanent waves.

HO LEAF OIL • *See* Fo-Ti.

HO SHOU WU • *See* Fo-Ti.

HOKKAIDO AKAN CLAY • Clay from the volcanic area of Hokkaido Akan Caldera, Japan, it is used in skin conditioners.

HOLLY • *Ilex aquifolium* Extract. A small evergreen, the leaves were used to increase perspiration, to treat inflammations of the mucous membranes, pleurisy, gout, and smallpox. The leaves contain theobromine (*see*). The berries were used to cause vomiting, and as a diuretic to remove excess fluid. The juice of the berries was used to treat jaundice.

HOMEOPATHIC REMEDIES • In the search for "natural" or "new," consumers are increasingly buying "old" remedies. Homeopathic remedies often use highly diluted plant extracts and therefore fit the natural trend. Homeopathic cosmetics also support the idea of holistic beauty with the emphasis being on health and well-being from the inside and out. For topical applications, products fall into a gray area where they are not seen as drugs but must nevertheless be labeled carefully when marketed as cosmetics.

HOMOSALATE • Heliphan. An organic compound used in some sunscreens. It is an ester formed from salicylic acid and 3,3,5-trimethylcyclohexanol, a derivative of cyclohexanol. It is found in many Coppertone products. Although it is approved in the European Union, Australia, and the United States, it has not been tested by the agencies involved. The salicylic acid portion of the molecule absorbs ultraviolet rays with a wavelength from 295 nm to 315 nm, protecting the skin from sun damage. The water-resistant cyclohexanol portion provides greasiness that prevents it from dissolving in water. *See o*-Cresol.

HOMO SALICYLATE • *See* Salicylates.

HONEY • Used as a coloring, flavoring, fragrance, and emollient in cosmetics. Formerly used in hair bleaches. The common, sweet, viscous material taken from the nectar of flowers and manufactured in the sacs of various kinds of bees. The flavor and color depend upon the plants from which it was taken. It is probably the most popular nonsugar sweetener used today in many applications. The darker the honey, the stronger the flavor, which means that less can be used to arrive at the same sweetness level. Additionally, honey is a self-preserving material. China is the world's largest producer of honey.

HONEYDEW MELON JUICE • Liquid expressed from fresh honeydew. Used in "organic" cosmetics.

HONEYSUCKLE • *Lonicera caprifolium* or *L. japonica.* The common fragrant tubular flowers, filled with honey, that are used in perfumes. Honeysuckle is employed for infectious and inflammatory conditions. It is particularly useful for poison oak and other rashes. The flowers are considered harmless, but the fruits are toxic when used to excess.

Cases of severe but not fatal poisoning have been reported in children as a result of eating berries from this plant. Symptoms of poisoning are drowsiness, dilated pupils, sensitivity to light, and extreme weakness.

HOPLOSTETHUS • Orange Roughy Oil. *See* Fish Oil.

HOPS • *Humulus lupulus.* Silent Night. Widely cultivated, this plant has been used in folk medicine for its calming effect on the body. Contains an estrogenlike ingredient as well as volatile oil, bitter principle, and tannin (*see all*). It is used to relieve gas and cramps, and to stimulate appetite. Also used in a poultice to relieve sciatica, arthritis, toothache, and other nerve pain. It has been used to induce sleep and as a tonic in wine. Both Abraham Lincoln and England's King George III reportedly relied on hops to promote a restful calm at bedtime. Hop flowers were listed in the United States Pharmacopeia (USP) for ninety years. Contraindicated in depressive illness because it may exacerbate the condition. Excessive doses or chronic use may cause dizziness and intoxication.

HOPS OIL • *See* Hops.

HORDEUM DISTICHON • *See* Barley Extract.

HOREHOUND • *Ballota nigra* (Black Horehound) and *Marrubium vulgare* (White Horehound). Madweed. Black horehound was used by the English colonists as a medicine for gout and arthritis. White horehound, native to Europe and imported to the United States, was used in an herbal tea for sore throat and bronchitis. Black horehound is used occasionally by herbalists to get rid of lice, and when soaked in boiling water, it is applied to the skin to relieve gout and arthritis. White horehound, used by ancient Egyptian doctors who dedicated it to the god Horus, and now native to Great Britain and the United States, is used in cough drops and cold medicines.

HORMONE DISRUPTORS • A variety of chemicals have been demonstrated to have effects on hormone systems in animals and humans. Some of the adverse effects observed in animals, and to a lesser extent in humans, include:

• Reproductive effects/birth defects

• Cancer

• Low sperm count/sexual dysfunction

• Heart disease

• Cognitive disorders

• Sex reversal

• Premature puberty

Some of these chemicals are used in plastics, food production and packaging, pesticides, cosmetics, pharmaceuticals, detergents, and wetting agents.

HORMONE CREAMS • The cosmetics manufacturers claim that hormone creams containing estrogen or progesterone are cosmetics, and many dermatologists and some staff members of the U.S. Food and Drug Administration maintain they are drugs. Cosmetics manufacturers, ever aware of the human desire to stay young forever, have advertised the hormone creams as wrinkle preventatives and youthful skin restoratives. According to the American Medical Association, there is little scientific evidence that locally applied hormones can thicken the thinning skin of aging and that simple emollient creams may do a better job. In a review of the experimental data on the use of sex steroids in cosmetics, there was some evidence that topically applied steroidal hormones, both active and inactive biologically, do cause a slight thickening of aged skin. However, the effects are negligible, and in the amounts considered safe to use in cosmetics, topically applied hormones have no effect on human oil glands and oil secretion. Estrogen may be added at not more than 10,000 international units per ounce. Progesterone content may not exceed 5 mg per ounce. Enlargement of the breast in boys using an estrogen-containing hair lotion has been reported in the *American Journal of the Diseases of Childhood.*

HORSE CHESTNUT • *Aesculus hippocastanum.* The seeds of *A. hippocastanum.* A tonic, natural astringent for skin, and fever-reducing substance that contains tannic acid. Traditionally used by herbalists to reduce fever, it is also used by modern herbalists to treat varicose veins and hemorrhoids. The powdered kernel of the nut causes sneezing. The nuts reputedly contain narcotic properties. The seeds contain escin, which is used today as a sunburn protective. Escin is also widely used in Europe as an anti-inflammatory ingredient for a variety of conditions, including varicose veins. Escin has also been found to be a powerful diuretic to reduce excess fluid. Contraindicated during pregnancy and in cases of acute kidney dysfunction. Cases of severe poisoning occur most in children who have eaten the seeds. Symptoms include vomiting, diarrhea, incoordination, dilated pupils, depression, and even paralysis.

HORSE FAT • Fats and oils used from horses in skin conditioners.

HORSE NETTLE • Solanum. Bull Nettle. Radical Weed. Air-dried ripe fruit of *Solanum carolinense,* a South American nightshade plant. It is also grown in Florida. It is used as a skin treatment, sedative, and anticonvulsant.

HORSE TISSUE EXTRACT • An extract from the tissue near the horse's mane.

HORSEMINT OIL • Monarda. Water Mint. A tall, erect, perennial herb with hairy leaves and purple-spotted creamy flowers. Used in flavorings.

HORSERADISH EXTRACT • *Amoracia lapathifolia.* Scurvy Grass. The grated root from the tall, coarse, white-flowered herb native to Europe. A condiment ingredient. It contains vitamin C and acts as an antiseptic, particularly in cosmetics. It is applied by herbalists as a poultice to accelerate the healing of stubborn wounds. It is used for arthritis to relieve pain by stimulating blood flow to inflamed joints. Potential adverse reactions include diarrhea and sweating if taken internally in large amounts.

HORSETAIL • *Equisetum arvense.* Shavegrass. Silica. The American Indians and the Chinese have long used horsetail to accelerate the healing of bones and wounds. Horsetail is rich in minerals the body uses to rebuild injured tissue. It facilitates the absorption of calcium by the body, which nourishes nails, skin, hair, bones, and the body's connective tissue. The herb helps eliminate excess oil from skin and hair. It is a mild diuretic and was used to promote urination in heart failure and kidney dysfunction. The FDA issued a notice in 1992 that horsetail has not been shown to be safe and effective as claimed in OTC digestive aid products.

HOT OIL TREATMENT • Used to restore luster to bleach-damaged hair. The hair is completely doused with oil and then heated by a lamp or an electric cap. Oils include mineral and vegetable.

HOUSELEEK • *Sempervivum tectorium.* Native to the mountains of Europe and to the Greek Islands. Its longevity led to its being named "sempervivum," which means "ever alive." It has been used to treat shingles and gout, and to get rid of bugs. Its pulp was applied to the skin for rashes and inflammation, and to remove warts and calluses. The juice was used to reduce fever and to treat insect stings. Houseleek juice mixed with honey was prescribed for thrush, and an ointment made from the plant was used to treat ulcers, burns, scalds, and inflammation.

HOUTTUYNIA CORDATA • A showy plant that grows in wet areas. A lily, it has heart-shaped leaves.

HOVENIA DULCIS • Japanese Raisin Tree. Used in flavorings and as a skin conditioner. The fruit is edible.

HUMAN CELLS, TISSUES, OR ANY PRODUCTS OF HUMAN ORIGIN • Primarily used in anti-aging products. Banned in cosmetics by ASEAN.

HUMAN FIBROBLAST CONDITIONED MEDIA • Human skin cells grown in a medium in the laboratory supplemented with calf serum and used in skin conditioners.

HUMAN PLACENTAL ENZYMES • Enzymes derived from human placentas obtained from normal afterbirth. Used in hair and skin conditioners.

HUMAN PLACENTAL LIPIDS • The fats obtained from human placentas obtained from normal afterbirth. Used in hair and skin conditioners.

HUMAN PLACENTAL PROTEIN • Protein derived from the sac that surrounds the fetus. Obtained from normal afterbirth. When placental materials were first used as cosmetic ingredients in the 1940s, manufacturers promoted the products as providing beneficial hormonal effects such as stimulating tissue growth and removing wrinkles, although newborns emerge from the womb with wrinkled skin. The hormone content and tissue-growth and wrinkle-removing claims classified the placenta-containing products as drugs, and the FDA declared them to be ineffective and therefore misbranded. The FDA's challenge caused placenta suppliers to change marketing strategies by claiming that hormones in their placenta ingredients have been extracted and were no longer in the product. They then offered placental raw materials without medical claims—only as a source of protein. Placenta is used in some anti-aging creams.

HUMAN UMBILICAL EXTRACT • Used in anti-aging creams.

HUMECTANT • A substance used to preserve the moisture content of materials, especially in hand creams and lotions. The humectant of glycerin and rose water, in equal amounts, is the earliest known hand lotion. Glycerin, propylene glycol, and sorbitol (*see all*) are widely used humectants in hand creams and lotions. Humectants are usually found in antiperspirants, baby preparations, beauty masks, dentifrices, depilatories, hair-grooming aids, and wave sets. *See* individual substances for toxicity.

HUMULUS LUPULUS • Widely used in cosmetics. *See* Hops.

HYACINTH • *Hyacinthus orientalis.* Used in perfumes and soaps. It is the extract of the very common fragrant flower. Also used as a flavoring for chewing gum. Dark green liquid with a penetrating odor, the juice of hyacinth is very irritating to the skin and can cause allergic reactions.

HYACINTHUS ORIENTALIS • *See* Hyacinth.

HYALURONAN • *See* Hyaluronic Acid.

HYALURONATE • The salt of hyaluronic acid (*see*), a natural protein found in umbilical cords, in sperm, in testes, and in the fluids around the joints. *See* Hyaluronidase.

HYALURONIC ACID • Hyaluronan. HA. A sugar compound present in all connective tissue in vertebrates. Its function is to cushion and lubricate. In humans, it is found in high concentrations in the skin, cartilage, in the umbilical cord, testes, and in synovial fluid. Used in "rejuvenating" skin products and in injections to puff out wrinkles. In gel form, hyaluronic acid binds up to a thousand times its weight in water and provides volume to fill in larger folds of skin around the mouth and cheeks. It is added to lipstick because it is claimed that it helps keep lips moist and supports tissue. If there is a lot of swelling, cosmetics containing this ingredient may help because it absorbs moisture, and according to some dermatologists, it helps reduce spider veins, deeply hydrates, and plumps fine lines in any climate. Maintaining levels of HA, whether it be through supplements, topical applications, or injections, is said to reduce wrinkles caused by dehydration and general aging. Many cosmetic companies in the United States have focused on launching beauty serums that incorporate HA into the formulations in an effort to maintain skin smoothness and elasticity. Because of the complexity of the extraction process, the costs associated with producing it mean that it is destined to remain a premium product. A nonanimal form of hyaluronic acid has been approved for use as a wrinkle-filling agent in Canada, Europe, and Australia.

HYALURONIDASE • Wydase. An enzyme used in topical skin preparations to reduce bruising and to increase the absorption of other drugs. Potential adverse reactions include rash, hives, and local irritation. Local anesthetics increase the potential for toxic local reaction. Should be used with caution in patients with blood-clotting abnormalities, and severe kidney or liver disease.

HYBRID SAFFLOWER OIL • The oil derived from the seeds of a genetic strain that contains mostly oleic acid triglyceride, as distinct from safflower oil.

HYDANTOIN • Derived from methanol (see), it is used as an intermediate in the synthesis of lubricants and resins. It caused cancer when injected into the abdomens of rats in doses of 1,370 mg per kg of body weight and when given orally to rats in doses of 1,500 mg per kilogram.

HYDRANGEA MACROPHYLLA • Seven Barks. Widely distributed shrubs with clusters of showy flowers. The roots contain glycosides, saponins, and resins (see all). It is used by herbalists to treat inflamed or enlarged prostate glands, and for urinary stones or gravel associated with infections such as cystitis. In 1992, the FDA proposed a ban on hydrangea extract in OTC oral menstrual drug products because it had not been shown to be safe and effective as claimed.

HYDRASTINE • Found together with berberine (see), it is used to stop uterine bleeding and as an antiseptic. On the Canadian Hotlist (see).

HYDRASTIS CANADENSIS • See Golden Seal.

HYDRATED • Combined with water.

HYDRATED ALUMINA • See Aluminum Hydroxide.

HYDRATED SILICA • An anticaking ingredient to keep loose powders free-flowing. See Silica and Hydrated.

HYDRAZIDE • Derived from hydrazine (see). On the Canadian Hotlist (see). Banned by the EU in cosmetics.

HYDRAZINE • Made from chloramine, ammonia, and sodium hydroxide. It is a reducing agent (see) in cosmetics. Toxic by ingestion, inhalation, and skin absorption. Strong irritant to the skin and eyes and it is a cancer-causing agent. The EU bans hydrazine and its salts in cosmetics.

HYDRIODIC ACID • Strong acid similar to hydrochloric acid (see).

HYDRO-, HYDR- • Prefixes from the Greek word *hydor,* meaning water.

HYDROABIETYL ALCOHOL • Abitol. Colorless, tacky, balsamic resins. These products are used when a combination of properties such as color, low tackiness, and oxidation resistance are desired. Derived from rosin (see) acids that have had hydrogen added to reduce unsaturation. Used in eyebrow pencils. The UK banned it in fragrances. A sensitivity problem. Contact dermatitis. See Abietic Acid.

HYDROBROMIC ACID • A pH adjuster. See Bromic Acid.

HYDROCARBONS • A large class of organic compounds containing only carbon and hydrogen. Petroleum, natural gas, coal, and bitumen are common hydrocarbon products. Hydrocarbons such as petrolatum, mineral oils, paraffin wax, and ozokerite have been used in sunscreens, hand creams, lotions, and nail polish They are believed to work by forming a water-repellent film that keeps water from evaporating from the skin.

HYDROCHLORIC ACID • Acid used in hair bleaches to speed up oxidation in rinses and to remove color. Used in hair products. Also a solvent. A clear, colorless, or slightly yellowish, corrosive liquid, it is a water solution of hydrogen chloride of varying concentrations. Inhalation of the fumes causes choking and inflammation of the respiratory tract. Ingestion may corrode the mucous membranes, esophagus, and stomach and cause diarrhea.

HYDROCHLOROFLUOROCARBON, 22, 142B, 152a • Propellants and refrigerants derived from chlorofluorocarbon, any of several compounds composed of carbon, fluorine, chlorine, and hydrogen. Though they are safer than many propellant gases, their use has diminished because of suspected effects on stratospheric ozone.

HYDROCORTISONE • An adrenal gland (*see*) corticosteroid (*see*) hormone introduced in 1952, used to decrease severe inflammation, as an adjunctive treatment for ulcerative colitis and proctitis, for shock, and to treat adrenal insufficiency. Also suppresses the immune response, stimulates bone marrow, and influences protein, fat, and carbohydrate metabolism. Most adverse reactions are the result of dose or length of time of administration. Sudden withdrawal may be fatal. Contraindicated in systemic fungal infections. Potential adverse reactions include burning, itching, irritation, dryness, inflammation of the hair follicles, streaking, acne, rash around the mouth, spots of pigment loss, hairiness, allergic contact dermatitis, and, if covered with a dressing, secondary infection, atrophy, streaks, and blisters. Should be used cautiously in skin problems caused by viruses such as herpes and in fungal or bacterial skin infections. Should not be applied near eyes or mucous membranes, under the arms, on the face or groin, or under the breast unless medically specified.

HYDROCOTYL EXTRACT • Extract from the leaves or roots of *Hydrocotyle asiatica.* Widely used in body and hand preparations, night skin care products, and face and neck creams.

HYDROGEN PEROXIDE • Peroxyl. A bleaching and oxidizing ingredient, detergent, and antiseptic. Used in skin bleaches, hair bleaches, cold creams, mouthwashes, toothpastes, and cold permanent waves. An unstable compound readily broken down into water and oxygen. It is made from barium peroxide and diluted phosphoric acid. Generally recognized as safe as a preservative and germ killer in cosmetics as well as in milk and cheese. A 3 percent solution is used medicinally as an antiseptic and germicide. A strong oxidizer, undiluted it can cause burns of the skin and mucous membranes. A skin antiseptic used to cleanse wounds, skin ulcers, and local infections, and used in the treatment of inflammatory conditions of the external ear canal. It is also used in mouthwash gargles. The FDA issued a notice in 1992 that hydrogen peroxide has not been shown to be safe and effective as claimed in OTC poison ivy, poison oak, and poison sumac products. Canada does not permit it in dentifrices, mouthwashes, or "other" purposes that involve long-term use in the oral cavity but says it may be used for tooth bleaching if safety data has been submitted and concentration is limited to 3 percent and labeled for use for no more than fourteen days unless under the supervision of a dentist. It is on the Canadian Hotlist (*see*).

HYDROGENATED AVOCADO OIL • Used as a skin conditioner. *See* Avocado.

HYDROGENATED BRASSICA CAMPESTRIS/ALEURITES • A film former. *See* Rapeseed Oil.

HYDROGENATED BUTYLENE/ETHYLENE/STYRENE COPOLYMER • Hydrogenated (*see*) butylene, ethylene, and styrene. Used as a thickener.

HYDROGENATED CANOLA OIL • *See* Hydrogenation and Canola Oil.

HYDROGENATED CAPRYLYL OLIVE ESTERS • *See* Olive Oil.

HYDROGENATED CASTOR OIL • Used as a wax. *See* Hydrogenation and Castor Oil.

HYDROGENATED COCO-GLYCERIDES • Widely used in makeup such as eyeliners, foundations, eye shadows, and blushers. *See* Hydrogenation, Coconut Oil, and Triglycerides.

HYDROGENATED COCONUT ACID • *See* Coconut Oil and Hydrogenation.

HYDROGENATED COCONUT OIL • *See* Hydrogenation and Coconut Oil.

HYDROGENATED COTTONSEED GLYCERIDE • *See* Cottonseed Oil and Hydrogenation.

HYDROGENATED COTTONSEED OIL • *See* Hydrogenation and Cottonseed Oil.

HYDROGENATED DECYL OLIVE OIL • Hair conditioner. *See* Olive Oil and Decanol.

HYDROGENATED DIDECENE • A skin-conditioning ingredient. *See* Hydrocarbons.

HYDROGENATED DITALLOW AMINE • An amine derived from hydrogenated tallow acid. *See* Tallow.

HYDROGENATED EGG OIL • An emollient. *See* Egg Oil and Hydrogenation.

HYDROGENATED ETHOXYLATED LANOLIN • *See* Hydrogenation and Lanolin.

HYDROGENATED ETHYLBICYCLOHEPTANE GUAIACOL • Fragrance ingredient. *See* Guaiacol.

HYDROGENATED FATTY OILS • Used in baby creams and lipstick. *See* Fatty Acids and Hydrogenation.

HYDROGENATED FISH OIL • Skin conditioner. *See* Fish Oil.

HYDROGENATED GLYCERYL DEHYDROABIETATE/TETRAHYDROA-BIETATE • A skin protectant. *See* Glycerol.

HYDROGENATED HONEY • Controlled hydrogenation (*see*) of honey. Used in cold creams and cleansing lotions.

HYDROGENATED JAPAN WAX • Skin conditioner and thickener. *See* Japan Wax.

HYDROGENATED JOJOBA OIL • *See* Jojoba Oil and Hydrogenation.

HYDROGENATED LANETH-5, -20, -25 • *See* Hydrogenated Lanolin.

HYDROGENATED LANOLIN • A light yellow to white, tacky solid that is soluble in ethyl ether but insoluble in water. It retains the emollient and adhering characteristics of lanolin but loses the latter's odor, taste, color, and tackiness. Widely used in eye makeup preparations; colognes and toilet water; manicuring preparations; waving preparations; skin care preparations such as creams, lotions, powders, and sprays; and suntan and sunscreen preparations. *See* Hydrogenation. On the basis of the available information, the CIR Expert Panel (*see*) found it safe in the early 1980s but is considering new information to determine if the final safety assessment should be reaffirmed, amended, or have an addendum.

HYDROGENATED LANOLIN ALCOHOL • The CIR Expert Panel (*see*) found it safe. *See* Hydrogenated Lanolin.

HYDROGENATED LARD GLYCERIDE • *See* Lard and Hydrogenation.

HYDROGENATED LECITHIN • Widely used in skin conditioners, face powders, skin care preparations, and eye shadows. *See* Lecithin and Hydrogenation.

HYDROGENATED MENHADEN ACID • The end product of hydrogenation of the fatty acids obtained from menhaden fish oil.

HYDROGENATED MENHADEN OIL • The hydrogenated oil from the fish menhaden.

HYDROGENATED MICROCRYSTALLINE WAX • Hydrogenated (*see*) crystalline wax.

HYDROGENATED MILK LIPIDS • Skin conditioner.

HYDROGENATED MINK OIL • Emollient and Moisturizer. No reported adverse effects. *See* Mink Oil and Hydrogenation.

HYDROGENATED OILS • Vegetable and animal and fish oils treated with hydrogen. The oil becomes partially converted from naturally polyunsaturated fats to saturated. Makes liquid oils partially solid.

HYDROGENATED C6–14 OLEFIN POLYMERS • Low-molecular-weight polymers of olefin monomers. Olefin is a class of unsaturated hydrocarbons obtained by "cracking" naphtha or other petroleum products, and they are used in the manufacture of surfactants (*see*).

HYDROGENATED ORANGE ROUGHY OIL • The hydrogenated oil (*see*) from the orange roughy fish.

HYDROGENATED PALM GLYCERIDES • Widely used emulsifier in makeup and moisturizers. *See* Palm Oil and Hydrogenation.

HYDROGENATED PALM-KERNEL OIL • Used as a skin conditioner in makeup, suntan products, and moisturizers. *See* Palm Kernel Oil and Hydrogenation.

HYDROGENATED PALM-KERNEL OIL PEG-6 COMPLEX • *See* Palm Kernel Oil, Hydrogenation, and Polyethylene Glycol.

HYDROGENATED PALM OIL • *See* Palm Oil and Hydrogenation.

HYDROGENATED PEANUT OIL • *See* Hydrogenation and Peanut Oil.

HYDROGENATED POLYDECENE • A synthetic polymer (*see*) used as a fragrance ingredient and emollient used in shampoos.

HYDROGENATED POLYISOBUTENE • A synthetic polymer from hydrocarbon (*see*) widely used as an emollient and skin conditioner in makeup and body and hand products. *See* Isobutyric Acid and Hydrogenation.

HYDROGENATED RICE BRAN WAX • *See* Hydrogenation and Rice Bran Oil.

HYDROGENATED SHARK-LIVER OIL • *See* Shark-Liver Oil and Hydrogenation.

HYDROGENATED SOY GLYCERIDE • *See* Soybean Oil and Hydrogenation.

HYDROGENATED SOYBEAN OIL • Widely used skin conditioner in body and hand preparations and moisturizers. *See* Soybean Oil and Hydrogenation.

HYDROGENATED STARCH HYDROLYSATE • The end product of the hydrogenation of corn syrup. *See* Hydrogenation and Corn Syrup.

HYDROGENATED SUNFLOWER SEED OIL • A skin conditioner. *See* Sunflower Seed Oil.

HYDROGENATED TALLOW • A binder (*see*) in cosmetics. *See* Hydrogenation and Tallow.

HYDROGENATED TALLOW ACID • *See* Tallow and Hydrogenation.

HYDROGENATED TALLOW BETAINE • *See* Hydrogenation and Betaine.

HYDROGENATED TALLOW GLYCERIDE • *See* Tallow and Hydrogenation.

HYDROGENATED TALLOWAMIDE DEA • Surfactant. A mixture of fatty acids derived from hydrogenated tallow. DEA products are under investigation and potential cancer-causing agents.

HYDROGENATED TALLOWETH-12–60 • Mixture of polyethylene glycol and hydrogenated tallow. The numbers signify the viscosity of the ingredient.

HYDROGENATED TALLOWTRIMONIUM CHLORIDE • *See* Quaternary Ammonium Compounds.

HYDROGENATED VEGETABLE GLYCERIDE • An emollient to prevent the skin from losing moisture. Used in hair dyes and makeup products. *See* Vegetable Oils and Hydrogenation.

HYDROGENATED VEGETABLE OIL • Widely used in moisturizing preparations, eye shadows, hair products, cold creams, night care preparations, and cleansing lotions. *See* Vegetable Oils and Hydrogenation.

HYDROGENATION • The process of adding hydrogen gas under high pressure to liquid oils. It is the most widely used chemical process in the edible fat industry. Used in the manufacture of petrol from coal, and in the manufacture of margarine and shortening. Used primarily in the cosmetics and food industries to convert liquid oils to semisolid fats at room temperature. Reduces the amount of acid in the compound and improves color. Usually, the higher the amount of hydrogenation, the lower the unsaturation in the fat and the less possibility of flavor degradation or spoilage due to oxidation. Hydrogenated oils still contain some unsaturated components that are susceptible to rancidity. Therefore, the addition of antioxidants is still necessary.

HYDROLYSATE • A product of hydrolysis in which hydrogen is added to a compound.

HYDROLYSIS • Decomposition that changes a compound into other compounds by taking up the elements of water. For example, hydrolysis of salt into an acid and a base or hydrolysis of an ester into an alcohol and an acid.

HYDROLYZED • Subject to hydrolysis or turned partly into water. Hydrolysis is derived from the Greek *hydro,* meaning "water," and *lysis,* meaning "a setting free." It occurs as a chemical process in which the decomposition of a compound is brought about by water, resolving into a simpler compound. Hydrolysis also occurs in the digestion of foods. The proteins in the stomach react with water in an enzyme reaction to form peptones and amino acids (*see*).

HYDROLYZED ACTIN • A protein in skin that is treated with acid, enzymes, or some other method of hydrolysis. Used in hair and skin products as a conditioner.

HYDROLYZED ALBUMEN • Skin-conditioning ingredient. *See* Hydrolyzed and Albumen.

HYDROLYZED ANIMAL PROTEIN • A flavor enhancer and hair and skin care product additive made from the bone material or carcasses of cows, pigs, or poultry. Pig blood and skin are the primary sources. The manufacturing process includes treating the animal parts with acid heat, and high pressure; "hydrolyzed" essentially means "treated with water." Most cosmetic companies have left out the word "animal" and substituted "hydrolyzed protein" or "hydrolyzed collagen."

HYDROLYZED CALF SKIN • Treated with enzymes, it is used in skin care products.

HYDROLYZED CASEIN • *See* Casein and Hydrolyzed.

HYDROLYZED COLLAGEN • The widely used hydrolysate of animal collagen derived by acid, enzyme, or other method of hydrolysis. It is used in many makeup products, bath preparations, and cuticle softeners. On the basis of the available data, the CIR Expert Panel (*see*) concludes that this ingredient is safe.

HYDROLYZED DNA • The hydrolysate of DNA (*see*). Used in hair products and skin conditioners.

HYDROLYZED EGG PROTEIN • Used in hair conditioners. *See* Egg and Hydrolyzed.

HYDROLYZED ELASTIN • The hydrolysate of animal connective tissue, particularly the ligaments, used in "youth" creams.

HYDROLYZED FIBRONECTIN • The hydrolysate of fibronectin, a fibrous link in connective tissue derived by acid, enzyme, or other method of hydrolysis.

HYDROLYZED GADIDAE PROTEIN • *See* Hydrolyzed and Fish Oil.

HYDROLYZED GLYCOSAMINOGLYCANS • Formerly called hydrolyzed mucopolysaccharides, it is a sugary substance used in emollients.

HYDROLYZED HAIR KERATIN • The hydrolysate of human hair keratin derived by acid, enzyme, or other method of hydrolysis.

HYDROLYZED HEMOGLOBIN • The hydrolysate of hemoglobin derived by acid, enzyme, or other method of hydrolysis.

HYDROLYZED HUMAN PLACENTAL PROTEIN • *See* Human Placental Protein and Hydrolyzed

HYDROLYZED KERATIN • The widely used hydrolysate of keratin derived by acid, enzyme, or other form of hydrolysis. The word *animal* was removed from this ingredient name. *See* Keratin.

HYDROLYZED MILK PROTEIN • The hydrolysate of milk protein derived by acid, enzyme, or other method of hydrolysis. Used in face creams.

HYDROLYZED MUCOPOLYSACCHARIDES • A mixture of polysaccharides derived from the hydrolysis of animal connective tissue.

HYDROLYZED OAT PROTEIN • The hydrolysate of oat protein.

HYDROLYZED PEARL • Pearls from oysters that have been treated with acid, enzyme, or some other method of hydrolysis. Used in face powders and mascara.

HYDROLYZED PLACENTAL PROTEIN • The hydrolysate of placental protein derived by acid, enzyme, or other method of hydrolysis.

HYDROLYZED POTATO PROTEIN • The potato protein derived by acid, enzyme, or other method of hydrolysis.

HYDROLYZED PROTEIN • Improves the ability to comb hair. The word *animal* was removed from this ingredient's name. *See* Proteins and Hydrolyzed.

HYDROLYZED PRUNUS DOMESTICA • *See* Prunes and Hydrolyzed.

HYDROLYZED RETICULIN • The hydrolysate of the reticulin portion of animal connective tissue derived by acid, enzyme, or other form of hydrolysis.

HYDROLYZED RICE PROTEIN • The hydrolysate of rice protein derived by acid, enzyme, or other method of hydrolysis.

HYDROLYZED RNA • The hydrolysate of RNA (*see*) derived by acid, enzyme, or other method of hydrolysis.

HYDROLYZED SERUM PROTEIN • The hydrolysate of serum protein derived by acid, enzyme, or other method of hydrolysis.

HYDROLYZED SILK • The hydrolysate (turned partly into water) of silk protein derived by acid, alkaline, or enzymatic hydrolysis.

HYDROLYZED SOY PROTEIN • Widely used in hair- and skin-conditioning products. *See* Soybean and Hydrolyzed.

HYDROLYZED SPINAL PROTEIN • The hydrolysate of animal spinal cord protein derived by acid, enzyme, or other method of hydrolysis. Used in hair and skin conditioners.

HYDROLYZED SWEET ALMOND PROTEIN • *See* Almond and Hydrolyzed.

HYDROLYZED ULVA LACTUCA • *See* Algae and Hydrolyzed.

HYDROLYZED VEGETABLE PROTEIN • The hydrolysate (liquefaction) of vegetable protein derived by acid, enzyme, or other method of hydrolysis.

HYDROLYZED WHEAT GLUTEN • Widely used in hair and skin and bath preparations. The hydrolysate of wheat gluten derived by acid, enzyme, or other method of hydrolysis.

HYDROLYZED WHEAT PROTEIN • The hydrolysate of wheat protein derived by acid, enzyme, or other method of hydrolysis.

HYDROLYZED YEAST • The hydrolysate of yeast (liquefaction) derived from acid, enzyme, or other method of hydrolysis.

HYDROLYZED YEAST PROTEIN • *See* Hydrolyzed Yeast.

HYDROLYZED ZEIN • The hydrolysate of corn. *See* Zein and Hydrolyzed.

HYDROPHILIC OINTMENT • An oil-in-water emulsion used as a base for skin preparations.

HYDROQUINOL • An alkaline solution that turns brown in air and is made up of white leaflets that are soluble in water. Used as an antiseptic and reducing agent (*see*) in cosmetics. Has caused skin cancer in mice.

HYDROQUINONE • Antioxidant used in bleach and freckle creams and in suntan lotions. It is also used in hair colorings. A white, crystalline phenol (*see*) that occurs naturally but is usually manufactured in the laboratory. Hydroquinone combines with oxygen very rapidly and becomes brown when exposed to air. Death has occurred from the ingestion of as little as 5 grams. Ingestion of as little as one gram (1/30th of an ounce) has caused nausea, vomiting, ringing in the ears, delirium, a sense of suffocation, and collapse. Industrial workers exposed to the chemical have suffered clouding of the eye lens. Application to the skin may cause allergic reactions. It can cause depigmentation in a 2 percent solution. In 1990, a report from South Africa showed a link between nail damage and this ingredient. It also causes mutations in laboratory tests. On the basis of the available data, the CIR Expert Panel (*see*) concluded that this ingredient is safe at concentrations of 1 percent and less for aqueous cosmetic formulations designed for discontinuous, brief use followed by rinsing from the skin and hair. Hydroquinone should not be used in leave-on nondrug cosmetic products. The European Union banned hydroquinone's use in skin lighteners. The EU said in 2003 that its use in nail systems does not pose a risk due to the very low exposure to the consumer; however, its applications should be done only by professionals. The EU also says it should not be used to dye eyelashes. On the Canadian Hotlist (*see*). Canada does not allow it to be applied on the skin of mucous membranes. The EU says if it is in a product, it must be printed on the label. Hydroquinone monoethyl ether is prohibited as a fragrance ingredient based on the depigmenting effect of this material.

HYDROQUINONE DIBENZYL ETHER • Tan powder insoluble in water. Used as a solvent and in perfumes, soap, plastics, and pharmaceuticals. *See* Hydroquinone.

HYDROQUINONE DIMETHYLETHER • White flakes with sweet clover odor used as a fixative in perfumes, dyes, cosmetics, and especially suntan preparations. *See* Hydroquinone.

HYDROQUINONE METHYLETHER • Used in artificial nails. The EU said in 2003 that its use in nail systems does not pose a risk due to the very low exposure to the consumer. White flakes with sweet clover odor used as a fixative in foods, perfumes, dyes, cosmetics, and especially suntan preparations. *See* Hydroquinone. ASP

HYDROSOL • Hydrolate. Floral Waters. Plant Waters. Distilled condensate of plant material usually used in aromatherapy (*see*).

HYDROTROPES • Water-soluble compounds used in cosmetics.

HYDROXY CETYLDIMONIUM CHLORIDE • A quaternary compound (*see*) used as an antistatic ingredient in hair products.

HYDROXY CITRONELLAL • Laurine. Colorless liquid obtained by the addition of water to citronellol (*see*). Used as a fixative (*see*) and a fragrance in perfumery for its sweet lilylike odor. It has been known to cause allergic reactions.

HYDROXYACETIC ACID • *See* Glycolic Acid.

***p*-HYDROXYANISOLE** • Used as an antioxidant in cosmetic products up to 1 percent. Undiluted, it is a severe skin and eye irritant in rabbits but a minimal skin irritant in humans. Because of the depigmenting action of this ingredient in black guinea pigs at reported concentrations approaching those used in cosmetics, it is concluded by the CIR

Expert Panel (*see*) that its use in cosmetics is unsafe because it causes skin depigmentation. It is on the Canadian Hotlist (*see*).

HYDROXYAPATITE • A mineral obtained from phosphate rock.

***o*-HYDROXYBENZOIC ACID** • *See* Salicylic Acid.

***p*-HYDROXYBENZOIC ACID** • Prepared from *p*-bromophenol. Used as a preservative and fungicide. *See* Benzoic Acid for toxicity.

HYDROXYBENZOMORPHOLINE • 4-Salicylomorpholine. A hair coloring. Used medically to stimulate the liver. No satisfactory data were available on the possible presence of nitrosamines (*see*). The CIR Expert Panel (*see*) advised that it should not be used in the presence of nitrosating (*see*) ingredients. On the basis of the available data, the panel concluded that this ingredient is safe at current levels of use. The EU has banned morpholine and its salts in cosmetics.

HYDROXYBUTYL METHYLCELLULOSE • *See* Methylcellulose.

HYDROXYCAPRIC ACID • Used in skin conditioners. *See* Capric Acid.

HYDROXYCAPRYLIC ACID • *See* Alpha-Hydroxy Acids.

HYDROXYCETETH-60 • *See* Polyethylene Glycol and Hexadecanoic Acid.

HYDROXYCETYL PHOSPHATE • Esters of phosphoric acid and cetyl alcohol (*see both*).

HYDROXYCITRONELLAL • Colorless liquid obtained by the addition of citronellol. Used as a fixative and a fragrance in perfumery for its sweet lilylike odor. It can cause allergic reactions. ASP

HYDROXYCITRONELLOL • Fragrance ingredient. A synthetic lemon, floral, and cherry flavoring additive for beverages, ice cream, ices, candy, baked goods, gelatin desserts, and chewing gum.

HYDROXYETHYL CARBOXYMETHYL COCAMINOPROPYLATE • *See* Coconut Oil.

HYDROXYETHYL CETYLDIMONIUM CHLORIDE • *See* Quaternary Ammonium Compounds.

HYDROXYETHYL CETYLDIMONIUM PHOSPHATE • *See* Quaternary Ammonium Compounds.

1-HYDROXYETHYL-4,5-DIAMINOPYRAZOLE SULFATE • Hair coloring. The Scientific Committee on Consumer Products (SCCP) said in 2006 that there is inadequate information to assess safety. It is known to cause skin sensitization. *See* Resorcinol.

HYDROXYETHYL-2,6-DINITRO-*p*-ANISIDINE • *See* Nitrophenol.

HYDROXYETHYL ERUCAMIDOPROPYL DIMONIUM CHLORIDE • Quaternary ammonium compound (*see*) used as an antistatic ingredient in hair products.

HYDROXYETHYL ETHYLCELLULOSE • *See* Cellulose.

HYDROXYETHYL ISOBUTYL PIPERIDINE CARBOXYLATE • A germicide.

HYDROXYETHYL-2-NITRO-*p*-TOLUIDINE • A coal tar hair coloring. *See* Coal Tar.

HYDROXYETHYL PEI-1000,-1500 • *See* PEI.

HYDROXYETHYL-*p*-PHENYLENEDIAMINE SULFATE • Hair coloring. The EU gave manufacturers until July 2005 to submit safety information. The substance was banned in 2006 because of insufficient safety data. *See* Resorcinol and *p*-Phenylenediamine.

HYDROXYETHYL PICRAMIC ACID • *See* Picramic Acid.

HYDROXYETHYL STEARAMIDE-MIPA • *See* Stearic Acid.

HYDROXYETHYL TALLOWDIMONIUM CHLORIDE • An antistatic ingredient used in hair conditioners. *See* Quaternary Ammonium Compounds.

HYDROXYETHYLAMINO-5-NITROANISOLE • *See* Ethanol.

HYDROXYETHYLCELLULOSE • Widely used modified cellulose (*see*) used as a binder, emulsion stabilizer, and thickener. It is in tanning products, hair rinses, makeup foundations, shampoos, mascara, body and hand lotions, and many other products. On the basis of the available animal and human data, the CIR Expert Panel (*see*) concludes that this ingredient is safe as used in cosmetics.

HYDROXYINDOLE • Hair coloring. *See* Phenols.

4-(4-HYDROXY-3-IODOPHENOXY)-3,5-DIIODOPHENYLACETIC ACID AND ITS SALTS • Suspected of affecting the thyroid gland. Banned in cosmetics by the EU.

HYDROXYISOHEXYL 3-CYCLOHEXENE CARBOXALEDEHYDE • A fragrance ingredient. *See* Aldehyde, Aliphatic.

HYDROXYLAMINE HCL • An antioxidant for fatty acids and soaps. May be slightly irritating to skin, eyes, and mucous membranes and may cause a depletion of oxygen in the blood when ingested. In the body it is reportedly decomposed to sodium nitrite. *See* Nitrite.

HYDROXYLAMINE SULFATE • A hair-waving component in permanent wave solutions, it is a crystalline ammonium sulfate compound. It is also used for dehairing hides, in photography, as a chemical reducing ingredient, and to purify aldehydes (*see*) and ketones (*see*).

HYDROXYLAPATITE • Hydroxyapatite. A mineral obtained from phosphate rock. Being studied as an injectable filler for wrinkles.

HYDROXYLATE • The process in which an atom of hydrogen and an atom of oxygen are introduced into a compound to make the compound more soluble.

HYDROXYLATED JOJOBA OIL • Hair and skin conditioner. *See* Jojoba Oil.

HYDROXYLATED LANOLIN • It is better than plain lanolin because the hydroxylation (*see*) makes it mix better with water and be more absorbable on the skin. It is widely used in makeup and skin care preparations. On the basis of the available information, the CIR Expert Panel (*see*) found it safe in the early 1980s but is considering new information to determine if the final safety assessment should be reaffirmed, amended, or have an addendum.

HYDROXYLATED LECITHIN • The product obtained by the hydroxylation of lecithin. Used in skin products as an emulsifier. *See* Lecithin and Hydroxylation.

HYDROXYLATED MILK GLYCERIDES • Used as an emulsifying ingredient and in skin conditioners. *See* Milk and Hydroxylate.

HYDROXYLATED POLYISOBUTENE • *See* Polyisobutene and Hydroxylate.

HYDROXYLATION • The process in which an atom of hydrogen and an atom of oxygen are introduced into a compound to make that compound more soluble.

HYDROXYLAURIC ACID • A skin conditioner. *See* Lauric Acid and Hydroxylation.

HYDROXYLAUROYL PHYTOSPHINGOSINE • A hair and skin conditioner. *See* Alkanolamides.

HYDROXYLYCINE • Lycine that has been hydroxylated to make it more soluble and to supposedly increase the protein content of a product. Used in tanning products. *See* Lysine and Hydroxylation.

HYDROXYMETHYLCELLULOSE • Thickener and bodying ingredient derived from plants. Used to thicken cosmetics and as a setting aid in hair products. On the basis of the available data, the CIR Expert Panel (*see*) concluded that this ingredient is safe. *See* Carboxymethyl Cellulose.

HYDROXYOCTACOSANYL HYDROXYSTEARATE • *See* Stearic Acid and Hydroxylation.

HYDROXYPALMITOYL SPHINGANINE • Alcohol used as a skin and hair conditioner. *See* Palmitic Acid.

HYDROXYPHENYL GLYCINAMIDE • Derived from the nonessential amino acid glycine (*see*) used as a buffering ingredient and as a violet scent.

11A-HYDROXYPREGN-4-ENE-3, 20-DIONE • With its esters, substances that produce endocrine activity levels in correlation with powerful hypertension effects. The EU says these substances should therefore be prohibited in cosmetic products.

HYDROXYPROLINE • L. Pronine. An amino acid (*see*). Used as a moisturizer to add protein to cosmetics in face, neck, hand, and body preparations. It is also used in eye makeup. *See* Hydroxylation and Proline.

HYDROXYPROPYL BIS-OLEYL-DIMONIUM CHLORIDE • *See* Quaternary Ammonium Compounds.

HYDROXYPROPYL GUAR • Guar Gum, 2-Hydroxypropyl Ether. *See* Guar Gum.

HYDROXYPROPYL METHYLCELLULOSE • Widely used ingredient in many hair and skin preparations as well as bubble bath and tanning preparations. On the basis of the available animal and human data, the CIR Expert Panel (*see*) concluded that this ingredient is safe as used in cosmetics. Reported to be a mild eye and skin irritant. *See* Cellulose Gums.

HYDROXYPROPYLAMINE NITRITE • *See* Isopropanolamine and Nitrite.

4-HYDROXYPROPYLAMINE-3-NITROPHENOL • Banned in the EU and Canada in 2006. *See* Resorcinol and Nitrophenol.

HYDROXYPROPYLCELLULOSE • A thickener. On the basis of the available animal and human data, the CIR Expert Panel (*see*) concluded that this ingredient is safe as used in cosmetics. *See* Hydroxymethylcellulose.

HYDROXYPROPYLTRIMONIUM HONEY • A quaternary ammonium compound (*see*) that is used as an antistatic ingredient in hair colors. *See* Honey.

HYDROXYPROPYLTRIMONIUM HYDROLIZED CASEIN • A quaternary ammonium compound formed from casein (*see*) used as an antistatic ingredient in hair conditioners and skin creams.

HYDROXYPROPYLTRIMONIUM HYDROLZYED COLLAGEN • *See* Hydrolyzed Collagen.

HYDROXYQUINOLINE • On the Canadian Hotlist (*see*). Permitted in Canada as a stabilizer for hydrogen peroxide in hair care preparations with a concentration equal to or less than 0.3 percent in rinse-off preparations and 0.03 percent in leave-on preparations. *See* Oxyquinoline Sulfate.

8-HYDROXYQUINOLINE SULFATE • Pale yellow powder with a slight saffron odor and burning taste. It is used as an antiseptic, antiperspirant, deodorant, and fungicide.

HYDROXYSTEARAMIDE MEA • Mixture of ethanolamide and hydroxystearic acid. *See* Stearic Acid.

HYDROXYSTEARIC ACID • A surfactant and cleansing ingredient in cosmetic products. Skin irritation has been produced by antiperspirant formulations in exaggerated conditions. On the basis of the available data, the CIR Expert Panel (*see*) concludes that this ingredient is safe. *See* Stearic Acid

HYDROXYSTEARYL METHYLGLUCAMINE • An amino sugar. *See* Glucose.

HYMENAEA COUBBARIL • *See* Locust Bean Gum.

HYOSCINE • Scopolamine. Acid reducer. On the Canadian Hotlist (*see*). Used as a "truth serum." *See* Atropa Belladonna.

HYPERICUM • Hypericin. St. John's Wort. Blue-black needles obtained from pyridine (*see*). The solutions are red or green with a red cast. Small amounts seem to be a tranquilizer and have been used as an antidepressant in medicine. It can produce a sensitivity to light.

HYPERKERATOSIS • Overgrowth of the top layer skin cells forming visible scales or flakes.

HYPERSENSITIVITY • The condition in persons previously exposed to an antigen in which tissue damage results from an immune reaction to a further dose of the antigen. Classically, four types of hypersensitivity are recognized, but the term is often used to mean the type of allergy associated with hay fever and asthma.

HYPNEA • Red alga that inhibits yeast. *See* Algae.

HYPO- • Prefix from the Greek, meaning "under" or "below," as in hypoacidity— acidity in a lesser degree than is usual or normal.

HYPOALLERGENIC • A term for cosmetics supposedly devoid of common allergens that most frequently cause allergic reactions. However, spokesmen for both the FDA and the AMA find the claims of scientific proof for their efficacy to be insufficient. When first marketed in the 1930s, these cosmetics were called nonallergic, which implied they could not cause an allergic reaction. The term was abandoned because there are always people who will be allergic to almost any substance. The term "hypoallergenic" means "least likely to cause a reaction." Not only the user, but his or her companion, may suffer an allergic reaction to cosmetics—for instance, a wife to her husband's shaving lotion or a child to its mother's hair spray.

HYPOPHOSPHORIC ACID • Crystals used in baking powder and sodium salt.

HYPOPHOSPHOROUS ACID • Phosphorus treated with a resin. White, or yellow, crystalline mass used as a reducing ingredient and for phosphite salts.

HYPTIS SUAVEOLENS • A plant that yields an essential oil used in fragrances.

HYSSOP OIL • *Hyssopus officinalis.* A liquor and spice flavoring. A historical and biblical herb whose name is derived from the Greek word *azob,* or holy herb, it has a pleasant mild fragrance that is used in aromatherapy. People with high blood pressure or seizures are warned not to ingest or smell this oil. EAF

HYSSOP EXTRACT • Extract of *Hyssopus officinalis.* A synthetic flavoring and fragrance ingredient from the aromatic herb. Used in bitters.

HYSSOPUS OFFICINALIS • *See* Hyssop Extract.

I

ICELAND MOSS EXTRACT • The extract of *Lichen islandicus.* A water-soluble gum that gels on cooling. Used to flavor alcoholic beverages, as a food additive, and in cosmetic gels. So named because Icelanders reputedly were the first to discover its benefits. It is high in mucilage, with some iodine, traces of vitamin A, and usnic acid. Herbalists use the lichen as a gentle laxative, and to treat dysentery, anemia, bronchitis, and upper respiratory problems associated with degenerative wasting.

ICHTHAMMOL • Ammonium Ichthosulfonate. Medicone Derma-HC. Pale yellow or brownish black, thick viscous liquid that smells like coal. It mixes with water, glycerol, fats, oils, and waxes, and is used medicinally as a topical antiseptic. It has slight bacteria-killing properties and is used in ointments for the treatment of skin disorders. Used in cosmetics as a germicide. May be a mild skin irritant.

IDOPROPYNYL BUTYLCARBAMATE • *See* Carbamate.

ILEX AQUIFOLIUM • *Ilex opaca.* European Holly. American Holly. A small evergreen, the leaves were used to increase perspiration, to treat inflammations of the mucous membranes, pleurisy, gout, and smallpox. The leaves contain theobromine (*see*). Used as a skin conditioner in cosmetics. The berries were used to cause vomiting and as a diuretic to remove excess fluid. The juice of the berries was used to treat jaundice.

ILEX PARAGUARIENSIS LEAF EXTRACT • Paraguay Tea. Yerba Maté. A hair and skin conditioner. *See* Ilex Aquifolium.

ILLICIIUM VERUM • *See* Anise.

ILLIPE BUTTER • The Illipe tree (*Shorea stenoptera*) that grows in the forests of Borneo. The first inhabitants of Borneo (the Dayaks) have been making a "butter" from illipe nuts for centuries for therapeutic and cosmetic purposes. Illipe butter has long-lasting moisturizing properties. It is used for its skin-softening quality. Illipe is similar to cocoa butter (*see*). Used in lipsticks, lip and body balms, creams, lotions, makeup foundations, hair conditioners, and bar soaps. It is claimed to help restore cells and prevent wrinkles. It is reputed to heal sores and mouth ulcers. Nontoxic.

ILLITE • Clays and micas used as abrasives and anticaking ingredients. *See* Mica.

IMIDAZOLE • Glyoxaline. 1,3-Diazole. Imidazol-4-ylacrylic acid and its ethyl ester (*see* Urocanic Acid). Derived from benzene (*see*). Consists of orange-colored needles. It is an antimetabolite and inhibitor of histamine and is used to control pests. In cosmetics, used as a pH (*see*) adjuster. Antifungal substance that works by killing fungus or preventing its growth. Vaginal products containing imidazoles are used to treat yeast infections. Among the imidazoles on the market are butoconazole, econazole, and miconazole.

IMIDAZOLIDINONE • Ethylene Urea. Prepared from ethylenediamine and carbon dioxide (*see both*). Used in pressure-sensitive adhesives, lacquers, and insecticides and for coatings.

IMIDAZOLIDINYL UREA • The most commonly used cosmetic preservative after the parabens, it is the second-most-identified cosmetic preservative causing contact dermatitis, according to the American Academy of Dermatology's Standards on Vehicle and Preservative Patch Testing Tray results. It is colorless, odorless, and tasteless and is employed in baby shampoos, lotions, oils, powders, eye shadows, permanent waves, rinses, fragrances, hair tonics, colognes, powders, creams, bath oils, blushers, rouges, moisturizers, and fragrances. On the basis of the available information, the CIR Expert Panel (*see*) found it safe in the early 1980s but is considering new information to determine if the final safety assessment should be reaffirmed, amended, or have an addendum. Reportedly may cause dermatitis (*see*).

IMIDAZOLINE • A derivative of imidazole (*see*); also called glyoxalidine.

IMIDAZOLINE AMPHOTERIC • Surfactant used in "no tears" shampoos. An "anti-irritant" that neutralizes the effects of a cosmetic. *See* Imidazolidinyl Urea.

3-IMIDAZOL-4-YLACRYLIC ACID AND ITS ETHYL ESTER • *See* Urocanic Acid.

IMIDUREA • *See* Urea.

IMINO-BIS-PROPYLAMINE • *See* Propylamine.

IMITATION • With reference to a fragrance, containing all or some portion of non-natural materials. For instance, unless a strawberry flavoring used in lipstick is made entirely from strawberries, it must be called imitation.

IMMORTELLE EXTRACT • Immortelle grows abundantly on the coast of the Mediterranean Sea and has an exceptionally long life; it never wilts, even after being picked. The name derives from the French *immortel*—"immortal" or "everlasting." Used for centuries, immortelle flowers produce an essential oil claimed to boost collagen synthesis, stimulate circulation, and enhance cell renewal. A natural flavoring extract from a red-flowered tropical tree. Used in raspberry, fruit, and liquor flavorings for beverages, ice cream, ices, baked goods, candy, gelatin desserts, and chewing gum. GRAS

IMPATIENS • *Impatiens glandulifera.* A large genus of widely distributed annual plants of the Balsaminaceae family. It has a watery juice and is used in "organic" cosmetics. Herbalists claim the flower can be used as a remedy against impatience. Used in skin moisturizers, for chapped skin, dandruff, and split hair ends. They are also used in skin lotions, creams, hair tonics, cosmetics, bath preparations, and detergents. The FDA issued a notice in 1992 that impatiens has not been shown to be safe and effective as claimed in OTC poison ivy, poison oak, and poison sumac products. It is used in cosmetics to reduce inflammation.

IMPERATA CYLINDRICA • Blady Grass. Grown in Fiji and Indonesia, it is used as a skin conditioner.

IMPERATORIN • A furocoumarin and a phytochemical that can be isolated from *Urena lobata* (Malvaceae). Synthesized from umbelliferone, a coumarin derivative. Has been used in skin-whitening creams. Banned in cosmetics by the EU and ASEAN (*see*) because it may interfere with blood clotting and the bioactivity of some pharmaceuticals. *See* Coumarins.

IMPETIGO • An acute skin infection, initially blisterlike in nature, which later becomes crusted after the blisters rupture; painless and often accompanied by itching.

INCI • Abbreviation for the International Nomenclature of Cosmetic Ingredients.

INDIAN CRESS EXTRACT • Phytelene of Capucine. The extract obtained from the flowers of *Tropaeolum majus,* a plant grown in Peru and imported to Europe. It is widely used in hair products today as a conditioner and in skin products as a moisturizer and stimulant.

INDIAN HEMP • *Apocynum cannabinum.* Dogbane. A North American dogbane that yields a tough fiber formerly used in rope.

INDIAN TRAGACANTH • *See* Karaya Gum.

INDIGO • Probably the oldest known dye. Prepared from various *Indigofera* plants native to Bengal, Java, and Guatemala. Dark blue powder with a coppery luster. No known skin irritation, but continued use on hair can cause hair to become brittle.

INDIGOFERA • *See* Indigo.

INDOLES • A white, lustrous, flaky substance with an unpleasant odor, occurring naturally in jasmine oil and orange flowers and used in perfumes. Also extracted from coal tar, kale, cabbage, and feces; in highly diluted solutions, the odor is pleasant. Large doses have been lethal to dogs.

INERT • A term used to indicate chemical inactivity in an element or compound. However, in drugs, food additives, cosmetics, and other chemical products, the term has come to mean ingredients added to mixtures chiefly for bulk and weight purposes. The chemicals still may have some activity of their own, although not for the product's specific purpose.

INFLAMMATION • Derived from the Latin word *inflammo,* meaning "flame," it is an immune reaction to tissue injury and generally involves redness, swelling, pain, and heat. The reddening results from increased blood flowing to the affected part. Many inflammatory conditions are designated by the suffix *-itis,* preceded by the name of the affected tissue. For example, appendicitis, otitis, and arthritis.

INGA EDULIS • Ice Cream Bean. Small tree native to Central and South America. Eaten as a vegetable and used by folk medicine practitioners to treat diarrhea and arthritis. Used in cosmetics as a flavoring and skin conditioner.

INK CAP • *Coprinus atramentarius.* A fungus with a white stem native to Europe and introduced to many moderate zones. It is a component of various health food products as a nutrient. In cosmetics, it is used as a covering and moisturizer with the combination of skin care and foundation. It contains disulfiram (*see*), which can have severe effects.

INN • Abbreviation for International Non-Proprietary Names.

INNER CELLULAR MEMBRANE COMPLEX • A vegetable-derived protein imitating cellular membrane complex (*see*). *See also* Hair.

INOSITOL • A dietary supplement of the vitamin B family used in emollients. Found in plant and animal tissues. Isolated commercially from corn. A fine, white, crystalline powder, it is odorless with a sweet taste. Stable in air.

INSOLUBLE METAPHOSPHATE • *See* Sodium Metaphosphate.

INTERMEDIATE • A chemical substance found as part of a necessary step between one organic compound and another, as in the production of dyes, pharmaceuticals, or other artificial products that develop properties only upon oxidation. For instance, it is used for hair-dye bases that have dyeing action only when exposed to oxygen.

INTERNATIONAL NON-PROPRIETARY NAMES • Abbreviation INN.

INTRA- • Prefix meaning within.

INTRADERMAL • Into or within the skin.

INULA HELENIUM • Elecampane. Scabwort. Horseheal. Wild Sunflower. Elfdock. Elfwort. Indigenous to Europe and Asia and is also grown in the United States. The name elecampane is derived from the Latin *campana,* meaning "country." The species name, *Helenium,* is said to be named after Helen of Troy, who was collecting elecampane when she was captured by Paris. It is used by folk medicine to treat digestive ills and in cosmetics as a germicide and skin conditioner. On the Canadian Hotlist (*see*). Banned in fragrances by the UK.

INULIN • Elecampane Extract. A sugar from plants. Used by intravenous injection to determine kidney function; also used in bread for diabetics. Used in cosmetics as a humectant and as a skin-conditioning ingredient. *See* Inula Helenium.

IN VITRO • Outside the body.

IN VIVO • Within the body.

IODIDE • The negative ion of iodine, it is made from iodine and water. *See* Iodine.

IODINE • Discovered in 1811 and classed among the rarer earth elements, it is found in the earth's crust as bluish black scales. Nearly two hundred products now contain this chemical. They are prescription and OTC medications. They can produce a diffuse red pimply rash, hives, asthma, and sometimes anaphylactic shock. Iodine is also used as an antiseptic and germicide in cosmetics. On the Canadian Hotlist (*see*). The EU bans it in cosmetics. In 1992, the FDA issued a notice that iodine had not been shown to be safe and effective as claimed in OTC digestive aid products.

IODIZED • The addition of iodine often used in compounds as a stabilizer and preservative.

IODIZED CORN PROTEIN • *See* Corn and Iodine.

IODIZED GARLIC • Powdered garlic to which iodine has been added. *See* Iodine and Garlic Extract.

IODIZED HYDROLYZED EXTENSIN • *See* Iodine and Extensin.

IODIZED ZEIN • *See* Iodine and Zein.

IODOFORM • Small, greenish yellow or lustrous crystals or powder with a penetrating odor. Derived from iodine (*see*). Used as a preservative and antiseptic. Can be irritating to the skin.

IODOPHOR • Tamed Iodine. A complex of iodine with certain surface-active ingredients that have detergent properties.

IODOPROPYNL BUTYLCARBAMATE • A preservative widely used in cosmetics. Its use in cosmetics was only provisionally permitted in the EU until June 1998. Although its safety was still unproven, its provisional status was extended. It is limited to a maximum of 0.1 percent of the finished product and is banned from oral care products and lip products. Has been shown to adversely affect livers in rats in feeding studies. It also affected their behavior. It was also mildly irritating in human testing. On the basis of the available animal and human data, the CIR Expert Panel (*see*) concludes that this ingredient is safe as used in cosmetics at concentrations up to 0.1 percent but it should not be used in aerosolized products. *See* Carbamates.

IOM • Abbreviation for the Institute of Medicine, one of the National Academies of the United States. The IOM conducts policy studies on health issues. For example, the IOM issued reports and recommendations in September 2001 on stem cell research and on the cancer risk from arsenic in drinking water.

ION • A molecule that carries an electrical charge. Ionic bonding is used in many cosmetic ingredients because they have a natural liking for water. They help to counteract static.

IONAX • *See* Benzalkonium Chloride.

IONIL • *See* Salicylic Acid.

IONONE • Used as a scent in perfumery and as a flavoring ingredient in foods, it occurs naturally in boronia, an Australian shrub, and in essential oils such as rose oil. Colorless to pale yellow, with an odor reminiscent of cedar wood or violets. It may cause allergic reactions.

IPBC • Abbreviation for iodopropynl butylcarbamate (*see*).

IPECAC • *Cephaelis ipecacuanha.* Ipecacuanha. From the dried rhizome and roots of a creeping South American plant with drooping flowers. Used by herbalists and sold in conventional pharmacies, ipecac is primarily used to induce vomiting when ingestion of noncaustic poisons has occurred. It may also be used in medicine to induce expulsion of mucus in lung congestion. Used as a denaturant in alcohol. Fatal dose in humans is as low as 20 milligrams per kilogram of body weight. Irritating when taken internally but okay on the skin. On the Canadian Hotlist (*see*). The EU bans it in cosmetics.

IPECACUANAH • *See* Ipecac.

IPOMOEA • A vinelike herb. Sweet potatoes and morning glories belong to this family. Used as a skin conditioner.

IRAKUSA EKISU • *Urtica thunbergiana. Urtica dioica.* Skin conditioner. *See* Nettles.

IRIS FLORENTINA, I. GERMANICA, AND I. PALLIDA • *See* Orris Root Extract.

IRIS VERSICOLOR • *See* Blue Flag.

IRISH MOSS • *Chondrus crispus.* Carrageenan. Seaweed used by herbalists for chronic lung and upper respiratory problems, and diseases associated with wasting. Contains iodine and a number of mucilaginous agents that soothe inflamed and ulcerated surfaces. Used to treat gastric and duodenal ulcers and as an expectorant. It was banned by the FDA in May 1992 for use in laxatives. *See* Carrageenan.

IRIS VERSICOLOR • *See* Blue Flag.

IRON OXIDES • Very widely used to color cosmetics. Any of several natural or synthetic oxides of iron (i.e., iron combined with oxygen), varying in color from red to brown, black to orange or yellow, depending on the degree of water added and the purity. Ocher, sienna, and iron oxide red are among the colors used to tint face powders, liquid powders, and foundation creams. Black iron oxide is used for coloring eye shadow. *See* Colors for toxicity. Permanently listed in 1977.

IRON PICOLINATE • Used in oral care products. *See* Iron Salts.

IRON SALTS • Iron sources: ferric, choline citrate, ferric orthophosphate, ferric phosphate, ferric sodium pyrophosphate, ferrous fumarate, ferrous gluconate, ferrous lactate, and ferrous sulfate. Widely used as enrichment for foods, they are used in cosmetics mainly for coloring and as astringents. Ingestion of large quantities can cause gastrointestinal disturbances, but there is no known toxicity in cosmetics.

IRONE • The fragrant principle of violets, usually isolated from the iris, and used in perfumery. A light yellow, viscous liquid, it gives off the delicate fragrance of violets when put in alcohol. It is also used to flavor dentifrices. *See* Orris Root Extract for allergy.

a-**IRONE** • A synthetic flavoring derived from the violet family and usually isolated from irises and orris oil. A light yellow, viscous liquid, it gives off the delicate fragrance of violets when put in alcohol. It is also used to flavor dentifrices and in perfumery. *See* Orris Root Extract for allergy.

IRVINGIA GABONENSIS • Dika Butter. Reduced stomach acid in medical experiments. Used as an emollient in cosmetics. *See* Mango.

ISATIN • A hair coloring. *See* Indoles.

ISATIS TINCTORIA • Woad. A biennial widely distributed in Europe, Asia, and North Africa, it is a member of the mustard family. The plant is used to treat St. Anthony's fire (gangrene and inflammation) and for plasters and ointments used to treat ulcers and inflammation.

ISO- • Greek for "equal." In chemistry, it is a prefix added to the name of one compound to denote another composed of the same kinds and numbers of atoms but different from each other in structural arrangement.

ISOAMIDOPROPYL ETHYLDIMONIUM ETHOSULFATE • *See* Quaternary Ammonium Compounds.

ISOAMYL ACETATE • A synthetic flavoring ingredient that occurs naturally in bananas and pears. Colorless, with a pearlike odor and taste, it is used in perfumery. Exposure to 950 ppm for one hour has caused headache, fatigue, shoulder pain, and irritation of the mucous membranes. It has been found to stimulate acetylcholine release in the nerve endings and act as a competitive inhibitor of acetylcholine in isolated nerves. Acetylcholine is a nerve messenger and plays a big part in memory functioning. It is used up to 10 percent in fingernail formulations. The CIR Expert Panel (*see*) concludes this is a safe ingredient in cosmetics. *See* Amyl Acetate. Acetylcholine and its salts are banned in cosmetics by ASEAN (*see*).

ISOAMYL ALCOHOL • A synthetic flavoring ingredient that occurs naturally in apples, cognac, lemons, peppermint, raspberry, strawberry, and tea. Used in chocolate, apple, banana, brandy, and rum flavorings for beverages, ice cream, ices, candy, baked goods, gelatin desserts, chewing gum, and brandy. A central nervous system depressant. Vapor exposures have caused marked irritation of the eyes, nose, and throat and headache. Amyl alcohols are highly toxic, and ingestion has caused human deaths from respiratory failure. Isoamyl alcohol may cause heart, lung, and kidney damage.

ISOAMYL LAURATE • The ester of isoamyl alcohol and lauric acid (*see both*) used as a synthetic fruit flavoring.

ISOAMYL *p*-METHOXYCINNAMATE • *See* Cinnamic Acid.

ISOBORNYL ACETATE • A synthetic pine odor in bath preparations. Also used as a synthetic fruit flavoring for beverages.

ISOBUTANE • A constituent of natural gas and illuminating gas, colorless and insoluble in water, used in refrigeration plants. A propellant used for cosmetic sprays. On the basis of the available information, the CIR Expert Panel (*see*) found it safe in the early 1980s but is considering new information to determine if the final safety assessment should be reaffirmed, amended, or have an addendum. *See* Paraffin and Propellant.

ISOBUTOXYPROPANOL • *See* Isopropyl Alcohol.

ISOBUTYL ACETATE • The ester of isobutyl alcohol and acetic acid used as a synthetic flavoring ingredient. A clear, colorless liquid with a fruity odor, it may be mildly irritating to mucous membranes, and in high concentrations it is narcotic.

ISOBUTYL METHYL TETRAHYDROPYRANOL • A fragrance ingredient.

ISOBUTYL MYRISTATE • Emollient and a moisturizer. The ester of isobutyl alcohol and myristic acid (*see*).

ISOBUTYL PALMITATE • *See* Palmitate.

ISOBUTYL PELARGONATE • The ester of isobutyl alcohol and pelargonic acid (*see*).

ISOBUTYL QUINOLINE • *See* Quinoline.

ISOBUTYL SALICYLATE • *See* Salicylates.

ISOBUTYL STEARATE • The ester of isobutyl alcohol and stearic acid. Used in waterproof coatings, polishes, face creams, rouges, ointments, soaps, dyes, and lubricants. Used as a skin-conditioning ingredient. On the basis of the available animal and human data, the CIR Expert Panel (*see*) concluded that this ingredient is safe as used in cosmetics. Has been linked to acne. *See* Fatty Alcohols.

ISOBUTYL TALLOWATE • The ester of isobutyl alcohol and tallow acid.

ISOBUTYLATED • A method to alkylate compounds to make them more soluble. *See* Butane.

ISOBUTYLATED BENZOATE • *See* Benzoic Acid and Isobutylated.

ISOBUTYLATED LANOLIN • The partial ester of lanolin oil (*see*).

ISOBUTYLATED LANOLIN OIL • *See* Lanolin and Isobutylated.

ISOBUTYLENE/ISOPRENE COPOLYMER • A copolymer of isobutylene and isoprene monomers derived from petroleum and used as a resin.

ISOBUTYLENE/MALEIC ANHYDRIDE COPOLYMER • A copolymer of isobutylene and maleic anhydride monomers derived from petroleum and used as a resin. Strong irritant.

ISOBUTYLENE/SODIUM MALEATE COPOLYMER • A synthetic polymer used as a film former.

ISOBUTYLPARABEN • Widely used in makeup, hair products, and skin conditioners as a preservative. On the basis of the available animal and human data, the CIR Expert Panel (*see*) concluded that this ingredient is safe as used in cosmetics. *See* Parabens.

ISOBUTYRIC ACID • A pungent liquid that smells like butyric acid (*see*). A mild irritant used chiefly in making fragrance materials.

ISOBUTYRYOYL C10–40 HYDROXYACID C10–40 ISOALKYL ESTERS • Skin-conditioning ingredient. *See* Esters and Alpha-Hydroxy Acids.

ISOCARBOXAZIDE • Marplan. An MAO inhibitor used to treat depression and nerve pain. Potential adverse effects include dizziness, weakness, headache, overactivity, tremors, muscle twitching, mania, insomnia, confusion, memory impairment, fatigue, a drop in blood pressure when rising from a sitting or prone position, irregular heartbeat, paradoxical high blood pressure, blurred vision, dry mouth, loss of appetite, nausea, diarrhea, constipation, rash, swelling, sweating, weight changes, and altered libido. Use with alcohol, barbiturates, and other sedatives and narcotics may cause unpredictable effects. Amphetamines, antihistamines, ephedrine, levodopa, meperidine, metaraminol, methotrimeprazine, methylphenidate, phenylephrine, and phenyl-propanolamine may raise blood pressure when used with isocarboxazide. The drug may also alter the necessary dosage of antidiabetic drugs. Contraindicated in elderly or debilitated patients, and in those with liver or kidney impairment, congestive heart failure, high blood pressure, heart disease, cerebrovascular disease, and severe or frequent headaches. Must also avoid foods containing tryptophan or tyramine, such as herring, cheese, and red wine. Alcohol, caffeine, over-the-counter medications for colds or hay fever, and other depressants should be avoided. Full effect may not be manifested until two to four weeks. Should not be withdrawn suddenly. Banned by ASEAN.

ISOCETEARETH-8 STEARATE • See Ethylene Oxide and Stearic Acid.

ISOCETETH-10, -20, -30 • Primarily emulsifiers. The polyethylene glycol ethers of isocetyl alcohol. See Cetyl Alcohol.

ISOCETETH-10 STEARATE • The ester of isoceteth-10 and stearic acid. See Stearic Acid.

ISOCETYL ALCOHOL • See Cetyl Alcohol.

ISOCETYL ISODECANOATE • See Cetyl Alcohol.

ISOCETYL ISOSTEARATE • A skin-conditioning ingredient. See Isostearic Acid.

ISOCETYL LAURATE • A skin-conditioning ingredient. See Lauric Acid.

ISOCETYL MYRISTATE • A skin-conditioning ingredient. See Myristic Acid.

ISOCETYL PALMITATE • Widely used emollient in hand and body products, fragrances, and makeup. See Cetyl Alcohol and Palmitate.

ISOCETYL STEARATE • See Cetyl Alcohol and Stearic Acid.

ISOCETYL STEAROYL STEARATE • The ester ofisocetyl alcohol, stearic alcohol, and stearic acid. Used in skin conditioners. See Fatty Acids.

ISODECANE • A gel. See Decanoic Acid.

ISODECETH-4, -5, -6 • Emollients. See Polyethylene Glycol and Decyl Alcohol.

ISODECYL HYDROXYSTEARATE • An emollient ingredient. See Decyl Alcohol and Stearic Acid.

ISODECYL ISONONANOATE • See Decyl Alcohol.

ISODECYL LAURATE • The ester of decyl alcohol and lauric acid (see both) used as a wetting ingredient (see).

ISODECYL MYRISTATE • See Decyl Alcohol and Myristic Acid.

ISODECYL NEOPENTANOATE • Emollient in makeup. See 1-Pentanol.

ISODECYL OCTANOATE • The ester of decyl alcohol and hexanoic acid.

ISODECYL OLEATE • An emollient in cleansing products. On the basis of the available information, the CIR Expert Panel (see) found it safe in the early 1980s but is considering new information to determine if the final safety assessment should be reaffirmed, amended, or have an addendum. See Decyl Alcohol and Oleic Acid.

ISODECYL PALMITATE • See Decyl Alcohol and Palmitic Acid.

ISODECYL SALICYLATE • The ester of decyl alcohol and salicylic acid.

ISODECYLPARABEN • The ester of decyl alcohol and p-hydroxybenzoic acid. See Propylparaben.

ISODONIS JAPONICUS • Perennial herb grown in Japan, Korea, and Russia. Yields essential oil. Contains terpenes (see). It can be a skin irritant. See Essential Oil.

ISODONIS TRICHOCARPUS • Enmeisou Ekisu. Isodonis Extract. Fragrant plant extract that contains terpenes. It can be a skin irritant. See Essential Oil.

ISOEICOSANE • See Eicosane.

ISOEUGENOL • An aromatic, liquid, phenol oil obtained from eugenol (see) by mixing with an alkali. Used chiefly in perfumes but also employed in hand creams and in making the flavoring vanillin. Strong irritant. Not recommended for use. The CIR Expert Panel (*see*) has listed this as top priority for review.

ISOFLAVONES • A family of plant estrogens found in soybeans. The FDA/National Center for Toxicological Research's Web page (November 15, 2007) says to avoid side effects of postmenopausal hormone treatment (HRT) many women are switching to alternative sources of estrogens, such as the isoflavone phytoestrogens, in the belief that naturally occurring substances may be safer. Two of the most commonly ingested isoflavones are daidzein (DZ) and genistein (GE) (*see both*). The two are major components of soy isoflavones and are presumed to be responsible for their health-promoting effects. However, the agency adds: It is possible that these compounds may also be toxic. In theory, the naturally occurring isoflavones can alter the metabolism of human hormones and, thus, influence hormone-dependent cancers. Early studies have shown that both DZ and GE are mutagenic, indicating that isoflavones may play some role in tumor mutagenesis.

ISOHEXADECANE • *See* Hexadecanoic Acid.

ISOHEXYL CAPRATE • An emollient. *See* Decanoic Acid.

ISOHEXYL LAURATE • *See* Lauryl Alcohol.

ISOHEXYL PALMITATE • *See* Palmitic Acid.

ISOJASMONE • *See* Jasomone

ISOLAURETH-3, -6, -10 • *See* Polyethylene Glycol and Lauric Acid.

ISOLEUCINE • An essential amino acid not synthesized within the human body. Isolated commercially from beet sugar, it is a building block of protein. Used as a hair- and skin-conditioning ingredient. GRAS

ISOLONGIFOLENE EXPOXIDE • An ingredient in fragrances.

ISOLONGIFOLENE KETON EXO • An ingredient in fragrances.

ISOMALT • A candidate for an artificial sweetener, it has 45 to 65 percent the sweetness of sugar. A component of bread obtained by the action of enzymes on starch. It contains calories and is physically similar to sugar. It is free-flowing, white, and crystalline. It has a sweet taste reportedly without any aftertaste. While it is not as sweet as sugar, it may be enhanced with an intense sweetener such as acesulfame. It is used in fifteen countries in candies, gums, ice cream, jams, and baked goods. Used in cosmetics as an anti-caking ingredient, thickener, and flavoring ingredient.

ISOMERIZED JOJOBA OIL • Used in emollients. *See* Jojoba Oil.

ISONONAMIDOPROPYL ETHYLDIMONIUM ETHOSULFATE • *See* Quaternary Ammonium Compounds.

ISONONYL FERULATE • An ester (*see*) of ferulic acid used in emollients.

ISONONYL ISONONANOATE • The ester (*see*) produced by the reaction of nonyl alcohol with nonanoic acid. Used in fruit flavorings for lipsticks and mouthwashes. Occurs in cocoa and oil of lavender.

ISOOCTYL THIOGLYCOLATE • Depilatory ingredient.EU. The ester of thioglycolic acid (*see*).

ISOPENTANAL • A flavoring and fragrance ingredient. *See* Aldehyde, Aliphatic.

ISOPENTANE • Volatile, flammable, liquid hydrocarbon found in petroleum and used as a solvent in cosmetics. A skin irritant. Narcotic in high doses. On the basis of the available information, the CIR Expert Panel (*see*) found it safe in the early 1980s but is considering new information to determine if the final safety assessment should be reaffirmed, amended, or have an addendum.

ISOPENTYL TRIMETHOXYCINNAMATE TRISILOXANE • Emollient and ultraviolet light absorber used in moisturizers. *See* Cinnamic Acid.

ISOPENTYLDIOL • A solvent. *See* Butyl Alcohol.

ISOPRENALINE. • Isoproterenol. • Aerolone. Dey-Dose Isoproterenol. Dispos-a-Med Isoproterenol. Isoprenaline. Isuprel. Vapo-Iso. Norisodrine Aerotrol. Medihaler-Iso. A skin stimulant and an experimental slimming cream. Used to treat bronchial asthma and reversible bronchospasm. Banned by the EU, UK, and ASEAN (*see*) in cosmetics. Potential adverse reactions reported in medical use include headache, mild tremor, weakness, dizziness, nervousness, insomnia, palpitations, rapid heartbeat, angina, a rise and then drop in blood pressure, sweating, nausea, vomiting, and high blood sugar.

ISOPRENE • A hydrocarbon formed naturally in plants and animals. Isoprene can be an important precursor of ozone. According to the U.S. Department of Health and Human Services Eleventh Edition Report on Carcinogens, isoprene is reasonably expected to be a human carcinogen. Tumors have been observed in multiple locations in multiple test species exposed to isoprene vapor. No adequate human studies of the relationship between isoprene exposure and human cancer have been reported.

Isoprene is the source of the pollution that U.S. president Ronald Reagan was speaking of in 1981, when he stated, "Trees cause more pollution than automobiles do." Banned in cosmetics by Canada in 2009.

ISOPRENE/PENTADIENE COPOLYMER • Thickener. *See* Rubber.

ISOPROPANOL • Legal name for isopropyl alcohol (*see*).

ISOPROPANOLAMINE • A water-soluble emulsifying ingredient with a light ammonia odor. It is used as a plasticizer and in insecticides, as well as in cosmetic creams as a solvent. Has been reported to cause allergies.

ISOPROPANOLAMINE LANOLATE • Cleanser. *See* Lanolin.

ISOPROPYL ACETATE • The ester of isopropyl alcohol and acetic acid, a colorless liquid with a strong odor, it is used as a solvent for resin, gums, and cellulose; for lacquers; and in perfumery. Flammable.

ISOPROPYL ALCOHOL • Isopropanol. An antibacterial, solvent, and denaturant (*see*). Solvent for the spice oleoresins. Used in hair-color rinses, body rubs, hand lotions, after-shave lotions, and many other cosmetics. It is prepared from propylene, which is obtained in the cracking of petroleum. Also used in antifreeze compositions and as a solvent for gums, shellac, and essential oils. Ingestion or inhalation of large quantities of the vapor may cause flushing, headache, dizziness, mental depression, nausea, vomiting, narcosis, anesthesia, and coma. The fatal ingested dose is about 1 fluid ounce. Isopropyl alcohol, also known as rubbing alcohol, is commonly used as a cleaning fluid, and is used to dissolve other ingredients in a variety of formulations as well as reducing the thickness of liquids and creams. California has tightened regulations. The significance of the Californian market means that cosmetics companies operating in the United States will have to adapt their procedures and practices to comply with tighter legislation. The Department of Toxic Substances Control unveiled various goals related to the elimination of toxic chemicals along with options as to how best to achieve them.

ISOPROPYL AVOCADATE • *See* Avocado.

ISOPROPYL BEHENATE • Emollient. *See* Behenic Acid.

ISOPROPYL CREOSOLS • *See* o-Cresol and p-Cresol.

ISOPROPYL ESTER OF PVM/MA COPOLYMER • Synthetic resin. *See* Polyvinyl Alcohol.

ISOPROPYL ISOSTEARATE • Widely used emollient in skin conditioners and cleansers. Undiluted, it is a skin irritant. On the basis of the available animal and human data, the CIR Expert Panel (*see*) concludes that this ingredient is safe as used in cosmetics. *See* Stearic Acid and Propylene Glycol.

ISOPROPYL JOJOBATE • Emollient. *See* Jojoba Oil.

ISOPROPYL TALLOWATE • *See* Fatty Acids.

ISOPROPYL LANOLATE • A mixture of isopropyl esters of lanolin acids. After purification, the acids are esterified (*see* Ester) with isopropyl alcohol (*see*). One of the more versatile lanolin derivatives because of its surfactant (*see*) properties and pigment-dispersing ability. It is used in combination with mineral oil and isopropyl palmitate (*see*) for pigments such as titanium dioxide, oxy red, and Red No. 9. In lipsticks, creams, lotions, and aerosol emulsions it acts as a lubricant and gives high gloss. It has been used for more than twenty years. May cause skin sensitization. Its effects on lung tissue have not been studied, although it is used as an aerosol. Used as a skin-conditioning ingredient. On the basis of the available information, the CIR Expert Panel (*see*) found it safe in the early 1980s but is considering new information to determine if the final safety assessment should be reaffirmed, amended, or have an addendum. *See* Lanolin.

ISOPROPYL LAURATE • *See* Lauric Acid.

ISOPROPYL LINOLEATE • An emollient. Used as a skin-conditioning ingredient. On the basis of the available animal and human data, the CIR Expert Panel (*see*) concluded that there is insufficient data to support the safety of this ingredient in cosmetics. *See* Linoleic Acid.

ISOPROPYL MYRISTATE • A widely used fatty compound derived from isopropyl alcohol and myristic acid. It causes blackheads and is being removed from many of the newer formulations. However, a more serious potential danger exists, since when nitrate compounds such as *n*-nitrosodiethanolamine (NDELA), an impurity in many cosmetic preparations, was applied in isopropyl myristate, its absorption was increased 230 times. NDELA may be a reaction product of di- or triethanolamine, used in many cosmetic formulations. Scientists are concerned that when isopropyl myristate is applied over large areas of the skin for long periods of time, such as in suntanning lotion, there will be a significant absorption of NDELA if the contaminant is present. On the basis of the available information, the CIR Expert Panel (*see*) found it safe in the early 1980s but is considering new information to determine if the final safety assessment should be reaffirmed, amended, or have an addendum. *See* Myristic Acid.

ISOPROPYL OLEATE • The ester of isopropyl alcohol and oleic acid (*see*).

ISOPROPYL PALMITATE • Widely used binder, skin-conditioning ingredient, and emollient. It is in makeup, moisturizers, hair products, baby lotions, colognes, and manicuring products. On the basis of the available information, the CIR Expert Panel (*see*) found it safe in the early 1980s but is considering new information to determine if the final safety assessment should be reaffirmed, amended, or have an addendum. *See* Palmitic Acid.

ISOPROPYL C12–15-PARETH-9 CARBOXYLATE • The ester of carboxylic acid (*see*).

ISOPROPYL RICINOLEATE • *See* Isopropyl Alcohol and Ricinoleic Acid.

ISOPROPYL STEARATE • An emollient. Used as a skin-conditioning ingredient. On the basis of the available animal and human data, the CIR Expert Panel (*see*) concluded that this ingredient is safe as used in cosmetics. *See* Stearic Acid.

ISOPROPYLAMINE DODECYLBENZENESULFONATE • *See* Quaternary Ammonium Compounds.

ISOPROPYLBENZYLSALICYLATE • *See* Salicylates.

ISOPROPYLPARABEN • On the basis of the available animal and human data, the

CIR Expert Panel (*see*) concluded that this ingredient is safe as used in cosmetics. *See* Parabens.

ISOPROTERENOL • Aerolone. Dey-Dose Isoproterenol. Dispos-a-Med Isoproterenol. Isoprenaline. Isuprel. Vapo-Iso. Norisodrine Aerotrol. Medihaler-Iso. Used in sun blockers. Potential adverse reactions include headache, mild tremor, weakness, dizziness, nervousness, insomnia, palpitations, rapid heartbeat, angina, a rise and then drop in blood pressure, sweating, nausea, vomiting, high blood sugar, and bronchial swelling and inflammation. It may turn sputum pink. Use with epinephrine increases the risk of irregular heartbeat. Propranolol and other beta-blockers make it less effective. Contraindicated in patients with rapid or irregular heartbeat, those having had a recent heart attack, and those with diabetes or overactive thyroids. If the drug causes a feeling of tightness in the chest or shortness of breath, it should be discontinued. If solution contains precipitate or is discolored, it should not be used.

ISOPTO ATROPINE • *See* Atropine, its salts and derivatives.

ISOPTO FRIN • *See* Phenylephrine.

ISOPTO HYOSCINE • *See* Scopolamine.

ISOPULEGYL ACETATE • Synthetic fragrance. ASP

ISOQUERCITRIN • An antioxidant. *See* Phenols.

ISOSORBIDE • A skin-conditioning ingredient. *See* Sorbic Acid. Isosorbide dinitrate is banned in cosmetics by the EU.

ISOSTEARAMIDE DEA • A mixture of fatty acids from stearic acid. The CIR Expert Panel (*see*) concluded that this ingredient is safe at maximum concentration of 40 percent. There is however a potential problem of producing nitrosamines (*see*), and it should not be used in products in which these cancer-causing ingredients may be formed.

ISOSTEARAMIDE MIPA • A mixture of isopropanolamides of isostearic acid.

ISOSTEARAMIDOPROPALKONIUM CHLORIDE • *See* Surfactants.

ISOSTEARAMIDOPROPYL BETAINE • *See* Surfactants.

ISOSTEARAMIDOPROPYL DIMETHYLAMINE GLYCOLATE • An antistatic ingredient used in hair products. *See* Surfactants.

ISOSTEARAMIDOPROPYL DIMETHYLAMINE LACTATE • *See* Surfactants.

ISOSTEARAMIDOPROPYL EPOXYPROPYLMORPHOLINIUM CHLORIDE • Used in hair conditioners. *See* Quaternary Ammonium Compounds.

ISOSTEARAMIDOPROPYL ETHYLDIMONIUM ETHOSULFATE • *See* Quaternary Ammonium Compounds.

ISOSTEARAMIDOPROPYL LAURYLACETODIMONIUM CHLORIDE • A quaternary ammonium compound (*see*) used as an antistatic ingredient in hair preparations.

ISOSTEARAMIDOPROPYL MORPHOLINE LACTATE • A hair conditioner. The CIR Expert Panel (*see*) concluded that it is safe for rinse-off formulations but there is insufficient data available to support safety in leave-on formulations. *See* Surfactants. EU has banned morpholine and its salts in cosmetics.

ISOSTEARAMIDOPROPYLAMINE OXIDE • *See* Surfactants.

ISOSTEARETH-2 THROUGH -20 • Primarily surfactants and emulsifiers. *See* Fatty Alcohols.

ISOSTEARIC ACID • A complex mixture of fatty acids similar to stearic acid (*see*). Used as a binder, solvent, surfactant, and emulsifier (*see all*). On the basis of the available information, the CIR Expert Panel (*see*) found it safe in the early 1980s but is considering new information to determine if the final safety assessment should be reaffirmed, amended, or have an addendum.

ISOSTEARIC HYDROLYZED COLLAGEN • The word *animal* was removed from the ingredient name. Used in creams. *See* Protein and Hydrolyzation.

ISOSTEARIC/MYRISTIC GLYCERIDES • Used in emollients. *See* Glycerides.

ISOSTEAROAMPHOGLYCINATE • *See* Surfactants.

ISOSTEAROAMPHOPROPIONATE • *See* Surfactants.

ISOSTEAROYL HYDROLYZED COLLAGEN • *See* Surfactants.

ISOSTEARYL ALCOHOL • *See* Stearyl Alcohol.

ISOSTEARYL AVOCADATE • A skin-conditioning ingredient. *See* Avocado.

ISOSTEARYL BENZOATE • A skin-conditioning ingredient. *See* Benzoic Acid.

ISOSTEARYL BENZYLIMIDONIUM CHLORIDE • *See* Surfactants.

ISOSTEARYL DIGLYCERYL SUCCINATE • *See* Surfactants.

ISOSTEARYL ERUCATE • *See* Surfactants.

ISOSTEARYL ETHYLIMIDAZOLINIUM ETHOSULFATE • Quaternary ammonium compound used as an antistatic ingredient in hair conditioners. *See* Quaternary Ammonium Compounds.

ISOSTEARYL GLYCERYL ETHER • A skin-conditioning ingredient. *See* Glycerin.

ISOSTEARYL GLYCERYL PENTAERYTHRITYL ETHER • A hair-conditioning ingredient. *See* Pentaerythritol.

ISOSTEARYL HYDROXYETHYL IMIDAZOLINE • *See* Surfactants.

ISOSTEARYL IMIDAZOLINE • *See* Surfactants.

ISOSTEARYL ISOSTEARATE • *See* Stearyl Alcohol.

ISOSTEARYL ISOSTEARYOL STEARATE • A skin-conditioning ingredient. *See* Stearic Acid.

ISOSTEARYL LACTATE • *See* Surfactants.

ISOSTEARYL MYRISTATE • The ester of isostearyl alcohol and myristic acid.

ISOSTEARYL NEOPENTANOATE • An emollient. On the basis of the available information, the CIR Expert Panel (*see*) concluded that it is safe as a cosmetic ingredient. *See* Surfactants.

ISOSTEARYL PALMITATE • *See* Surfactants.

ISOSTEAROYL PG-TRIMONIUM CHLORIDE • An antistatic ingredient in hair preparations. *See* Quaternary Ammonium Compounds.

ISOSTEARYL STEAROYL STEARATE • *See* Surfactants.

ISOTHIAZOLINONES • 5-chloro-2-methyl-4-isothiazolin-3-one (MCI) Kathon. Broad-spectrum biocides used as preservatives in shampoos and many other household and industrial products. Unlike the preservatives DMDM hydantoin and imidazolidinyl urea also commonly used in these products, isothiazolinones do not release formaldehyde, to which some people are sensitive. However, some people are sensitive to isothiazolinones. Most of those who do show a reaction are also allergic to nickel.

ISOTHIOCYANATES • Found in mustard, horseradish, radishes, they seem to induce protective enzymes.

ISOTRETINOIN • Accutane. Introduced in 1979, it is a derivative of vitamin A that decreases the size of the oil glands and alters the composition of sebum, making it less likely to plug hair outlets. Used to treat severe cystic acne unresponsive to conventional therapy. Potential adverse reactions include nausea, vomiting, anemia, headache, fatigue, pressure on the brain, red eyes, dry eyes, high blood sugar, gum bleeding and inflammation, liver dysfunction, sore lips, rash, dry skin, peeling of palms and toes, skin infection, decreased libido, impotence, decreased vaginal secretions, irregular menstruation, sensitivity to light, high blood fats, muscle and bone pain, and thinning of hair. Contraindicated in women of childbearing age unless the patient has had a negative pregnancy test within two weeks before beginning therapy. It is definitely harmful to the fetus. It must never be taken by a pregnant or likely-to-be-pregnant woman. Also contraindicated in patients with hypersensitivity to parabens, which are used as preservatives. If used with other photosensitivity-causing agents, it may compound the effect. Abrasives, medicated soaps and cleansers, acne preparations containing peeling agents, topical alcohol preparations (including cosmetics, after-shave, and cologne) may cause increased irritation or excessive drying of the skin. Alcohol ingested increases the risk of high blood fats. Tetracyclines increase the risk of brain pressure. Vitamin A and vitamin supplements containing A increase isotretinoin's toxic effects. Should be taken with or shortly after meals to ensure adequate absorption.

ISOTRIDECYL ISONONANOATE • *See* Tridecyl Alcohol.

ISOVALERIC ACID • Occurs in valerian, hop oil, tobacco, and other plants. Colorless liquid with a disagreeable taste and odor, used in flavors and perfumes. *See* Valeric Acid.

IV • Abbreviation for intravenous medicine administered through the veins.

IVY EXTRACT • Extract of climbing plant with evergreen leaves native to Europe and Asia, *Hedera helix.* Widely used in body and hand products, bubble bath, bath soaps, mudpacks, and moisturizers. Produces a color that ranges from dark grayish green to yellowish. All parts of the plants are poisonous. Contact with a fresh plant can cause skin rash in sensitive adults.

J

JABORANDI • *Pilocarpus pennatifolius.* A tincture from the leaves of the pilocarpus plant, grown in South America. It supposedly stimulates the sebaceous glands and scalp, and was formerly used to induce sweating. Used in hair tonics. A source of pilocarpine (*see*). Poisonous when ingested on the skin. The EU bans it in cosmetics.

JAGUAR GUM • *See* Guar Gum.

JALAP RESIN • *Ipomoea purga.* A resin (*see*) used in cosmetics. The dried purgative tuberous root of a Mexican plant. Was once used as a drastic cathartic.

JAMBUL EXTRACT • Jamboo. Java Plum. An extract of the roots of *Syzyglum jambolanum.* The bark, resin, and oil contain volatile oils, fat, gallic acid (*see*), and albumen. It is used medically as an antidiarrheal. Extracts of the bark are used in cosmetics to soothe the skin.

JANIA RUBENS • Red Algae. Coral Weed. Moisturizer and protective ingredient. Has been found by scientific researchers to have some antitumor activity.

JAPAN WAX • *Rhus succedanea.* Vegetable Wax. Japan Tallow. A fat squeezed from the fruit of a tree grown in Japan and China. Pale yellow, flat cakes, disks, or squares with a fatlike rancid odor and taste. Used as a substitute for beeswax in cosmetic ointments. It is related to poison ivy and may cause allergic contact dermatitis. The CIR Expert Panel (*see*) concluded this is a safe ingredient.

JAPANESE ANGELICA • *Angelica acutiloba.* A shrub or small Japanese tree. Used in bath products. *See* Angelica.

JAPANESE COLORS

Colors with parentheses are not permitted by the FDA at present.

Japanese name		CI Number	Color Index name
Brown #201	D & C Brown No.1	C.I. 20170	Acid Orange 24
Black #401	(D & C Black No.1)	C.I. 20470	Acid Black 1
Violet #201	D & C Violet No.2	C.I. 60725	Solv. Violet 13
Violet #401	EXT. D & C Violet No.2	C.I. 60730	Acid Violet No.43
Bleu #1	FD & C Blue No.1	C.I. 42090	Food Blue 2
Bleu #2	FD & C Blue No.2	C.I. 73015	Acid Blue 74
Bleu #201	D & C Blue No.6	C.I. 73000	Vat Blue 1
Bleu #202		C.I. 42052	Acid Blue 5
Bleu #203		C.I. 42052	Acid Blue 5
Bleu #204	D & C Blue No.9	C.I. 69825	Vat Blue 6
Bleu #205	D & C Blue No.4	C.I. 42090	Acid Blue 9
Bleu #403		C.I. 61520	Solv. Blue 63
Bleu #404	mPhthalocyaninato(2-)ncopper	C.I. 74160	Pig. Blue 15
Green #201	D & C Green No.5	C.I. 61570	Acid Green 25
Green #202	D & C Green No.6	C.I. 61565	Solv. Green 3
Green #204	D & C Green No.8	C.I. 59040	Solv. Green 7
Green #205		C.I. 42095	Acid Green 5
Green #3	FD & C Green No.3	C.I. 42053	Food Green
Green #401	(EXT. D & C Green No.1)	C.I.10020	Acid Green 1
Green #402		C.I. 42085	Acid Green 3
Yellow #201	D & C Yellow No.7	C.I. 45350	Acid Yellow 73
Yellow #202-(1)	D & C Yellow No.8	C.I. 45350	Acid Yellow 73
Yellow #202-(2)		C.I. 45350	Acid Yellow 73
Yellow #203	D & C Yellow No.10	C.I. 47005	Acid Yellow 3
Yellow #204	D & C Yellow No.11	C.I. 47000	Solv. Yellow 33
Yellow #205		C.I. 21090	Pig. Yellow 12
Yellow #4	FD & C Yellow No.5	C.I. 19140	Acid Yellow 23
Yellow #401	(EXT. D & C Yellow No.5)	C.I. 11680	Pig. Yellow 1
Yellow #402	(not permitted by FDA or EU)	C.I. 18950	Acid Yellow 40
Yellow #403-(1)	EXT. D & C Yellow No.7	C.I. 10316	Acid Yellow 1
Yellow #404		C.I. 11380	Solv. Yellow 5
Yellow #405		C.I. 11390	Solv. Yellow 6
Yellow #406	(EXT. D & C Yellow No.1)	C.I. 13065	Acid Yellow 36
Yellow #407	(EXT. D & C Yellow No.3)	C.I. 18820	Acid Yellow 11
Yellow #5	FD & C Yellow No.6	C.I. 15985	Food Yellow 3
Orange #201	D & C Orange No.5	C.I. 45370	Solv. Red 72
Orange #203	(D & C Orange No.17)	C.I. 12075	Pig. Orange 5
Orange #204		C.I. 21110	Pig. Orange 13
Orange #205	D & C Orange No.4	C.I. 15510	Acid Orange 7
Orange #206	D & C Orange No.10	C.I. 45425	Solv. Red 73

Japanese name		CI Number	Color Index name
Orange #207	D & C Orange No.11	C.I. 45425	Acid Red 95
Orange #401		C.I. 11725	Pig. Orange 1
Orange #402	(EXT. D & C Orange No.3)	C.I. 14600	Acid Orange 20
Orange #403	(EXT. D & C Orange No.4)	C.I. 12100	Solv. Orange 2
Red #102		C.I. 16255	Acid Red 18
Red #104-(1)	D & C Red No.28	C.I. 45410	Acid Red 92
Red #105-(1)		C.I. 45440	Acid Red 94
Red #106		C.I. 45100	Acid Red 52
Red #2	(FD & C Red No.2)	C.I.16185	Acid Red 27
Red #201	D & C Red No.6	C.I. 15850	Pig. Red 57–1
Red #202	D & C Red No.7	C.I. 15850	Pig. Red 57
Red #203	(D & C Red No.8)	C.I. 15585	Pig. Red 53
Red #204	(D & C Red No.9)	C.I. 15585	Pig. Red 53(Ba)
Red #205	(D & C Red No.10)	C.I. 15630	Pig. Red 49(Na)
Red #206	(D & C Red No.11)	C.I. 15630	Pig. Red 49(Ca)
Red #207	(D & C Red No.12)	C.I. 15630	Pig. Red 49(Ba)
Red #208	(D & C Red No.13)	C.I. 15630	Pig. Red 49(Sr)
Red #213	(D & C Red No.19)	C.I. 45170	Basic Violet 10
Red #214		C.I. 45170	Solv. Red 49
Red #215	(D & C Red No.37)	C.I. 45170	Solv. Red 49
Red #218	D & C Red No.27	C.I. 45410	Solv. Red 48
Red #219	D & C Red No.31	C.I. 15800	Pig. Red 64
Red #220	D & C Red No.34	C.I. 15880	Pig. Red 63(Ca)
Red #221	(D & C Red No.35)	C.I. 12120	Pig. Red 3
Red #223	D & C Red No.21	C.I. 45380	Solv. Red 43
Red #225	D & C Red No.17	C.I. 26100	Solv. Red 23
Red #226	D & C Red No.30	C.I. 73360	Vat Red 1
Red #227	D & C Red No.33	C.I. 17200	Acid Red 33
Red #228		C.I. 12085	Pig. Red 4
Red #230-(1)	D & C Red No.22	C.I. 45380	Acid Red 87
Red #230-(2)		C.I. 45380	Acid Red 87
Red #231		C.I. 45410	Acid Red 92
Red #232		C.I. 45440	Acid Red 94
Red #3	FD & C Red No.3	C.I. 45430	Acid Red 51
Red #401	(EXT. D & C Red No.3)	C.I. 45190	Acid Violet 9
Red #404		C.I. 12315	Pig. Red 22
Red #405		C.I. 5865	Pig. Red 48
Red #501		C.I. 26105	Solv. Red 24
Red #502		C.I. 16155	Food Red 6
Red #503		C.I. 16150	Acid Red 26
Red #504	FD & C Red No.4	C.I.14700	Food Red 1
Red #505		C.I. 12140	Solv. Orange 7
Red #506		C.I. 15620	Acid Red 88

JAPANESE QUINCE EXTRACT • Extract of the seeds of *Chaenomeles japonica*. *See* Quince Seed.

JASMINE • *Jasminum officinale*. Used in perfumes. The essential oil extracted from the extremely fragrant white flowers of the tall, climbing, semi-evergreen jasmine shrub. May cause allergic reactions. Synthetic jasmine contains cinnamic aldehyde (*see*).

JASMINE ABSOLUTE • Oil of jasmine obtained by extraction with volatile or non-volatile solvents. Sometimes called the "natural perfume" because the oil is not subjected to heat and distilled oils. For centuries, the jasmine flower has been brewed in tea to aid relaxation. May cause allergic reactions. The rhizomes and roots contain the alkaloid gelsemine, a very potent analgesic that is used to treat the severe pain in the face known as tic douloureux, or trigeminal neuralgia (*see*). Herbalists claim that jasmine oil rubbed on the body increases sexual interest. Jasmine can be highly toxic and can cause death by respiratory arrest. *See* Absolute.

JASMINUM OFFICINALE • The EU name for jasmine (*see*).

JASOMONE • Derived from the oil of jasmine flowers, it is used in flavorings and perfumery.

JAVA JUTE EXTRACT • Extract of the flowers of *Hibiscus sabdariffa*. *See* Hibiscus.

JECFA • Abbreviation for Joint Expert Committee on Food Additives under FAO/WHO (*see*).

JELLYFISH EXTRACT • The collagen extract is used in skin care. In South Korea, it is used for weight loss. Also is being studied for its anticancer properties and prevention of heart disease.

JEN SHANG • *See* Ginseng.

JESUIT'S TEA • *See* Maté Extract.

JEWELWEED • *See* Impatiens.

JIOU EKISU • *Rehmannia chinensis*. Chinese Foxglove. Used as a moisturizer.

JOB'S TEARS • *Coix lacryma-jobi*. Tear Grass. Asiatic grass now widely cultivated. A skin-conditioning ingredient. *See* Yokuinin.

JOCK ITCH • Tinea Cruris. Ringworm of the groin; a fungus infection of the skin of the upper thighs near the genital organs. It is caused by the same group of organisms that causes athlete's foot.

JOE-PYE WEED • *Eupatorium maculatum* and *E. purpureum*. A member of the daisy (Compositae) family. A North American perennial, it is found in moist woods and meadows. It was named after a New England medicine man who was renowned for his cures for typhus and other fevers with his decoctions from this plant. Learning from Indian women, who bathed their ailing children in an infusion of the root, white settlers gathered joe-pye weed for all kinds of medicinal purposes. Its astringent (*see*) and diuretic properties made it a dependable medicine for arthritis, backache, pain, edema, and urinary problems. It is used by homeopaths to treat aching bones. Botanical additive to lotions and creams.

JOJOBA ALCOHOL • Fatty alcohol from Jojoba. *See* Jojoba Oil.

JOJOBA BUTTER • Obtained from jojoba oil (*see*).

JOJOBA OIL • *Buxus chinensis*. Widely used in cosmetics, it is the oil extracted from the beanlike seeds of the desert shrub *Simmondsia chinensis*. A liquid wax used as a lubricant and as a substitute for sperm oil, carnauba wax, and beeswax. Mexicans and American Indians have long used the bean's oily wax as a hair conditioner and skin lubricant. U.S. companies are now promoting the ingredient in shampoos, moisturizers, sunscreens, and conditioners as a treatment for "crow's feet," wrinkles, stretch marks, and dry skin. May cause allergic reactions. On the basis of the available information, the CIR Expert Panel (*see*) concluded that it is safe as a cosmetic ingredient.

JOJOBA WAX • The semisolid fraction of jojoba oil (*see*). On the basis of the available information, the CIR Expert Panel (*see*) concluded it is safe as a cosmetic ingredient.

JOJOBA WAX PEG 80, 120 ESTERS • Used as surfactants, cleansing ingredients, and solubilizing ingredients.

JONQUIL EXTRACT • Extract of *Narcissus jonquilla*, a member of the daffodil (Amaryllidaceae) family. Fragrance ingredient. May cause skin irritation.

JUGLANS • *See* Walnut Extract.

JUGLANS MANDSHURICA • The EU name for walnut.

JUGLONE • A coloring for hair dyes. Yellow needles, slightly soluble in hot water but soluble in alcohol. It is the active coloring principle in walnuts. When mixed in solution with an alkali, it gives a purplish red color. It has antihemorrhaging activity. The lethal oral dose in mice is only 2.5 milligrams per kilogram of body weight. No known skin toxicity.

JU HUA • *See* Chrysanthemum.

JUJUBE EXTRACT • Da T'sao. Extract of the fruit of *Ziziphus jujuba*. The Chinese jujube date is commonly used in a wide variety of herbal formulas. It is found dried in most oriental markets. It is used to enhance the taste and benefits of soups and stews and to energize the body. Chinese herbalists believe it relieves nervous exhaustion, insomnia, apprehension, forgetfulness, dizziness, and clamminess.

JUNIPER BERRY • *Juniperus communis*. Viscum. Mistletoe. The berries are used by herbalists to treat urinary problems. According to herbalists, it acts directly on the kidneys, stimulating the flow of urine. Juniper berries and extracts are in several OTC drugstore diuretic and laxative preparations. In fact, gin was created in the 1500s by a Dutch pharmacist using juniper berries to sell as an inexpensive diuretic. The berries have long been used by herbalists to treat gout caused by high uric acid in the blood. The berries are high in vitamin C. It is used in "organic" cosmetics. Juniper is also used to lower cholesterol and to treat arthritis. Large amounts may irritate the kidneys. The FDA issued a notice in 1992 that juniper has not been shown to be safe and effective as claimed in OTC digestive aid products and oral menstrual drugs. The EU banned it in cosmetics.

JUNIPER TAR • Oil of Cade. The volatile oil from the wood of a pine tree. Dark brown, viscous, with a smoky odor and acrid, slightly aromatic taste. Used as a skin peeler and anti-itching factor in hair preparations and as a scent in perfumes. Less corrosive than phenol (*see*).

JUNIPERUS • *See* Juniper Berry.

JUNIPERUS OXYCEDRUS TAR • Obtained from the wood of the juniper bush. Used to scent hair products. *See* Juniper Berry.

K

K+ 10 • *See* Potassium Chloride.

KAEMPFERIA GALANGA • The EU name for Cekur. A member of the ginger family used to reduce swelling. Reportedly protects the skin against UV damage, according to research published in *Experimental Dermatology* in 2008. The researchers, led by Emanuela Camera from the San Gallicano Dermatology Institute in Rome, compared the protection provided by astaxanthin (AX) to that of canthaxanthin (CX) and beta-carotene (*see all*). Out of the three, it was astaxanthin that provided the most effective protection when human dermal fibroblasts underwent UV radiation. UVA radiation is known to both trigger the creation of reactive oxygen species (ROS) and deplete the antioxidant defense system of the fibroblasts by affecting antioxidant enzymes.

KALANCHOE PINNATA • An African and Australian herb. *See* Cedar.

KALAYA OIL • *See* Emu Oil.

KALLIKREIN • An enzyme isolated from pancreatic tissue used as conditioner for skin and hair.

KANGAROO PAW FLOWER • *Anigozanthos flavidus.* An Australian sedgelike spring-flowering herb related to the amaryllis. It has clustered flowers covered with greenish wool. Used in Australian-imported hair sprays.

KANOKOSOU EKISU • Skin conditioner. *See* Valerian.

KANZOU • Skin conditioner. *See* Licorice.

KAOLIN • China Clay. Aids in the covering ability of face powder and in absorbing oil secreted by the skin. Used in baby powders, bath powders, face masks, foundation cake makeups, liquid powders, face powders, dry rouges, and emollients. Originally obtained from Kaolin Hill in Kiangsi Province in southeast China. Essentially a hydrated aluminum silicate (*see*). It is a white or yellowish white mass or powder, insoluble in water and absorbent. Used medicinally to treat intestinal disorders, but in large doses it may cause obstructions, perforations, or granuloma (tumor) formation. May clog the skin. It is also used in the manufacture of color lakes (*see*).

KAPPAPHYCUS ALVAREZII • Brown Licorice. Euchema. Tambalang. A seaweed that contains carrageenan (*see*).

KARAYA GUM • Kaday. Katilo. Kullo. Kuterra. Sterculia Gum. Indian Tragacanth. Mucara. The exudate of a tree found in India. The finely ground white powder is used in gelatins and gumdrops. The vegetable gum is used as a bulk-forming laxative. *See* Gum Karaya.

KASSOU • Brown algae. Phaeophyta. Used as a skin conditioner.

KATHON CG • Octhilinone. A fungicide used in cosmetics and shampoos and for leather preservation. It has been extensively studied in cosmetics and toiletries. It is effective in low concentration and is very useful against bacteria, yeasts, and fungi. Although toxicity has not been a problem at usual use levels, sensitization, particularly among women, has been reported. The main source of sensitization has been kathon in cosmetics. Researchers in the United States and Europe are reporting an increase in patients becoming sensitized to the preservative.

KATSU201 • The Japanese name for Acid Orange or Brown 1.

KAVA KAVA • *Piper methysticum.* Kawa. Ava. The Polynesian herb's root is used by herbalists as a remedy for insomnia and nervousness. A compound in kava is marketed in Europe as a mild sedative for the elderly. Other ingredients in kava have been shown to have antiseptic properties in the laboratory, and it is used in "organic" cosmetics. It is also a reputedly potent analgesic and antiseptic that may be taken internally or applied directly to a painful wound.

KAWA EXTRACT • The extract of the roots, stems, and leaves of *Piper methysticum.* *See* Kava Kava.

KEFIRAN • A skin conditioner and humectant made from glucose and galactose (*see both*).

KEIHI EKISU • A fragrance ingredient. *See* Cinnamon

KELP • Recovered from the giant Pacific marine plant *Macrocystis pyriffrae,* it is used by herbalists to supply the thyroid gland with iodine, to help regulate the texture of the skin, and to help the body burn off excess fat. In Japan, where kelp is a large part of the diet, thyroid disease is almost unknown. Kelp was banned from OTC diet pills by the FDA on February 10, 1992. Kelp does contain many minerals, and herbalists claim that it has anticancer, antirheumatic, anti-inflammatory, and blood pressure–lowering properties. Contraindicated in those with overactive thyroids or sensitivity to iodine.

KERATIN • Animal Keratin. Protein (*see*) obtained from the horns, hoofs, feathers, quills, and hairs of various creatures. Yellowish brown powder. Insoluble in water, alcohol, or ether but soluble in ammonia. Used in permanent-wave solutions and hair rinses. On the Canadian Hotlist (*see*).

KERATIN AMINO ACIDS • Animal Keratin Amino Acids. The cosmetics manufacturers took out as many "animals" in the labels as possible. A mixture of amino acids from the hydrolysis of keratin (*see*). *See also* Hydrolyzed Keratin.

KERATOLYTICS • Products that appear to loosen skin flakes and allow them to be more easily washed away. Lotions containing salicylic acid (*see*) are used for this purpose.

KERION • A fungal infection of the beard or scalp.

KEROSENE • *See* Deodorized Kerosene.

KEROTOSIS • Any lesion on the skin marked by the presence of an overgrowth of the horny layer. Among such lesions are those due to the sun, age, and hair follicles. *See* Actinic Kerotoses.

KETOCONAZOLE • Nizoral. Introduced in 1981, it inhibits the growth of fungi and is used to treat systemic candidiasis, chronic mucocandidiasis, oral thrush, candiduria, coccidioidomycosis, histoplasmosis, chromomycosis, and paracoccidioidomycosis—severe skin infections resistant to therapy with topical or oral griseofulvin. In topical applications, the potential adverse reactions include itching, stinging, or irritation. A ketoconazole shampoo is fairly harsh on the hair shafts, so it is often recommended by dermatologists that a conditioner be used after cleansing the hair with ketoconazole shampoos.

KETOGLUTARIC ACID • A deodorant. *See* Carboxylic Acid.

KETONES • Acetone, Methyl, or Ethyl. Aromatic substances obtained by the oxidation of secondary alcohols. Ethereal or aromatic odor, generally insoluble in water but soluble in alcohol or ether. Solvents used in nail polish and nail polish removers. When injected into the abdomens of rats, intermediate dosages are lethal. *See* Acetone for skin toxicity.

KHAYA SENEGALENSIS • The EU name for African mahogany. Used as a fungicide and germicide. Africans used it to lower fever.

KI • *See* Potassium Iodide.

K-IDE • *See* Potassium Bicarbonate and Potassium Citrate.

KIDACHI ALOE EKISU • Emollient. *See* Aloe Vera.

KIDNEY BEAN EXTRACT • Extract of *Phaseolus vulgaris,* the beans were used as a nutrient and a laxative by the American Indians.

KIE • *See* Ephedrine and Potassium Iodide.

KIGELIA AFRICANA • Sausage Tree. Often cultivated in tropical countries for its brownish red, bell-shaped flowers and long sausage-shaped fruits. Used in skin care products.

KINA EKISU • *See* Cinchona Extract.

KINETIN • Found in many yeast plants. Used as a plant growth regulator. In cosmetics, it is employed in skin care and "age-defying" products.

KINGINKA EKISU • *Lonicera japonica. See* Honeysuckle.

KINO • *Pterocarpus marsuipun. P. indicus. P. echinatus.* Gummi. Narra. Bibla Prickly Narra. Padauk. The exudate from the trunk of this large tree is used as an astringent (*see*) for the treatment of wounds, scrapes, diarrhea, and skin ulcers. It contains a tanninlike substance. It was also used as an aphrodisiac in Africa.

KIWI EXTRACT • Extract of the fruit named for the kiwi bird, *Actinidia chinensis.* It is used in cosmetic flavorings and in emollients. Kiwi fruit extract combines high essential fatty acids with antioxidant properties. A New Zealand company is promoting it as an anti-aging ingredient both through topical application and oral use. The extract contains antioxidants more powerful than green tea, a common anti-aging ingredient in cosmetics applications, according to the Auckland-based company Kiwifruit Extract Ventures (KEVL). "We discovered a range of powerful antioxidants in the undigested parts of the kiwifruit that appear to be many times more potent than green tea and equal to the most powerful antioxidant ingredients on the market today," said Spratt, CEO of the company. In addition, the company references studies that suggest the extract has other important beneficial effects on the skin. "Studies have shown that kiwifruit extract improves skin radiance, reduces the appearance of fine lines, and reduces the dark circles under the eyes," said Spratt. He added that kiwi's antioxidant properties, in combination with a selection of essential fatty acids, make the extract a good anti-aging ingredient.

K-LOR • *See* Potassium Chloride.

KLOR-CON • *See* Potassium Chloride.

KLOR-CON/EF • *See* Potassium Bicarbonate and Potassium Citrate.

KLOROMIN • *See* Chlorpheniramine.

KLORVESS • *See* Potassium Chloride.

KLOTRIX • *See* Potassium Chloride.

KNIPHOFIA UVARIA • Red Hot Poker. Torch Lily. Used as a skin protectant.

KNOTWEED EXTRACT • Extract of *Polygonum aviculare.* A common weed, the FDA issued a notice in 1992 that knotgrass, a member of the family, has not been shown to be safe and effective as claimed in OTC digestive aid products. As of this writing, no such caution has been made about its use in cosmetics.

KOHL • Cohol, Kahl, Kajal, Sorma. Used in some parts of the world for enhancing the appearance of the eyes. But kohl is unapproved for cosmetic use in the United States. It contains salts of heavy metals such as antimony and lead. Reports have linked the use of kohl to lead poisoning in children. Some eye cosmetics may be labeled with the word *kohl* only to indicate the shade, not because they contain true kohl. A preparation of antimony or soot mixed with other ingredients used especially in Arabia and Egypt to darken the edges of the eyelids. In Israel, it is used even on the eyes of some babies. The application to the eyes of babies or their mothers increases the blood lead levels in the infants. The incidence of adverse reactions is high, according to the FDA—about 25 percent if applied daily and 18 percent if applied occasionally. Third World–manufactured kohls have been purchased in the United States and Britain, suggesting that this hazard is no longer confined to the Third World. The kohls that contain lead are being sold in violation of U.S. and British law.

KOJIC ACID • A skin lightener produced from a fungus. *Aspergillus* (*see*) *oryzae.* Kojic acid works by blocking the formation of pigment by the deep cells on the skin. It is used to counteract age spots, pregnancy marks, and freckles as well as general skin pigmentation disorders of face and body.

KO KEN • *See* Kudzu.

KOKUM BUTTER • Obtained from the fruit kernel of *Garcinia indica,* which grows in the savanna areas in parts of the Indian subcontinent. It has very high content of stearic-oleic-stearic triglycerides (*see all*). Kokum butter has been used as an astringent, and for local application to ulceration and fissures of lips, hands, and soles. Used in skin and hair products, acne products, and skin tonics.

KOLA NUT • *Cola acuminata.* Cola. Guru Nut. Collected from a tree that grows in tropical Africa and is cultivated in South America, the seeds contain caffeine, theobromine, tannin, and volatile oil (*see all*). It is used in "organic" cosmetics. It is used for stimulation to counteract fatigue and as a diuretic. Herbalists use it to treat some types of migraine headache and diarrhea caused by anxiety. It is also used to treat emotional depression.

KOMBUCHKA • The product of the fermentation of sweet black tea by the symbiosis of two microorganisms. Historically, kombucha was considered the "fungus of long life" because it was believed to confer longevity. It is new and patented but aimed at reducing skin roughness in cosmetic creams.

KOU-CHA EKISU • Extract of black tea leaves of *Camelia sinensis* used as an antioxidant and skin conditioner. *See* Tea.

KOUSOU • Red Algae. *See* Algae.

KRAMERIA EXTRACT • Khatany Extract. A synthetic flavoring derived from the dried root of either of two American shrubs. Used in raspberry, bitters, fruit, and rum flavorings. Used in cosmetics as an astringent. Low oral toxicity. Large doses may produce gastric distress. Can cause tumors and death after injection, but not after ingestion.

KUDZU • A wild weed taking over the U.S. South. When taken internally, it can dilate capillaries. Source of isoflavone and the plant estrogens, genistein, and daidzein. It is claimed that the skin becomes firmer and the appearance of wrinkles is reduced if kudzu is used. It supposedly "energizes and revitalizes" the skin.

KUKUI NUT OIL • *Aleurites moluccana.* Candlenut Oil. Varnish Tree. Lumbang Oil. The oily seed of a tropical tree widely distributed in the tropics and used locally to make candles and commercially as a source of oil for making soap. Has been used by native Hawaiians for thousands of years to treat dry skin, psoriasis, acne, and other common skin problems.

KULLO • *See* Karaya Gum.

KURO401 • Japanese name for a diazo color for Acid Black 1, Disodium Salt. *See* Acid Black 1.

KURUMI KAKU • An abrasive. *See* Walnut Shell Powder.

KUTERRA • *See* Karaya Gum.

KYOUNIN EKISU • *See* Apricot.

L

LABDANUM • *Cistus labdanifer.* Synthetic Musk. Used in perfumes, especially as a fixative, it is a volatile oil obtained by steam distillation from gum extracted from various rockrose shrubs. Golden yellow, viscous, with a strong balsamic odor and a bitter taste. Also used as a synthetic flavoring in foods.

LABRADOR TEA EXTRACT • Hudson's Bay Tea. Marsh Tea. The extract of the dried flowering plant or young shoots of *Ledum palustre* or *L. groenlandicum,* a tall, resinous evergreen shrub found in bogs, swamps, and moist meadows. Brewed like tea, it has a pleasing antiscorbutic and stimulating quality. It was used by the American Indians and settlers as a tonic supposed to purify blood. It was also employed to treat wounds. *L. palustre* contains, among other things, tannin and valeric acid (*see both*).

LAC • A substance secreted by the lac insect and used chiefly in the form of shellac.

LAC • *See* Milk.

LACCAIC • A pigment found in a sticky substance produced by the insect *Coccus laccae* on certain trees in India. *See* Phenols.

LACCASE • An enzyme produced by the fermentation of *Aspergillus oryzae. See* Aspergillus.

LACQUER • A Japanese lacquer tree contains a lacquer related to poison ivy. *See* Shellac.

LACRIMAL • Pertaining to tears.

LACTAMIDE DEA • Skin-conditioning ingredient and humectant.

LACTAMIDE MEA • A mixture of ethanolamines (*see*) of lactic acid (*see*). Used as a conditioner and thickener in hair products and moisturizers.

LACTAMIDOPROPYL TRIMONIUM CHLORIDE • Antistatic ingredient. *See* Quaternary Ammonium Compounds.

LACTIC ACID • Used in skin fresheners. Odorless, colorless, usually a syrupy product normally present in blood and muscle tissue as a product of the metabolism of glucose and glycogen. Present in sour milk, beer, sauerkraut, pickles, and other food products made by bacterial fermentation. Also an acidulant. Caustic in concentrated solutions when taken internally or applied to the skin. In cosmetics, it may cause stinging in sensitive people, particularly in fair-skinned women. The FDA issued a notice in 1992 that lactic acid has not been shown to be safe and effective as claimed in OTC digestive aid products. *See* Alpha-Hydroxy Acids.

LACTIC YEASTS • Obtained from milk. *See* Lactic Acid and Faex.

LACTICARE • An oil-in-water emulsion of lactic acid (*see*) and sodium-PCA. Used as a base for skin care products.

LACTIS LIPIDA • Milk fat.

LACTIS PROTEINUM • Milk protein.

LACTITOL • Obtained from lactose (*see*) and used as a flavoring ingredient and humectant.

LACTOBACILLUS • Lactobacilli are any of the various rod-shaped bacteria of the genus *Lactobacillus*. These versatile bacteria ferment lactic acid (*see*). Because of their ability to derive lactic acid from glucose, these bacteria create an acidic environment that inhibits growth of many bacterial species that can lead to urogenital infections. *Lactobacillus* is generally harmless to humans, rarely inciting harmful infections or diseases. Yogurt contains lactobacilli.

LACTOBACILLUS/GLYCERIN/HYDROLYZED SOY PROTEIN • Skin conditioner. *See* Lactobacillus.

LACTOBIONIC ACID • A pH adjuster. *See* Carboxylic Acid.

LACTOFERRIN • A substance found in the milk of mammals believed to be involved in the transport of iron to the red blood cells. Used in hair and skin conditioners.

LACTOFLAVIN • Vitamin B_2. The nutrient riboflavin approved by the EU as a colorant but not in the United States.

LACTOGLOBULIN • Protein isolated from milk. Used in hair- and skin-conditioning products.

LACTOPEROXIDASE • An enzyme obtained from milk used as a moisturizer.

LACTO PEROXIDE • Reported to have antimicrobial activity. *See* Milk and Peroxide.

LACTOSE • Milk Sugar. Used widely as a base in eye lotions. Present in the milk of mammals. Stable in air but readily absorbs odors. Used in preparing food for infants, in tablets, and as a general base and diluent in pharmaceutical and cosmetic compounding. In large doses it is a laxative and diuretic. It was found to cause tumors when injected under the skin of mice in 50-milligram doses per kilogram of body weight. Generally nontoxic. In 1992, the FDA issued a notice that lactose had not been shown to be safe and effective as claimed in OTC digestive aid products.

LACTOYLGLUTATHIONE • A skin conditioner. *See* Carboxylic Acid and Glycine.

LACTOYL METHYLSILANOL ELASTINATE • The ester (*see*) of lactic acid and the salt of elastin (*see*). Used in emollients.

LACTOYL PHYTOSPHINGOSINE • A skin and hair conditioner. *See* Sphingolipids.

LACTUCA SATIVA • *See* Lettuce Extract.

LACTUCA SCARIOLA SATIVA • The EU name for lettuce extract (*see*).

LACTULOSE • A humectant and skin conditioner. *See* Fructose.

LADY'S MANTLE EXTRACT • From the dried leaves and flowering shoots of *Alchemilla vulgaris.* A common European herb covered with spreading hairs, it has been used for centuries by herbalists to concoct love potions.

LADY'S SLIPPER • *Cypripedium calceolus.* The root is used to treat anxiety, stress, insomnia, neurosis, restlessness, tremors, epilepsy, and palpitations. Herbalists claim it is also useful for depression. It is used in "organic" cosmetics. It contains volatile oils, resins, glucosides, and tannin (*see all*).

LADY'S THISTLE EXTRACT • *Silybum marianum.* A class of substances, flavon-lignans, produced by the plant are being studied for their liver-protecting capacity. *See* Thistle.

LAGENARIA VULGARIS • The EU name for gourd. The extract is used as a moisturizer.

LAGERSTROEMIA INDICA • Crape Myrtle. The deciduous crape myrtle is among the longest-blooming trees in existence with flowering periods lasting from 60 to 120 days. Originally from Asia, crape myrtle has been naturalized throughout the United States.

LAKES, COLOR • A lake is an organic pigment prepared by precipitating a soluble color with a form of aluminum, calcium, barium potassium, strontium, or zirconium, which then makes the colors insoluble. Not all colors are suitable for making lakes.

LAMINARIA • *See* Algae.

LAMIUM • White Nettle. A troublesome weed, with stingers, it has a long history and was used in folk medicine. Its flesh is rich in minerals and plant hormones, and it supposedly stimulates hair growth and shines and softens hair. Also used to make tomatoes resistant to spoilage, to encourage the growth of strawberries, and to stimulate the fermentation of humus. Hemp belongs to the nettle family.

LAMPBLACK • Used in eye makeup pencils. It is a bluish black, fine soot deposited on a surface by burning liquid hydrocarbons (*see*) such as oil. It is duller and less intense in color than other carbon blacks and has a blue undertone. It is also used in pigments for paints, enamels, and printing inks. *See* Carbon Black for toxicity.

LANDOPHIA OWARIENSIS • The EU name for an African plant that belongs to the dogbane family. Has been used to stop bleeding. It contains tannin (*see*). Some species of dogbane are poisonous.

LANETH • Derivatives of lanolin (*see*) widely used in cosmetics.

LANETH-5 THROUGH -40 • Emulsifiers. On the basis of the available information the CIR Expert Panel (*see*) found them to be safe in the early 1980s but is considering new information to determine if the final safety assessment should be reaffirmed, amended, or have an addendum. *See* Lanolin Alcohols.

LANETH-9 AND -10 ACETATE • Emulsifiers. On the basis of the available information, the CIR Expert Panel (*see*) concluded that they are safe as a cosmetic ingredient. *See* Lanolin Alcohols.

LANOLIN • Wool Fat. Wool Wax. A product of the oil glands of sheep. Used in lipsticks, liquid powders, mascaras, nail polish removers, protective oils, rouges, eye shadows, foundation creams, foundation cake makeups, hair conditioners, eye creams, cold creams, brilliantine hairdressings, ointment bases, and emollients. A natural emulsifier, it absorbs and holds water to the skin. Chemically a wax instead of a fat. Contains about 25 to 30 percent water. Advertisers have found that the words *contains lanolin* help to sell a product and have promoted it as being able to "penetrate the skin better than other oils," although there is little scientific proof of this. Lanolin has been found to be a common skin sensitizer, causing allergic contact skin rashes. It will not prevent or cure wrinkles and will not stop hair loss. It is not used in pure form today because of its allergy-causing potential. Products derived from it are less likely to cause allergic reactions. The CIR Expert Panel (*see*) found it safe. The FDA issued a notice in 1992 that lanolin has not been shown to be safe and effective as claimed in OTC poison ivy, poison oak, and poison sumac products.

LANOLIN ACID • On the basis of the available information, the CIR Expert Panel (*see*) found it safe in the early 1980s but is considering new information to determine if the final safety assessment should be reaffirmed, amended, or have an addendum. *See* Lanolin.

LANOLIN ALCOHOLS • Sterols. Triterpene Alcohols. Aliphatic Alcohols. Derived from lanolin (*see*), lanolin alcohols are available commercially as solid waxy materials that are yellow to amber in color or as pale to golden-yellow liquids. They are widely used as emulsifiers and emollients in hand creams and lotions, and while they are less likely to cause an allergic reaction than lanolin, they still may do so in the sensitive. Have been linked to acne. On the basis of the available information, the CIR Expert Panel (*see*) found them safe in the early 1980s but is considering new information to determine if the final safety assessment should be reaffirmed, amended, or have an addendum.

LANOLIN CERA • Lanolin Wax. *See* Lanolin.

LANOLIN LINOLEATE • *See* Lanolin.

LANOLIN OIL • Widely used in cosmetics including eyeliners, cold creams, suntan gels, bath soaps, hair conditioners, fragrance preparations, skin care products, moisturizers, face powders, and baby oils, it consists of 15 to 17 percent cholesterol, with the remainder liquid lanolin. On the basis of the available information, the CIR Expert Panel (*see*) found it safe in the early 1980s but is considering new information to determine if the final safety assessment should be reaffirmed, amended, or have an addendum. *See* Lanolin for toxicity.

LANOLIN RICINOLEATE • *See* Lanolin Alcohols.

LANOLIN WAX • Lanolin Cera. An emollient. On the basis of the available information, the CIR Expert Panel (*see*) found it safe in the early 1980s but is considering new information to determine if the final safety assessment should be reaffirmed, amended, or have an addendum. *See* Lanolin.

LANOLINAMIDE DEA • The ethanolamides of lanolin acid. *See* Lanolin.

LANOSTEROL • A widely used skin softener in hand creams and lotions, it is the fatty alcohol derived from the wool fat of sheep. *See* Lanolin.

LANTANA CAMARA • The EU name for verbena (*see*).

LANTHANUM CHLORIDE • An inorganic salt. A rare earth mineral that occurs in cerite, monazerite, orthite, and certain fluorspars. Used as a reingredient (*see*) and catalyst (*see*) in cosmetic preparations. No known toxicity from topical use, but a very small oral dose is lethal in rats.

LAPACHO EXTRACT • *Tabecuia heptaphylla* or *T. impetiginosa.* Pau d'arco Lapacho. The inner bark of a tree in the forests of Brazil, it was used by Brazilian Indians for the treatment of cancer. Contains quinones and lapachol. It also is used to treat fungal and parasitic infections, and to aid digestion. Also reportedly lowers blood sugar. Pau d'arco is now being studied in Brazil to treat cancers, including leukemia. Related structurally to vitamin K.

LAPIS LAZULI • No longer authorized for use in cosmetics. *See* Colors.

LAPPA EXTRACT • Burdock Extract. The extract of the roots of *Arctium lappa,* it contains tannic acid (*see*) and is used to soothe the skin.

LAPYRIUM CHLORIDE • Germ killer and antistatic ingredient. *See* Quaternary Ammonium Compounds.

LARD • Easily absorbed by the skin, it is used as a lubricant, emollient, and base in shaving creams, soaps, and various cosmetic creams. It is the purified internal fat from the abdomen of the hog. It is a soft, white, unctuous mass, with a slight characteristic odor and a bland taste. Insoluble in water.

LARD GLYCERIDE • *See* Lard.

LARIX EUROPEAEA • The EU name for European larch, a member of the pine family. It has astringent properties and is used to treat psoriasis and eczema.

LARKSPUR • *Consolida regalis.* The seeds are used to treat nits and lice on the skin and hair. It is a poison and should not be taken internally.

LARREA DIVARICATA • *See* Chaparral Extract.

LATEX • Synthetic Rubber. The milky, usually white juice or exudate of plants obtained by tapping. Used in beauty masks (*see* Face Masks and Packs) for its coating ability. Any of various gums, resins, fats, or waxes in an emulsion of water and synthetic rubber or plastic are now considered latex. Ingredients of latex compounds can be poisonous, depending upon which plant products are used. Can cause skin rash. Has, in rare cases, caused fatal allergic reactions when surgeons wear latex gloves.

LATHER • Produced by action of air bubbles in a soap solution. For satisfactory shaving, a lather must be dense. The air bubbles must be fine and stable for the duration of the shave. In bubble baths the air bubbles must be large and light.

LATISSE • *See* Eyelash Enhancer.

LAURALKONIUM BROMIDE • *See* Quaternary Ammonium Compounds.

LAURALKONIUM CHLORIDE • May form nitrosamines (*see*). Based on the available data, the CIR Expert Panel (*see*) concluded that this ingredient is safe as a cosmetic ingredient. However, it should not be used in cosmetic products containing nitrosating ingredients. *See* Quaternary Ammonium Compounds.

LAURAMIDE DEA • A widely used mixture of ethanolamides of lauric acid, the principal fatty acid of coconut oil, it is widely used in cosmetic soaps and detergents as a softener, thickener, and foam booster. *See* Lauric Acid.

LAURAMIDE MEA • *See* Lauric Acid.

LAURAMIDE MIPA • A mixture of isopropanolamides of lauric acid widely used as a wetting ingredient in soaps and detergents. *See* Lauric Acid.

LAURAMIDOPROPYL ACETAMIDODIMONIUM CHLORIDE • *See* Quaternary Ammonium Compounds.

LAURAMIDOPROPYL BETAINE • *See* Quaternary Ammonium Compounds.

LAURAMIDOPROPYL DIMETHYLAMINE • *See* Lauric Acid and Dimethylamine.

LAURAMIDOPROPYL HYDROXYSULTAINE • Antistatic ingredient and emollient. *See* Betaines.

LAURAMINE OXIDE • Widely used as a cleansing ingredient and conditioner in hair products such as shampoos and dressings. Can form nitrosamines (*see*). In rats up to 40 percent was absorbed through the skin. On the basis of the available information, the CIR Expert Panel (*see*) concluded that it is safe as a cosmetic ingredient for rinse-off products, but for leave-on products it should be limited to 5 percent. *See* Lauric Acid.

LAURAMINOPROPIONIC ACID • *See* Propionic Acid.

LAURDIMONIUM HYDROXYPROPYL HYDROLYZED SOY PROTEIN • An antistatic ingredient in hair conditioners. *See* Quaternary Ammonium Compounds.

LAURDIMONIUM HYDROXYPROPYL HYDROLYZED WHEAT PROTEIN • An antistatic ingredient in hair conditioners. *See* Quaternary Ammonium Compounds

LAUREL • The fresh berries and leaf extract of the laurel tree *Laurus nobilis.* The berries are used as a flavoring for beverages, and the leaf extract is a spice flavoring for vegetables. *See* Laurel Leaf Oil. GRAS

LAUREL ALCOHOL • Extract of *Laurus nobilis* used as a water softener.

LAUREL GALLATE • An antioxidant, the laurel ester of gallic acid (*see*).

LAUREL LEAF OIL • Derived from steam distillation of the leaves of *Laurus nobilis,* it is a yellow liquid with a spicy odor used as a flavoring ingredient. Moderately toxic by ingestion. A skin irritant. GRAS

LAURETH-1, -30 • Surfactants. On the basis of the available information, the CIR Expert Panel (*see*) concluded that this ingredient is safe as a cosmetic. On the basis of the available information, the CIR Expert Panel found -4,-23 safe in the early 1980s but is considering new information to determine if the final safety assessment should be reaffirmed, amended, or have an addendum. *See* Lauryl Alcohol.

LAURETH PHOSPHATE • A complex mixture of esters of phosphoric acid and ethoxylated lauryl alcohol. *See* Surfactants.

LAURIC ACID • *n*-Dodecanoic Acid. A common constituent of vegetable fats, especially coconut oil and laurel oil. Its derivatives are widely used as a base in the manufacture of soaps, detergents, and lauryl alcohol (*see*) because of their foaming properties. Has a slight odor of bay and makes copious large bubbles when in soap. A mild irritant but not a sensitizer. The CIR Expert Panel (*see*) concluded that this ingredient is safe for use in cosmetic products.

LAURIC ALDEHYDE • *See* Lauric Acid.

LAURIC DEA • Creates a good, long-lasting foam in shampoos. *See* Lauric Acid.

LAURIC/PALMITIC/OLEIC TRIGLYCERIDE • Turtle Oil. A mixture of glycerin with lauric, palmitic, and oleic acids used as a skin moisturizer.

LAUROAMPHOACETATE • A preservative. *See* Imidazole.

LAUROAMPHODIACETATE • A preservative. *See* Imidazole.

LAUROAMPHODIPROPIONATE • *See* Propionic Acid and Lauric Acid.

LAUROAMPHODIPROPIONIC ACID • Preservative. *See* Lauric Acid and Propionic Acid.

LAUROAMPHODROXYPROPYLSULFONATE • *See* Imidazole.

LAUROAMPHOPROPINOATE • *See* Lauric Acid and Propionic Acid.

LAUROYL COLLAGEN AMINO ACIDS • A condensation product of lauric acid chloride and hydrolyzed (*see*) animal protein used in soaps. The word *animal* has been removed from this ingredient name.

LAUROYL ETHYL GLUCOSIDE • An emulsifier. *See* Laurel.

LAUROYL HYDROLYZED COLLAGEN • A condensation product of lauric acid chloride and hydrolyzed collagen (*see*). The word *animal* has been removed from this ingredient name. Used in hair products as a cleanser and conditioner.

LAUROYL HYDROLYZED ELASTIN • Used in hair and skin conditioners. *See* Laurel and Elastin.

LAUROYL LYSINE • Widely used in makeup such as blushers and lipsticks. *See* Lauric Acid and Lysine.

LAUROYL METHYL BETA-ALANINE • A skin conditioner. *See* Alanine.

LAUROYL SARCOSINE • *See* Sarcosines.

LAUROYL SILK AMINO ACIDS • Made from silk and lauric acid (*see both*) used in hair products as a cleanser and conditioner.

LAURTRIMONIUM CHLORIDE • *See* Quaternary Ammonium Compounds.

LAURUS NOBILIS • On the Canadian Hotlist (*see*). *See* Laurel.

LAURYL ALCOHOL • 1-Dodecanol. A colorless, crystalline compound that is produced commercially from coconut oil. Used to make detergents because of its sudsing ability. Has a characteristic fatty odor. It is soluble in most oils but is insoluble in glycerin. Used in perfumery. *See* Lauric Acid for toxicity.

LAURYL AMINE • *See* Lauric Acid.

LAURYL AMINOPROPYLGLYCINE • *See* Lauryl Alcohol.

LAURYL BEHENATE • Used as a skin-conditioning ingredient and as a cover-up. The ester (*see*) of lauric acid and behenic acid (*see both*).

LAURYL BETAINE • Widely used in bath products. *See* Lauric Acid.

LAURYL DIETHLENDIAMINEGLYCINE • *See* Lauryl Alcohol.

LAURYL DIMETHYLAMINE ACRYLINOLATE • *See* Lauric Acid and Dimethylamine.

LAURYL DIMETHYLAMINE ACRYLINOLEATE • *See* Lauric Acid.

LAURYL DIMONIUM HYDROXYPROPYL HYDROLYZED COLLAGEN • *See* Quaternary Ammonium Compounds.

LAURYL DIMONIUM HYDROXYPROPYL HYDROLYZED KERATIN • Protein derivative from skin. *See* Quaternary Ammonium Compounds.

LAURYL DIMONIUM HYDROXYPROPYL HYDROLYZED SOY PROTEIN • *See* Soy and Quaternary Ammonium Compounds.

LAURYL GLUCOSIDE • Widely used surfactant in hair dyes and shampoos. A wetting ingredient that lowers water's surface tension, permitting it to spread out and penetrate more easily. *See* Lauryl Alcohol and Glucose.

LAURYL GLYCOL • *See* Lauryl Alcohol and Glycol.

LAURYL HYDROSULTAINE • A salt of lauric acid (*see*) used as a softener.

LAURYL HYDROXYETHYL IMIDAZOLINE • A preservative. *See* Imidazoline.

LAURYL HYDROXYSULTAINE • An antistatic ingredient used in shampoos. *See* Betaines.

LAURYL ISOQUINOLINIUM BROMIDE • Quaternary ammonium compound (*see*) active against a microorganism believed to cause a type of dandruff. Used in hair tonics and cuticle softeners. Slightly greater toxicity than benzalkonium chloride in rats. No skin irritation or sensitization in concentrations of 0.1 percent and lower. Used also as an agriculture fungicide.

LAURYL ISOSTEARATE • The ester of lauryl alcohol and isostearic acid (*see both*).

LAURYL LACTATE • *See* Lauric Acid and Lactic Acid.

LAURYL LAURATE • Binder and stabilizer in hair products. *See* Lauric Acid.

LAURYL METHACRYLATE • *See* Lauric Acid and Acrylates.

LAURYL PALMITATE • The ester (*see*) of lauryl alcohol and palmitic acid (*see both*).

LAURYL PHOSPHATE • An emulsifier. *See* Phosphoric Acid and Lauric Acid.

LAURYL PYRIDINUM CHLORIDE • *See* Quaternary Ammonium Compounds.

LAURYL PYRROLIDONE • Hair conditioner. *See* Lauric Acid and Pyrrolidone.

LAURYL STEARATE • The ester of lauryl alcohol and stearic acid (*see both*).

LAURYL SULFATE • Derived from lauryl alcohol (*see*). Its potassium, zinc, magnesium, sodium, calcium, and ammonium salts are used in shampoos because of their foaming properties. *See* Sodium Lauryl Sulfate.

LAURYL SULTAINE • *See* Lauryl Alcohol and Betaine.

LAVANDIN OIL • *Lavandula hybrida.* Used in soaps and perfumes. It is the essential oil of a hybrid related to the lavender plant. Fragrant, yellowish, with a camphor-lavender scent.

LAVANDULA • *See* Lavender Oil.

LAVENDER • *Lavandula vera.* An evergreen of the mint family, it is native to the Mediterranean coast and is cultivated in France, Italy, and England. The name is derived from the Latin word *lavare,* which means "to wash." Lavender flower contains large amounts of essential oils that have antispasmodic, antiseptic, and carminative activity.

LAVENDER OIL • *Lavandula angustifolia.* Widely used in skin fresheners, powders, shaving preparations, mouthwashes, dentifrices, and perfumes. The volatile oil from the fresh flowering tops of lavender. Also used in a variety of food flavorings. It can cause allergic reactions and has been found to cause adverse skin reactions when the skin is exposed to sunlight. Related to the lavender plant. Fragrant, yellowish, with a camphor-lavender scent.

LAWSONE • Derived from the leaves of *Lawsonia inermia,* it is used as a sunscreen ingredient. *See* Henna.

LAWSONIA INERMIA • *See* Henna.

L-CARNITINE • *See* Carnitine.

LEAD ACETATE • Sugar of Lead. Colorless crystals or grains with an acetic odor. Bubbles slowly. It has been used as a topical astringent but is absorbed through the skin, and therefore might lead to lead poisoning. Also used in hair dyeing and printing colors and in the manufacture of chrome yellow (*see* Colors). Still used to treat bruises and skin irritations in animals. Not recommended for use because of the possibility of lead buildup in the body. Permission was given in 1981 by the FDA to use this in progressive hair dyes, although it is a proven carcinogen. Permanently listed as a color component of hair dye in 1969 with a caution that it "should not be used on cut or abraded scalp." Permitted in Canada and EU only in hair-dye preparations at concentrations equal to or less than 0.6 percent. On the Canadian Hotlist (*see*). The EU requires the label to read: "Keep away from children; avoid contact with eyes; wash hands after use; contains lead acetate; do not use to dye eyelashes, eyes, or moustaches; if irritation develops, discontinue." *See* Lead Compounds.

LEAD COMPOUNDS • Used in ointments and hair dye pigments. Lead may cause contact dermatitis. It is poisonous in all forms. It is one of the most hazardous of toxic metals because its poison is cumulative and its toxic effects are many and severe. Among them are leg cramps, muscle weakness, numbness, depression, brain damage, coma, and death. Ingestion and inhalation of lead cause the most severe symptoms. On the Canadian Hotlist (*see*).

LECITHIN • From the Greek, meaning "egg yolk." A natural antioxidant and emollient used in eye creams, lipsticks, liquid powders, hand creams and lotions, soaps, and many other cosmetics. Also a natural emulsifier and spreading ingredient. It is found in all living organisms and is frequently obtained from common egg yolk and soybeans for commercial purposes. Egg yolk is 8 to 9 percent lecithin. Nontoxic. The final report to the FDA of the Select Committee on GRAS Substances stated in 1980 that it should continue its use.

LECITHINAMIDE DEA • Antistatic ingredient. A reaction product of lecithin and diethanolamine with ammonia. *See* Quaternary Ammonium Compounds. DEA products are cancer suspects.

LEDUM GROENLANDICUM • Labrador Tea. *See* Labrador Tea Extract.

LEMON • *Citrus medica. C. limon.* The common fresh fruit and fruit extract is the most frequently used acid in cosmetics. It is 5 to 8 percent citric acid. Employed in cream rinses, hair color rinses, astringents, fresheners, skin bleaches, and for reducing alkalinity of many other products. Do-it-yourselfers can squeeze two lemons into a strainer, add the juice to 1 cup of water, and use it as a rinse after shampooing to remove scum and to leave a shine on the hair. Lemon can cause allergic reactions.

LEMON BALM • Sweet Balm. Garden Balm. Used in perfumes and as a soothing facial treatment. An Old World mint cultivated for its lemon-flavored, fragrant leaves. Often considered a weed, it has been used by herbalists as a medicine and to flavor foods and medicines. It reputedly imparts long life. Also used to treat earache and toothache.

LEMON BIOFLAVONOIDS • *See* Lemon and Bioflavonoids.

LEMON EKISU • Japanese name for lemon juice. *See* Lemon.

LEMON EXTRACT • *See* Lemon Oil.

LEMON JUICE • *See* Lemon.

LEMON OIL • Cedro Oil. Used in perfumes and food flavorings, it is the volatile oil expressed from the fresh peel. A pale yellow to deep yellow, it has a characteristic odor and taste of the outer part of fresh lemon peel. It can cause an allergic reaction, especially when exposed to sunlight, and has been suspected of being a co-cancer-causing ingredient. The International Fragrance Association (IFRA) has made specific recommendations for its use in cosmetics and recommends that "for applications on areas of skin exposed to light, excluding bath preparations, soaps and other products which are washed off the skin, lemon oil cold pressed should not be used such that the level in the consumer products exceeds 2%." Recent research reports it may be a beneficial antioxidant on the skin.

LEMON PEEL • From the outer rind, the extract is used as a flavor in medicines and in beverages, confectionery, and cooking. *See* Lemon for toxicity.

LEMON VERBENA EXTRACT • Extract of *Lippia citriodora*. *See* Lemongrass Oil.

LEMONGRASS OIL • *Cymbopogon schoenanthus*. Indian Oil of Verbena. Used in perfumes, especially those added to soap. It is the volatile oil distilled from the leaves of lemon grasses. A yellowish or reddish brown liquid, it has a strong odor of verbena. Also used in insect repellents and in fruit flavorings for foods and beverages. Death was reported when taken internally, and autopsy showed lining of the intestines was severely damaged. Skin toxicity unknown.

LENS ESCULENTA • *See* Lentil Extract.

LENTIL EXTRACT • The extract of the fruit of *Lens culinaris* or *L. esculenta*. A widely grown annual plant. Used as a skin conditioner.

LENTINUS EDODES • The EU name for shiitake mushroom. Used as a skin conditioner.

LEONTOPODIUM ALPINUM • The EU name for edelweiss (*see*).

LEONURUS SIBIRICUS EXTRACT • Lion's Tail. Marahuanella. Little Cannabis. Yi-mu-cao. Siberian Motherwort. Used by the Chinese to treat infections and circulatory problems. Skin conditioner. May have hormonal action since it stimulates the uterus when used as a medicine.

LEOPARD'S BANE • *See* Arnica.

LEPTOSPERMUM PETERSONII OIL • Fragrance ingredient. *See* Lemon Oil.

LEPTOSPERMUM SCOPARIUM • *See* Tea Tree Oil.

LESPEDEZA • An herb or shrub named for a Spanish governor of Florida. It is a member of the legume family. Some cosmetic sellers say it whitens skin and others say it prolongs tanning. It is also being sold in "slimming" and "anti-aging" products. Its safety has not been identified.

LESQUERELLA OIL • The oil expressed from the seed of *Lesquerella fendleri*. A genus of low annual or perennial American herbs with yellow flowers and puffy pods. Used as a hair and skin conditioner.

LETTUCE EXTRACT • *Lactuca elongata*. An extract of various species of *Lactuca*. Used in commercial toning lotions and by herbalists to make soothing skin decoctions. During the Middle Ages, lettuce was used as a valuable narcotic, and its milky juice was used with opium to induce sleep.

LEUCINE • An essential amino acid (*see*) for human nutrition not manufactured in the body. It is isolated commercially from gluten, casein, and keratin (*see all*) and used in permanent waves and hair conditioners.

LEUKOCYTE EXTRACT • Extract of white blood cells used in anti-aging products.

LEUKODERMA • *See* Vitiligo.

LEUKOTRIENES • Substances issued by cells that have physiologic activity, such as playing a part in inflammation and allergic reactions.

LEVISTICUM OFFICINALE • The EU name for lovage (*see*), used as a fragrance ingredient.

LEVULINIC ACID • Crystals used as an intermediate for plasticizers, solvents, resins, flavors, and pharmaceuticals. Also used as a fragrance ingredient and skin conditioner.

LEVULOSE • *See* Fructose.

LIATRIS • *See* Deer's Tongue Leaves.

LICE • *Pediculus humanus capitis,* head lice. *P. humanus corporis,* body lice. *Phthirus pubis,* genital lice. The head louse and pubic (crab) louse prefer hairy places; the body louse likes to live in undergarments. Body lice can spread typhus. Crab and head lice are less dangerous but still annoying.

LICHEN EXTRACT • *Usnea barbata.* Old Man's Beard. Usnea. Beard Lichen. The plant, which is a lichen growing on branches of trees, is used internally and externally for fungus infections and for viral and bacterial infections. When combined with echinacea (*see*), it is used as a general antibiotic and antifungal medication. Used externally for fungal infections.

LICORICE • Liquorice. Glycyrrhizin. *Glycyrrhiza glabra.* Sweet Wood. A perennial shrub, it is native to Europe and Asia (China and Mongolia). It was introduced into Britain in the sixteenth century by Black Friars. A black substance derived from a plant, *Glycyrrhiza glabra,* "sweet root," belonging to the Leguminosae family and cultivated from southern Europe to Central Asia. It is used in fruit, licorice, anise, maple, and root beer flavorings. The dried root contains sugars, glycosides (*see*) with adrenocortical-like activity, flavonoids, coumarins, bitter principle, and estrogen (*see all*). Glabridin licorice extract is used for its effects on the skin due to its skin whitening and anti-inflammatory properties. The skin-lightening property is due to its ability to inhibit the skin's manufacture of melanin (*see*). Another of its major derivatives, glycyrrhetic acid, has been found to have substantial antiarthritic activity. Modern scientists report licorice has an anti-inflammatory action and suppresses coughs as well as codeine does. It stimulates the production of two steroids, cortisone and aldosterone. It has also been found to produce sodium and water retention with subsequent loss of potassium in some instances. Scientists in the United States and Japan are studying extracts of licorice to inhibit cancer. Licorice may cause allergic reactions, and it can be toxic if taken in large amounts. It is used in allopathic medicine to treat peptic ulcers. Some people known to have eaten licorice candy regularly and generously have suffered high blood pressure, headaches, and muscle weakness. In 1992, the FDA proposed a ban on licorice root in oral menstrual drug products because it has not been shown to be safe and effective for its stated claims.

LIDOCAINE • Xylocaine. LidoPen Auto-Injector. Bactine Antiseptic. Caine-2. Dalcaine. Dilocaine. DuoTrach Kit. Mycitracin Plus Pain Reliever. Nervocaine. Octocaine. Unguentine Plus First Aid. Xylocaine Ointment. Derived from benzene or alcohol, it is a local anesthetic introduced in 1949. It relieves itching, pain, soreness, and discomfort due to rashes, including eczema, and minor burns. Can cause an allergic reaction. It is on the Canadian Hotlist (*see*).

LIGHT • Sensitivity to light may be caused by drugs, cosmetics, or foods or may be an allergy itself. When some people are exposed to sunlight, their skins erupt with eczema, hemorrhages, hives, and scales. In severe sunlight allergy, the person may break out all over in large hives, feel dizzy, and fall into shock. The allergy may appear suddenly, last for years, and then disappear, or it may remain for a lifetime. Some people allergic to sunlight are also sensitive to fluorescent light.

LIGNOCERIC ACID • Obtained from beechwood tar or by distillation of rotten oak wood. Occurs in most natural fats. Used in shampoos, soaps, and plastics.

LIGNOL • *See* Lignoceric Acid.

LIGUSTRUM LUCIDIUM EXTRACT • A common plant used as a hedge in many yards, its fruits contain mannitol and glucose (*see both*), as well as oleanolic acid, and fatty oil. It is used to treat liver, kidney, and adrenal gland problems. Herbalists also claim that it can prevent premature graying of the hair or loss of vision.

LILAC • *Syringa vulgaris.* Used in perfumes. Derived from the plant, especially the European shrub variety. It has fragrant bluish to purple-pink flowers.

LILIUM • Tiger Lily. White Lily. Grown in China and Japan, the plant flowers in July and August. The bloom is orange and spotted. In cosmetics used as a moisturizer and cleanser. A tincture is made from the fresh plant and is used by herbalists to treat uterine and nerve problems, congestion, and irritation. It is poisonous.

LILY OF THE VALLEY • Convallaria Flowers. A perfume ingredient extracted from the low perennial herb. It has oblong leaves and fragrant, nodding, bell-shaped, white flowers. Has been used as a heart stimulant.

LIME • *Citrus aurantifolia. Tilia cordata.* A perfume ingredient from the small, greenish yellow fruit of a spicy tropical tree. Its very acid pulp yields a juice used as a flavoring ingredient and as an antiseptic. A source of vitamin C. Can cause an adverse reaction when skin is exposed to sunlight.

LIME BLOSSOM • *Tilia europea.* Linden. The flowers contain essential oils, mucilage, flavonoids, coumarin, and vanillin (*see all*). Herbalists use it for relaxation from nervous tension and to lower blood pressure. In 1992, the FDA issued a notice that linden had not been shown to be safe and effective as claimed in OTC digestive aid products. Widely used in emollients, body creams, and fragrances. *See* Lime.

LIME OIL • A natural flavoring extracted from the fruit of a tropical tree. Colorless to greenish. Used in grapefruit, lemon, lemon-lime, lime, orange, cola, fruit, rum, nut, and ginger flavorings. May cause a sensitivity to light. The International Fragrance Association (IFRA) has made specific recommendations for its use in cosmetics. The IFRA recommends that "for applications on areas of skin exposed to light, excluding bath preparations, soaps and other products which are washed off the skin, lime oil cold pressed should not be used such that the level in the consumer products exceeds 0.7%."

LIME SULFUR • Topical antiseptic. A brown, clear liquid prepared by boiling sulfur and lime with water. Can cause skin irritation.

LIMEWATER • An alkaline water solution of calcium hydroxide that absorbs carbon dioxide from the air, forming a protective film of calcium carbonate (*see*) on the surface of the liquid. Used in medicines, as an antacid, and as an alkali in external washes, face masks, and hair-grooming products.

LIMNANTHES ALBA • Meadowfoam. A family of North American herbs. Has succulent leaves. Skin conditioner used in moisturizers and lipsticks.

LIMONENE • D, L, and DL forms. A synthetic flavoring ingredient that occurs naturally in star anise, buchu leaves, caraway, celery, oranges, coriander, cumin, cardamom, sweet fennel, common fennel, mace, marigold, oil of lavandin, oil of lemon, oil of mandarin, peppermint, petitgrain oil, pimento oil, orange leaf, orange peel (sweet oil), origanum oil, black pepper, peels of citrus, macrocarpa bunge, and hops oil. Used in lime, fruit, and spice flavorings. A skin irritant and sensitizer.

LIMONIUM VULGARE • *See* Lavender.

LINALOE OIL • Bois de Rose Oil. An ingredient in perfumes that is the colorless to yellow, volatile, essential oil distilled from a Mexican tree. It has a pleasant flowery scent and is soluble in most fixed oils. May cause allergic reactions.

LINALOOL • Linalol. Used in perfumes and soaps instead of bergamot or French lavender. It is a fragrant, colorless liquid that occurs in many essential oils such as linaloe, Ceylon cinnamon, sassafras, orange flower, and bergamot. May cause allergic reactions. Has been linked to eczema (*see*). ASP

LINALOOL OXIDE • Linalool oxide offers a floral woody earthy note with a camphoraceous undertone. Found in 60 to 80 percent of personal-hygiene products, it's a key component of lavender, lavandin, and geranium-type fragrances. Studies have shown that it is the third most common cause of allergic contact skin rashes, including eczema. It is used in fragrances and hair care products as well as household cleaning products. ASP

LINALYL ACETATE • A colorless, fragrant liquid, slightly soluble in water, it is the most valuable constituent of bergamot and lavender oils, which are used in perfumery. It occurs naturally in basil, jasmine oil, lavandin oil, lavender oil, and lemon oil. It has a strong floral scent. Also used as a synthetic flavoring in food.

LINALYL ESTERS • *See* Linalool and Ester.

LINDANE • Gamma Benzene Hexachloride. Hexachlorocyclohexane. G-well. Bio-Well. GBH. Kildane. Kwell. Kwildane. Scabene. Thionex. An insecticide in a cream, lotion, or shampoo introduced in 1952 to treat parasitic infestation such as scabies or lice (*see*). Lindane is poisonous. Can be absorbed through the skin. Potential adverse reactions include dizziness, seizures, rash, or irritation with repeated use. Contraindicated when skin is raw or inflamed. Should not be applied to open areas, acutely inflamed skin, face, eyes, or mucous membranes. Must be kept away from the mouth because it is poisonous and may be fatal if swallowed. Do not use unless there is no safer alternative.

LINDEN • *See* Lime Blossom.

LINDEN EXTRACT • *Tilia cordata.* A natural flavoring ingredient from the flowers of the tree grown in Europe and the United States. Widely used in fragrances, skin fresheners, moisturizers, cold creams, shampoos, and many other products. It is also used in raspberry and vermouth flavorings. GRAS. ASP

LINDERA STRYCHNIFOLIA • Chinese herb that is antibacterial and is used in Chinese medicine to warm and relieve pain.

LINEAR POLYSILOXANES • *See* Methicone and Dimethicone.

LINGONBERRY • Has the nutritional value similar to cranberry or bilberry. Like most superfruits, the lingonberry has elevated levels of phytonutrients such as flavonoids and phenolic acids. It is being marketed on its heart health, immunity, and anti-aging benefits as well as the cranberry-dominated urinary tract infection (UTI) area. The food supplements industry will be the first target on both sides of the Atlantic, with functional foods and beverages potential to be explored at some later date along with China, the rest of Asia, and Latin America.The company's testing revealed lingonberry extract contained five times the level of type-A procyanidins as cranberry as well as being high in resveratrol and other polyphenols (*see both*).

LINLUM USITATISSIMUM • *See* Linseed Oil.

LINOLEAMIDE • *See* Linoleic Acid.

LINOLEAMIDE DEA • Alkyl amides produced by a diethanolamine (*see*) condensation of linoleic acid. Used as a foaming ingredient in soaps and shampoos. May form nitrosamines (*see*). Based on the available data, the CIR Expert Panel (*see*) concluded that this ingredient is safe as a cosmetic ingredient. However, it should not be used in cosmetic products containing nitrosating ingredients. *See* Quaternary Ammonium Compounds and Coconut Acids.

LINOLEAMIDE MEA • A mixture of ethanolamides of linoleic acid (*see*). Used as a surfactant (*see*).

LINOLEAMIDE MIPA • A mixture of isopropanolamides of linoleic acid. Used as an emulsifier. *See* Linoleic Acid.

LINOLEAMIDOPROPALKONIUM CHLORIDE • *See* Quaternary Ammonium Compounds.

LINOLEAMIDOPROPYL-PG-DIMONIUM CHLORIDE • *See* Quaternary Ammonium Compounds.

LINOLEAMIDOPROPYL ETHYDIMONIUM ETHOSULFATE • *See* Quaternary Ammonium Compounds.

LINOLEIC ACID • Used as an emulsifier. An essential fatty acid (*see*) prepared from edible fats and oils. Component of vitamin F and a major constituent of many vegetable oils, for example, cottonseed and soybean. Used in emulsifiers and vitamins. Used in hair and skin conditioners. Large ingested doses can cause nausea and vomiting. No known skin toxicity and, in fact, may have emollient properties.

LINOLELEYL LACTATE • Skin-conditioning ingredient. *See* Linolenic Acid and Lactic Acid.

LINOLENIC ACID • Colorless, liquid glyceride found in most oils. Insoluble in water, soluble in organic solvents. Xylocaine. LidoPen Auto-Injector. Bactine Antiseptic. Caine-2. Dalcaine. Dilocaine. DuoTrach Kit. Mycitracin Plus Pain Reliever. Nervocaine. Octocaine. Unguentine Plus First Aid. Xylocaine Ointment. Derived from benzene or alcohol, it is a local anesthetic introduced in 1949. It relieves itching, pain, soreness, and discomfort due to rashes, including eczema, and minor burns. It is also used to make nail polishes dry faster. Slightly irritating to mucous membranes.

LINSEED ACID • *See* Linseed Oil.

LINSEED OIL • *Linum usitatissimum.* Oil used in shaving creams, emollients, and medicinal soaps. Soothing to the skin. It is the yellowish oil expressed or extracted from flaxseed. Gradually thickens when exposed to air. It has a peculiar odor and a bland taste and is also used in paint, varnish, and linoleum. Can cause an allergic reaction.

LINUM USITATISSIMUM • Emollient and moisturizer. May promote acne. *See* Linseed Oil.

LIP BRUSH • A brush to trace a sharp outline of the lips with lipstick.

LIP CREAM • A mixture of oils that melt on contact with the skin to soften and soothe the lips. Almost identical to night creams or moisturizers. *See* Emollients.

LIP GLOSS • Usually comes in jars, sticks, sometimes in tubes. Contains different proportions of the same ingredients as lipstick but usually has less wax and more oil to make the lips shinier. Used alone or with lipstick and applied with the fingertip.

LIP PENCIL • A colored wax mixture in wood or metal casing for the same purpose as a lip brush (*see*).

LIP PRIMER • A stick similar to lipstick but containing less wax, used to soften the lips and to serve as a base for lipstick. Makes the lips shinier.

LIPASE • Used to describe various enzymes that split fats (lipids) into their constituents, glycerine and a variety of fatty acids. Lipases also can transform certain fatty acids or rearrange them within a larger molecule. An enzyme that breaks down fat, it is widely distributed in plants and animal tissues, especially in the pancreas. Isolated from castor beans. Employed to make synthetic vitamin derivatives for skin care and the production of aromas through the splitting off of specific esters (*see*) from the fats themselves. The FDA issued a notice in 1992 that lipase has not been shown to be safe and effective as claimed in OTC digestive aid products. Food-product enzymes are not regarded as ingredients and are not included on the list of ingredients. Therefore, producers, at this writing, are not worried about labeling in regard to their production using genetically modified microorganisms.

LIPIDS • Fatty acids, sebum, and fats found in plants and skin. In cosmetics, lipids are used as emollients and thickening ingredients.

LIPO • Glyceryl, ethylene glycol, and propylene glycol esters used as emulsifiers and stabilizers. Widely used as emollients and thickeners in creams and lotions, and as opacifying and pearling ingredients in surfactants.

LIPO- • Fat.

LIPOCOL • Polyoxyethylene ethers used as nonionic surfactants in antiperspirants, depilatories, creams, lotions, and pigment dispersions. Also used as emulsifiers, defoamers, wetting ingredients, solubilizers, and conditioning ingredients in shampoos, detergents, bleaches, and dyes.

LIPOGEN PS • Used in anti-aging creams. Found in fish, green leafy vegetables, soy beans, and rice. Its effects are now being tested in relation to Alzheimer's disease–related memory loss. *See* Phosphatidylserine.

LIPOLAN • *See* Lanolin.

LIPOMA • A benign fatty tumor.

LIPONATE • Emollient used to give a velvety feel to creams, lotions, and bath preparations. Also used for thickening, viscosity control, and pigment.

LIPONIC • Humectant to control the moisture exchange between a product and the atmosphere, thus helping to retard drying of the product in the package.

LIPOPEG • Mild, fatty, polyoxyethylene glycol esters used in bath oils, creams, and lotions for solubilizing, spreading, emulsifying, dispersing, and lubricating.

LIPOSOMES • Microscopic sacs, or spheres, manufactured from a variety of fatty substances, including phospholipids. The material for cosmetics may be obtained either from natural or synthetic sources. When properly mixed with water, phospholipids form liposome spheres, which can "trap" any substance that will dissolve in water or oil. Manufacturers claim liposomes act like a delivery system. They say that, when present in a cream or lotion, liposomes can more easily penetrate the surface skin to underlying layers, "melt," and deposit other ingredients of the product. *See also* Phytosomes.

LIPOSORB • Sorbitan esters used as emulsifying, thickening, and lubricating ingredients. *See* Sorbitan Fatty Acid Esters.

LIPOVOL • Emollient oils for use as lubricants and conditioners in skin products, hair care products, makeups, fine soaps, and bath oils.

LIPOWAX • Emulsifying waxes.

LIPPIA CITRIODORA • Lemon Verbena. *See* Lemongrass Oil.

LIPSTICK • Regular, Frosted, Medicated, Sheer. Primarily a mixture of oil and wax in a stick form with a red-staining certified dye dispersed in oil, red pigments similarly dispersed, flavoring, and perfume. Bromo acid, D & C Red No. 21, and related dyes are most often used. Among other common lipstick dyes are D & C Red No. 27 and insoluble dyes known as lakes, such as D & C Red, No. 34 Calcium Lake, and D & C Orange No. 17 Lake. Pinks are made by mixing titanium dioxide with various reds. Among the oils and fats used are olive, mineral, sesame, castor, butyl stearate, polyethylene glycol, cocoa butter, lanolin, petrolatum, lecithin, hydrogenated vegetable oils, carnauba and candelilla waxes, beeswax, ozokerite, and paraffin. Colors of lipsticks on the market remain essentially the same, but the names, such as "strawberry rose," are frequently changed to induce customers to buy. A typical lipstick formula contains castor oil, about 65 percent; beeswax, 15 percent; carnauba wax, 10 percent; lanolin, 5 percent; certified dyes, soluble; color lakes, insoluble; and perfume. Frosted lipstick includes a pearling ingredient that adds luster to the color. Such an ingredient may be a bismuth compound or guanine. Medicated lipstick is used to treat or prevent chapped or sun-dried lips. It may or may not combine coloring with ingredients but usually contains petrolatum, mineral wax, and oils. It may or may not contain menthol or a sunscreen. Sheer lipsticks include transparent coloring and no indelible dyes so as to give a more natural look to the lips. A Japanese company has come up with a lipstick that shines while reducing the appearance of those age lines above the lips and wrinkles. Shiseido, the developer, says it is the first time these two features have been combined in the same product. If it works well, you can be sure there will be a parade of other companies following the Japanese lipstick-anti-aging, antiwrinkle idea. The main difficulty with lipsticks, in general, results from allergy to the dyes or to specific ingredients. Traces of lead have been found in lipstick. Reportedly, there is more lead in lipstick than the maximum permitted in toys. European and American trade associations have dismissed claims from a consumer group that some lipsticks on the U.S. market contain unacceptably high levels of lead. The Campaign for Safe Cosmetics released the results of independent research claiming that 61 percent of tested lipsticks contained detectable levels of lead. *See* Cheilitis.

LIPSTICK HOLDER • *See* Nickel.

LIQUEFYING CREAM • Cleansing cream designed to liquefy when rubbed into the skin. It usually contains paraffin, a wax, stearic acid, sodium borate, liquid petrolatum (54 percent), and water (26 percent). *See* Sodium Borate.

LIQUID MAKEUP • *See* Foundation Makeup.

LIQUID PETROLATUM • *See* Mineral Oil.

LIQUID POWDER • *See* Foundation Makeup.

LIQUIDAMBAR STYRACIFLUA • American Sweet Gum. Used as a fragrance ingredient. *See* Witch Hazel.

LISTERINE ANTISEPTIC • *See* Eucalyptol.

LISTERMINT WITH FLUORIDE • *See* Sodium Fluoride.

LITARGIRIO • Used as a deodorant. It is sold in two-inch by three-inch clear packets by convenience and specialty stores catering to Spanish-speaking customers—particularly those from the Dominican Republic. Children using it have been found to have blood lead levels as high as four times the level known to cause behavioral and cognitive problems even after abatement of household lead sources and medical treatment. Their blood lead levels began to decline only after use of this substance was discontinued. The FDA warns against its use.

LITHIUM • A metal that has been used as a medicine since ancient Greece, when it was prescribed for gout, rheumatism, and kidney stone. Lithium has a very narrow margin of safety and may have severe side effects. *See* Lithium Chloride and Lithium Hydroxide.

LITHIUM CHLORIDE • A crystalline salt of the alkali metal, used as a scavenger in purifying metals, to remove oxygen, and in soap and lubricant bases. The crystals absorb water and then become neutral or slightly alkaline. It is also used in the manufacture of mineral waters. Formerly used as a salt substitute.

LITHIUM HYDROXIDE • Used in making cosmetic resins and esters (*see both*). A granular, free-flowing powder, acrid, and strongly alkaline. It is the salt of the alkaline metal that absorbs water from the air and is soluble in water. Hair straightener. Used in photo developers and in batteries. Very irritating to the skin, and flammable in contact with the air. Can cause blindness.

LITHIUM MAGNESIUM SILICATE • A synthetic clay used as a thickener. *See* Magnesium and Lithium.

LITHIUM STEARATE • White, fatty, solid, and soluble in water and alcohol. A metallic soap used as an emulsifier, lubricant, and plasticizer in various cosmetic creams and lotions. Also a coloring ingredient. On the basis of the available information, the CIR Expert Panel (*see*) found it safe in the early 1980s but is considering new information to determine if the final safety assessment should be reaffirmed, amended, or have an addendum. *See* Aluminum Distearate.

LITHIUM SULFIDE • Depilatory ingredient. Toxic and irritating.

LITHOSPERMUM EXTRACT • Pucoon. An extract of the roots of *Radix lithospermi,* an herb with polished, white, stony nutlets. The extract is supposed to be soothing to the mucous membranes.

LITHOTHAMNIUM • Red Seaweed. An abrasive claimed to smooth cellulite. A source of calcium, it is used in bath products.

LITSEA CUBEBA • Small plum tree with evergreen leaves. Essential oil used in fragrances.

LIVE YEAST CELL DERIVATIVE • Preparation H. Wyanoids Relief Factor. Yeast is a one-celled organism that occurs in sugary liquids such as fruit juices or malt liquids. It is used for fermentation by enzymes, which convert sugar and other carbohydrates into carbon dioxide and water in the presence of oxygen, alcohol, carbon dioxide, or lactic acid. Live yeast cell derivative reportedly acts by increasing the oxygen uptake of skin tissue and facilitating the action of collagen (*see*). It is used in preparations for hemorrhoids.

LIVER EXTRACT • Extract of bovine livers used in antiwrinkle creams.

LIVER LILY • *See* Blue Flag.

LOCUST BEAN GUM • *Ceratonia siliqua.* St. John's Bread. Carob Bean Gum. A natural flavor extract from the seed of the carob tree cultivated in the Mediterranean area. The history of the carob tree dates back more than two thousand years, when the ancient Egyptians used locust bean gum as an adhesive in mummy binding. Used in cosmetics as a thickener and stabilizer. Also used in depilatories and in facial moisturizer/treatments, anti-aging products, around-eye cream, foundation, moisturizer, facial powders, masks, breath fresheners, sunscreens SPF 15 and above, and nail treatments. The carob pods are used as feed for stock today because of their high protein content. It is on the FDA list for study of side effects. It is suspected of causing tumors and toxicity.

LOESS • An abrasive and absorbent. Believed to be deposited by the wind, it consists of shells, bones, and teeth of mammals as well as sand.

LOGWOOD • *Haematoxylum campechianum.* An active ingredient known as hematoxylin from the very hard brown, or brownish red, heartwood of a tree common to the West Indies and Central America. It was widely used as a liquid or as a solid extract obtained by evaporation in black hair colorings and for neutralizing red tones in dyed hair. It is also a mild astringent. May cause an allergic reaction in the hypersensitive. No longer authorized for use in cosmetics.

LONICERA CAPRIFOLIUM • *See* Honeysuckle.

LONITEN • *See* Minoxidil.

LOOFAH • Luffa. Dish Cloth Sponge. A material obtained from the fruit of the sponge *Luffa cylindrica.* The fibrous skeleton of the loofah is used as a sponge and to exfoliate (*see*) the skin. When used, the sponges should be allowed to dry completely because they have been found to support the growth of numerous bacteria. When skin flakes are trapped in the fibers of the loofah, sponges can become a rich breeding ground for pathogens.

LOOSESTRIFE, PURPLE • *Lythrum salicaria.* A perennial herb grown in many parts of the world, in damp, marshy places. It is used as an astringent and tonic. Also used in Europe to treat fevers and in Ireland for diarrhea and the healing of wounds. Used by herbalists in soothing eyedrops and in salves for skin ulcers.

LOQUAT • *Eriobotrya japonica.* The leaves and fruit are used by herbalists to treat coughs and lung inflammations. It contains amygdalin (*see*), which is also found in cherry bark and apricot kernel, both of which are used to treat coughs.

LOTION • Liquid applied to large areas of the skin.

LOTUS • The name of several water lilies. It grows in marshes from Egypt to China, and its leaves and pink flowers grow on stalks rising several feet from the water. The fruit, the sacred bean of Asia, is eaten, and the large rhizomes yield a starchy powder. Lotus is used in "organic" cosmetics.

LOVAGE • An ingredient in perfumery from an aromatic herb, *Levisticum officinale.* Native to southern Europe and grown in monastery gardens centuries ago for medicine and food flavoring. It has a hot, sharp, biting taste. The yellow-brown oil is extracted from the root or other parts of the herb. It has a reputation for improving health and inciting love; Czech girls reportedly wear it in a bag around their necks when dating boys. It supposedly has deodorant properties when added to bathwater. Has been used by herbalists as an eye wash, a cure for colds, and to treat arthritis. Contraindicated in pregnancy and for patients with kidney dysfunction.

LOVE-IN-WINTER • *See* Pipsissewa Leaves Extract.

LOVE-LIES-BLEEDING • *See* Amaranth.

LUBRICATING CREAM • *See* Emollients.

LUFFA CYLINDRICA • Sponge Gourd Powder. *See* Loofah.

LU HUI • *See* Aloe Vera.

LUNGWORT • *Pulmonaria officinalis.* Black Hellebore. Mullein. Wall Hawkweed. Virginia Cowslip. Lungworts are used by herbalists to treat diarrhea. The leaves contain mucins, silicic acid, tannin, saponin, allantoin, quercetin, and vitamin C (*see all*). Externally, this plant is used to heal wounds. It is used in "organic" cosmetics.

LUPIN EXTRACT • Lupine. Extract of *Lupinus albus.* Used as a hair and skin conditioner as well as a humectant. Produces a light blue dye.

LUPINUS ALBUS • A member of the legume family, it has white, yellow, or blue flowers. A skin conditioner. *See* Lupin Extract.

LUPULIN • From the hop plant *Humulus lupulus,* it contains lupulone, which is active against fungus and bacteria, and humulone, which is an antibiotic.

LU RONG • *See* Deer Antler.

LYCHEE FRUIT • *Litchi sinensis.* Juicy and sweet subtropical fruit native to China. Lychee nut extract used as a skin conditioner. May cause an allergic reaction.

LYCIUM CHINENSE • Wolfberry. Ko-Chi-Kuko. A member of the nightshade family that includes potatoes and tomatoes, folk practioners claim it is good for sore backs, knees, and legs as well as impotence. It is said to be good for insect bites. The USDA has found it does contain a number of active chemicals. It is used as an antioxidant in cosmetics.

LYCOPENE • Red crystals, insoluble in water. The main pigment of paprika, grapefruit, and rose hips. Used as an antioxidant in cosmetics. Being studied as a compound to prevent heart disease and cancer.

LYCOPODIUM • Ground Pine. Ground Fir. A dusting powder derived from erect, or creeping, evergreen plants grown in North America, Europe, and Asia. The plant's spores create a fine yellow powder that sticks to the fingers when touched. It is odorless and absorbent. It may cause a form of inflammatory reaction in wounds or exposed tissues and can cause allergic reactions such as a stuffy nose and hay fever.

LYCOPSIS ARVENSIS • Bugloss Extract. *See* Bugloss Extract.

LYSIMACHIA • Creeping Charlie. *See* Loosestrife.

LYSINE • An essential amino acid (*see*) isolated from casein, fibrin, or blood. It is used to improve the protein quality of a product.

LYSOLECITHIN • The product obtained from treating lecithin with enzymes. Used as a base for creams.

LYSOZYME • An enzyme isolated from egg white used as a skin conditioner. A natural antibacterial substance contained in many bodily secretions, such as tears.

LYSOZYME BETA-GLUCAN • Made up of lysozyme (*see*) mixed with betaglucan. *See* Betaglucans.

LYTHRUM SALICARIA • *See* Loosestrife.

M

MA • Abbreviation for maleic anhydride (*see*).

MACADAMIA NUT OIL • Queensland Nut Oil. Derived from the nut of a small evergreen tree, it is widely cultivated. Used in emollients. Contains magnesium and thiamine.

MACADEMIA TERNIFOLIA SEED OIL • Fats and oils from the nuts of *Macademia ternifolia* widely used as an emollient and occlusive in makeup, cleansers, and suntan gels.

MACE • Oil and Oleoresin. Obtained by steam distillation from the ripe, dried seed of the nutmeg. Colorless to pale yellow, with the taste and odor of nutmeg. It is used in cosmetics and toiletries because of its aromatic properties, especially in men's fragrances.

MACELA • *See* Achyrocline Satureoides.

MACERATION • Extraction of flower-oil production by immersion in warm fats.

MACROCYSTIS PYRIFERA • *See* Kelp.

MACROTOMIA EUCHROMA • *Lithspermum euchroma* Royale. A plant used for eczema and burns in folk medicine and as an emollient and humectant in cosmetics.

MAD WEED • *See* Skullcap.

MADDER • *Rubia tincorum.* Dyers' Madder. A shrub that is a member of the Rubiaceae family, it is widely distributed in Europe. In medicine it is used as a mild tonic and has astringent properties. Was once used for treating edema. The root was boiled in wine or water to treat palsy, jaundice, sciatica, and bruises. The leaves and roots were beaten and applied externally to remove freckles and other skin blemishes. Contraindicated in kidney dysfunction, peptic ulcer, and albuminuria.

MADECASSIC ACID • Brahmic Acid. Extracted from *Centella asiatic,* an herb widely used in Europe to treat keloids, leg ulcers, and slow-healing wounds. It penetrates the skin easily. It is used in conditioner in cosmetics. May cause allergic reaction.

MADECASSICOSIDE • An antioxidant and skin conditioner. *See* Madecassic Acid.

MAGNESIA • A skin freshener and dusting powder ingredient. Slightly alkaline, white powder taken from any one of several ores, such as periclase. Named after Magnesia, an ancient city in Asia Minor. An antacid.

MAGNESIUM • A silver-white, light malleable metal that occurs abundantly in nature and is widely used in combination with various chemicals as a powder. It was reevaluated by the FDA in 1976 and found not harmful at presently used levels. The World Health Organization recommended further studies because of kidney damage found in dogs that ingested it.

MAGNESIUM ACETATE • A buffering ingredient. *See* Magnesium.

MAGNESIUM ACETYLMETHIONATE • The magnesium salt of *n*-acetyl-methionine. *See* Magnesium and Methionine.

MAGNESIUM ALGINATE • *See* Magnesium and Alginic Acid.

MAGNESIUM ALUMINUM SILICATE • Fuller's Earth. A silver-white, light malleable metal that occurs abundantly in nature and is widely used in combination with various chemicals as a powder. It is used primarily as a thickener in cosmetics. It was reevaluated by the FDA in 1976 and found not harmful at presently used levels. The World Health Organization recommended further studies because of kidney damage found in dogs that ingested it.

MAGNESIUM/ALUMINUM/ZINC/HYDROXIDE/CARBONATE • A combination of magnesium, aluminum, and zinc (*see all*), it is used as an antidandruff ingredient and a deodorant.

MAGNESIUM ASCORBATE • An antioxidant and skin-conditioning ingredient. *See* Magnesium and Ascorbic Acid.

MAGNESIUM ASCORBYL PHOSPHATE • An antioxidant used in suntan products. *See* Magnesium and Ascorbic Acid.

MAGNESIUM ASPARTATE • Used widely as a skin-conditioning ingredient. *See* Magnesium and Aspartic Acid.

MAGNESIUM BENZOATE • A preservative. *See* Benzoic Acid.

MAGNESIUM BROMIDE • The inorganic salt of magnesium (*see*). It is used in dusting powders and toothpastes.

MAGNESIUM CAPRATE • An anticaking agent and emulsifier. NUL

MAGNESIUM CAPRYLATE • An anticaking agent and emulsifier. NUL

MAGNESIUM CARBONATE • CI 77713. Gaviscon. Kanalka. Maalox. Marblen. Perfume carrier, anticaking ingredient, and coloring ingredient. Used in baby powder, bath powder, tooth powders, face masks, liquid powders, face powders, and dry rouges. It is a silver-white, very crystalline salt that occurs in nature as magnetite or dolomite. Used as an absorbent, bulking ingredient, pH adjuster, and opacifying ingredient in makeup and hand and body products. Not approved as a colorant in the United States but is in the European Union. May cause irritation when applied to abraded skin. GRAS. ASP. E

MAGNESIUM CHLORIDE • The inorganic salt of magnesium (*see*) used in shampoos.

MAGNESIUM CITRATE • Magnesium salt of citric acid. Used in hair sets or hair-bodying products. It leaves a glossy film after drying.

MAGNESIUM COCOATE • The magnesium salt of coconut acid (*see*) used in soaps.

MAGNESIUM DNA • Used as a skin conditioner. *See* Magnesium and DNA.

MAGNESIUM FLUORIDE • Used in toothpastes. The EU requires it to be listed on the label and restricts it to 0.15 percent when mixed with other fluoride compounds. *See* Fluoride and Magnesium.

MAGNESIUM FLUOROSILICATE • Used in toothpastes. The EU calculates at 0.15 percent when mixed with fluorine compounds. Fluorine concentration must not exceed 0.15 percent. The EU label says, "Contains Magnesium fluorosilicate." *See* Fluoride and Silicates.

MAGNESIUM GLUCONATE • Magonate. The inorganic salt of gluconic acid (*see*) taken from sea salt. A buffering agent used as an antacid and in vitamin tablets. A dietary supplement for treatment of magnesium deficiencies. In cosmetics and personal care products, gluconic acid and its derivatives may be used in the formulation of mouthwashes, bath products, cleansing products, skin care products, and shampoo. *See* Magnesium.

MAGNESIUM GLYCEROPHOSPHATE • Used in toothpaste. *See* Magnesium and Glycerol.

MAGNESIUM HYDROXIDE • Used as an alkali in dentifrices and skin creams.

Slightly alkaline, crystalline compound obtained by hydration of magnesia (*see*) or precipitation of seawater by lime. Toxic when inhaled. Harmless to skin and in fact soothes it.

MAGNESIUM LANOLATE • Magnesium salt of lanolin. *See* Magnesium and Lanolin.

MAGNESIUM LAURETH-11 CARBOXYLATE • A cleansing ingredient. *See* Magnesium and Polyethylene Glycol.

MAGNESIUM LAURETH SULFATE • Widely used as a surfactant because of its low irritation potential in shampoos. *See* Anionic Surfactants.

MAGNESIUM LAURETH-5 SULFATE • Used in eye makeup removers. *See* Sulfuric Acid and Lauric Acid.

MAGNESIUM LAURYL SULFATE • A detergent. *See* Sodium Lauryl Sulfate.

MAGNESIUM METHYL COCOYL • Used as a surfactant and a cleansing ingredient. *See* Coconut Oil.

MAGNESIUM MONTMORILLONITE • *See* Montmorillonite.

MAGNESIUM MYRETH SULFATE • Inorganic salt of myristyl alcohol (*see*).

MAGNESIUM MYRISTATE • The magnesium salt of myristic acid (*see*).

MAGNESIUM NITRATE • Used in shampoos. *See* Nitrates.

MAGNESIUM OLEATE • Salt of magnesium used in liquid powders as a texturizer. It is a yellowish powder of mass that is insoluble in water.

MAGNESIUM OLETH SULFATE • Used in eye makeup removers and shampoos. *See* Oleyl Alcohol.

MAGNESIUM OXIDE • White Charcoal. The inorganic salt of magnesium (*see*) used in bath products and hair bleaches.

MAGNESIUM PALMITATE • The inorganic salt of magnesium and palmitic acid (*see both*) used in soap as an anticaking ingredient.

MAGNESIUM PCA • Used as a skin-conditioning ingredient and a humectant.

MAGNESIUM PEG-3 COCAMIDE SULFATE • A magnesium salt of coconut oil used as an emulsifier.

MAGNESIUM PEROXIDE • An oxidizing ingredient. It is on the Canadian Hotlist (*see*). Canada does not allow it in dentifrices, mouthwashes, or "other" purposes that involve long-term use in the oral cavity. May be used as a tooth bleaching agent if safety data is submitted. *See* Peroxide.

MAGNESIUM PHOSPHATE (OTC) • Made from magnesium oxide and phosphoric acid (*see both*). It is used as a dentifrice polishing agent, an antacid, a food additive, and a dietary substance. *See* Phosphate.

MAGNESIUM POTASSIUM FLUOROSILICATE • An abrasive. *See* Mica.

MAGNESIUM PROPIONATE • A preservative. *See* Propionic Acid.

MAGNESIUM SALICYLATE • The EU has banned its use in children under three years except in shampoos. Related to aspirin, it is used as a preservative in cosmetics. May cause allergic reactions.

MAGNESIUM SILICATE • An insoluble, effervescent, white powder that is slowly decomposed by acids to form a soluble salt and an insoluble silica, which has strong absorptive properties. Used to opacify shampoos and in mud packs; also medicinally to reduce stomach acidity, with slow neutralizing action. Toxic by inhalation.

MAGNESIUM SODIUM FLUOROSILICATE • Used as an abrasive (*see*).

MAGNESIUM STEARATE • Coloring ingredient used in face powder, protective creams, and baby dusting powders. It is a white soapy powder, insoluble in water. Also used for tablet making. On the basis of the available information, the CIR Expert Panel (*see*) found it safe in the early 1980s but is considering new information to determine if the final safety assessment should be reaffirmed, amended, or have an addendum. Magnesium stearate, a soft, white powder, tasteless, odorless, and insoluble in water, is used as a dietary supplement, in food packaging, and as an emulsifying additive in cosmetics. *See* Aluminum Distearate.

MAGNESIUM SULFATE • Epsom Salts. A magnesium salt used to treat deficiency during stress and to decrease the release of certain nerve impulses in the brain to prevent or control seizures. Used in cosmetics as a thickener in creams and lotions and bath products. In 1992, the FDA proposed a ban on magnesium sulfate in oral menstrual drug products because it has not been shown to be safe and effective for its stated claims. *See* Magnesium.

MAGNESIUM SULFIDE • A depilatory ingredient. On the Canadian Hotlist. *See* Sulfides.

MAGNESIUM TALLOWATE • The magnesium salt of tallow (*see*).

MAGNESIUM/TEA-COCO-SULFATE • Cleanser. *See* Coconut Oil.

MAGNESIUM THIOGLYCOLATE • Used in depilatories. *See* Thioglycolic Acid Compounds.

MAGNESIUM TRISILICATE • Abrasive, absorbent, and anticaking ingredient in dusting powder and talcums. *See* Magnesium Aluminum Silicate.

MAGNOLIA • Sweet Bay. *Magnolia glauca.* White Bay. Beaver Tree. Used in perfumery and emollients. A genus of North American and Asian shrubs and trees named after the French botanist Pierre Magnol. The plants have evergreen or deciduous leaves and usually snowy white, yellow, rose, or purple flowers appearing in early spring. The dried bark is used in folk medicine to induce sweating and as a bitter tonic. Also employed to treat rheumatism and as a tonic. The Chinese prize magnolia as an aphrodisiac. In Mexico, the plant is used to treat scorpion stings.

MAHONIA AQUIFOLIUM • *Berberis aquifolium.* Oregon Grape Root. Holly Barberry. Evergreen shrub with a long history of medicinal use. It is used to treat chronic skin diseases such as psoriasis and eczema. Used in cosmetics today as an astringent (*see*). Pregnant women are cautioned not to use it because it can stimulate the uterus.

MAIDENHAIR FERN EXTRACT • *Adiantum capillus-veneris.* Venus Hair. Extract of the leaves of the fern *A. capillus-veneris.* Used in herbal creams to soothe irritated skin.

MAIZE OIL • *See* Corn Oil.

MAKEUP BASE, FOUNDATION • *See* Foundation Makeup.

MALACHITE • A green hydrous copper carbonate mineral. It occurs both in the Eastern Desert of Egypt and in Sinai. In predynastic burials, lumps of ore have been found beside palettes and grinding pebbles, presumably for grinding into powder to be used as green eye-paint. Malachite is also employed to treat rheumatism and as a tonic. At this writing, there is a promotion of mineral makeups that include this semiprecious stone. It is primarily being used around the eyes. However, one site says of the stone: "The dark bands found in malachite are said to allow expansion of the creative ideas in your mind. For many malachite is protective and soul mirroring. It attests to the truth within you and aids you in your quest for true self expression." The regulating agencies, in the meantime, are seeking information on malachite's possible cancer-causing potential.

MALEATED SOYBEAN OIL • Modified soybean oil in which some of the unsaturation has been converted to carboxylic acid. *See* Maleic Acid and Soybean Oil.

MALEIC ACID • Colorless crystals with a bad taste. Toxic by ingestion. Used as a preservative for oils and fats and as a pH adjuster in cosmetics.

MALEIC ANHYDRIDE • Colorless needles derived from oxidation of benzene. Used in the manufacture of polyester resins, pesticides, as a preservative for oils and fats, and in permanent-press resins. Irritating to tissue.

MALIC ACID • A colorless, crystalline compound with a strong acid taste that occurs naturally in a wide variety of fruits, including apples and cherries. An alkali in cosmetics, foods, and wines. Also used as an antioxidant for cosmetics and as an ingredient in hair lacquer. Irritating to the skin and can cause an allergic reaction when used in hair lacquers. *See* Alpha-Hydroxy Acids.

MALLOTUS JAPONICUS • A Japanese herb used to treat hemorrhoids and swelling. Used in cosmetics as a skin conditioner.

MALLOW EXTRACT • *Malva sylvestris.* From the herb family. A moderate purplish red that is paler than magenta rose. Used in coloring and also as a source of pectin (*see*). May have anti-inflammatory properties.

MALONIC ACID • An antioxidant prepared synthetically. Occurs naturally in many plants. Used in cosmetics as a pH adjuster. The colorless crystals obtained from the oxidation of malic acid are used in the manufacture of barbiturates. It is a strong irritant. Large doses injected into mice are lethal.

MALPIGHIA GLABRA • *See* Acerola.

MALT EXTRACT • Extracted from barley that has been allowed to germinate, then heated to destroy vitality and dried. It contains sugars, proteins, and salts from barley. The extract is mixed with water and allowed to solidify. It is used as a nutrient and in cosmetics as a texturizer.

MALTITOL • Obtained from maltose (*see*). Used as a moisturizer.

MALTODEXTRIN • The sugar obtained by hydrolysis of starch. Used as a film former, a hair and skin conditioner, and an absorbent (*see*).

MALTOL • A white, crystalline powder with a butterscotch odor, found in the bark of young larch trees, pine needles, chicory, wood tars, and roasted malt.

MALTOSE • Malt Sugar. Colorless crystals derived from malt extract and used as a nutrient, sweetener, culture medium, and stabilizer. Used in cosmetics as a humectant (*see*), an emollient, and a flavoring.

MALTOSYL CYCLODEXTRAIN • Skin conditioner. *See* Maltose.

MALVA MOSCHATA • Malvacae. An erect European perennial herb with rosy purple flowers. Contains mucilage, essential oil, and a trace of tannin. The herb is used to soothe inflammation in the mouth and throat and to treat earache. Also used in bathwater or in a compress to heal boils, abscesses, and minor burns.

MALVA SYLVESTRIS • Used as a skin conditioner in many moisturizers and lotions including baby products. Also used in suntan products. *See* Mallow.

MAMMARIAN HYDROLYSATE • The hydrolysate (*see*) of animal mammarian tissue derived by acid, enzyme, or other method of hydrolysis. Used as a source of protein in cosmetic products. *See* Mammary Extract.

MAMMARY EXTRACT • The extract of cow's mammary tissue. Claimed by some cosmetic companies as an anti-aging or cellular supporting ingredient. There is always a caution about using animal extracts without specific testing for contaminants.

MAMUSHI OIL • Oil from the Japanese mamushi snake used as an emollient.

MANDARIN ORANGE OIL • Obtained by expression of the peel of a ripe mandarin orange, *Citrus nobilis.* Clear, dark orange to reddish yellow, with a pleasant orange-like odor. It is an orange, tangerine, cherry, and grape flavoring. GRAS

MANDELIC ACID • Amygdalic Acid. Large white crystals or powder with a faint odor. Used in cosmetics as a germicide. Toxic by ingestion.

MANDRAGORA OFFICINARUM • *See* Mandrake.

MANDRAKE • Mayapple. Devil's Apple. Alraun. Satan's Apple. Mandragora. Devil's Testicles. The oldest known narcotic plant, it is native to southern Europe and the Mediterranean, it belongs to the potato family. According to legend, mandrake shrieks when it is pulled out of the ground. It contains ingredients similar to belladonna. Homeopaths use it to treat coughs, asthma, and hay fever. In the Middle Ages, mandrake was believed to be an aphrodisiac. Used to treat skin inflammation. The FDA considers the plant a poisonous narcotic.

MANGANESE ACETYLMETHIONATE • *See* Manganese Sources and Methionine.

MANGANESE ASPARTATE • *See* Aspartic Acid, DL & L Forms, and Manganese Sources.

MANGANESE CARBONATE • Rose-colored crystals derived from manganese. Used as a pigment.

MANGANESE GLUCONATE • Used in skin fresheners and cold creams. *See* Gluconic Acid and Salts and Manganese Sources.

MANGANESE GLYCEROPHOSPHATE • Used in oral care products. *See* Glycerol and Phosphate.

MANGANESE PCA • Used in skin conditioners. *See* Manganese Sources and Carboxylic Acid.

MANGANESE SOURCES • Manganese acetate, manganese carbonate, manganese chloride, manganese citrate, manganese sulfate, manganese glycerophosphate, manganese hypophosphite, and manganese oxide. Used in cosmetics as emollients, oral care ingredients, and as cleansers. A mineral supplement first isolated in 1774, it occurs in minerals and in minute quantities in animals, plants, and water. Many forms are used in dyeing. Manganous salts are activators of enzymes, and are necessary to the development of strong bones. They are used as nutrients and as dairy substitutes. Toxicity occurs by inhalation. Symptoms include languor, sleepiness, wakefulness, emotional disturbances, and Parkinsonlike symptoms. *Manganese chloride, citrate, glycerophosphate,* and *hypophosphite* are all considered GRAS according to the final report of the Select Committee on GRAS Substances and should continue their GRAS status as nutrients with no limitations other than good manufacturing practices. However, *manganese oxide,* according to the Select Committee, does not have enough known about it upon which to base an evaluation when it is used as a food ingredient.

MANGANESE STEARATE • *See* Stearic Acid and Manganese Sources.

MANGANESE SULFATE • Usually prepared by dissolving dolomite (*see*) or magnetite in acid. It is the salt of the element manganese, a metal ore. Its pale red crystals are used in red hair dye. Apparently nontoxic to the hair or scalp, but very small doses injected into mice are lethal.

MANGANESE VIOLET • CI 77742. Burgundy Violet. Permanent Violet. Ammonium Manganese Pyrophosphate. A moderate purple that is redder and duller than heliotrope and bluer than amethyst. Toxic when inhaled. Permanently listed in 1976 for cosmetic coloring, including around the eyes.

MANGIFERA INDICA • *See* Mango.

MANGO • *Mangifera indica* is an evergreen native to India and the tropics. It produces a rich, juicy fruit with a hard pit that is eaten in many parts of the world. Mango butter is obtained from deshelled fruit kernels of the mango tree. It reportedly helps wound healing and is protective against UV radiation. It is a soft solid with a very slight sweet scent and can be a replacement for paraffin-based (*see*) emollient. It is used in skin care products, lotions, massage creams, and hair products.

MANIHOT UTILISSIMA • Cassava. A tropical herb. Contains glycosides (*see*) and vitamin E. It is used as a thickener.

MANJAKANI • *See* Oak Gall.

MANNAN • *See* Glucose.

MANNITAN LAURATE • The monoester of lauric acid and mannitol (*see both*) used as an emulsifier.

MANNITOL • A humectant in hand creams and lotions and used in hair-grooming products as an emulsifier and antioxidant. It is widespread in plants but mostly prepared from seaweed. White, crystalline solid, odorless, and sweet tasting. In cosmetics, it is used as a flavoring ingredient, humectant, and skin conditioner. Its use as a food additive is under study by the FDA because it can cause gastrointestinal disturbances.

MANNOSE • Used as a humectant. *See* Glucose.

MARANTA ARUNDINACEA • *See* Arrowroot.

MARE MILK • Milk from female horses used as a skin conditioner.

MARGOSA OIL • *See* Neem Oil and Neem Leaves Extract.

MARIGOLD • *See* Calendula Extract and Oil.

MARIS AQUA • Seawater.

MARIS LIMUS • Sea silt.

MARIS SAL • Sea salt.

MARITIME PINE EXTRACT PYCNOGENOL • Extract of the bark and pine buds of *Pinus maritima*. Water extract from the bark of the French maritime pine is being highly promoted at this writing for a number of ailments, including aging skin. The extract has four basic properties, according to its producer. "It's a powerful antioxidant, acts as a natural anti-inflammatory, selectively binds to collagen and elastin, and finally, it aids in the production of endothelial nitric oxide which helps to vasodilate blood vessels." Pycnogenol is certified kosher and halal and has earned generally regarded as safe (GRAS) status in the United States for its applications in foods and beverages. Additionally, Pycnogenol is a proprietary extract and is protected by several U.S. and international patents. *See* Pine Tar.

MARJORAM OIL • Used in hair preparations, perfumes, and soaps, it is the essential oil from sweet marjoram. Insoluble in water, soluble in alcohol and chloroform. Can irritate the skin. Redness, itching, and warmth experienced when applied to the skin are caused by local dilation of the blood vessels or by local reflex. May produce allergic reactions. Essential oils such as marjoram are believed to penetrate the skin easily and produce systemic effects.

MARMOT OIL • Oil from a short-legged rodent. Related to the woodchuck or prairie dog. Used in hair- and skin-conditioning products. It is occlusive.

MARROW EXTRACT • Extract from bovine bone marrow used as a humectant and emollient.

MARROW LIPIDS • The soft, spongy center of the bone that acts like a factory to produce white blood cells, the primary ingredients of the body's immune system. The fatty substance contained in bovine bone marrow is used in cosmetics as a skin conditioner and emollient.

MARRUBIUM VULAGRE • *See* Horehound.

MARSDENIA CONDURANGO • *See* Condurango Extract.

MARSHMALLOW ROOT • *Althea officinalis*. A demulcent containing up to 35 percent mucilage, it is an old-time remedy for digestive disorders. It soothes mucous membranes and has been used externally for hundreds of years as a wound healer. Marshmallow ointments and creams are used on chapped hands and lips. It is used as a mouthwash and gargle and to soothe teething infants. Herbalists claim it has a general calming effect on the body.

MARSILEA MINUTA • Water Clover. A small herb that grows in swamps and ponds and is used to soothe gums and to stop nosebleeds.

MASCARA • A cosmetic for coloring the eyelashes and eyebrows. Contains insoluble pigments, carnauba wax, triethanolamine stearate, paraffin, and lanolin. Pigments in eye makeup must be inert and are usually carbon black, iron oxides, chromium oxide, ultramarine, or carmine. Coal tar dyes are not permitted. The excipients may contain beeswax, cetyl alcohol, glyceryl monostearate, gums such as tragacanth, mineral oil, perfume, preservatives such as *p*-hydroxybenzoic acid, propylene glycol, spermaceti, and synthetics such as isopropyl myristate, as well as vegetable oils. The newer lash extenders may carry certain tiny fibers of rayon or nylon. Almost any one of the ingredients may cause an allergic reaction in the susceptible. Do not apply while driving in a car. Do not lend to or use someone else's mascara. Do not moisten it with your spit. Mascara is easily contaminated and must be used carefully. Some experts suggest you change yours every three months.

MASKING FRAGRANCE • A small amount of fragrance used literally to mask the unpleasant odors in a product such as soaps.

MASSOY BARK OIL • *Cryptocarya massoy.* Fragrance ingredient.

MATÉ EXTRACT • *Chamomilla recutita.* Paraguay Tea Extract. St. Bartholomew's Tea. Jesuit's Tea. A natural flavoring extract from small gourds grown in South America, where maté is a stimulant beverage. Among its constituents are caffeine, purines, and tannins. The FDA data bank, PAFA, has not yet done a search of the toxicology literature concerning maté. However, it was reported in the February 1, 1995, issue of the *Journal of the American Medical Association* to be toxic to the liver. GRAS

MATILJA POPPY • *Romneya coulteri. See* Poppy Oil.

MATRICARIA EXTRACT • Wild Chamomile Extract. Extract of the flower heads of *Matricaria chamomilla.* Used internally as a tonic and externally as a soothing medication for contusions and other inflammation. Widely used in cold creams, cleansing lotions, shampoos, suntan gels, hair care products, skin fresheners, and eye makeup. *See* Tannic Acid.

MATRICARIA OIL • Chamomile Oil. The volatile oil distilled from the dried flower heads of *Matricaria chamomilla. See* Matricaria Extract.

MATRIX PROTEINS • A spongy and feltlike support material, consisting of an insoluble collagen matrix containing releaseable soluble collagen, is used as a cosmetic carrier for the application of moisturizing collagen to the skin. The structure and function of these proteins are not well understood, but they are being promoted as understructures supporting sagging, aging skin. The connective tissue found in skin is an intricate mesh of interacting protein molecules that constitute the extracellular matrix. The main types of proteins that make up the matrix include collagens, elastin, fibronectin, and laminin. Another consideration affecting the use of proteins such as elastin as cosmetic ingredients concerns the degree to which the proteins produce unwanted allergic responses in the skin. This is particularly troublesome since the elastin used in most cosmetics is derived from the neck tendons of young calves or other mammals. Nonhuman sources of many proteins are potent allergens and cannot be used in unmodified form in humans. The use of human extracellular matrix proteins in cosmetics could avoid these problems, cosmetic chemists say. A biotechnology-based process to manufacture human elastin or tropoelastin is said to provide a functional source of this matrix protein for cosmetic compositions. The material displays several properties that are said to make it superior to conventional sources of this material.

MATTE FINISH MAKEUP • Designed to be an all-in-one makeup combining foundation and powder. It is a more concentrated version of standard makeup and contains more powder, pigment, and emollient than standard makeup. Effective in covering blemishes. Skin toxicity depends upon ingredients used.

MAURITIA FLEXUOSA • Belonging to the palm family, its fruit oil is used as an emollient and is being studied by pharmaceutical companies.

MAYAPPLE • *Podophyllum peltatum.* Duck's Foot. Hogapple. Mandrake. A perennial plant of the barberry family, it is native to North America. Used by early American settlers as a laxative and to treat diarrhea, arthritis, and kidney problems. American Indians reportedly used it as a poison to commit suicide. *See* Mandrake.

MAYBLOSSOM • *See* Hawthorn Berry.

MAYONNAISE • The common salad dressing. Semisolid, made with eggs, vegetable oil, and vinegar or lemon juice. Used by natural cosmeticians as a dry hair conditioner. The hair is rubbed liberally with mayonnaise, a hot towel is wrapped around the hair and kept on for fifteen minutes, and then it is removed. Two soapings and plenty of rinsing follow. As effective as any of the more expensive commercial products.

MDM • Abbreviation for monomethyl dimethyl.

MDM HYDANTOIN • Monomethylol Dimethyl Hydantoin. Used as a preservative in cosmetic preparations, the compound liberates an allergen steadily at a slow rate in the presence of water. The resin is used in hair lacquers. Has been linked to contact dermatitis (*see*).

MEA • The abbreviation for monoethanolamine.

MEA-BENZOATE • A preservative. Benzoates have been linked to health issues. *See* Benzoic Acid.

MEA-BIOTINATE • Used as an emollient. *See* Biotin.

MEABORATE • Enzyme stabilizer used in detergents. The ester ofethanolamine borate. Low toxicity. Borates have been linked to fetal malformations. *See* Boric Acid.

MEA-DICETEARYL PHOSPHATE • An emulsifier. *See* Cetearyl Alcohol.

MEA-HYDROLYZED COLLAGEN • The monoethanolamine salt of hydrolyzed animal protein. The word *animal* has been removed from this ingredient's name.

MEA-O-PHENYOLPHENATE • Preservative. E

MEA-SULFITE • Preservative. May cause contact dermatitis and contact allergies. Not on the EU list. *See* Sulfites.

MEADOW BUTTERCUP • *Ranunculus acris.* An erect perennial native to Europe, Asia, and the eastern United States, it is used in homeopathic medicines to treat arthritis, sciatica, and skin disease. All parts of the plant are very toxic. It strongly irritates the mucous membrane of the stomach and can also cause severe skin irritation.

MEADOW SAFFRON • *Colchicum autumnale.* A perennial plant native of the temperate parts of Europe where it grows wild in meadows. All parts of the meadow saffron plant contain colchicine (*see*), which is used to treat the inflammation of gout. Used as a skin conditioner and coloring. Meadow saffron can be toxic and may even be fatal if ingested. On the Candian Hotlist (*see*).

MEADOWFOAM • *Limnanthes alba.* Developed as an agricultural crop for its oil in the late 1950s. Added to cosmetics and creams as a moisturizer. In shampoos and soaps, it is used to add shine and moisture to hair and scalp. In lipsticks and balms, it is used to moisturize dry, cracked lips. Used as a humectant in suntan lotions, eye shadows, eyeliners, mascara, hand and face creams, cuticle repair lotions, body oils and creams, shaving creams, foundations, rouges, face powders, and lipsticks.

MEADOWROOT • *See* Meadowsweet.

MEADOWSWEET • *Spiraea ulmaria.* A perennial common to Europe, eastern United States, and Canada, it grows in meadows. It was used to treat diarrhea and stomach upsets. It was also given for gout, arthritis, and flu. It is rich in vitamin C and contains salicylic acid and citric acid (*see both*). Widely used in "organic" cosmetics as a skin-conditioning ingredient.

MEA-IODINE • *See* Iodine.

MEA-LAURETH-6 CARBOXYLATE • *See* Polyethylene Glycol.

MEA-LAURETH SULFATE • The monoethanolamine salt of ethylated lauryl sulfate. *See* Quaternary Ammonium Compounds.

MEA-PPGP6P-LAURETH-7-CARBOXYLATE • *See* Quaternary Ammonium Compounds.

MEA-SALICYLATE • A preservative. The EU has banned it for children under three years except in shampoos. *See* Salicyclic Acid.

MEA-THIOLACTATE • Used in hair-straightening and hair-curling products. *See* Thiolactic Acid.

MEDICAGO SATIVA • *See* Alfalfa Extract.

MEDICATED MAKEUP • Cosmetics manufacturers advertise medicated makeup that both "covers" and treats the skin simultaneously. Such cosmetics contain antibacterials such as bithionol and tribromsalan. The American Medical Association frowns on such preparations because such anti-infective ingredients are useful in medical preparations for the treatment of minor cuts and abrasions, but in cosmetics and toilet preparations they serve merely to limit the bacterial contamination of the product during use. Furthermore, their potential harm often outweighs their benefit because such ingredients may cause allergic reactions and sensitivity to sunlight or bright lights; when the skin is exposed, it breaks out or reddens.

MEHNDI BODY ART • A tradition of India and other Middle Eastern nations, it is growing in popularity in the United States and elsewhere. Intricate "tattoos" are applied to the surface of the skin using a paintlike henna paste. The paste stays on the skin for several hours and when it is removed, a stain remains that darkens over the following twenty-four hours. Mehndi body art can last one to two weeks or longer. In India, mehndi is a form of beautification much like makeup or jewelry. How long mehndi body art lasts on the skin depends on the quality of the henna paste, the amount of time it stays on the skin, the area of the body decorated with mehndi body art, and skin type. Henna stains the top layers of skin, so as the skin naturally exfoliates or loses cells, the mehndi body art fades. Mehndi tends to last longer on areas that generate more heat, like the hands and feet, though washing with harsh soaps will cause mehndi body art to fade sooner. Oils, other natural ingredients, and the application of heat can increase the depth of color to dark brown, deep coffee, or a brownish black. Darker stains are desirable, as they create more contrast and can last longer. However, so called "black henna" is sometimes made from black hair dye containing para-phenylenediamine (*see*) (PPD). The black dye can cause blistering and other serious problems, and it is illegal to apply to the skin. If considering mehndi body art, be sure to avoid paste that contains PPD. *See* Temporary Tattoos.

MEK • Methyl Ethyl Ketone. A flammable, colorless liquid compound resembling acetone and most often made by taking the hydrogen out of butyl alcohol. Used chiefly as a solvent. Similar to, but more irritating than, acetone; its vapor is irritating to mucous membranes and eyes. Central nervous system depression in experimental animals has been reported, but the irritating odor usually discourages further inhalation in humans. No serious poisonings reported in humans, except for skin irritation when nail polish was applied with MEK as a solvent. Large doses inhaled by rats are lethal.

MEL • *See* Honey.

MELALEUCA • *See* Tea Tree Oil and Cajeput.

MELAMINE • White, free-flowing, powdered resin. Used in nail enamel. First introduced into industry in 1939, it is now used in a wide variety of products, including boil-proof adhesives and scratch-resistant enamel finishes. Combined with urea resins, it forms the heat-resistant amino plastics. It may cause skin rashes, but that is believed to be caused by the formaldehyde component rather than the melamine. *See* Urea-Formaldehyde Resin.

MELAMINE/FORMALDEHYDE RESIN • A film former. Respiratory distress, bleeding in the lungs, significant weight loss, and other lung problems were observed during inhalation studies in rats. Feeding studies in animals did not show toxicity. Human sensitization to this has been reported in medical literature. The safety of this ingredient has not been documented and substantiated according to the CIR Expert Panel (*see*). *See* Melamine.

MELAN- • Prefix meaning black, as in melanin.

MELANOMA • A cancer made up of pigmented skin cells. A potentially fatal disease.

MELANIN • The pigment that is responsible for the color of skin, hair, feathers, and fur. Use of this ingredient is prohibited in the United States and may be restricted in other countries but is found in some foundations, suntan gels, creams and liquids, and mascara.

MELASYN • A synthetic melanin (*see*) that protects against ultraviolet light.

MELATONIN • A hormone secreted in the night by humans. First isolated in the late 1950s, it plays a key role in the transmittal of light information and modulates a variety of endocrinological, neurophysiological, and behavioral functions, including the regulation of reproduction, sleep, seasonal disorders, depression and aging, and modulation of retina of the eye. Low doses of melatonin are considered harmless, but the dosage, purity, and usefulness of OTC preparations with melatonin are the subject of controversy. The University of Texas Health Science Center claimed evidence that melatonin is a very potent antioxidant and it may be among the natural agents protecting organisms from oxygen radical damage. Accumulated free radical damage is one of the main factors responsible for DNA modification and carcinogenic changes in tissues influencing the rate of aging. It has been suggested that the role of melatonin in the protection against radical-induced damage is mainly based on its ability to scavenge hydroxyl radicals. The cosmetics companies are producing melatonin-containing products isolated from the pineal glands of beef cattle. The producers claim it is effective to combat anti-aging skin in humans.

MELIA AZADIRACHTA • *See* Neem Tree.

MELIBIOSE • A skin conditioner. *See* Glucose.

MELILOT OIL • Esberiven. Sweet Clover. Dried leaves and flowering tops of *Melilotus officinalis*. Contains coumarin, resins, and volatile oils (*see all*).

MELILOTUS OFFICINALIS • *See* Sweet Clover Extract.

MELISSA OFFICINALIS EXTRACT • *See* Melissa Oil.

MELISSA OIL • *Melissa officinalis*. Lemon Balm. Sweet Balm. A sweet-tasting herb introduced into Britain by the Romans, it has been used from early times in England for nervousness, menstrual irregularity, and surgical dressings. Widely used in cosmetics as a moisturizer and fragrance ingredient in bath oils and hair sprays. The Greeks used it for fevers and to treat scorpion stings and the bites of mad dogs. A hot tea made from it causes perspiration and is said to stop the early symptoms of a cold. *See* Lemon Balm and Balm Mint Oil.

MELISSIC ACID • *See* Bayberry.

MELON EXTRACT AND JUICE • *Cucumis melo*. Honey Dew. Used in products for dry hair and as a skin conditioner.

MELOTHRIA HETEROPHYLLA • A weed belonging to the cucumber family. Used as an emollient and skin protectant.

MENADIOL • Vitamin K_4. A water-soluble vitamin converted to menadione (*see*) after ingestion. It is about half as potent as menadione. *See* Vitamin K.

MENADIONE • Vitamin K₃. Used as a preservative in emollients. A synthetic with properties of vitamin K. Bright yellow crystals that are insoluble in water. They are used medically to prevent blood clotting and in food to prevent souring of milk products. Can be irritating to mucous membranes, respiratory tract, and the skin.

MENHADEN OIL • Pogy Oil. Mossbunker Oil. Obtained along the coast of Africa from the menhaden fish, which are a little larger than herrings. The fish glycerides of menhaden are reddish and have a strong fishy odor. Used in soaps and creams.

MENTHA • *See* Mint.

MENTHA AQUATICA • Water mint. *See* Mint.

MENTHA ARVENSIS • *See* Wild Mint Extract.

MENTHA PIPERITA • May cause allergic skin reaction. *See* Peppermint.

MENTHA PULEGIUM • *See* Pennyroyal Extract.

MENTHA VIRIDIS • *See* Spearmint Oil.

P-MENTHAN-7-OL • A fragrance ingredient. *See* Mint.

MENTHANEDIOL • *See* Turpentine.

MENTHENAMINE • Preservative. Skin irritant. Limited to 0.2 percent of the finished product.

MENTHOL • Used in perfumes, emollient creams, hair tonics, mouthwashes, shaving creams, preshave lotions, after-shave lotions, body rubs, liniments, and skin fresheners. It gives that "cool" feeling to the skin after use. It can be obtained naturally from peppermint or other mint oils and can be made synthetically by hydrogenation (*see*) of thymol (*see*). It is a local anesthetic in low doses, but in concentrations of 3 percent or more it exerts an irritant action that can, if long continued, induce changes in all layers of the mucous membranes. The Food and Drug Administration issued a notice in 1992 that menthol had not been shown to be safe and effective for stated claims in OTC products, including those for the treatment of fever blisters and cold sores, poison ivy, poison oak, poison sumac, and insect bites and stings, as well as in astringents. Also used in grooming aids, skin fresheners, mouthwashes, fragrances, creams, cleansing lotions, bath soaps, and many other cosmetic products.

MENTHONE GLYCERIN ACETAL • A flavoring ingredient. *See* Mint.

MENTHOXYPROPANEDIOL • A cooling ingredient. *See* Menthol and Propylene Glycol.

MENTHYL ACETATE • A flavoring ingredient. The ester (*see*) of menthol and acetic acid (*see both*).

MENTHYL ANTHRANILATE • Ester of menthol (*see*) used in sunscreens.

MENTHYL LACTATE • Flavoring and fragrance ingredient in hand and body products. *See* Menthol and Lactic Acid.

MENTHYL PCA • A skin conditioner. *See* Menthol.

MENTHYL SALICYLATE • The ester of menthol and salicylic acid used in medicines and sunscreen preparations. *See* Salicylic Acid.

MENYANTHES TRIFOLIATA • *See* Buckbean Extract.

MERBROMIN • Mercurochrome. Derived from dibromofluorescein and mercuric acetate, it is used as a topical antiseptic. Toxic by ingestion. In 1992, the FDA issued a notice that merbromin had not been shown to be safe and effective as claimed in OTC poison ivy, poison oak, and poison sumac products.

MERCAPTANS • Quicksilver. Used in depilatories. A class of compounds that contain sulfur and have a disagreeable odor. Depilatories containing mercaptans can cause irritation and allergic reactions, as well as infections of hair follicles.

MERCAPTOPROPIONIC ACID • *See* Mercaptans.

MERCURIALIS ANNUA • A weed, it is used to treat wounds and is being investigated as a treatment for breast cancer since it is believed to inhibit the milk-producing hormone prolactin.

MERCURIALIS EXTRACT • Dog Rhythmitised dilution of *Mercurialis perennis,* or "dog's mercury." It has dark green leaves that are purported to contain natural wound-cleansing substances that support the skin's own healing capabilities and stimulate the skin's metabolism. It also has anti-inflammatory properties. Mercurialis grows primarily in the shady forests of Europe and is hermaphroditic, meaning it forms plants that carry pollen and ovaries. It is hand harvested in early spring, just as its greenish flowers appear. This spring flower is found across Europe, but is almost absent from Ireland, Orkney, and Shetland. It is a hairy dioecious perennial with erect stems bearing simple, serrate leaves. The inflorescence is green, bearing inconspicuous flowers in March and April. It is frequently found covering large areas in dense stands as an understory plant in woodlands, especially, but not exclusively, on calcareous soils. Dog's mercury is a poisonous plant; however, boiling or drying can destroy the toxins.

MERCURIC CHLORIDE • A highly toxic mercury that has been used as a topical antiseptic. In 1992, the FDA issued a notice that mercuric chloride had not been shown to be safe and effective as claimed in OTC poison ivy, poison oak, and poison sumac products.

MERCURIC OXIDE • Red Mercuric Oxide. Yellow Mercuric Oxide. Derived by heating mercurous nitrate, it is used in perfumery as a topical disinfectant and as a fungicide. Highly toxic.

MERCURY COMPOUNDS • Quicksilver. Until July 5, 1973, mercury was widely used in cosmetics, including wax face masks, hair tonics, medicated soaps, and bleach and freckle creams. Mercury compounds are heavy, silver liquids from the metal that occurs in the earth's crust. Mercury is potentially dangerous by all portals of entry, including the skin. It may cause a variety of symptoms, ranging from chronic inflammation of the mouth and gums to personality changes, nervousness, fever, and rash. If ingested in small amounts, it may be fatal. The ban on mercury was brought about because it was found that its use in bleaching creams and other products over a long period of time caused mercury buildup in the body. Mercury is still used in eye preparations as a preservative to inhibit growth of germs. It is now the only use permitted. Because the prevention of eye infection warrants the use of mercury, eye makeup contains up to 0.0065 percent. On the Canadian Hotlist (*see*). *See also* Calomel.

MEROXAPOL-105, -108, -171, -172, -174, -178, -251, -252, -254, -255, -258, -311, -312, -314 • Pluronic. The polyoxypropylene block polymer that is derived from petroleum. It is a liquid nonionic—resists freezing and shrinkage—surfactant used in hand creams. The numbers after the name identify the liquidity of the compound: the higher the number, the more solid.

MESOPHYLLUM LICHENOIDES • Red Algae. *See* Alginates.

METABROMSALAN • Banned by the FDA because it may cause sensitivity to sunlight. *See* Bromates.

METALLIC HAIR DYES • Metals such as copper are used to change the color of hair. They are not used very often because they tend to dull the hair. However, they are used in products that are designed for daily application over a week or so to effect color changes gradually. Combs impregnated with dye or hair lotions may contain metals for this purpose. *See* Hair Coloring for further information, including toxicity.

METHACRYLATES • Methacrylates and cyanoacrylates are used in fake nails and can cause irritation, trauma, and infection. Allergic itchy rashes can occur around the eyes and there may be burning and tenderness of the nail bed, cuticle area, and areas of the face and neck. According to the American Academy of Dermatology experts, although the liquid form of methacrylate is banned by twenty-three states and the FDA has issued warnings about its hazards, the substance is still used in some discount salons because it costs so much less than the safer compounds.

METHACRYLIC ACID • The Methacrylate Producers Association, Inc. (MPA) believes that methacrylic acid and its esters (including methyl methacrylate, ethyl methacrylate, *n*-butyl methacrylate, isobutyl methacrylate, lauryl methacrylate, and 2-ethylhexyl methacrylate) in unreacted monomeric liquid form are not appropriate for use in cosmetics. The known corrosive properties of the acid and skin sensitization properties of the esters, as underscored by recent reports of injury due to their use in some nail products, indicates their use in cosmetics should be restricted. Nail builders (elongators, extenders) have been involved in numerous reports of irritation, inflammation, and infection of nail bed and nail fold as well as complaints of discoloration, splitting, and loss of fingernails. The methacrylate monomers currently used in nail builders are mostly ethyl, hydroxyethyl, butyl, isobutyl, hydroxypropyl, or other esters of methacrylic acid. Methyl methacrylate is now rarely used. The currently used esters of methacrylic acid may be as harmful as methyl methacrylate. The FDA's belief that MMA is rarely used has proven not to be the case in recent years. Numerous reports of its increasing use in nail products have led to a flurry of articles in the beauty salon trade press and national media. On the Canadian Hotlist (*see*). The inner and outer label of a cosmetic in liquid form that contains more than 5 percent methacrylic acid shall carry a warning that it is poisonous and should be kept out of reach of children.

METHACRYLOYL ETHYL BETAINE/METHACRYLATES COPOLYMER • *See* Methacrylic Acid.

METHANOL • Methyl Alcohol. Wood Alcohol. A solvent and denaturant obtained by the destructive distillation of wood. Flammable, poisonous liquid with a nauseating odor. Better solvent than ethyl alcohol. Has been associated with eczema (*see*). Methanol is highly toxic and readily absorbed from all routes of exposure. It is on the Canadian Hotlist (*see*). The EU restricts it to 5 percent calculated a percentage of ethanol and isopropyl alcohol.

METHENAMINE • An odorless, white, crystalline powder made from formaldehyde and ammonia. Used as an antiseptic and bacteria killer in deodorant creams and powders, mouthwashes, and medicines. It is one of the most frequent causes of skin rashes in the rubber industry and is omitted from hypoallergenic cosmetics. Skin irritations are believed to be caused by formic acid, which occurs by the action of perspiration on the skin. On the basis of the available information, the CIR Expert Panel (*see*) concludes that it is safe as a cosmetic ingredient.

METHENAMMONIUM CHLORIDE • Busan 1500. A water-soluble bactericide active over a wide pH range. *See* Ammonia.

METHICONE • Widely used as a skin-conditioning ingredient in foundations, eye shadows, face powders, lipsticks, blushers, eyeliners, moisturizers, masacara, makeup bases, and powders. Also after-shave lotions. *See* Silicones.

METHIONINE • An essential amino acid (*see*) that occurs in protein. Used as a texturizer in cosmetic creams. Also used as a dietary substance and is attracted to fat.

METHOCARBAMOL • A skeletal muscle relaxant prepared from phenol. The EU bans it in cosmetics.

METHOTREXATE • Amethopterin. Folex. Mexate. MTX. Rheumatrex. Belongs to the group of medicines known as antimetabolites. It is used to treat psoriasis, purities, and rheumatoid arthritis. Methotrexate blocks an enzyme needed by the cell to live. This interferes with the growth of certain cells, such as skin cells in psoriasis that are growing rapidly. It was introduced in the 1950s to treat cancer and a cosmetic company quietly experimented with it for an anti-aging cream. This drug has a high incidence of serious side effects. Now banned in cosmetics by the EU and ASEAN (*see*).

3-METHOXYBUTANOL • A solvent. *See* Butyl Alcohol.

o-METHOXY CINNAMIC ALDEHYDE • *See* Cinnamic Aldehyde.

7-METHOXYCOUMARIN • *See* Coumarins. The UK banned it in fragrances because it induces allergic and photo-allergic reactions.

METHOXYDIGLYCOL • Fragrance ingredient, solvent. *See* Glycols.

METHOXY PEG 10–40 • Humectants. *See* Polyethylene Glycol.

METHOXY PEG-22/DODECYL GLYCOL • *See* Polymers.

METHOXY PROPANOL • *See* Propylene Glycol.

p-METHOXYACETOPHENONE • *p*-Acetanisole. Crystalline solid with a pleasant odor. Soluble in alcohol and fixed oils and derived from the interaction of anisole and acetyl chloride with aluminum chloride and carbon disulfide. Used in perfumery as a synthetic floral odor and in flavoring.The permissible human exposure levels of this ethylene glycol ether is 25 ppm to 5 ppm, and a further reduction has been proposed. It is both a reproductive and developmental toxicant. May cause birth defects. Carbon disulfide is banned in cosmetics by the EU. FEMA (*see*), however, judged the substance is GRAS. On the Canadian Hotlist (*see*). *See* Ethylene Glycol. EAF

METHOXYINDANE • Phoralid. A synthetic fragrance.

METHOXYISOPROPANOL • A solvent used in nail polish. *See* Propylene Glycol.

2-METHOXYMETHYL-p-AMINOPHENOL • *See* Phenols.

4-METHOXYPHENOL • Prohibited. Should not be used as a fragrance ingredient based on its depigmenting effect.

METHOXYPHENYL • Used in sunscreens and skin-conditioning creams. The UK has banned the compound in fragrances. It may be toxic.

2- AND 4-METHOXY-m-PHENYLENEDIAMINE • *See* p-Phenylenediamine.

4-METHOXY-m-PHENYLENEDIAMINE • Hair-dye ingredient. On the basis of the available information, the CIR Expert Panel (*see*) concluded that it is unsafe as a cosmetic ingredient. It is on the Canadian Hotlist (*see*). *See* Phenylenediamine.

4-METHOXY-m-PHENYLENEDIAMINE-HCL • A hair-dye ingredient. On the basis of the available information, the CIR Expert Panel (*see*) concluded that it is unsafe as a cosmetic ingredient. It is on the Canadian Hotlist (*see*). *m*-Phenylenediamine has been banned in cosmetics by the EU.

4-METHOXY-m-PHENYLENEDIAMINE SULFATE • A hair-dye ingredient. On the basis of the available information, the CIR Expert Panel (*see*) concluded that it is unsafe as a cosmetic ingredient. On the Canadian Hotlist (*see*). *m*-Phenylenediamine has been banned in cosmetics by the EU. *See* Phenylenediamine.

2-METHOXY-p-PHENYLENEDIAMINE SULFATE • It is on the Canadian Hotlist (*see*). *See* Phenylenediamine.

6-METHOXY-2–3-PYRIDINEDIAMINE • *See* Pyridine.

METHOXYSALEN • 8-Methoxypsoralen. White to cream-colored, odorless crystalline solid; slightly soluble in alcohol and almost insoluble in water. Used as a suntan accelerator and a sunburn protectant.

4-METHOXYTOLUENE-2, 5-DIAMINE HCL • A colorless liquid used in perfumery and flavorings. *See* Toluene.

METHOXYTRIMETHYLPHENYL DIHYDROXYPHENYL PROPANOL • An alcoholic antioxidant and skin-conditioning ingredient. *See* Propanol.

2-METHOXY-4-VINYLPHENOL • Spicy, vanilla flavoring also used in fragrances to add spicy notes. ASP

METHYACRYLIC ACID • 2-Methylpropenoic Acid. Occurs in Roman chamomile oil. Has a bad odor and is corrosive. It is used to make clear plastic.

METHYL ACETAMIDE • *See* Methyl Acetate.

METHYL ACETATE • Acetic Acid. Colorless liquid that occurs naturally in coffee, with a pleasant apple odor. Used in perfume to emphasize floral notes (*see* Floral Bouquet), especially that of rose, and in toilet waters having a lavender odor. Also occurs naturally in peppermint oil. Used as a solvent for many resins and oils. May be irritating to the respiratory tract, and in high concentrations may be narcotic. Since it has an effective fat solvent drying effect on skin, it may cause skin problems such as chafing and cracking.

METHYL ACETOACETATE • 3-Oxobutanoic Acid. Methyl Ester. *See* Butanoic Acid.

METHYL ACETYL RICINOLEATE • *See* Ricinoleic Acid.

METHYL ACRYLATE • 2-Propanoic Acid. Methyl Ester. Derived from ethylene chlorohydrin, it is transparent and elastic. Used as a film former. Can be highly irritating to the eyes, skin, and mucous membranes. Convulsions occur if vapors are inhaled in high concentrations. The liquid form of methyl acrylate has been banned in twenty-three states. *See* Acrylates.

METHYL ALCOHOL • On the Canadian Hotlist (*see*). *See* Methanol.

METHYL ANTHRANILATE • Used as an "orange" scent for ointments, in the manufacture of synthetic perfumes, and in suntan lotions. Occurs naturally in neroli, ylang-ylang, bergamot, jasmine, and other essential oils. Colorless to pale yellow liquid with a bluish fluorescence and a grapelike odor. It is made synthetically from coal tar (*see*). Can irritate the skin. The CIR Expert Panel (*see*) has listed this as top priority for review.

METHYL ASPARTIC ACID • *See* Aspartic Acid.

METHYL BEHENATE • Skin-conditioning ingredient. *See* Behenic Acid.

METHYL BENZOATE • Essence of Oil of Niobe. Made from methanol and benzoic acid (*see both*). Used in perfumes. Colorless, transparent liquid with a pleasant fruity odor. Also used as a flavoring in foods and beverages.

METHYL BUTENE • Solvent. *See* Butene.

METHYL CAPROATE • Methyl Hexanoate. The ester produced by the reaction of methyl alcohol and caproic acid. Used as a stabilizer and plasticizer for hand and face creams.

METHYL CAPRYLATE • *See* Methyl Caproate.

METHYL CHLORIDE • Chloromethane. Colorless gas or colorless liquid with a sweet taste, it is used as a methylating agent for products such as cellulose, quaternary ammonium compounds, and silicones (*see all*).

METHYL CINNAMATE • White crystals, strawberrylike odor, and soluble in alcohol. Derived by heating methanol, cinnamic acid, and sulfuric acid. Used in perfumes and flavoring. *See* Cinnamic Acid.

METHYL COCOATE • Emollient. *See* Coconut Oil.

6-METHYL COUMARIN • A synthetic compound once used in suntan products. Used in fragrances. A potent photosensitizer. Not recommended for use in fragrance ingredients. The EU restricts it to zero in oral hygiene products. The FDA does not ban its use in cosmetics but has expressed caution about it.

METHYL CYCLODEXTRIN • *See* Dextrin.

METHYL DEHYDROABIETATE • An emollient. *See* Abietic Acid.

METHYLDIBROMO GLUTARONITRILE • Preservative. Can cause allergic contact dermatitis and contact eczema. It is limited to 0.1 percent of the finished product or 0.025 percent in suntan and sunscreen products. It is activated by sunlight and can cause damage to skin cells and can destroy the UV-absorbing compounds in the suntan lotions rendering them ineffective as sunscreens. Listed by both the European Union and the United States.

METHYL DICOCOAMINE • Antistatic ingredient for hair preparations. *See* Coconut Oil.

METHYL DIISOPROPYL PROPIONAMIDE • A fragrance ingredient. *See* Propionic Acid.

METHYL ETHYL KETONE • *See* MEK.

METHYL EUGENOL • Eugenol. Methyl Ether. The UK has banned this except for normal content in the natural essences used, provided that the concentration does not exceed 0.01 percent in fine fragrances; 0.004 percent in eau de toilette; 0.002 percent in fragrance cream; 0.002 percent in rinse-off products; and 0.0002 percent in other leave-on products and oral hygiene products. *See* Eugenol and Ether.

METHYL GLUCETH-10 OR -20 • The polyethylene glycol ether of methyl glucose. *See* Glucose Glutamate.

METHYL GLUCETH-20 SESQUISTEARATE • Glucamate. Used in moisturizers. *See* Glucose Glutamate.

METHYL GLUCOSE SESQUIOLEATE • A mixture of diesters of methyl glucoside and oleic acid. *See* Glutamic Acid.

METHYL GLUCOSE SESQUISTEARATE • A mixture of diesters of methyl glucoside and stearic acid. *See* Glutamic Acid.

METHYL HYDROGENATED ROSINATE • The ester of methyl alcohol and hydrogenated acids derived from rosin (*see*).

METHYL *p*-HYDROXYBENZOATE • *See* Methyl Paraben.

2-METHYL-5-HYDROXYETHYLAMINOPHENOL • Hair coloring.

METHYL HYDROXYETHYLCELLULOSE • *See* Methylcellulose.

METHYL HYDROXYMETHYL OLEYL OXAZOLINE • A synthetic wax. *See* Oxazoline.

METHYL HYDROXYSTEARATE • The ester of methyl alcohol and hydroxystearic acid used in cosmetic creams. *See* Methanol and Stearic Acid.

METHYL JASMONATE • Found in jasmine and green tea. Used as a flavor and fragrance in apple, floral, gardenia, grease, herbal, honeysuckle, jasmine, lilac, lily, melon, watermelon, muskmelon, cantaloupe, lily of the valley, pea, petal flower, petal plum, and tutti-frutti. *See* Jasmine. ASP

METHYL LACTATE • The ester of menthol and lactic acid (*see both*).

METHYL LAURATE • The ester of methyl alcohol and lauric acid. Derived from coconut oil, it is used in detergents, emulsifiers, wetting ingredients, stabilizers, resins, lubricants, plasticizers, and flavorings.

METHYL LINOLEATE • The ester of methyl alcohol and linoleic acid, it is a colorless oil derived from safflower oil and used in detergents, emulsifiers, wetting ingredients, stabilizers, resins, lubricants, and plasticizers. It is used in skin conditioners.

METHYL METHACRYLATE CROSSPOLYMER • *See* Methacrylic Acid and Polymer.

METHYL METHACRYLATE MONOMER • Banned in nail products because of adverse effects.

METHYL 3-METHYLRESORCYLATE • *See* Resorcinol.

METHYL MYRISTATE • A skin-conditioning ingredient. *See* Myristic Acid.

METHYL NICOTINATE • Derived from nicotinic acid (*see*) and used as a rubefacient (*see*).

METHYL OLEATE • An emollient ingredient. *See* Oleic Acid.

METHYL PALMITATE • The ester of methyl alcohol and palmitic acid. Colorless liquid derived from palm oil. Used in detergents, emulsifiers, wetting ingredients, stabilizers, resins, lubricants, and plasticizers. Low toxicity.

METHYL PARABEN • Methyl *p*-Hydroxybenzoate. One of the most widely used preservatives in cosmetics, it has a broad spectrum of antimicrobial activity and is relatively nonirritating, nonsensitizing, and nonpoisonous. It is stable over the acid-alkalinity range of most cosmetics and is sufficiently soluble in water to produce the effective concentration in the water phase. Can cause allergic reactions. In 1992, the FDA issued a notice that methyl paraben alum had not been shown to be safe and effective as claimed in OTC products.

METHYL PELARGONATE • Nonanoic Acid. Methyl Ester. The ester of ethyl alcohol and pelargonic acid (*see*) used as an emollient in perfume and flavorings.

METHYL PHENYLACETATE • Colorless liquid with a honeylike odor used in perfumery and as a flavoring. *See* Phenylacetic Acid.

2-METHYL 4-PHENYL-2-BUTANOL METHYL CELLULOSE • A grayish-white powder prepared from cellulose (*see*) that swells to a highly viscous colloidal solution in water. Used as a food additive and in water paints, leather tanning, and cosmetics. It is sold under a variety of trade names and is used as a thickener and emulsifier in various foods. Like cellulose, it is nondigestible, nontoxic, and nonallergenic. ASP

2-METHYL-*m*-PHENYLENEDIAMINE • Banned in cosmetics by ASEAN. *See* Phenylenediamine.

METHYL PHTHALYL ETHYL GLYCOLATE • *See* Phthalic Acid and Polyethylene Glycol.

METHYLPREDNISOLONE • Mar-Pred. Medrol. Medrol Enpak. Medrol Oral. Mepred. Meprolone. Methylone. A-Metha-Pred. Solu-Medrol. A hormone secreted by the adrenal gland that affects carbohydrate and protein metabolism. It was introduced as a medication in 1957 to treat severe inflammation, for immunosuppression, and to decrease residual damage following spinal cord trauma. Most adverse reactions are the result of dosage or length of time between administration.

METHYL RICINOLEATE • The ester of methyl alcohol and ricinoleic acid. A colorless liquid used as a plasticizer, lubricant, cutting oil, and wetting ingredient. *See* Castor Oil, Methanol, and Ricinoleic Acid.

METHYLROSANILINE CHLORIDE CRYSTAL VIOLET • *See* Gentian.

METHYL ROSINATE • Rosin Acid. Methyl Ester. The ester of acids recovered from rosin (*see*). *See* Methanol.

METHYL SALICYLATE • Salicylic Acid. Oil of Wintergreen. Arum Analgesic. Ben-Gay. Ger-O-Foam. Icy Hot Balm. Listerine Antiseptic. Theragold Analgesic Lotion. Found naturally in sweet birch, cassia, and wintergreen, it is used as an analgesic in rubefacient (*see*) preparations to relieve muscle and joint pain. A counterirritant (*see*), local anesthetic, and disinfectant used in perfumes, toothpaste, tooth powder, and mouthwash. The volatile oil obtained by maceration and subsequent steam distillation in a species of leaves, including those of sweet birch, cassia, and wintergreen. A strong irritant to the skin and mucous membranes, it may be absorbed readily through the skin. Used as a flavor in foods, beverages, and pharmaceuticals, and used as an odorant in perfumery and as an ultraviolet absorber in sunburn lotions. Toxic by ingestion. Use in foods restricted by the FDA. Lethal dose 30 cc in adults, 10 cc in children. Canada limits it to concentration of 1 percent or less and expresses concern about absorption if used as a counterirritant in sports creams. It is on the Canadian Hotlist (*see*). Toxic by ingestion. The FDA proposed that liniments and other liquid preparations containing more than 5 percent methyl salicylate be marketed in special child-resistant containers. In 1992, the FDA proposed a ban for the use of methyl salicylate to treat fever blisters and cold sores, and in astringent (*see*) drugs because it had not been shown to be safe and effective as claimed in OTC products. *See* Salicylates. ASP

METHYLSILANOL ELASTINATE • Antistatic ingredient. Derived from elastin (*see*).

METHYL SILICONE • Prepared by hydrolyzing (*see*) dimethyldichlorosilane or its esters, it is used to help compounds resist oxidation. *See* Silicones.

METHYL STEARATE • *See* Stearic Acid and Methyl Alcohol.

METHYLTESTOSTERONE • Android. Metandren. Oreton Methyl. Testred. Virilon. A prescription testosterone drug.

METHYL THIOGLYCOLATE • Hair-straightening and hair-waving ingredient. *See* Thioglycolic Acid Compounds.

METHYLAMINES • Occur in herring brine, in the urine of dogs, in certain plants such as mints, and in methanol. Used in tanning and in organic processing. Irritating to the eyes, skin, and respiratory tract.

3-METHYLAMINO-4-NITROPHENOXYETHANOL • Semipermanent hair coloring. The EU set a deadline of July 2005 for manufacturers to submit data on this substance or it will be proposed for a ban. In 2005, it was found it could combine with other chemicals to form nitrosamines (*see*). The EU said it can be used in nonoxidative (semipermanent) hair-coloring products at a maximum concentration of 0.15 percent. This risk assessment relates to the use of 3-methylamino-4-nitrophenoxy-ethanol in nonoxidative hair dye formulations only. The EU's Scientific Committee on Consumer Products (SCCP) in 2007 met and ruled it was of the opinion that the use of 3-methylamino-4-nitrophenoxy-ethanol as a nonoxidative hair dye at a maximum concentration of 0.15 percent on the head does not pose a risk to the health of the consumer. Although it did not irritate the skin of rabbits, it did cause a high death toll in mice and damage to the fetus. There was only one human test and that was of tissue: A piece of human skin from four female donors, dermatomed skin thickness set at 500 μm was used. After thirty minutes of exposure, the hair dye remaining on the skin surface was removed by washing. Twenty-four hours after application, skin samples were removed and analyzed by liquid scintillation counting to assess the cutaneous distribution of 3-methylamino-4-nitrophenoxy-ethanol. The mean total dermal absorption (sum of the amounts measured in the living epidermis, dermis, and receptor fluid) of B058 under the conditions of the experiment represented 0.14 ± 0.05 μgeq/cm^2 or (0.45 ± 0.15 percent of the applied dose).

p-**METHYLAMINOPHENOL SULFATE** • Crystals that discolor in air and are soluble in water. Used in hair dyes. May cause skin irritation, allergic reactions, and a shortage of oxygen in the blood. In solution applied to the skin, restlessness and convulsions have been produced in humans.

METHYLATE • To mix with methanol (*see*).

METHYLATED SPIRITS • Toilet Quality. Alcohol denatured with methanol (*see*). Used in fragrances and other cosmetic products in amounts of over 85 percent ethyl alcohol, 5 percent methyl alcohol, and 5 percent water. *See* Ethanol for toxicity.

METHYLATION • Treating substances to create esters (*see*), often with hot methanol (*see*) in the presence of hydrochloric acid (*see*).

METHYLBENZETHONIUM CHLORIDE • Diaparene Chloride. A quaternary ammonium compound used as a germicide in cosmetics and baby products such as baby oils. Also used as a topical disinfectant. *See* Quaternary Ammonium Compounds for toxicity.

4-METHYLBENZYLIDENE CAMPHOR • *See* Camphor Oil.

METHYLCELLULOSE • Cellulose Methyl Ether. Citrucel. Cologel. A binder, thickener, and emulsifying ingredient used in wave-setting lotions, bath oils, and other cosmetic products. Introduced in 1947, this compound is prepared from wood pulp or chemical cotton by treatment with alcohol. It swells in water and increases bulk. It is not absorbed systemically. On the basis of the available animal and human data, the CIR Expert Panel (*see*) concludes that this ingredient is safe as used in cosmetics.

METHYLCHLOROISOTHIAZOLINONE • A preservative used in shampoos, hair, skin, and after-shave and bath products that was taken from industry to replace formaldehyde. While it has been shown to be a sensitizer in animals, it has not been shown to be a sensitizer in humans. *See* Imidazole.

METHYLDIBROMO GLUTARONITRILE • A preservative used in bubble baths, indoor tanning preparations, and hair conditioners. Application to the skin of rats for twenty-one days at a level of 4.0 g/kg produced severe irritation, whereas skin studies in rabbits showed only slight to moderate irritation. It is readily absorbed through the skin. Based on available data, the CIR Expert Panel (*see*) concluded it is safe as used in rinse-off products and safe up to 0.025 percent in leave-on products. Has been linked to eczema (*see*). *See* Bromates and Glutaric Acid.

METHYLDIHYDROJASMONATE • *See* Jasomone.

METHYLENE-BIS-6-(2H-BENZOTRIAZOL-2-YL-4-TETRAMETHYLBUTYL-1,1,3,3,-PHENOL • Used as a sunscreen and according to the EU, "is not likely to produce harmful effects."

METHYLENE CHLORIDE • A solvent for nail enamels and for cleansing creams. A colorless gas that compresses into a colorless liquid of pleasant odor and sweet taste. High concentrations are narcotic. Damage to the liver, kidneys, and central nervous system can occur, and persistent postrecovery symptoms after inhalation include headache, nervousness, insomnia, and tremor. Can be absorbed through the skin and converted to carbon monoxide, which can cause stress on the cardiovascular system. It is also a skin irritant. In 1988, the CIR Expert Panel (*see*) determined it was safe in cosmetics designed for brief use. Not permitted in aerosols in Canada. It is on the Canadian Hotlist (*see*). Methylene chloride has been used as an ingredient of aerosol cosmetic products, principally hair sprays, at concentrations generally ranging from 10 to 25 percent. In a two-year animal inhalation study sponsored by the National Toxicology Program, methylene chloride produced a significant increase in benign and malignant tumors of the lung and liver of male and female mice. Based on these findings and on estimates of human exposure from the customary use of hair sprays, the FDA concludes that the use of methylene chloride in cosmetic products poses a significant cancer risk to consumers, and that the use of this ingredient in cosmetic products may render these products injurious to health. Any cosmetic product that contains methylene chloride as an ingredient is deemed adulterated and is subject to regulatory action under the Federal Food, Drug, and Cosmetic Act. Banned by the FDA.

METHYLENEDIOXYPHENOL • *See* Phenols.

METHYLETHANOLAMINE • *See* Ethanolamines and Methanol.

5-METHYL-2,3-HEXANEDIONE • Banned in fragrances by the UK.

2-METHYL-5-HYDROXYETHYLAMINOPHENOL • A hair dye ingredient. Only slight absorption was observed in mice skin studies. On the basis of the available data, the CIR Expert Panel (*see*) concluded that it is safe as a cosmetic ingredient. *See* Phenols.

2-METHYL-4-HYDROXYPYRROLINE • A plasticizer derived from acetylene and formaldehyde. *See* Formaldehyde for toxicity.

METHYLISOTHIAZOLINONE • Widely used with methylchloroisothiazolinone as a preservative in shampoos to replace formaldehyde. Although it is a sensitizer in animals, it has not been shown to be a sensitizer in shampoos. Also used in baby products, moisturizers, body and hand preparations, and cleansing creams as well as makeup removers and suntan preparations. On the Canadian Hotlist (*see*). In Canada, it is permitted up to a maximum of 0.0015 percent in rinse-off products and 0.000075 percent in leave-on products. *See* Kathon CG.

METHYLISOTHIAZOLINONE/METHYLCHLOROISOTHIAZOLINONE • Used in cosmetics as a broad spectrum preservative. It is highly toxic in rats and rabbits orally but only moderately toxic when applied to the skin. Can be a skin sensitizer in humans. On the basis of the available data, the CIR Expert Panel (*see*) concluded that it can be safely used in rinse-off products at a concentration not to exceed 15 ppm and in leave-on products at concentrations not to exceed 7.5 ppm. The stated safe use concentration refers to a mixture containing 23.3 percent methylisothiazolinone and 76.7 percent methylchloroisothiazolinone.

N-METHYL-3-NITRO-*p*-PHENYLENEDIAMINE • Coal tar (*see*) hair coloring.

METHYLPHENYLPOLYSILOXANE • Cresol (*see*) with a blend of silicone (*see*) oils. An oily, fluid resin, stable over a wide temperature range, used in lubricating creams.

2-METHYLRESORCINOL • Orcin. An aromatic compound with white crystalline prisms derived from lichen and used in medicine and as a reingredient for sugars and starches. A mild skin irritant. On the basis of the available data, the CIR Expert Panel (*see*) concluded that it is safe as a cosmetic ingredient. In 2008, the EU said it was a moderate sensitizer. Recommended that pregnant women and people with skin diseases not use it. *See* Resorcinol.

METHYLSILANOL • *See* Silicones.

METHYLSILANOL ELASTINATE • A product of methylsilanol and elastin. *See* Silicones and Elastin.

METHYLSTYRENE/VINYLTOLUENE COPOLYMER • The polymer of methylstyrene and vinyltoluene monomers. Used as a wax. *See* Styrene.

MI DIE XIANG • *See* Rosemary.

MIBK • Methyl Isobutyl Ketone. Colorless liquid with a pleasant odor that is used as a solvent for paints, varnishes, and nitrocellulose lacquers, and as a denaturant for alcohol. Hazardous by either ingestion or inhalation.

MICA • Pearls. Any of a group of minerals that are found in crystallized, thin, elastic sheets that can be separated easily. They vary in color from pale green, brown, or black to colorless. Ground and widely used as a lubricant, coloring in cosmetics, and to create a glow in makeup. Irritant by inhalation; may be damaging to the lungs. Coloring permanently listed for cosmetic use in 1977.

MICROBES • Microscopic organisms including fungi, bacteria, and viruses as well as other members of the biological group.

MICROCOCCUS LYSATE • A catalase is an enzyme in plant and animal tissues. It exerts a chemical reaction that converts hydrogen peroxide into water and oxygen. Derived from bacteria by a pure culture fermentation process, bacterial catalase may be used safely, according to the FDA, in destroying and removing the hydrogen peroxide that has been used in the manufacture of cheese—providing "the organism *Micrococcus lysodeikticus* from which the bacterial catalase is to be derived, is demonstrated to be non-toxic and non-pathogenic." The organism is removed from the bacterial catalase prior to the use of the catalase, the catalase to be used in an amount not in excess of the minimum required to produce its intended effect.

MICROCRYSTALLINE CELLULOSE • Abrasive, anticaking, and bulking ingredient in emulsions. It is the colloid crystalline portion of cellulose fibers. *See* Cellulose Gums.

MICROCRYSTALLINE WAX • Any of various plastic materials that are obtained from petroleum. They are different from paraffin (*see*) waxes in that they have a higher melting point, higher viscosity, and much finer crystals that can be seen only under a microscope. Widely used in nail polishes and in cake cosmetics. *See* Ceresin.

MICROENCAPSULATION • Microscopic particles of an ingredient are encased in gelatin like bubbles that are dissolvable, allowing the particles to be suspended and isolated within a product so they arrive at the skin in the purest form released by heat, solution, or other means.

MICROFINE ZINC OXIDE • Zinc oxide is one of the best sunblockers, but it is not "esthetic" to wear. Microfine is a zinc oxide that has been synthesized at a specific particle size to make it more acceptable, and it is expected to replace other sunblockers that are not as effective or that have more unwanted side effects.

MICRO-K • *See* Potassium Chloride.

MICROMERIA CHAMISSONIS • Trailing Evergreen. Yerba Buena. A member of the mint family used in fragrances and flavorings.

MICROORGANISMS • Tiny organisms that can only be seen under a microscope—such as bacteria and viruses.

MIDORI3 • Japanese coal tar hair color called Green 3 Lake in the United States. EU 640053.

MIDORI201 • A Japanese name for a coal tar color used in hair dye. Called Green 5 or Acid Green 25 in the United States. EU CI 61570.

MIDORI202 • Japanese name for a coal tar color used in hair dye called Green 6 or Solvent Green in the United States. EU CI 61565.

MIDORI204 • Japanese name for a coal tar hair dye called Green 8 or Solvent Green 7 in the United States. EU CI 59040.

MIDORI205 • Japanese name for aluminum or zirconium lake color not permitted for use in the European Union or United States.

MIDORI401 • Japanese name for coal tar color not approved for use in the United States. Acid Green 1. EU CI 10020.

MIDORI402 • Japanese coal tar color not approved for use in the United States or European Union. Food Green 1.

MILFOIL • *See* Yarrow.

MILK • Used in bath preparations and face masks as a soothing skin cleanser. Also used by natural cosmeticians as a face wash: for dry skin, cream is used; for oily skin, skim milk. It is as effective as many more expensive products, but if not rinsed thoroughly from the skin with water, rancidity sets in and becomes a focus of bacteria. Consequently, the skin may break out in pimples.

MILK AMINO ACIDS • Derived from milk protein, used as a hair and skin conditioner in shampoos and skin products.

MILK FERMENT • Produced by the fermentation of milk with yeasts and bacilli to produce a skin conditioner.

MILK LIPIDS • Fats from milk used in skin-conditioning ingredients for emollients.

MILK OF MAGNESIA • *See* Magnesium Hydroxide.

MILK PROTEIN • Obtained from cows' milk and used in skin- and hair-conditioning products.

MILK SUGAR • *See* Lactose.

MILK THISTLE • *Silybum marianum. Carduus marianus.* St. Mary's Thistle. In cosmetics, it is used in bath products. The seeds and stems are used to treat liver problems and mushroom poisoning. Milk thistle is reported by herbalists to lower fat deposits in the liver and to act against cirrhosis, necroses, and hepatitis, conditions affecting the liver. Recent studies have shown that a compound in thistle, sylmarin, increases the content of liver glutathione, a nutritive that plays an important role in the activation of some liver enzymes and in oxygen metabolism. Liver enzymes detoxify many potentially harmful chemicals.

MILKAMIDOPROPYL AMINE OXIDE • A fatty acid derived from milk used in hair-conditioning products and as a foam booster.

MILKAMIDOPROPYL BETAINE • A fatty acid derived from milk used as an anti-static ingredient in hair products. *See* Betaines.

MILLET • *Panicum miliaceum.* A cereal and forage grass used in "natural cosmetics."

MIMOSA • Reddish yellow solid with a long-lasting, pleasant odor resembling ylang-ylang, used in perfumes. Derived from trees, shrubs, and herbs native to tropical and warm regions. Used in tanning and in skin care products. May produce allergic skin reactions.

MINERAL • Inorganic matter found in the earth's crust. Cosmetic companies are promoting minerals as one of the newest ingredients for face powders and makeup.

MINERAL OIL • White Oil, Liquid Petrolatum, Agoral Plain, Aquaphor, Aqua Care Lotion, Duolube Eye Ointment, Eucerin Lotion. Widely used in baby creams, baby lotions, bay oil, brilliantine hairdressings, cleansing creams, cold creams, emollients, moisturizing creams, eye creams, foundation creams and makeup, hair conditioners, hand lotions, lipsticks, mascaras, rouge, shaving creams, compact powders, makeup removers, suntan creams, oils, and ointments. Also a cosmetic lubricant, protective ingredient, and binder. It is a mixture of refined liquid hydrocarbons (*see*) derived from petroleum. Colorless, transparent, odorless, and tasteless. When heated, it smells like petroleum. It stays on top of the skin and leaves a shiny protective surface. Propylene glycol, another cosmetic form of mineral oil, is sometimes found in high concentrations (up to 50%) in baby lotions and pre- and after-shave lotions. Mineral oil is one of the most common ingredients in skin care products and colored cosmetics. It is a lightweight inexpensive oil that is odorless and tasteless. One of the common concerns regarding the use of mineral oil is its presence on several lists of comedogenic (*see* Comedogen) substances. These comedogenic lists were developed many years ago, yet remain frequently quoted in the dermatologic literature. Different grades of mineral oil are available. Industrial-grade mineral oil is used as a machine lubricant and is not of the purity required for skin application. Cosmetic-grade mineral oil reputedly is the purest form without contaminants.

MINERAL SALTS • Used as a skin conditioner.

MINERAL SPIRITS • Ligroin. A refined solvent of naphtha. Contains naphthenes and paraffin (*see*). Used as a solvent in cosmetic oils, fats, and waxes. *See* Kerosene for toxicity.

MINERAL SUPPLEMENT • A tablet, capsule, or liquid that provides additional inorganic nutrients from sources outside the diet.

MINERAL WAX • Aquaphor Healing Ointment. Used to soothe dry, cracked skin and minor burns. Used as an eyebrow wax. *See* Ceresin.

MINK OIL • Used in emollients, it supposedly softens the skin. It became popular as a cosmetic ingredient when a mink farmer noticed his hands were softer after handling minks. According to the American Medical Association, mink oil is no more effective than other oils in minimizing the evaporation of moisture from the skin and smoothing the surface scales of excessively dry skin. The CIR Expert Panel (*see*) concluded there is not enough data to conclude that it is safe as a cosmetic ingredient.

MINK WAX • The solid fraction derived from mink oil (*see*).

MINKAMIDO • Fatty acids derived from mink oil (*see*). Used as a thickener and foam booster.

MINKAMIDOPROPALKONIUM CHLORIDE • A quaternary ammonium compound (*see*) used as an antistatic ingredient in hair products.

MINKAMIDOPROPYL DIETHYLAMINE • Fatty acids derived from mink oil. *See* MIPA.

MINODYL • *See* Minoxidil.

MINOXIDIL • 6-(Piperidinyl)-2,4-pyrimidiamine-3-oxide. Only over-the-counter, topical pharmaceutical whose claims regarding hair regrowth have been approved by the FDA. Minoxidil, at one time available only under the trade name Rogaine, is now available under different names from several different companies and can increase hair growth by a statistically significant percentage in both men and women. It dilates the blood vessels around the hair follicles. It takes about four months before any results appear. According to the *Mayo Clinic's Women's Health Report* in 1998, minoxidil is successful for 44 percent to 63 percent of women who try it. It is actually far less effective for men, working in only about 20 percent of men who use it. The best results for this use are in patients with balding areas smaller than four inches that occurred within ten years. Extensive research and statistics suggest that this fairly inexpensive treatment works well for some people, although for women it may grow hair where they don't want it. The EU says minoxidil and its salts are substances that produce powerful systemic vasodilating effects. Furthermore, a special scientific assessment needs to be made of minoxidil derivatives in order to determine their possible effects on health. The EU says minoxidil and its salts should therefore be prohibited in cosmetic products. Can cause allergic reactions. One company has developed a nano version of the hair treatment. Nanosomes are tiny organic microspheres that penetrate into the lowest levels of the skin and gradually release the ingredients over a fifteen-hour period. Discontinuing the drug may result in the loss of new hair, which is usually very fine in texture. Potential adverse effects include edema, irregular heartbeat, congestive heart failure, skin rash, hair growth, and breast tenderness. When used topically, it may cause headache, dizziness, faintness, fluid retention, chest pain, increased or decreased blood pressure, palpitations, increased or decreased pulse rate, sinusitis, urinary tract infection, kidney stones, inflammation of the urine channel, irritation, upper respiratory tract infection, allergic contact dermatitis, local scalp redness, itching, dry skin or scalp, flaking, hair loss, back pain, and inflammation of the tendons.

MINT • Mentha. Peppermint and spearmint are alike in their actions but peppermint is the stronger of the two. They are both used as flavorings, and in herbal teas to aid digestion. Peppermint also is used for headaches, vomiting, and insomnia, as a bath additive for general aches and pains, and as a salve for massage. Spearmint is used in folk medicine for "women's complaints." See Spearmint Oil, Peppermint Oil, Wintergreen Oil, and Sassafras Oil.

MIPA • Abbreviation for monoisopropanolamine.

MIPA-BORATE • Boric acid (*see*) mixed with propanol isopropanolamine.

MIPA-DODECYLBENZENESULFONATE • *See* Quaternary Ammonium Compounds.

MIPA-HYDROGENATED COCOATE • *See* Coconut Oil.

MIPA-LANOLATE • *See* Lanolin.

MIPA-LAURYL SULFATE • The monoisopropanolamine salt of lauryl sulfate. *See* Quaternary Ammonium Compounds.

MISTLETOE • *Viscum album* (European Mistletoe); *Phoradendron flavescens* (American Mistletoe). A parasitical plant with a root firmly attached to the wood of the tree on which it grows, it was sacred to the Druids and reputedly used by them to cure sterility and epilepsy and as an antidote for poisons. Hippocrates and Galen used it as an external remedy and internally to treat sleep disorders. It is also used in "organic" cosmetics. *See also* Juniper Berry.

MITOSIS • Cell division.

MITRACARPUS SCABER • A South American vine.

MIXED CRESOLS • A preservative. *See* Cresols.

MIXED IONONES • Fragrance ingredients.

MIXED ISOPROPANOLAMINES MYRISTATE • A mixture of amine salts formed by neutralizing myristic acid with mixed isopropanolamines. Can induce acne. *See* Myristic Acid and Isopropyl Alcohol.

MIXED TERPENES • Terpenes are a class of organic compounds widely distributed in nature. They are components of volatile or essential oils and are found in substantial amounts in cedar wood oil, camphor, thymol, eucalyptol, menthol, turpentine, and pure oil. They are used in cosmetics as wetting ingredients and surfactants. Can cause local irritation.

MODERN BLENDS • One of the basic perfume types, it has indefinable top notes (*see*) that cannot be linked to either the floral or the oriental. These blends contain aldehydes (*see*), meaning that whether they are basically floral or woody, they have a sparkle in their more insistent notes that enhances all the others.

MODIFIED SEA SALT • Salt derived from seawater with a reduced sodium chloride content.

MODIFIED STARCH • Ordinary starch that has been altered chemically to modify such properties as thickening or jelling. Among chemicals used to modify starch are succinic anhydride, aluminum sulfate, and sodium hydroxide (*see all*). On the FDA top priority list for reevaluation since 1980. Nothing new reported by the FDA since.

MODIFIER • A term in cosmetics to describe a substance that induces or stabilizes certain shades in hair coloring.

MOISTURIZERS • Emollients. Skin Softeners. Creams. Lotions. The selection of a night cream, hand cream, eye cream, skin softener, moisturizer, and so on, is really the selection of an emollient. They all perform the same function—to make the skin feel softer and smoother and to reduce the roughness, cracking, and irritation of the skin. Most are a mixture of oils. The most common ingredients are: mineral oil, stearic acid, lanolin, beeswax, sorbitol, and polysorbates. Among the other ingredients added may be natural fatty oils such as olive, coconut, corn, peach, and sesame; natural fats such as stearate and diglycol laurate; hydrocarbon solids such as paraffin; alcohols such as cetyl, stearyl, and oleyl; emulsifiers, preservatives, and antioxidants, including vitamin E and paraben; antibacterials and perfumes, especially menthol and camphor. As you can see from the preceding list, many of the ingredients are common allergens described in this book.

MOLASSES EXTRACT • Molasses is a very dark syrupy liquid that is a by-product of the production of sugar. It is higher in vitamins and minerals than regular table sugar. In cosmetics, it is used as a skin conditioner and flavoring.

MOLECULE • The smallest amount of a specific chemical substance that can exist alone.

MOLYBDENUM ASPARTATE • Skin-conditioning ingredient. The molybdenum salt of aspartic acid (*see*).

MOLYBDIC ACID • White or slightly yellow powder, used in ceramic glazes and as a clarifying ingredient.

MONARDA DIDYMA • Bee Balm. Oswego Tea. Used in fragrances because of its mintlike aroma. May be harmful in large amounts.

MONASCUS/RICE FERMENT • The fermentation of rice by the organism *Monascus purpureus*. Used as an antioxidant.

MONK'S PEPPER BERRIES • Chaste Tree. A large shrub native to the Mediterranean area. The ingredient was found to significantly stimulate the proliferation of human epidermal cells in laboratory cultures. Monk's pepper berries have traditionally been used as plant medicine, mainly to regulate women's menstrual cycles and PMS. There are scientific publications that have found a beta-endorphin-like effect of monk's pepper berries. This effect is thought to come from berry compounds that bind to the human beta-endorphin receptor or berry compounds that stimulate the production of beta-endorphins (*see*) in humans.

MONO AMMONIUM GLYCYRRHIZINATE • *See* Ammonia and Glycyrrhizic Acid.

MONOAZO COLOR • A dye made from diazonium and phenol, both coal tar derivatives. *See* Coal Tar.

MONOBENZONE • Hydroquinone Monobenzyl Ether. Prepared synthetically and used as an antioxidant and to retard melanin production. Used also in bleach and freckle creams. It may cause blotchiness and allergic skin reactions.

MONOGLYCERIDES • Produced synthetically by treating fats with glycerol and alcohol. Used as emulsifiers, cosmetics, and lubricants. *See* Glycerol.

MONOMER • A molecule that by repetition in a long chain builds up a large structure, or polymer (*see*). The gas ethylene, for instance, is the monomer of polyethylene (*see*).

MONOPOTASSIUM GLUTAMATE • Flavor enhancer and salt substitute used on meat. Mildly toxic by ingestion. May cause headaches. *See* Glutamate.

MONOSACCHARIDE LACTATE CONDENSATE • The condensation product of sodium lactate and the sugars glucose, fructose, ribose, glucosamine, and deoxyribose. Skin conditioner.

MONOSODIUM CITRATE • Used to adjust pH (*see*).

MONOTERPENES • Found in parsley, carrots, broccoli, cabbage, cucumbers, squash, yams, tomatoes, eggplant, peppers, mint, basil, citrus fruits, they have some antioxidant properties. Used as fragrance ingredients. They reportedly aid protective enzyme activity. Five monoterpenes (carvacrol, *p*-cymene, linalool, α-terpinene, and thymol) derived from the essential oil of thyme (*Thymus vulgaris*) were examined for their repellency against the mosquito *Culex pipiens pallens*. All five monoterpenes effectively repelled mosquitoes based on a human forearm bioassay. α-Terpinene and carvacrol showed significantly greater repellency than a commercial formulation, N,N-diethyl-*m*-methylben-zamide (deet), whereas thymol showed similar repellency to that of deet. The duration of repellency after application for all these monoterpenes was equal to or higher than that of deet. These findings indicate that a spray-type solution containing 2 percent α-terpinene may serve as an alternative mosquito repellent.

MONTAN CERA • *See* Montan Wax.

MONTAN WAX • Lignite Wax. White, hard earth wax derived from extraction of lignite, which is coal made from wood. Its physical properties vary with the source of lignite. It is used as a substitute for carnauba and beeswax (*see both*). Binder, thickener used in lipsticks and foundations.

MONTMORILLONITE • A type of clay that is the main ingredient of bentonite and fuller's earth. In cosmetics, it is used as an abrasive, absorbent, thickener, and stabilizer, particularly in mud packs. Widely used in the petroleum industry. It is used in the manufacture of many chemical compounds. Inhalation of the dust can cause respiratory irritation. *See* Fuller's Earth.

MORDANTS • Chemicals that are insoluble compounds that serve to fix a dye, usually a weak dye, to hasten the development of the desired shade or to modify it in hair colorings. Toxicity depends upon specific ingredients.

MORINDA CITRIFOLIA • Indian Mulberry. A small evergreen tree that yields an astringent and emollient.

MORINGA OIL • Ben Oil. Oil from the seeds of the tropical tree *Moringa oleafera*. *See* Horseradish Extract.

MOROCCAN LAVA CLAY • Mined in Morocco, it is used as an abrasive, absorbent, thickener, and stabilizer in cosmetics.

MORPHOLINE • A salty fatty acid used as a surface-active ingredient (*see*) and an emulsifier in cosmetics. Prepared by taking the water out of diethanolamine (*see*). A mobile, water-absorbing liquid that mixes with water. It has a strong ammonia odor. A cheap solvent for resins, waxes, and dyes. Also used as a corrosion inhibitor, antioxidant, plasticizer, viscosity improver, insecticide, fungicide, local anesthetic, and antiseptic. Irritating to the eyes, skin, and mucous membranes. It may cause kidney and liver injury and can produce sloughing of the skin. The safety of this ingredient has not been documented and substantiated. The CIR Expert Panel (*see*) "cannot conclude that it is safe for use in cosmetic products until such time that the appropriate safety data has been obtained and evaluated." On the Canadian Hotlist (*see*). The EU has banned morpholine and its salts in cosmetics.

MORPHOLINE STEARATE • A coating and preservative. *See* Morpholine.

MORTIERELLA OIL • Oil from the seeds of *Mortierella isabellina*. Used in emollients.

MORUS ALBA • *See* Mulberry Extract.

MOSCHUS MOSCHIFERUS • A musk from an Asian deer. *See* Musk.

MOSKENE • Pentamethyl-4,6-dinitroindane. A perfume and bleach combination. Can cause pigmented dermatitis. Prohibited in cosmetics by ASEAN and EU.

MOTHER OF PEARL • *See* Calcium Carbonate.

MOUNTAIN ASH EXTRACT • The extract from the berries of the European tree or shrub *Sorbus aucuparia*. High in vitamin C. Used in cosmetics as an antioxidant.

MOUNTAIN GRAPE • *See* Oregon Grape Root.

MOUNTAIN MAPLE EXTRACT • Extract from a tall shrub or bushy tree found in the eastern United States. Used in chocolate, malt, and maple flavorings.

MOURERA FLUVIATILIS • A plant high in sugar and amino acids. Used as a moisturizer in skin creams.

MOUSE-EAR • *Pilosella officinarum*. Hawkweed. Named for the shape of its leaves, its ingredients include coumarin, flavones, and flavonoids. Used as an antispasmodic, expectorant, and astringent. Also used for respiratory problems where there is inflammation and a quantity of mucus being formed. Used by herbalists to treat bronchitis and bronchial asthma. Has been used in poultices for wound healing.

MOUTHWASH • Promoted as a method to cleanse the mouth and overcome objectionable odors. Claims for such abilities have not been proven. Among ingredients used in mouthwashes are sodium bicarbonate, alcohol, mixed flavoring oils, cinnamon, methyl salicylate, menthol, anethole, thyme, certified colors, resorcinol, sorbitol, urea, methyl salicylate, boric acid, benzalkonium chloride, benzoic acid, propylene glycol, cetylpyridinium chloride, and chlorophyllin. Several of the preceding, particularly the colorings and the flavorings, are common allergens. Resorcinol is a resin (*see*), and methyl salicylate is related to aspirin and other salicylates.

MUCILAGE • A solution in water of the sticky principles of vegetable substances. Used as a soothing application to the mucous membranes.

MUCINS • Any of a group of proteins found in various secretions and tissues of humans and lower animals such as saliva, lining of the stomach, and skin. They are white or yellowish powders when dry and thick when moist.

MUCOPOLYSACCHARIDES • A complex of proteins (*see*). Used in moisturizers.

MUCOSA • *See* Mucous Membranes.

MUCOUS MEMBRANES • The thin layers of tissue that line the respiratory and intestinal tracts and are kept moist by a sticky substance called mucus. These membranes line the nose and other parts of the respiratory tract and are found in other parts of the body that have communication with air.

MUCUNA BIRDWOODIANA • Asian plant being studied for medical properties. It is used in cosmetics as a skin conditioner.

MUD PACKS • Long in use as a facial treatment. Today, they consist of a paste for the face composed chiefly of fuller's earth and astringents (*see both*). There is no evidence that mud packs are effective.

MUGWORT • The extract of the flowering herb *Artemisia absinthium*. Can have antibacterial properties but may irritate the skin. *See* Wormwood and Sesquiterpene Lactones.

MUIRA PUAMA EXTRACT • *Liriosma ovata*. A wood extract used as an aromatic resin and fat. This Brazilian herb is used primarily to treat impotence, frigidity, and diarrhea.

MULBERRY EXTRACT • An extract of the dried leaves of various species of *Morus*, which produces a purplish black dye.

MULLEIN EXTRACT • *Verbascum thapsus*. The extract of common mullein. Used in henna dyes. A perennial of the figwort family, native to Europe, Asia, Africa, and the United States, it grows wild. Its dried leaves were smoked to treat asthma. The ashes were made into soap to restore gray hair to its former color. The crushed flowers reputedly cured warts and a cloth dipped in hot mullein tea was used for inflammation.

MULLEIN FLOWERS • The flowers from common mullein, *Verbascum thapsis*. Used as a flavoring in alcoholic beverages only and in henna hair coloring.

MUNG BEAN • *See* Vigna Radiata.

MURASAKI201 • A Japanese coal tar color called Violet 2 or Solvent Violet 13. EU CI 60725.

MURASAKI401 • Japanese name for coal tar hair coloring called Violet 2 or Acid Violet 43 in the United States. EU CI60730.

MURRAYA EXOTICA • Used as an emollient and in oral care products. *See* Myrtle.

MUSA NANA • Dwarf Bananas. Lady Fingers. Used as a hair and skin conditioner. *See* Banana.

MUSA SAPIENTUM • Banana (*see*).

MUSCLE EXTRACT • The oil extracted from cow muscle.

MUSHROOM EXTRACT • *Fomes officinalis. Polyporus umbellatus*. The extract of various species of mushrooms used as an oil and plasticizer.

MUSK • Ambrettolide, Civetone, Muscone, Exaltolide. An unctuous, brownish semiliquid when fresh; dried, in grains or lumps with color resembling dried blood and it has the characteristic odor. The odoriferous principles of natural musk, civet, and musky type plants. It is the dried secretion from preputial follicles of the northern Asian small hornless deer, which has musk in its glands. Musk is a brown, unctuous, smelly substance associated with attracting the opposite sex and that is promoted by stores for such purposes. Used in perfumes, and used in cosmetics as a fixative in perfumery. Also used in food flavorings and at one time as a stimulant and nerve sedative in medicine. It can be made synthetically. Can cause allergic reactions.

MUSK AMBRETTE • Found to have neurotoxic properties. This was first discovered in 1967 when mice were fed varying levels of musk ambrette. Since dietary consumption of musk ambrette is generally very low, the impact was discounted and no assessment was made of exposures from fragranced products. In 1985, after studies were published on the neurotoxic effect and it was determined that the musk ambrette was readily absorbed through the skin, the fragrance industry recommended that musk ambrette not be used in direct skin contact products. Musk ambrette had been used in fragranced products before the 1920s. It reportedly damages the myelin, the covering of nerve fibers. It can cause photosensitivity (*see*) and contact dermatitis. Musk ambrette is still used in food but not in cosmetics. Although not banned by the FDA, the agency cautions that this compound may cause photocontact sensitization.

MUSK KETONE • MK. A synthetic compound with a typical musk odor is widely used in cosmetics and is permitted as a food additive. Exposure to it, experiments in animals and with human cells indicate, might increase the susceptibility to health hazards caused by carcinogens in humans. ASP

MUSK MOSKENE • A soft, sweet fragrance resembling musk ambrette. It is a creamy powder and is used in fragrances. It costs less than other musks and is not as sensitive to sunlight. It is therefore being increasingly used. Rouges and perfumes containing musk moskene have been reported to cause hyperpigmentation of the skin of some patients. The hyperpigmentation slowly disappeared after discontinuation of the products.

MUSK ROSE OIL • Delta Rose. The oil obtained from *Rosa rubiginosa*. Used in fragrances.

MUSK TIBETENE • Fragrance. On the Canadian Hotlist (*see*). Banned in cosmetics by ASEAN and UK.

MUSKMELLON EXTRACT • Extract of the common mullein, *Verbascum thapsis.*

MUSSEL EXTRACT • The extract from sea mussels used to soothe aching muscles and joints. The cosmetic companies that include it in their products claim that it improves the elasticity and firmness of the skin as well as making it feel softer and silkier.

MUSTARD, BLACK • *Brassica nigra.* Koch. Boiss. A native of Europe and the Americas, it is cultivated in Holland, Italy, and Germany as a condiment. Mustard seed is used to stimulate appetite. Mustard is used medicinally to treat arthritis, sciatica, and other pain. It is also used as an emetic to counteract ingested poisons. Mustard plasters were a popular treatment for pain and swelling. Mustard is used in footbaths and to treat colds. Mustard is rapidly absorbed and is used as a counterirritant (*see*) in cosmetics.

MUSTARD OIL • Allyl isothiocyanate. The greenish yellow, bland fatty oil expressed from the seeds of the mustard plant. Used in soaps, liniments, and lubricants. It has an intensely pungent odor that can be irritating. It is a strong skin blisterer and is used diluted as a counterirritant (*see*) and rubefacient (*see*). Can cause allergic reactions. On the Canadian Hotlist (*see*) and ASEAN (*see*).

MUSTARD SEED • *See* Mustard Oil.

MUSTELA • *See* Mink Oil.

MUTAGEN • A substance (such as a chemical) that damages the inner workings of the cell. Mutagens that cause cancer are carcinogens. Those that cause birth defects are called teratogens or mutagens. Some of the cosmetic ingredients listed in this dictionary are labeled mutagens or teratogens or carcinogens.

MUTAGENIC • Having the power to cause mutations. A mutation is a sudden change in the character of a gene that is perpetuated in subsequent divisions of the cells in which it occurs. It can be induced by the application of such stimuli as radiation, certain food and cosmetic chemicals, or pesticides.

MUTATION • A permanent change in the genetic material that will be passed on to new generations of cells.

MYO- • Prefix meaning related to muscle, as in myography, the recording of muscle movements.

MYOSOTIS SYLVATICA • Forget-Me-Not Extract. A perennial herb that has blue and white flowers.

MYRCENOL • An alcohol used as a fragrance ingredient.

MYRCIA • *See* Bay Rum.

MYRETH-3 • The polyethylene glycol ether of myristyl alcohol (*see*).

MYRETH-3 CAPRATE • Myristic Ethoxy Caprate. *See* Capric Acid.

MYRETH-3 MYRISTATE • Emollient in cleansers, hand and face creams, and makeup bases. *See* Myristic Acid.

MYRETH-4 • The polyethylene glycol ether of myristyl alcohol (*see*).

MYRICA CERIFERA • *See* Bayberry.

MYRICA GALE • Sweet Gale. Fragrance ingredient. *See* Myrtle.

MYRICACEAE • *See* Bayberry.

MYRICYL ALCOHOL • Triacontanol. Emollient and Moisturizer. Waxy alcohol used as a substitute for bayberry wax.

MYRISTALKONIUM CHLORIDE • *See* Quaternary Ammonium Compounds.

MYRISTAMIDE DEA • Myristic Diethanolamide. *See* Myristic Acid and Diethanolamide.

MYRISTAMIDE MIPA • A mixture of isopropanolamides of lauric acid (*see*).

MYRISTAMIDOPROPYL BETAINE • *See* Surfactants.

MYRISTAMIDOPROPYL DIETHYLAMINE • *See* Quaternary Ammonium Compounds.

MYRISTAMIDOPROPYLAMINE OXIDE • *See* Quaternary Ammonium Compounds.

MYRISTAMINE OXIDE • Cleanser used in shampoos and hair wave sets. *See* Myristic Acid.

MYRISTAMINOPROPIONIC ACID • *See* Propionic Acid and Myristic Acid.

MYRISTATE • The ester of myreth-3 and myristic acid (*see both*).

MYRISTIC ACID • Used in shampoos, shaving soaps, and creams. A solid, organic acid that occurs naturally in butter acids (such as nutmeg butter to the extent of 80 percent), oil of lovage, coconut oil, mace oil, cire d'abeille in palm seed fats, and in most animal and vegetable fats. Also used in food flavorings. When combined with potassium, myristic acid soap gives a very good copious lather. The CIR Expert Panel (*see*) concluded that this ingredient is safe for use in cosmetic products. *See* Lauric Acid.

MYRISTICA FRAGRANS • *See* Nutmeg and Mace.

MYRISTIMIDE MEA • A mixture of ethanolamide of myristic acid (*see*).

MYRISTOAMPHOACETATE • *See* Surfactants.

MYRISTOYL GLUTAMIC ACID • An emulsifying ingredient in hair conditioners and skin creams. *See* Myristic Acid and Lactic Acid.

MYRISTOYL HYDROLYZED PROTEIN • The condensation product of myristic acid and hydrolyzed animal protein (*see both*). Used as a setting ingredient and film former, it allows the incorporation of protein into non-water-based cosmetics. The "animal" was taken out of the ingredient name but not out of the ingredient.

MYRISTOYL SARCOSINE • *See* Myristic Acid and Sarcosines.

MYRISTYL ALCOHOL • Used as an emollient in hand creams, cold creams, and lotions to give them a smooth velvety feel. White crystals prepared from fatty acids (*see*). Has been reported to cause allergic reactions. *See* Behenyl Alcohol.

MYRISTYL BETAINE • *See* Myristyl Alcohol.

MYRISTYL LACTATE • Widely used emollient in lipsticks, makeup, indoor tanning products, cleanliness products, and body and hand preparations. *See* Myristyl Alcohol and Lactic Acid.

MYRISTYL MYRISTATE • Widely used skin conditioner and occlusive used in moisturizers, makeup, skin care preparations, after-shave lotions, eyebrow pencils, bath oils, foot powders, and baby lotions. On the basis of the available information, the CIR Expert Panel (*see*) found it safe in the early 1980s but is considering new information to determine if the final safety assessment should be reaffirmed, amended, or have an addendum. *See* Myristic Acid.

MYRISTYL PROPIONATE • A fatty acid used in cosmetics. May cause acne. *See* Myristric Acid.

MYRISTYL STEARATE • Emollient. On the basis of the available animal and human data, the CIR Expert Panel (*see*) concluded that this ingredient is safe as used in cosmetics. *See* Myristic Acid.

MYROCARPUS FASTIGIATUS • *Myristica fragrans,* a South American plant used in fragrances.

MYROTHAMNUS FLABELLIFOLIA • Resurrection Plant. Contains high levels of arbutin (*see*). It is an effective antioxidant and used as a skin conditioner.

MYROXYLON BALSAMUM • *See* Balsam Tolu.

MYROXYLON PEREIRAE • *See* Balsam Peru.

MYRRH EXTRACT • *Commiphora abyssinica.* Used in perfumes, dentifrices, and skin topics. One of the gifts of the Magi, it is a yellowish to reddish brown, aromatic, bitter gum resin that is obtained from various trees, especially from East Africa and Arabia. Used by the ancients as an ingredient of incense and perfumes and as a remedy for localized skin problems. The gum resin has been used to break up intestinal gas and as a topical stimulant.

MYRRH GUM • *Commiphora molmol* or *myrrha.* Guggul. One of the gifts of the Magi, it is a yellowish to reddish brown, aromatic, bitter gum resin that is obtained from various myrrh trees, especially from East Africa and Arabia. The gum resin has been used to break up intestinal gas and as a topical stimulant. The Chinese for centuries used the herb to treat menstrual problems and bleeding. In Asia and Africa, it was used as an antiseptic for mucous membranes. It is also used as a stimulant tonic; there are constituents in myrrh that stimulate gastric secretions and relax smooth muscles. In modern studies, myrrh has been shown to inhibit bacteria such as *Staphylococcus aureus.* The herb contains volatile oils, including limonene, eugenol, and pinene, which have been found helpful in easing breathing during colds, and increasing circulation. It also contains tannin, which is thought to be the reason that myrrh allays the pain and speeds the healing of mouth ulcers and sore gums. In 1992, the FDA issued a notice that myrrh fluid extract had not been shown to be safe and effective as claimed in OTC digestive aid products.

MYRRHIS ODORATA • *See* Myrrh Extract.

MYRTENOL • Flavoring. A constituent of myrtle oil, it is the unsaturated primary alcohol. The FAO/WHO said it has no safety concern. *See* Myrtle. ASP

MYRTIMONIUM BROMIDE • A quaternary ammonium compound (*see*).

MYRTLE • *Myrtus communis.* A native of the Mediterranean, the attractive plant has been a symbol of innocence for many centuries. In fact, Aphrodite, the Greek goddess of beauty and love, apparently found refuge in a myrtle bush after she was created as a beautiful nude woman. Association with purity and chaste beauty becomes more apparent when one smells the clean, uplifting fragrance of myrtle and the oil extracted from its flowers. The leaves and flowers were a major ingredient of "angel's water," a sixteenth-century skin care lotion. Plant parts used: leaves, twigs, and flowers. Method: steam distillation. The most important constituents of myrtle oil (up to 0.8 percent in the leaves) are myrtenol, myrtenol acetate, limonene (23 percent), linalool (20 percent). It is used in folk medicine and reportedly relieves cramps, is relaxing in a bath, and helps combat acne. EAF

MYRTUS COMMINUS • *See* Myrtle.

N

NAIL, ARTIFICIAL • *See* Artificial Nails.

NAIL BLEACHES • Compounds designed to remove ink, nicotine, vegetable, and other stains from fingernails. They consist mainly of an oxidizing ingredient and chlorinated compounds. A typical formula includes titanium dioxide, 20 percent; talc, 20 percent; zinc peroxide, 7.5 percent; petrolatum, 26 percent; mineral oil, 26.5 percent; and perfume (*see all*). Toxicity depends upon ingredients used.

NAIL COSMETICS • Nail cosmetics may induce side effects such as sensitization. The most common side effect is allergic contact dermatitis from nail lacquer caused by toluene sulfonamide formaldehyde resin. Other causes are allergy to methacrylates and cyanoacrylates from acrylic nails. Irritation, trauma, and infection can occur. Allergic itchy rashes can occur around the eyes and there may be burning and tenderness of the nail bed, cuticle area, and areas of the face and neck. According to the American Academy of Dermatology experts, although the liquid form of methacrylate (*see*) is banned by twenty-three states and the FDA has issued warnings about its hazards, the substance is still used in some discount salons. This occurs because it costs so much less than the safer acrylate alternatives such as ethylmethacrylate, according to Phoebe Rich, MD, clinical associate professor of dermatology, Oregon Health Sciences University, Portland, OR.

NAIL ENAMEL • *See* Nail Polish.

NAIL (FAKE) REMOVER • Contains acetonitrile. Contact with skin and eyes should be avoided, as well as prolonged breathing of vapors. Flammable. Poisonous if swallowed. Skin and eye contact requires flushing thoroughly with water and medical attention. Must be kept out of the reach of children. Acetonitrile is on the Canadian Hotlist (*see*). *See* Artificial Nail Remover.

NAIL FINISHES • Top Coat. Usually a colorless nail polish (*see*) or it can be slightly pink. Contains celluloid, amyl acetate, and acetone (*see all*). Protects the nail by strengthening it physically, helps to keep the nail polish from chipping, and produces a shiny surface.

NAIL GLUE • May contain cyanoacrylate, which may cause an allergic reaction and/or separation of the nail from the nail bed.

NAIL HARDENERS • Keep the nails from breaking or chipping. Most nail hardeners formerly contained formaldehyde but now contain polyesters, acrylics, and polyamides. Sensitization rarely occurs.

NAIL MENDING • There are kits that contain glue, enamel, and pieces of silk or paper to mend broken nails. Some suggest using a piece of a tea bag covering or coffee filter paper and then using nail glue or enamel to seal it on the nail. May have acrylic adhesives, which are sensitizers. Can be an eye irritation. Also, when a nail tip falls off, and you glue it back on, if you leave a space, you may get a fungus growing there. *See* Nail Glue.

NAIL POLISH • Used to paint the nails with colors, usually some shade of red. Polishes contain cellulose nitrate (nitrocellulose), butyl acetate, ethyl acetate, toluene, dibutyl phthalate, alkyl esters (amyl, acetate, ethyl acetate), dyes, glycol derivatives, gums, hydrocarbons (aromatic and aliphatic), ketones (acetone, methyl, ethyl), lakes, and phosphoric acid. Common colors used are D & C Red No. 19 or 31 (*see*). Skin rashes of the eyelids and neck are common in those allergic to nail polish. Among recent complaints to the FDA about nail polishes were irritation of the nail area, discolored nails, nails permanently stained black, splitting of nails, and nausea. A spilled bottle of nail polish onboard an aircraft prompted emergency services to rush into action at an airport in northern Germany in April 2004. Ambulances and security officials were summoned and part of the Bremen airport closed off after police were alerted that passengers onboard a flight from Amsterdam that was about to land were complaining of nausea for unknown reasons. After the plane landed, the roughly forty-five passengers onboard were taken off by officials using breathing apparatus, police said. But doctors found that none was injured or ill, and the passengers soon felt better. Police then determined that a female passenger's nail polish had leaked and its pungent odor was circulated by the aircraft's air conditioning system.

NAIL POLISH REMOVER • Usually a liquid, it is used to remove nail polish. It contains acetone, toluene, alcohol, amyl acetate, butyl acetate, benzene, and ethyl acetate. It also contains castor oil, lanolin, cetyl alcohol, olive oil, perfume, spermaceti, synthetic oil (ethyl oleate, butyl stearate) (*see all*). Many components are very toxic and can cause central nervous system depression, especially the toluene and aliphatic acetates. A report to the FDA described a "tight smothering feeling in the chest" after use of a nail polish remover.

NAILS, PRESS-ON • Fake nails made of resins and acrylic glues. The acrylic glues may sensitize.

NAIL STRENGTHENERS • *See* Nail Hardeners.

NAIL WHITENERS • The cream nail whiteners may contain titanium dioxide, beeswax, cetyl alcohol, petrolatum, cocoa butter, sodium borate, tincture of benzoin (*see all*), and water. The liquid nail whites may contain titanium dioxide, glyceryl monostearate, beeswax, almond oil, petrolatum (*see all*), and water. Toxicity is dependent upon ingredients.

NALORPHINE AND ITS SALTS AND ETHERS • Derived from morphine and is used in the form of its hydrochloride as a respiratory stimulant to counteract poisoning by morphine and similar narcotic drugs. There was interest by cosmetic companies to use it in antiwrinkle creams, but it has been banned in cosmetics by most authorities.

NANOCOCOA • A nanoemulsion of oil extracted from the nibs of the "Criollo" cocoa bean. According to Mibelle's, its manufacturer, the neurotransmitter anandamide is one of the active chemicals within the extract, which produces a feeling of euphoria and relaxation. The Switzerland-based company, which is employing one of the country's largest exporters, says the hopes are the ingredient will tap into the trend for merging food and cosmetics. The cannabinoid receptors that are targeted by NanoCocoa are not only found in the central nervous system, the company claims they have also been identified in the mast cells, hair follicles, and nerve cells of the skin, leading the company to investigate anandamide's potential as a skin care ingredient. According to the company, an in vitro study using human muscle fibers illustrated that application of the anandamide decreased the frequency of muscle contractions after a twenty-four-hour period. The effect was completely reversible and normal muscle fiber behavior resumed after forty-eight hours, according to the company's test. They are investigating their ingredient to determine if it has an antiwrinkle benefit.

NANOPARTICLES • There is great difficulty for researchers, manufacturers, and consumers to define nanoparticles. The definition that seems to be the most popular is: "any microscopic particle less than about 100 nanometers (nm) in diameter. In aerosol science, the term is often reserved for particles less than 50 nm in diameter; the term 'ultrafine particles' is used for particles less than 100 nm in diameter." Tiny particles of materials that can be natural or manufactured so that they are smaller than normal. The limit of the human eye's capacity to see without a microscope is about 10,000 nm.

Urgent action is needed to develop the testing and regulation of nanomaterials, according to a report from the UK Royal Commission on Environmental Pollution. According to the Commission, the pace at which new nanomaterials are reaching the market is beyond the capacity of existing testing and regulatory arrangements. Although the report is careful to point out that there is no evidence that nanomaterials harm either human health or the environment, it does state that the amount of testing on such materials has been limited and must be increased. "In the Royal Commission study we looked hard for evidence of nanomaterials causing harm to human health or to the environment, and found no such evidence," the report reads. For this reason, the Commission concluded that there were no grounds for a blanket ban or moratorium on nanoparticles. However, laboratory tests on some nanoscale particles suggest they could pose dangers, said the Commission. Therefore, it has concluded that existing regulations are inadequate and new arrangements "are vital to deal with the challenges posed by current and future innovation in this sector."

The FDA's Nanotechnology Task Force got more than just a mixed message when it convened experts and stakeholders in 2007 to get advice as to whether the agency should regulate nanotechnology products. Some said current regulations are sufficient, whereas others said safety testing is long overdue, especially for products like cosmetics. But they also disagreed as to how to define a nanoparticle, and even if there should be such a definition in the first place. Some progress can be made by extending the current REACH (*see*) regulations to successfully cover nanoparticles. REACH imposes a responsibility on those who import and manufacture chemicals to identify, and provide information on, any potential health threats. REACH does not discount nanomaterials, but the Commission noted that the nanoform of a material may be treated in the same way as its non-nano counterpart. In addition, the limit of one ton (under which the chemicals are exempt from regulation) may be too high, as nanoparticles are often used in very small quantities. The UK suggested a checklist system for materials not covered by the REACH system, where manufacturers would be obliged by law to provide information about the potential risks posed by the materials throughout the product life cycle, including disposal by the consumer. Manufacturers could be offered legal protection if they filled in this checklist to the best of their abilities given the knowledge available. According to the report, an environmental monitoring system is also needed, along with the development of techniques to detect nanomaterials in the environment and living organisms. Regardless of the testing or regulations implemented, the report was clear that a material's potential toxicity should be judged on its functionality and not on its size. In other words, although the behavior of a material in the nanoscale may well differ from the macro, this does not mean that all nanoparticles will behave in the same way. By making this distinction, the report highlights the need to address nanomaterials depending on what they do and are capable of doing, rather than assuming they are a single class of materials with unifying properties.

The FDA must recognize that the size of a particle may affect its behavior and call for compulsory safety testing and labeling of nanoparticles in cosmetics, according to a U.S. consumer group.The Consumers Union wrote to the FDA asking that it require a full safety assessment on the use of nanoparticles in cosmetics, sunscreens, and sunblocks before a product is allowed to market. In addition, the Consumers Union called for the labeling of nanoparticles in products so that consumers can make an informed choice. The letter was in response to a series of investigations by the Consumers Union that highlighted both widespread use of nanoparticles and widespread misinformation regarding their use. Back in July 2007 the consumer group tested eight mineral-based sunscreens and found all eight contained nanoparticles of zinc oxide and/or titanium dioxide, although only one disclosed this fact on the label. This prompted the group to test an additional five products that the companies' representatives said did not contain nanoparticles. Four out of the five products contained nanoparticles. According to Michael Hansen, chief scientist at the Consumers Union and author of the letter, these investigations show that use of nanoparticles is widespread and that consumers are not being informed of their presence. At present, the FDA does not recognize that the size of a material affects its behavior, Hansen told CosmeticsDesign.com. This means that manufacturers can include nano-scale particles of materials that have already been approved on the macro scale, he explained.

NANOTECHNOLOGY • The ability to measure, see, manipulate, and manufacture things usually between 1 and 100 nanometers (nm). A nanometer is one billionth of a meter. A human hair is roughly 100,000 nanometers wide. *See* Nanoparticles.

NA PCA • *See* Sodium PCA.

NAPHTHALENE • A coal tar (*see*) derivative, it is used to manufacture dyes, solvents, and lubricants; as a moth repellent; and as a topical and internal antiseptic. It has been used as a dusting powder to combat insects on animals. Can cause allergic contact dermatitis.

2,3-NAPHTHALENEDIOL • A hair coloring. The EU banned it in 2006. *See* Naphthas.

2, 7-NAPHTHALENEDIOL • The EU banned it in hair dyes in 2006. *See* Naphthas.

NAPHTHAS • Obtained from the distillation of petroleum, coal tar, and shale oil. It is a common diluent (*see*) found in nail lacquer. Among the common naphthas that are used as solvents are coal tar/naphtha and petroleum/naphtha. *See* Kerosene for toxicity.

NAPHTHAZOLINE HYDROCHLORIDE • Privine Hydrochloride. Prepared from acids, it is composed of bitter-tasting crystals, which are soluble in water. Used as a nasal and eye decongestant. It may cause sedation in infants, and high blood pressure and central nervous system excitement followed by depression in adults. On the Canadian Hotlist (*see*).

NAPHTHOL • *a*-Naphthol. A coal tar (*see*) derivative, it is used as an antiseptic, in hair dyes, and to treat eczema, ringworm, and psoriasis. May cause allergic contact dermatitis. On the Canadian Hotlist (*see*).

1-NAPHTHOL • *a*-Naphthol. Used in hair dyes and treatment of skin diseases, as an antiseptic, and as an antioxidant for fats and oils. Also used in perfumery. White crystals with phenolic odor and disagreeable burning taste. Toxic by ingestion and skin absorption. Hair dyes containing this ingredient when applied to the skin were neither teratogenic nor carcinogenic. On the basis of the available data, the CIR Expert Panel (*see*) concluded that it is safe as a cosmetic ingredient. However, it has been reported to cause severe skin and eye irritation. Maximum amount allowed by the European Union and the United States is 0.5 percent, and its presence must be on the list of ingredients. The EU gave manufacturers to July 2005 to submit safety information or the substance will be proposed for a ban. In September 2005, the 1-naphthol proposal was submitted for use in an oxidative hair product at a concentration up to a maximum level of 4 percent (2% on-head level). Submission III presented updated scientific data on the above-mentioned substance in line with the second step of the strategy for the evaluation of hair dyes.

2-NAPHTHOL • *b*-Naphthol. Used as an antiseptic and modifier in hair preparations, with tendency to darken gray hair. Sometimes used in treatment of eczema, ringworm, and psoriasis. *See* 1-Naphthol for toxicity.

B-NAPHTHYL ETHYL ETHER • White crystals with an orange-blossom odor. It is used in perfumes, soaps, and flavorings. *See* Nerol.

B-NAPHTHYL METHYL ETHER • White crystals with a menthol odor. Used to perfume.

NARCISSUS OIL • Anarylidiaceae. Poeticus Extract. Jonquilla Extract. Genus of Old World bulbous herbs. Used as a fragrance. Can numb skin.

NARCOTICS, NATURAL AND SYNTHETIC • Banned by ASEAN in cosmetics.

NASTURTIUM EXTRACT • The extract of the leaves and stems of *Tropaeolum majus*. A member of the mustard family, it has pungent and tasty leaves. It is very rich in vitamins A and C, as well as containing vitamins B and B$_2$. It is soothing to the skin and supposedly has blood-thinning factors and increases the flow of urine.

NATIONAL RESEARCH COUNCIL • The NRC functions under the auspices of the National Academy of Sciences (NAS), the National Academy of Engineering (NAE), and the Institute of Medicine (IOM). The NAS, NAE, IOM, and NRC are part of a private, nonprofit institution that provides science, technology, and health policy advice under a congressional charter signed by President Abraham Lincoln that was originally granted to the NAS in 1863. Under this charter, the NRC was established in 1916, the NAE in 1964, and the IOM in 1970. The four organizations are collectively referred to as the National Academies. The mission of the NRC is to improve government decision making and public policy, increase public education and understanding, and promote the acquisition and dissemination of knowledge in matters involving science, engineering, technology, and health. The institution takes this charge seriously and works to inform policies and actions that have the power to improve the lives of people in the United States and around the world. The NRC is committed to providing elected leaders, policymakers, and the public with expert advice based on sound scientific evidence. The NRC does not receive direct federal appropriations for its work. Individual projects are funded by federal agencies, foundations, other governmental and private sources, and the institution's endowment. The work is made possible by six thousand of the world's top scientists, engineers, and other professionals who volunteer their time without compensation to serve on committees and participate in activities.

NATIONAL TOXICOLOGY PROGRAM • NTP. Tests chemicals for all federal agencies.

NATTO GUM • The fermentation product of soy protein by *Bacillus nato*. Used as a thickener.

NATURAL • There is no official designation for "natural." It generally means that the ingredients are extracted directly from plants or animal products as opposed to being produced synthetically. According to the 2008 Pink Report, *The Age of Naturals,* 72 percent of women who buy natural/organic beauty products believe in the concept of inside/out beauty, compared with 49 percent of women who buy only traditionally made beauty products. The study found that natural/organic beauty buyers are more likely than traditional beauty brand buyers to engage in activities that are good for the body and mind. *See* Organic Cosmetics.

NATURAL RED 26 • Carthamic Acid. A red, crystalline, glucoside coloring constituting the coloring matter of the safflower (*see*).

NEATSFOOT OIL • Bubulum. Lubricant used in creams and lotions. A pale yellow,
fatty oil made by boiling the feet and shinbones of cattle. Used chiefly as a leather dressing and waterproofing. In cosmetics it is used as a cover-up in skin care products. Can
cause allergic reactions in the hypersensitive.

NECTARINE • *Prunus persica nectarina.* The leaves or bark from young trees native
to China, but widely cultivated, are used by herbalists to make sedatives, diuretics,
expectorants, and soothing compounds.

NEEM OIL AND NEEM LEAVES EXTRACT • *Melia azadirachta* neem oil or
neem seed oil is a brownish yellow color. A liquid, with smell of a garlic. The seed oil
at concentration of 0.3 percent on agar plates was active against *Staphylococcus aureus*
and at 0.4% was active against *Salmonella typhosa.* The seed oil at concentration of 3
percent on agar plate was active against *E.coli* and *Proteus* species, a concentration of
6.0 percent was active against *Klebsiella pneumoniae.* Methanol and butyl methyl ether
extracts showed antifungal activity against a number of fungi. Neem oil is used for preparation of various cosmetics and toiletries including all-purpose cream, hair oils, toothpastes, bath soaps, hair shampoos, and face packs. *See* Neem Tree.

NEEM TREE • *Azadirachta indica.* Nim. Margosa. Traditionally labeled as "The
Village Pharmacy" because of its multifaceted healthful properties. The bark, leaves, and
seeds are used in India as a treatment for many skin diseases. The extract of the leaves
has been shown to have antibacterial and antiviral activity. Neem is also taken internally
to eliminate worms. The branches of the tree are chewed and used to clean the teeth and
to prevent gum inflammation. *See* Neem Oil and Neem Leaves Extract.

NELUMBIUM SPECIOSUM • *See Lotus.*

NELUMBO NUCIFERA FLOWER EXTRACT • Sacred Lotus. *See* Lotus.

NENOLONE HEMISUCCINATE • *See Succinic Acid.*

NEODECANOIC ACID • Colorless liquid used in plasticizers and lubricants. *See*
Decanoic Acid.

NEOFOLINONE • Occurs naturally in oil of lavender, orange leaf (absolute), palmarosa oil, rose, neroli, and oil of petitgrain. Used in citrus, honey, and neroli flavorings
and fragrances.

NEOHESPERIDINE DIHYDROCHALCONE • Flavoring. *See* Dihydrochalcones.

NEOMYCIN • Used in underarm deodorants, it is a product of the growth of microorganisms inhabiting the soil. It inhibits the growth of bacteria and, therefore, the odor from
sweat. It can cause the skin to swell, redden, or break out when exposed to light. It produces allergic reactions in many people. Highly toxic to the eighth nerve, which involves
hearing, and to the kidneys. The FDA does not believe the use of neomycin in deodorants is justified because it caused resistant strains of staphylococci to develop. Such staph
infections are extremely difficult to treat and could be lethal. Available only by prescription in United Kingdom. U.S. cosmetics with antibiotics banned in the EU.

NEOMYCIN SULFATE • Introduced in 1951, it is one of the most widely used
antibiotics for humans. In a cream or ointment, it is used to treat skin infections, minor
burns, wounds, skin grafts, itching, inflammation of the outer ear, and skin ulcers.
Potential adverse skin reactions include rashes, contact dermatitis, hives, and possible
kidney, ear, and nerve toxicity when absorbed systemically. The skin product should not
be used on more than 20 percent of the body surface and should not be used to treat deep
wounds, puncture wounds, or serious burns without medical advice.

NEOPENTYL ALCOHOL • Peppermint odor. Used in sunscreens to protect against
UV radiation.

NEOPENTYL GLYCOL • White, crystalline solid from propanediol that is used in polyester foams, insect repellents, plasticizers, and lubricants. Used in expensive anti-aging cream.

NEOPENTYL GLYCOL DICAPRATE • The diester of glycol dicaprate is the diester of neopentyl glycol and decanoic acid (*see*). Used in lipsticks, eye makeup removers, and body and hand products.

NEOPENTYL GLYCOL DICAPRYLATE/DIPELARGONATE/DICARPRATE • The esters of neopentyl glycol and caprylic, pelargonic, and capric acids. Used in creams and lotions.

NEOPENTYL GLYCOL DIOCTANOATE • The ester of neopentyl glycol and octanoic acid (*see*).

NEOPENTYL GLYCOL DISTEARATE • The ester of neopentyl glycol and stearic acid (*see*).

NEORUSCOGENIN • Fatty alcohol used as a skin conditioner. *See* Butcher's Broom.

NEPETA • *See* Catnip.

NEPHELIUM LAPPACEUM • Rambutan. Skin conditioner.

NERIUM OLEANDER • *See* Oleander.

NEROL • A primary alcohol used in perfumes, especially in rose and orange blossom scents. Occurs naturally in oil of lavender, orange leaf, palmarosa oil, rose, neroli, and oil of petitgrain. It is colorless, with the odor of rose. Similar to geraniol (*see*) in toxicity.

NEROLI BIGARADE OIL • Used chiefly in cologne and in perfumes. Named for the putative discoverer, Anna Maria de La Trémoille, princess of Nerola (1670). A fragrant, pale yellow essential oil obtained from the flowers of the sour orange tree. It darkens upon standing. Also used in food flavorings.

NEROLIDOL • A sesquiterpene alcohol. A straw-colored liquid with an odor similar to rose and apple. Occurs naturally in balsam Peru and oils of orange flower, neroli, sweet orange, and ylang-ylang. Also made synthetically. Used in perfumery and flavoring. *See* Nerol.

NEROSOL • *See* Nerol

NERYL ACETATE • A synthetic citrus, fruit, and neroli flavoring. *See* Nerol.

NERYL BUTYRATE • A synthetic berry, chocolate, cocoa, citrus, and fruit flavoring. *See* Nerol.

NERYL FORMATE • Formic Acid. A synthetic berry, citrus, apple, peach, and pineapple flavoring. *See* Formic Acid for toxicity. *See* Nerol.

NERYL ISOBUTYRATE • A synthetic citrus and fruit flavoring and fragrance. *See* Nerol.

NERYL ISOVALERATE • A synthetic berry, rose, and nut flavoring ingredient for fragrances. *See* Nerol.

NERYL PROPIONATE • A synthetic berry and fruit flavoring and fragrance. *See* Nerol.

NETTLES • *Urtica dioica* and Lamium Album (White Nettle) Flower Extract. Used in hair tonics, shampoos, facial moisturizer/treatments, facial cleansers, conditioners, masks, styling mousses/foams, exfoliants/scrubs, and for pain relief and around-eye cream. White nettle contains components that can have both anti-irritant as well as inflammatory properties. The serrated leaves and stems are covered with stinging hairs that contain histamine, serotonin, and acetylcholine. Stinging nettle also includes protein, B vitamins and vitamins A and C, high amounts of chlorophyll, formic, caffeic and malic acids, serotonin, glucoquinones, high amounts of iron, silica, potassium, calcium, magnesium, copper, manganese, phosphorus, selenium, sulfur, zinc, tannins, histamine, mucilage, ammonia (which causes the stinging), lecithin, lycopene, essential fatty and other acids, folate, beta-carotene, and choline. Netttles have a long history and were used in folk medicine. Nettle tea was one of the most popular of all springtime medicines in the 1700s. In modern laboratories, it has been shown to have anti-inflammatory activity and to lower sugar levels in the blood. As an astringent, stinging nettle has been effective in stopping external (with topical use) bleeding. The herb's astringency also shrinks inflamed tissues and helps to alleviate hemorrhoids. Used externally, modern herbalists use stinging nettle as a hair tonic and growth stimulant and also an antidandruff shampoo. Nettle tea is also considered an effective hair tonic that may bring back the natural color of the hair. A poultice made of the leaves alleviates pain due to inflammation, and the dried powdered leaf is said to stop nosebleed. As a wash, stinging nettle is good for burns, eczema, insect bites, and wounds. Ironically, although stinging nettle is a stinging plant, it is sometimes used in cosmetics as a facial. The uncooked plants can cause kidney damage and poisoning. The bristly hairs can be irritating to the skin. In 1992, the FDA issued a notice that nettle had not been shown to be safe and effective as claimed in OTC digestive aid products. When the stinging hairs are touched, they can cause local irritation and a burning sensation that may last for several hours. Fortunately, the stinging hairs on the plant are inactivated by drying or cooking the plant.

NEURAL EXTRACT • The extract of animal nerve tissue.

NEURALGIA • Severe pain in a nerve or along its route.

NEURITIS • Inflammation of the nerve or its parts due to infection, toxins, compression, or trauma.

NEURON • The basic nerve cell of the central nervous system.

NEUROPATHY • Disease, inflammation, or damage to the peripheral nerves, which connect the central nervous system to the sense organs, muscles, glands, and internal organs.

NEUROPEPTIDES • Any of the molecules composed of amino acids found in brain tissue. Some are both neurotransmitters (*see*) and hormones. They are believed to be involved in carbohydrate craving, as well as in many other physical and emotional functions.

NEUROTENSIN • A peptide of thirteen amino acid derivatives that helps regulate blood sugar by its effects on a number of hormones, including insulin and glucagon. It also is thought to play a part in pain suppression.

NEUROTRANSMITTERS • Molecules that carry chemical messages between nerve cells. Neurotransmitters are released from nerve cells, diffuse across the minute distance between two nerve cells (synaptic cleft), and bind to a receptor at another nerve site.

NEUT • *See* Sodium Bicarbonate.

NEUTRACEUTICAL • A product between a drug and a food; any substance that may be considered a food or part of a food and provides medical or health benefits, including the prevention and treatment of disease. An example is L-carnitine, which is sold over the counter as a dietary supplement and as the drug, Carnitor, to treat an inborn error of metabolism.

NEUTRA-PHOS • *See* Potassium Phosphate and Sodium Phosphate.

NEUTRA-PHOS-K • *See* Potassium Phosphate.

NEUTROGENA T/GEL • *See* Coal Tar.

NEUTROPHIL • Infection-fighting white blood cell.

NGDA • *See* Nordehydroguaiaretic Acid.

NGO • International Working Group for Safer Chemicals and Sustainable Materials.

NIAC • *See* Niacin.

NIACELS • *See* Niacin.

NIACIN • Nia-Bid. Niacels. Niacor. Niaplus. Nicotinic Acid. Nicotinamide. Niac. Nico-400. Nicobid. Nicolar. Nicotinex. Span-Niacin. Ni-Span. Endur-Acin. Slo-Niacin. Tega-Span. Introduced as a nutritional supplement in 1937, it is an essential nutrient that participates in many energy-yielding reactions and aids in the maintenance of a normal nervous system. A component of the vitamin B complex, it releases energy from foods, maintains healthy skin, and helps in the normal functioning of the nervous system and digestive tract. Deficiency symptoms include nervous disorders and skin problems. In 1992, the FDA proposed a ban on niacinamide in oral menstrual drug products because it had not been shown to be safe and effective as claimed.

NIACINAMIDE • Nicotinamide. Vitamin B_3. Used as a skin stimulant and hair conditioner in cleansing products including shampoos and cold creams. It has also been reported to be an effective skin lightener, especially for skin conditions where hyperpigmention may occur on the face or other visible parts of the body.

NIAPLUS • *See* Niacin.

NICKEL • Metal that occurs in the earth. May be present in eyelash curlers or tweezers, causing a skin reaction. *See* Nickel Sulfate.

NICKEL SULFATE • Used in hair dyes and astringents. Occurs in the earth's crust as a salt of nickel. Obtained as green or blue crystals and is used chiefly in nickel plating. It has a sweet astringent taste and acts as an irritant and causes vomiting when swallowed. Its systemic effects include blood vessel, brain, and kidney damage and nervous depression. Frequently causes skin rash when used in cosmetics. It is used in eye pencils and some containers.

NICKEL SULFATE (OTC) • Occurs in the earth's crust as a salt of nickel. Obtained as green or blue crystals. It has a sweet, astringent taste. Used chiefly in nickel plating. Also used in hair dyes and astringents. Used as a mineral supplement, up to 1 mg. per day.

NICO-400 • *See* Niacin.

NICOBID • *See* Niacin.

NICOLAR • *See* Niacin.

NICOMETHANOL HYDROFLUORIDE • Used in oral hygiene products. The EU restricts it to 0.15 percent calculated as fluorine when mixed with other fluorine compounds. Must have on the label "contains nicomethanol hydroflouride." Swallowing the toothpaste is discouraged. Fluorides are toxic and may discolor teeth. *See* Fluoride.

NICOTIANA TABACUM • Tobacco Extract. *See* Nicotinyl Alcohol.

NICOTINAMIDE • Skin conditioner. *See* Niacin.

NICOTINE REMOVERS • *See* Nail Bleaches.

NICOTINEX • *See* Niacin.

NICOTINIC ACID • *See* Niacin.

NICOTINYL ALCOHOL • Used as a skin-conditioning ingredient reportedly for its ability to dilate blood vessels. It is also a solvent.

NICOTINYL TARTRATE • Skin conditioner. *See* Pyridium Compounds.

NIGELLA SATIVA • *See* Caraway Seed and Oil.

NIGHTSHADE, BLACK • *Solanum nigrum.* Garden Nightshade. Common Nightshade. Morelle. An annual plant, the leaves were used by North American Indians as a treatment for TB and to expel worms. Many cultures have used the plant to induce sleep. Ancient Greek and Arab physicians used the leaves to treat burns, itching, hemorrhoids, and arthritis. The leaves and berries are poisonous, especially in the unripe state. The juice of the fresh herb is sometimes used for fever and to allay pain. In large doses, black nightshade can cause serious, but usually not fatal, poisoning. Externally, the juice or an ointment prepared from the leaves can be used for skin problems and tumors. The berries are poisonous, but boiling apparently destroys the toxic substances and makes them usable for preserves, jams, and pies. The fruit is used as a cosmetic by rubbing the seeds on the cheeks to remove freckles. Decoctions of stalk, leaves, and roots are good for wounds and cancerous sores.

NIMH • Abbreviation for National Institute of Mental Health.

NINDOU EKISU • *See* Honeysuckle.

NISIN • Crystals from *Streptococcus lactis* used as a preservative and antimicrobial ingredient in cosmetics. The European Parliament said in 2003 that nisin should not be used because it could cause resistance to antibiotics in humans. GRAS

NITRATES • Potassium and Sodium. Potassium nitrate, also known as saltpeter and niter, is used as a color fixative in cured meats. Sodium nitrate, also called Chile saltpeter, is used as a color fixative in cured meats. Both nitrates combine with natural stomach saliva and food substances (secondary amines) to create nitrosamines—powerful cancer-causing additives. Strontium nitrate is reportedly used in some product types such as toners/astringents, facial moisturizer/treatments, anti-aging products, facial cleansers, and acne treatments. The EU and the Japanese have banned its use in cosmetics. The U.S. EPA Toxic Release Inventory list shows one or more animal studies produce broad systemic effects at moderate exposure. Some animals suffered endocrine-system disruption at high doses (*see* Endocrine Disrupter Chemicals). Neurotoxicity occurred at high doses. More well known is the development of nitrosamine in cosmetic and food products because of the presence of nitrates. Researchers at the Michael Reese Medical Center's Department of Pathology in Chicago induced cancer in mice by giving single doses of one three-thousandth (0.3 microgram) of a gram of nitrosamine for each gram of the animal's weight. This is in contrast to the way other researchers have induced cancer in laboratory animals with nitrosamines by using repeated small doses or single large doses. The tumors that developed were analogous to human liver tumors. The color additive, silver, is a crystalline powder of high purity silver prepared by the reaction of silver nitrate with ferrous sulfate. Nitrate is used in hair coloring and fingernail polish, which the FDA restricts to only 1 percent of the final product. It is exempt from certification of the color. Nitrosamines caused pancreatic cancer in hamsters, similar to human pancreatic cancers. Nitrates have caused deaths from methemoglobinemia (it cuts off oxygen to the brain). Because nitrates are difficult to control in processing, they are being used less often.

NITRICUM ACIDUM • Nitric Acid. Aqua Fortis. A homeopathic remedy made from a mineral acid. It is used for bad breath, anger, anxiety, the common cold, earache, joint pain, insomnia, headache, gas, eye inflammation, sore throat, piles and thrush. *See* Nitrates.

NITRILOTRIACETIC ACID • NTA. Chelating and sequestering ingredient. Used in detergents. Can be irritating.

NITRITE • Potassium and Sodium. Used as color fixatives and preservatives. The question about nitrites concerns their combining with substances in organic substances in cosmetics called amines. This combination known as nitrosamines (*see*) has been found to be a potential cancer-causing ingredient. On the Canadian Hotlist (*see*). *See* diethanolamine (DEA) and DEA-related ingredients.

NITRO- • A prefix denoting one atom of nitrogen and two of oxygen. Nitro also denotes a class of dyes derived from coal tars. Nitro dyes can be absorbed through the skin. When absorbed or ingested they can cause a lack of oxygen in the blood. Chronic exposure may cause liver damage. *See* Colors.

3-NITRO-4-AMINOPHENOXYETHANOL • An aromatic ether alcohol used as a fungicide. *See* o-Phenylphenol.

NITROBENZENE • Essence of Mirabane. A colorless to pale yellow, oily, poisonous liquid (nitric acid and benzene). It is used to scent cheap soaps and in the manufacture of aniline. It is also a solvent for cellulose, an ingredient of metal polishes, shoe polishes, and many other products. It is rapidly absorbed through the skin. Workers are warned not to get it in their eyes, or on their skin, and not to breathe the vapor. Exposure to essence of mirabane may cause headaches, drowsiness, nausea, vomiting, lack of oxygen in the blood (methemoglobinemia), and cyanosis. On the Canadian Hotlist (*see*). The EU bans the use of nitrobenzene in cosmetics.

NITROCELLULOSE • Any of several esters (*see*) obtained as white fibrous flammable solids by adding nitrate to cellulose, the cell walls of plants. Used in skin protective creams, nail enamels, and lacquers.

3-NITRO-*p*-CRESOL • A hair coloring. On the Canadian Hotlist (*see*). *See* Coal Tar and Colors. The EU bans its use in cosmetics.

NITROGEN • A gas that is 78 percent of the atmosphere by volume and essential to all living things. Odorless. Used as a preservative for cosmetics. In high concentrations, it can asphyxiate. Toxic concentration in humans is 90 ppm; in mice, 250 ppm. GRAS. ASP. E

2-NITRO-5-GLYCERYL METHYLANILINE • *See* Aniline Dyes.

4-NITROGUAIACOL • Hair coloring. *See* Phenols.

3-NITRO-*p*-HYDROXYETHYLAMINOPHENOL • *See* o-Phenylphenol.

2-NITRO-*n*-HYDROXYETHYL-*p*-ANISIDINE • *See* Azo Dyes.

NITROMETHANE. • The principal use is as a stabilizer for chlorinated solvents, which are used in dry cleaning, semiconductor processing, and degreasing. It is also used most effectively as a solvent or dissolving agent for acrylate monomers, such as cyanoacrylates (more commonly known as "super-glue"). It is also a rust inhibitor.

NITROPHENOL • A hair coloring. *See* Coal Tar.

4-NITRO-*m*-PHENYLENEDIAMINE • A hair coloring. The safety has not been documented and substantiated. The CIR Expert Panel (*see*) "cannot conclude that this ingredient is safe for use in cosmetic products until the appropriate safety data have been obtained and evaluated." *m*-Phenylenediamine has been banned in cosmetics by the EU. *See* p-Phenylenediamine.

4-NITRO-*o*-PHENYLENEDIAMINE • A hair coloring. The safety has not been documented and substantiated. The CIR Expert Panel (*see*) "cannot conclude that this ingredient is safe for use in cosmetic products until the appropriate safety data have been obtained and evaluated." *See* Phenylenediamine.

2-NITRO-*p*-PHENYLENEDIAMINE • *See* Phenylenediamine.

4-NITROPHENYL AMINOETHYLUREA • *See* Phenols and Urea.

6-NITRO-2, 5-PYRIDINEDAMINE • *See* Coal Tar.

6-NITRO-O-TOLUIDINE • *See* Coal Tar.

NITROSAMINES • Compounds formed when chemicals containing nitrites react with amine, natural chemicals found in foods and in the body. Nitrosamines may be formed in cosmetics containing amines and amino derivative ingredients (e.g., diethanolamine (DEA) combined with a nitrosating agent (e.g., 2-bromo-2-nitropropane-1,3-diol [BronopolTM, Onyxide 500], 5-bromo-5-nitro-1,3-dioxane [Bronidox C] or tris(hydroxymethyl)nitromethane [Tris Nitro]); or they may become contaminated with a nitrosating agent (e.g., sodium nitrite). Many nitrosamines are among the most potent cancer-causing ingredients found. Because there are numerous chemicals capable of reacting with nitrite, nitrosamines have been found in air, water, tobacco smoke, cured meats, cosmetics, pesticides, and alcoholic beverages. It is also believed that they may be formed in our bodies. Some epidemiological studies have associated increased incidence of human cancer with the presence of nitrosamines. *See* Diethanolamine (DEA) and DEA-related ingredients, for example.

NITROSATING • The introduction of a nitrogen and oxygen (nitroso) of molecules into a compound that may cause the compound to form cancer-linked nitrosamines (*see*).

NITROUS OXIDE • Laughing Gas. A whipping ingredient for whipped cosmetic creams and a propellant in pressurized cosmetic containers. Slightly sweetish odor and taste. Colorless. Used in rocket fuel. Less irritating than other nitrogen oxides but narcotic in high concentrations, and it can asphyxiate.

NIX • *See* Permethrin.

NOBELITIN • A substance found in citrus fruit that has been found to have anticancer properties in laboratory studies.

NONACNEGENIC • Used to indicate a cosmetic that does not produce acne. Anyone can claim it regardless of proof. *See* Noncomedeogenic.

g-NONALACTONE • *See* Coconut Oil.

NONANAL • Colorless liquid with an orange-rose odor. Used in perfumery and flavoring. *See* Aldehyde, Aliphatic.

NONANE-1, 3-DIOL MONOACETATE • Colorless to slightly yellow mixture of isomers used in perfumery and flavoring. *See* Nonanoic Acid and Acetic Acid.

NONANOIC ACID • A colorless, oily liquid that is insoluble in water, it occurs in the oil of pelargonium plants such as the geranium. It is practically insoluble in water and is used in producing salts and in the manufacture of lacquers. Can be very irritating to the skin.

NONCOMEDOGENIC • Does not cause pimples and blackheads by blocking pores.

NONETH-8 • The polyethylene glycol ether of nonyl alcohol (*see*).

NONFAT DRY COLOSTRUM • The residue produced by the dehydration of defatted colostrum, the first milk secreted after the birth of a baby.

NONFAT DRY MILK • The solid residue produced by removing the water from defatted cow's milk. Hair and skin conditioner. *See* Milk.

NONIONIC • A group of emulsifiers used in hand creams. They resist freezing and shrinkage. Toxicity depends upon specific ingredients.

NONOXYNOL-1, -2, -3, -4, -5, -6, -7, -8, 9, -10, -12, -14, -15, -30, -40 and -50 • Can be liquids, paste-like liquids, or waxes. In cosmetics and personal care products, Nonoxynols are used in hair and skin care products, bath and shaving products, and personal cleanliness products. Nonoxynols-1, -2, -3, -4, -5, -6, -7, and -8 (lower molecular weight Nonoxynols) are used principally in hair dyes and colors. Safety of the Nonoxynols has been assessed by the CIR Expert Panel (*see*). The CIR Expert Panel evaluated scientific data and based concluded that Nonoxynols 9, -10, -12, -14, -15, -30, -40 and -50 are safe as cosmetic ingredients in the present practices of concentration and use. In 1999, the CIR Expert Panel considered available data on the lower molecular weight Nonoxynols and concluded that Nonoxynol-1, -2, -3, -4, -5, -6, -7, and -8 are safe as used in rinse-off products and safe at concentrations of 5 percent or less in leave-on.

NONOXYNYL HYDROXYETHYLCELLULOSE • Thickener. Used as a skin and hair conditioner. *See* Hydroxyethylcellulose.

NONSTEROIDAL ANTI-INFLAMMATORY DRUGS • NSAIDs. Aspirin was the first fever-reducing, painkilling, nonsteroidal anti-inflammatory drug. The first nonaspirin NSAID was introduced in 1964. Today these include diclofenac, etodolac, ibuprofen, indomethacin, naproxen, piroxicam, sulindac, and nabumetone. They inhibit arachidonic acid, a fatty acid precursor of leukotrienes, prostaglandins, and thromboxanes, all involved in inflammation. NSAIDs are now widely used to treat the pain of arthritis, menstruation, postsurgery, and many other aches.

NONYL ACETATE • Used in perfumery. An ester produced by the reaction of nonyl alcohol and acetic acid (*see*). Pungent odor, suggestive of mushrooms, but when diluted, it resembles the odor of gardenias. Insoluble in water.

NONYL ALCOHOL • Nonalol. A synthetic flavoring, colorless to yellow with a citronella oil odor. Occurs in oil of orange. Used in butter, citrus, peach, and pineapple flavorings for beverages, ice cream, ices, candy, and chewing gum. Also used in the manufacture of artificial lemon oil. In experimental animals it has caused central nervous system and liver damage.

***y*-NONYL LACTONE** • Yellowish to almost colorless liquid with a coconut-like odor. Used in perfumery and flavors. *See* Nonyl Alcohol.

NONYL NONANOATE • Nonyl Pelargonate. Liquid with a floral odor used in flavors, perfumes, and organic synthesis. *See* Nonyl Alcohol.

NONYL NONOXYNOL-5 THROUGH -100 • The ethoxylated (*see*) alcohol. *See* Phenols.

NOOTKA • *See* Cedar.

NOPYL ACETATE • A fragrance ingredient.

NORDIHYDROGUAIARETIC ACID • NGDA. An antioxidant used in brilliantines and other fat-based cosmetics. Occurs in resinous exudates of many plants. White or grayish white crystals. Lard containing .01 percent NGDA stored at room temperature for nineteen months in diffuse daylight showed no appreciable rancidity or color change. Canada banned the additive in food in 1967, after it was shown to cause cysts and kidney damage in a large percentage of rats tested. The FDA removed it from the GRAS list of food additives in 1968 and prohibited its use in products over which it has control. The U.S. Department of Agriculture, which controls antioxidants in lard and animal shortenings, banned it in 1971.

NORVALINE • A protein amino acid (*see*), soluble in hot water and insoluble in alcohol. *See* Valeric Acid.

NORWAY SPRUCE EXTRACT • The extract of the buds of *Picea abies*. A widely cultivated pine tree. *See* Pine Oil.

NOTE • A distinct odor or flavor. "Top" note is the first note normally perceived when a flavor is smelled or tasted; usually volatile and gives "identity." "Middle" or "main" note is the substance of the flavor, the main characteristic. "Bottom" note is what is left when top and middle notes disappear. It is the residue when the aroma or flavoring evaporates.

NTA • Abbreviation for nitrilotriacetic acid (*see*).

NTP • Abbreviation for National Toxicology Program (*see*).

NUCLEIC ACIDS • Vital chemical constituents of living things; a class of comolex threadlike molecules comprising two main types of acids—DNA and RNA. DNA is found almost exclusively in the nucleus of living cells where it forms the chief material of the chromosomes.

NUPHAR JAPONICUM • Skin conditioner. This plant grows in shallow pond or marsh. Japanese name is Kou-hone (river-bone). This is an aquatic plant and its root looks like white bone.

NUTMEG • A natural flavoring extracted from the dried ripe seed of *Myristica fragrans*. Used as a flavoring. Can cause flushing of the skin, irregular heart rhythm, and contact dermatitis.

NUTRACOSMECEUTICALS OR NUTRICOSMETICS • The newest push in cosmetic products at this writing is the growing link between what we eat and how well our skin appears. A typical slogan is: "What's good for a healthy body is also good for a beautiful skin." In dietetics as in cosmetics, it is essential to follow a good, balanced diet based on the fundamental beauty/health ingredients: carbohydrates, lipids, proteins, minerals, and vitamins. Polyunsaturated fatty acids (*see*) are part of the mix. *See* page 10 for more on the new trend.

NYLON • The commonly known synthetic material used as a fiber in eyelash lengtheners and mascaras and as a molding compound to shape cosmetics. Also used as a thickener and opacifier (*see*). Comes in clear or white opaque plastic for use in making resins. Can cause allergic reactions.

NYLON-6 THROUGH -66 • Thickeners and opacifiers.

NYMPHAEA ALBA • Water Lily. Water Rose. Nenuphar. Candock. Cultivated in pools, this beautiful and romantic flower was used in folk medicine to depress sexual function. Externally, white and yellow water lilies were used to treat various skin disorders such as boils, inflammations, tumors, and ulcers. Used as a skin conditioner in cosmetics.

NYMPHAEA LOTUS ROOT EXTRACT • Used as an astringent.

NYMPHAEA ODORATA • Extract of the root of *Nymphaea alba*. Used in fragrances. *See* Water Lily.

NYSTATIN • Mycostatin. Nilstat. Yellow to light-tan powder with a cereal-like odor. Antifungal medication introduced in 1954. It is used in human medicine to treat oral, vaginal, and intestinal infections caused by *Candida albicans* (Monilia) and other *Candida* species. In cream or ointment, it is used to treat infant eczema, itching around the anus or vagina, and localized forms of candidiasis. Skin applications may cause occasional contact dermatitis from preservatives in some formulations. Nystatin is in the Environmental Protection Agency's Genetic Toxicology Program to determine its effects on DNA. Causes birth defects in experimental animals. Moderately toxic by ingestion.

O

OAK BARK EXTRACT • *Quercus alba*. Oak Chip Extract. The extract from the white oak used in bitters and whiskey flavorings for beverages, ice cream, ices, candy, whiskey (1,000 ppm), and baked goods. Contains tannic acid (*see*) and is exceedingly astringent. The Indians used it in a wash for sore eyes and as a tonic. ASP

OAK GALL • Manjakani. An herbal remedy from Bali containing tannin, calcium, iron, and vitamins A, B and E, used for centuries in traditional medicine. The presence of the oak gall is said to strengthen and tighten weak vaginal muscles due to its astringent and antioxidant properties, which may help to reverse the loss of elasticity due to aging and childbirth. It is also said to be antimicrobial and antiseptic, therefore combating infection and odors.

OAKMOSS, ABSOLUTE • Any one of several lichens, *Evernia* spp., that grow on oak trees and yield a resin for use as a fixative (*see*) in perfumery. Stable green liquid with a long-lasting characteristic odor. Used in fruit, honey, and spice flavorings. A common allergen in after-shave lotions. Found in fragrances to be high on the list of ingredients that cause photosensitivity.

OAKMOSS, CONCRETE • *Evernia prunastri*. Strong sensitizing potential. Oakmoss concrete is prepared by hydrocarbon solvent extraction of the lichen *Evernia prunastri*, collected mainly from oak trees in Yugoslavia, France, Italy, Corsica, Morocco, Hungary, and various central European countries. The lichen is often soaked in lukewarm water twenty-four hours prior to extraction. Oakmoss concrete is a solid, waxy, dark green mass with a phenolic woody, slightly tarlike but delicate and pleasant odor, reminiscent of seashore, forest, bark, wood, green foliage, and tannery. Should not be used on the body because of its sensitivity potential.

OAT BRAN • The broken coat of oats, *Avena sativa. See* Oat Flour.

OAT EXTRACT • The extract of the seeds of oats, *Avena sativa. See* Oat Flour.

OAT FLOUR • Flour from the cereal grain that is an important crop grown in the temperate regions. Light yellowish or brown to weak greenish or yellow powder. Slight odor; starchy taste. Makes a bland ointment for cosmetic treatments, including soothing baths.

OAT GUM • A plant extract used as a thickener and stabilizer. It can cause an allergic reaction, including diarrhea and intestinal gas.

OAT ROOT EXTRACT • The extract of the roots of the oak tree species *Quercus,* grown in the eastern United States and Canada. The bark contains tannic acid, oak-red resin, pectin, levulin, and quercitol. The extract is used as an astringent.

OATMEAL • *Avena sativa.* Meal obtained by the grinding of oats from which the husks have been removed. Used through the ages by women as a face mask. Here is a modern version: In a blender put 4 tablespoons quick-cooking or regular oatmeal and 1 teaspoon dried mint leaves and turn to high until the mix is finely ground; add enough hot water to make a spreadable paste; smooth and pat on the face gently. When the paste is dry, remove with lukewarm water, then rinse well with cool water. Apply chilled witch hazel. Soothing.

OCHRONOSIS • A disturbance of metabolism in which the skin of the face, the whites of the eyes, and other tissues such as muscle and cartilage become discolored brown. The urine is also dark brown. Exogenous ochronosis is a condition characterized by hyperpigmentation of the face secondary to the long-term use of hydroquinone-containing bleaching creams. It is characterized by yellowish brown bumps, coarsening of the skin, and eventually scars. It is epidemic in South African blacks. *See also* Hydroquinone.

OCIMENE • A terpene obtained from sweet basil oil. Used in flavors and perfumes.

OCIMUM • *See* Basil Extract.

OCTACOSANOL • A constituent of vegetable wax. Isolated from the green blades of wheat and from carnauba wax.

OCTACOSANYL • An emulsifier and stabilizer. *See* Octanoic Acid.

OCTADECANE • A solvent for emollients. *See* Octadecanoic Acid.

OCTADECANOIC ACID • A waxy, saturated fatty acid; occurs widely as a glyceride in animal and vegetable fats.

OCTADECENE/MA COPOLYMER • An emulsion stabilizer and film former. *See* Octanoic Acid.

OCTADECYL-AMMONIUM FLUORIDE • Oral hygiene product. The EU calculates at 0.15 percent when mixed with other fluorine compounds. Fluorine concentration must not exceed 0.15 percent, and the EU label must say, "Contains octadecyl-ammonium fluoride monofluorophosphate." *See* Fluoride.

OCTANE • Used as a solvent.

OCTANOIC ACID • Colorless, oily liquid with a bad odor, derived from coconut, it is used as an antimicrobial ingredient and flavoring. Mildly toxic by ingestion and a skin irritant, it has caused mutations in experimental animals.

1-OCTANOL • Caprylic Alcohol. Used in the manufacture of perfumes. Occurs naturally in oil of lavender, oil of lemon, oil of lime, oil of lovage, orange peel, and coconut oil. It has a penetrating, aromatic scent. May cause skin rash.

2-OCTANOL • Caprylic Alcohol. An oily aromatic liquid with a somewhat unpleasant odor. For use in the manufacture of perfumes and disinfectant soaps. *See* 1-Octanol.

OCTENE • A hydrocarbon (*see*) used as a solvent.

OCTOCRYLENE • An absorbent. *See* Phenols.

OCTODODECANOL • 2-Octyl Dodecanol. *See* Stearyl Alcohol.

OCTODODECETH-16, -20, -25 • Polyethylene ethers of octyldodecanol and stearic acid (*see both*).

OCTODODECYL MYRISTATE • *See* Myristic Acid.

OCTODODECYL NEODECANOATE • The ester of octyl dodecanol and neodecanoic acid (*see both*).

OCTODRINE AND ITS SALTS • Viscous liquid with a fishy odor used as a decongestant. Banned in cosmetics by the EU, UK, and ASEAN (*see*).

OCTOXYGLYCERYL BEHENATE • An ester of glycerin and behenic acid (*see both*). Used in lipsticks.

OCTOXYGLYCERYL PALMITATE • *See* Glycerin and Palmitic Acid.

OCTOXYNOL-1, -3, -10, -13, -40, -70 • Waxlike emulsifiers, dispersing ingredients, and detergents used in hand creams, lotions, and lipsticks. Derived from phenol (*see*). The number signifies the viscosity.

OCTOXYNOL-9 OR -20 CARBOXLYLIC ACID • *See* Octoxynols and Carboxylic Acid.

OCTRIZOLE • An absorbent derived from phenol (*see*).

OCTYL ACETOXYSTEARATE • *See* Stearic Acid.

OCTYL COCOATE • *See* Coconut Acids.

OCTYL DIMETHYL PABA • Used in sunscreens and makeup. *See* Para-aminobenzoic Acid and Sunscreen Preparations.

OCTYL DODECANOL • Widely used emulsifier, opacifying ingredient, hair conditioner, emollient, and surfactant. *See* Stearyl Alcohol.

OCTYL HYDROXYSTEARATE • *See* Ester and Stearic Acid.

OCTYL ISONONANOATE • *See* Ester and Nonanoic Acid.

OCTYL ISOPALMITATE • An ester of palmitic acid (*see*), it is used as a skin-conditioning ingredient in body and hand products, eye shadows, skin care products, blushers, and fragrances.

OCTYL METHOXYCINNAMATE • Widely used as an ultraviolet light absorber in makeup bases, foundations, suntan lotions, and hair preparations. *See* Ester and Methyl Cinnamate.

OCTYL MYRISTATE • *See* Ester and Myristic Acid.

OCTYL OCTANOATE • *See* Ester and Octanoic Acid.

OCTYL PALMITATE • Widely used as an emollient in makeup, cold creams, lipsticks, and shaving creams. On the basis of the available information, the CIR Expert Panel (*see*) found it safe in the early 1980s but is considering new information to determine if the final safety assessment should be reaffirmed, amended, or have an addendum. *See* Ester and Palmitate.

OCTYL PELARGONATE • *See* Ester and Pelargonic Acid.

OCTYL SALICYLATE • A sunscreen widely used in makeup, lipsticks, hair sprays, and hand creams. *See* Salicylates.

OCTYL STEARATE • Widely used as an emollient in makeup bases, skin care products, eye shadows, cold cream, and indoor tanning preparations. Used as a skin-conditioning ingredient. On the basis of the available animal and human data, the CIR Expert Panel (*see*) concluded that this ingredient is safe as used in cosmetics. *See* Stearic Acid.

OCTYL TRIAZONE • A PABA-derivative not approved as an active ingredient in the United States. Used as a colorant and in sunscreens. Reportedly causes skin reactions in sunlight and can be harmful to plants and animals in the wild. May be restricted in other countries.

OCTYLACRYLAMIDE/ACRYLATES/BUTYLAMINOETHYL METHACRYLATE COPOLYMERS • Used in hair products as a fixative. *See* Acrylates.

OCTYLACRYLAMIDE/ACRYLATES COPOLYMER • *See* Acrylates and Polymer.

OCTYLDECANOL • Widely used as a skin-conditioning ingredient in hair products, body and hand products, moisturizing preparations, cold creams, cleansing lotions, eyebrow pencils, blushers, suntan gels, makeup, deodorants, and preshave lotions. *See* Decanal.

OCTYLDECYL PHOSPHATE • Emulsifier. *See* Phosphoric Acid.

OCTYLDODECETH-16, -20, -25 • Emulsifiers and surfactants. Polyethylene ethers of octyl dodecanol (*see*).

OCTYLDODECYL BEHENATE • The ester (*see*) of octyl dodecanol and behenic acid (*see*). Used in skin creams.

OCTYLDODECYL BENZOATE • The ester (*see*) of octyl dodecanol and benzoic acid (*see*).

OCTYLDODECYL MYRISTATE • Widely used as a skin-conditioning ingredient in moisturizers and body and hand cosmetics. *See* Ester and Myristic Acid.

OCTYLDODECYL NEODECANOATE • *See* Ester and Neodecanoic Acid.

OCTYLDODECYL NEOPENTANOATE • *See* Ester and Pentanoic Acid.

OCTYLDODECYL OLEATE • *See* Ester and Oleic Acid.

OCTYLDODECYL OLIVATE • The ester (*see*) of olive oil used as a skin-conditioning ingredient.

OCTYLDODECYL RICINOLEATE • Skin conditioner. *See* Ricinoleic Acid.

OCTYLDODECYL STEARATE • The ester of octyl dodecanol and stearic acid (*see both*).

OCTYLDODECYL STEAROYL STEARATE • A skin-conditioning ingredient widely used in face powders, eye shadows, foundations, blushers, eye makeup, makeup bases, and moisturizers. *See* Stearic Acid.

OCTYLDODECYLTRIMONIUM CHLORIDE • A quaternary ammonium compound (*see*) used as an antistatic hair product ingredient.

OCTYLISOTHIAZOLINONE • A preservative.

ODONTELLA • Oil extracted from algae. Used as an emollient.

ODORIKOSOU EKISU • *Lamium album.* White Nettle. *See* Lamium.

OENOTHERA BIENNIS • *See* Evening Primrose.

OIL OF SASSAFRAS, SAFROLE FREE • This flavoring without the safrole is permitted in foods. Oil of sassafras that is used to correct disagreeable odors in cosmetics is 80 percent safrole. May produce allergic reactions in sensitive persons. Banned in foods.

OLAFLUR • A dentifrice. *See* Fluoride.

OLAX • An evergreen tree that yields an essential oil used in fragrances. It grows in Asia, Africa, and Australia.

OLEA EUROPAEA • May cause acne. *See* Olive Oil.

OLEALKONIUM CHLORIDE • *See* Quaternary Ammonium Compounds.

OLEAMIDE • Oleylamide. *See* Oleic Acid.

OLEAMIDE DEA • Oleic Diethanolamide. Widely used as a foam booster and thickener in hair products and bubble baths. May form nitrosamines (*see*). Based on available data, the CIR Expert Panel (*see*) concluded that this ingredient is safe as a cosmetic ingredient. However, it should not be used in cosmetic products containing nitrosating ingredients. *See* Quaternary Ammonium Compounds, Oleic Acid, and Diethanolamide.

OLEAMIDE MIPA • *See* Oleic Acid and MIPA.

OLEAMIDOPROPYL BETAINE • *See* Quaternary Ammonium Compounds.

OLEAMIDOPROPYL DIMETHYLAMINE • Emulsifier. Has been reported to cause allergic reactions. *See* Quaternary Ammonium Compounds.

OLEAMIDOPROPYL DIMETHYLAMINE GLYCOLATE • Antistatic ingredient in hair products. *See* Quaternary Ammonium Compounds.

OLEAMIDOPROPYL DIMETHYLAMINE HYDROLYZED COLLAGEN • Antistatic ingredient in hair products. Hydrolyzed animal protein (*see*).

OLEAMIDOPROPYL DIMETHYLAMINE LACTATE • *See* Lactic Acid and Quaternary Ammonium Compounds.

OLEAMIDOPROPYL DIMETHYLAMINE PROPIONATE • *See* Quaternary Ammonium Compounds.

OLEAMIDOPROPYL HYDROXYSULTANE • *See* Quaternary Ammonium Compounds.

OLEAMIDOPROPYL PG-DIMONIUM CHLORIDE • *See* Quaternary Ammonium Compounds.

OLEAMIDOPROPYLAMINE OXIDE • *See* Quaternary Ammonium Compounds.

OLEAMIDOPROPYLDIMONIUM HYDROXYPROPYL HYDROLYZED COLLAGEN • Hair- and skin-conditioning ingredient. *See* Quaternary Ammonium Compounds.

OLEAMIDOPROPYLETHYLDIMONIUM ETHOSULFATE • *See* Quaternary Ammonium Compounds.

OLEAMINE • Oleyl Amine. A fatty amine derived from oleic acid (*see*) and used as a stabilizer and plasticizer in creams, lotions, lipsticks, and perfumes. Not as greasy as oil-type stabilizers and plasticizers.

OLEAMINE BISHYDROXYPROPYLTRIMONIUM CHLORIDE • *See* Quaternary Ammonium Compounds.

OLEAMINE OXIDE • Hair-conditioning and hair-cleansing ingredient. *See* Oleamine.

OLEANDER • Oleandrin. The extract of *Nerium oleander.* The extract is used medically as a diuretic. It is used in cosmetic fragrances. The seeds are poisonous. More than two thousand people in Sri Lanka, according to the June 5, 2003, *Lancet,* die each year from oleander poisoning. On the Canadian Hotlist (*see*).

OLEANDRIN • The EU bans it in cosmetics. *See* Oleander.

OLEIC ACID • Obtained from various animal and vegetable fats and oils. Colorless. On exposure to air, it turns a yellow to brown color and develops a rancid odor. Used in preparations of Turkey-red oil (*see*), soft soap, permanent wave solutions, vanishing creams, brushless shave creams, cold creams, brilliantines, nail polish, toilet soaps, and lipsticks. Possesses better skin-penetrating properties than vegetable oils. Also employed in liquid makeup, liquid lip rouge, shampoos, and preshave lotions. Low oral toxicity but is mildly irritating to the skin. The CIR Expert Panel (*see*) concluded this ingredient is safe for use in cosmetic products.

OLEIC/PALMITIC/LAURIC/MYRISTIC/LINOLEIC TRIGLYCERIDE • The mixed esters (*see*) of fatty acids used in skin creams.

OLEOAMPHODIPROPIONATE • *See* Surfactants.

OLEOAMPHOHYDROXYPROPYLSULFONATE • *See* Surfactants.

OLEORESIN • A natural plant product consisting of essential oil and resin extracted from a substance, such as ginger, by means of alcohol, ether, or acetone. The solvent—alcohol, for example—is percolated through the ginger. Although the oleoresin is very similar to the spice from which it is derived, it is not identical because not all the substances in the spice are extracted. Oleoresins are usually more uniform and more potent than the original product. The normal use range of an oleoresin is from one-fifth to one-twentieth the corresponding amount for the crude spice. Certain spices are extracted as oleoresins for color rather than for flavor. Examples of color-intensifying oleoresins are those from paprika and turmeric.

OLEOSTEARINE • *See* Tallow and Fatty Acids.

OLEOYL HYDROLYZED COLLAGEN • Used as a hair- and skin-conditioning ingredient as well as a cleanser. The condensation product after oleic acid chloride and hydrolyzed animal protein have been processed. The word *animal* was taken out of the ingredient name but not out of the ingredient. *See* Hydrolyzed Protein.

OLEOYL HYDROXYETHYL IMIDAZOLINE • *See* Imidazoline.

OLEOYL PG-TRIMONIUM CHLORIDE • *See* Quaternary Ammonium Compounds.

OLEOYL SARCOSINE • The condensation product of oleic acid with *n*-methyl glycine, widely used in polishing compounds, soaps, and lubricating oils. Can be mildly irritating to the skin.

OLETH-2 AND -3 • Emulsifiers. The polyethylene glycol (*see*) esters of oleyl alcohol. They are surfactants and emulsifiers, and cleansing ingredients. Limited data is available. The CIR Expert Panel (*see*) concluded that this ingredient is safe for use in cosmetic products. *See* Oleyl Alcohol.

OLETH-5 AND -10 • *See* Oleyl Alcohol.

OLETH-20 • Widely used in hair preparations, moisturizers, bath products, colognes, makeup, and deodorants. An oily liquid derived from fatty alcohols. Used as an emulsifier and surfactant (*see*).

OLETH-25 AND -50 • *See* Oleyl Alcohol.

OLETH-3, -6, -10 CARBOXYLIC ACID • *See* Oleic Acid and Carboxylic Acid.

OLETH-2, -3, -4, -10, -20 PHOSPHATE • *See* Phosphoric Acid and Oleic Acid.

OLEUROPEIN • *Olea europaea. See* Olive Leaves.

OLEYL ACETATE • Acetyl ester of oleyl alcohol (*see*). *See also* Acetylated.

OLEYL ALCOHOL • Widely used cosmetic ingredient found in fish oils. Oily and usually pale yellow. Gives off an offensive burning odor when heated. Chiefly used in the manufacture of detergents and wetting ingredients and as an antifoam ingredient; also a plasticizer for softening and lubricating fabrics and as a carrier for medications.

OLEYL ARACHIDATE • The ester of oleyl alcohol and arachidic acid (*see both*) used as a wax.

OLEYL BETAINE • *See* Oleamine.

OLEYL ERUCATE • A skin-conditioning ingredient. The ester of erucic acid and oleyl alcohol (*see both*).

OLEYL HYDROXYETHYL IMIDAZOLINE • *See* Oleyl Alcohol and Imidazoline.

OLEYL IMIDAZOLINE • *See* Oleyl Alcohol and Imidazoline.

OLEYL LACTATE • The ester of lactic acid and oleyl alcohol (*see both*).

OLEYL LANOLATE • *See* Lanolin.

OLEYL MYRISTATE • *See* Myristic Acid.

OLEYL OLEATE • *See* Oleic Acid.

OLEYL PALMITAMIDE • *See* Quaternary Ammonium Compounds.

OLEYL STEARATE • *See* Oleic Acid and Stearic Acid.

OLIBANUM EXTRACT • Frankincense Extract. The extract of *Boswellia carterri* of various species. The volatile, distilled oil from the gum resin of a plant found in Ethiopia, Egypt, and Arabia. It was one of the gifts of the Magi. It is used in flavorings and fragrances.

OLIVAMIDE DEA • Thickener and surfactant. *See* Olive Oil.

OLIVAMIDOPROPYL BETAINE • The salt of olive oil used as a quaternary ammonium compound (*see*).

8-OLIVAMIDOPROPYL DIMETHYLAMINE • *See* Quaternary Ammonium Compounds.

OLIVAMIDOPROPYLAMINE OXIDE • Fatty acids derived from olive oil (*see*).

OLIVE ACID • Mixture of fatty acids from olives used as a cleansing ingredient.

OLIVE HUSK OIL • The solvent extraction of olive oil (*see*).

OLIVE LEAVES • The olive tree, *Olea europaea,* was known in biblical times as the "Tree of Life." Oleuropein is the major phenolic constituent extracted from the olive leaf, constituting about 19 percent from virgin olive oil. Oleuropein is reported to be hydrolyzed to another biologically active compound, hydroxytyrosol, in vivo. A variety of anitimicrobial actions of oleuropein and its associated compounds have been demonstrated in the laboratory. The inhibitory action of oleuropein against the growth and toxin production of *Staphylococcus aureus, Bacillis cerus, Pseudomonas syringae,* and several other bacterial strains has been reported in the scientific literature, although the precise mechanism of antimicrobial action has as yet to be elucidated. Oleuropein and related compounds appear to have surface-active properties that interfere with microbial cell membranes. Oleuropein could also interfere with the synthesis of amino acids (*see*) crucial to viral replication and, in the case of retroviruses, neutralize the production of reverse transcriptase and protease. Additionally, oleuropein is also reported to stimulate the immune response to infection (phagocytosis). *See* Olive Oil.

OLIVE OIL • *Olea europaea.* Superior to mineral oils in penetrating power. Used in brilliantine hairdressings, emollients, eyelash oils, lipstick, nail polish removers, shampoos, soaps, face powders, and hair colorings, and antiwrinkle and massage oils. It is a pale yellow or greenish fixed oil obtained from ripe olives grown around the Mediterranean Sea. May cause allergic reactions.

OLIVE OIL PEG-6 ESTERS • A complex mixture of the esterification (*see* Ester) of olive oil and polyethylene glycol (*see both*).

OLIVE OIL UNSAPONIFIABLES • *See* Olive Oil and Saponification.

OLIVOYL HYDROLYZED WHEAT PROTEIN • Hair and skin conditioner. *See* Olive Oil and Wheat Germ Oil.

OLUS • Black Lovage. Similar to angelica (*see*), it is a perennial herb with globular fruit. When ripe it is almost black. It is used in skin care products and makeup. *See* Lovage.

OMEGA 3 CERAMIDE • Used in skin moisturizers. *See* Flaxseed.

OMEGA 9 CERAMIDE • Derived from olives to firm the skin.

OMENTAL LIPIDS • Fats obtained from bovine omentum, a fold of tissue that connects a cow's stomach to the intestines. Used in skin conditioners.

ONION EXTRACT • Extract of the bulbs of the onion, *Allium cepa.* Used in flavorings and as a skin-conditioning ingredient.

ONONIS • *See* Restharrow Extract.

ONSEN-SUI • Water obtained from hot spring in Japan. Used as a skin-conditioning ingredient.

OPACIFIERS • Substances such as the fatty alcohols stearyl and cetyl (*see both*) that make shampoos and other liquid cosmetics impervious to light.

OPHIOGON JAPONICUS • Allheal. An herb related to celery. A fragrance ingredient.

OPOPNAX OIL • An odorous gum resin formerly used in medicine and believed to be obtained from *Hercules allheal.* A fragrance ingredient.

OPUNTIA • Prickly Pear. *See* Cactus.

OPUNTIA FICUS-INDICA EXTRACT • An extract from the Indian fig or prickly pear cactus. Used as an emollient.

ORANGE 4 • A coal tar color called Acid Orange 7 in the United States and Daidai205 by the Japanese. EU CI 15510. Used in face powders and blushers.

ORANGE 4 LAKE • A coal tar color. Used in lipsticks, blushers, and makeup except for around the eye. Called Daidai205 in Japan. EU CI 15510.

ORANGE 5 • Solvent Red 72 in the United States; Daidai201 in Japan; CI 45370 in the EU.

ORANGE 5 LAKE • Used in lipsticks and makeup preparations except around the eye. In the United States called Orange 5 Lake. EU CI 45370.

ORANGE 10 • A coal tar color. Also Orange 11 and Solvent Red 73. The Japanese call it Daidai206; the EU calls it CI 45425.

ORANGE 10 LAKE • EU name CI 45425.

ORANGE 11 • The EU calls it CI 45425. Japanese call it Daidai207.

ORANGE-FLOWER OIL • *See* Nerol.

ORANGE-FLOWER WATER • The watery solution of the sweet-smelling principles of the flowers of *Citrus sinensis*.

ORANGE OIL • *Citrus sinensis*. Sweet Orange Oil. Yellow to deep orange, highly volatile, unstable liquid with a characteristic orange taste and odor expressed from the fresh peel of the ripe fruit of the sweet orange plant species. Once used as an expectorant, it is now employed in perfumery, soaps, and flavorings. Inhalation or frequent contact with oil of orange may cause severe symptoms such as headache, dizziness, and shortness of breath. Perfumes, colognes, and toilet water containing oil of orange may cause allergic reaction in the hypersensitive. Omitted from hypoallergenic cosmetics. ASP

ORANGE PEEL WAX • The wax obtained from the peel of the orange and used as a skin-conditioning ingredient.

ORANGE ROUGHY OIL • The oil obtained from the fat under the skin of the deep sea fish *Hoplostethus atlanticus*. Used as a skin-conditioning ingredient.

ORANGE YU • A fragrance and skin-conditioning ingredient. *See* Orange Oil.

ORBIGNYA OLEIFERA • *See* Babassu.

ORCHID • *Orchis morio. Cymbidium grandiflorum*. A very large family of plants that produce colorful and elaborate flowers. Orchids produce minute seeds that are devoid of stored food and thus require the aid of fungi to supply the nourishment needed for germination. They are used in "organic" cosmetics.

ORCHIS • *See* Orchid.

OREGON GRAPE ROOT • *Berberis aquifolium*. Wild Oregon Grape. Rocky Mountain Grape. Trailing Mahonia. Berberis. Employed by early American physicians to treat skin diseases or other illnesses that dried out the skin or produced sores, including syphilis and chronic hepatitis. Oregon grape root contains hydrastine, used to stop uterine bleeding, and berberine (*see both*), used today as an antiseptic and decongestant in eye lotions. Modern studies have found that Oregon grape also contains oxyacanthine chloride and columbine chloride, which show antibacterial properties. Herbalists have also used the root to treat hepatitis, arthritis, cancer, and heart problems.

ORGANIC COSMETICS • There are no federal standards for the term, but "organic" usually means produce grown without pesticides, herbicides, or synthetic fertilizers, on land that has been free of such chemicals from one to seven years. Cosmetics made from only animal or vegetable products. Used as a gimmick to sell some cosmetics to those who believe "natural" is better, although most cosmetic ingredients are derived from natural sources. The leading natural and organic certification bodies in Europe have published a harmonized standard that promises to break down trade barriers. The details of the proposed standard can be viewed by clicking on the link http://www.cosmos-standard.org/docs/Cosmetics_Organic_Standard_Consultation.pdf.

The Cosmos standard was drawn up by more than a thousand companies offering an estimated eleven thousand certified products. Standards have been developed at the international level by ICEA (Italy), BDIH (Germany), Bioforum (Belgium), Cosmebio/Ecocert (France), and the Soil Association (UK) in order to define minimum requirements and definitions for organic and/or natural cosmetics. They added a "green" element to their standards asking participating companies to substitute "natural" products for petrochemicals. Under most of the varying proposals put forth so far, to qualify for the *natural* standard, no more than 5 percent of the total product may be synthetic.

ORIENTAL BLENDS • One of the basic perfume types, this group gives an impression of subtlety and warmth, with an intense note of spices and incense. They usually include amber, musk, and civet. They vary between heavily floral and richly resinous. They are more insistent in their predominating notes than any other type and usually are worn at night.

ORIGANUM OIL • The volatile oil is obtained by steam distillation from a flowering herb. Yellowish red to dark brown, with a pungent odor. Used in flavorings. A teaspoonful can cause illness, and less than an ounce has killed adults. GRAS

ORIZANOL • *See* Oryzanol.

ORMENIS MULTICAULIS • Fragrance ingredient. *See* Chamomile.

ORNITHINE • An amino acid (*see*) used as a skin-conditioning ingredient.

ORNITHOGALUM UMBELLATUM • Star of Bethlehem. A lily with white, green, or yellow flowers. Used in fragrances.

OROBANCHE RAPUM • Bitter Vetch. Broomrape. Chick Pea. Plant native to western America. Used in cosmetics as a thickening agent and emollient.

OROTIC ACID • Pyrimidecarboxylic Acid. Found in milk and certain molds, it is a growth factor for certain microorganisms. Skin-conditioning ingredient.

ORRIS ABSOLUTE • *Iris germanica* or *I. pallida.* One of the most widely used perfume ingredients, it is the oldest and most expensive of all natural perfume materials. It is twice the price of rose Bulgarian (*see*) and three times that of French jasmine (*see*). The so-called oil is produced by steam distillation from the underground stems of the iris. The rhizomes are washed, dried, and then stored for three years to acquire their fragrance. Prior to distillation, they are pulverized, and the absolute is distinctly violetlike with a fruity undertone—sweet, floral, warm, and lasting. The bulk of the material is produced in Italy, distillation taking place mostly in France and sometimes in England and Italy. Can cause allergic reactions.

ORRIS ROOT EXTRACT • Obtained from dried orris root. Has an intense odor and is used in perfumery. Causes frequent allergic reactions.

ORRIS ROOT OIL • *Iris germanica* or *I. pallida.* White Flag. Love Root. Distilled for use in dusting powders, perfumes, dry shampoos, toothpastes, and sachets. Made from the roots of the plant. Yellowish, semisolid, and fragrant oil. Discontinued in the United States because of frequent allergic reactions to orris, including infantile eczema, hay fever, stuffy nose, red eyes, and asthma. It is, however, used in raspberry, blackberry, strawberry, violet, cherry, nut, and spice flavorings.

ORTHOSIPHON STAMINEUS • A perennial herb with thick wood. There are about forty-five species. There are three in China and others in Africa, Asia, and Australia. It contains essential oils and resins that are used in fragrances.

ORYZA SATIVA • Widely used in cosmetics, soaps, and bath products. Contains fatty acids used in emollients. *See* Rice Starch.

ORYZANOL • Orizanol. The ester of ferulic acid and terpene alcohol widely found in plants used in flavorings and perfumes. Also an antistatic ingredient. *See* Cinnamate.

OSMANTHUS • Osmanthus is an evergreen shrub with attractive foliage and clusters of small, very fragrant flowers. These flowers are also used in some of the world's most famous and expensive fragrances. May be a skin irritant.

OSTREA • Oyster Shell Extract. Used as an abrasive.

OSTRICH OIL • Used in hair conditioners and skin emollients.

OTC • Abbreviation for over-the-counter, referring to nonprescription medicine.

OTOGIRISOU EKISU • Skin conditioner. *See* Hypericum.

OUBAKU • Abrasive. Obtained from the bark of phellodendron (*see*).

OUREN EKISU • An extract of the roots of *Copis japonica* or other species of Ranunculaceae. Used as a skin conditioner.

OURICURY WAX • The wax exuded from the leaves of the Brazilian palm tree. Hard, brown wax has the same properties and uses as carnauba wax (*see*).

OVALISS • Newer creams containing a complex of ingredients that are claimed to burn fat and inhibit the formation of new fat cells. In a recent study, topically applied Ovaliss "noticeably reduced chin fat by more than 10% in 7 out of 25 women." The other eighteen saw less than a 6 percent improvement.

OVARIAN EXTRACT • The extract of cow ovaries.

OVINE • Sheep. The spleen and ingredients therefrom are banned by ASEAN in cosmetics with the exception of tallow (*see*) that has been "used and strictly certified by the producer."

OVUM • *See* Egg Yolk.

OX BILE • Oxgall. Emulsifier from the fresh bile of male castrated bovines. Brownish green or dark green; viscous. Characteristic odor. Bitter, disagreeable taste. Used in dried egg whites up to 0.1 percent. The final report to the FDA of the Select Committee on GRAS Substances for food additives stated in 1980 that it should continue its GRAS status with no limitations other than good manufacturing practices.

OXALIC ACID • Occurs naturally in many plants and vegetables, particularly in the *Oxalis* genus; also in many molds. Used in freckle and bleaching cosmetic preparations as well as hair products. The EU says it should be applied by professionals only. Caustic and corrosive to the skin and mucous membranes; may cause severe intestinal upsets and kidney damage if ingested. Used industrially to remove paint, varnish, rust, and ink stains. Used in dentistry to harden plastic models. Fingernails exposed to it have turned blue, become brittle, and fallen off.

OXAZOLIDINE • Curing agent and an ingredient of pesticides. Listed as a potential cancer-causing agent.

OXAZOLINE • A series of synthetic waxes that are versatile and miscible with most natural waxes and can be applied to the same uses.

OXGALL • *See* Ox Bile.

OXIDIZED BEESWAX • Used as a thickener. *See* Beeswax.

OXIDIZED POLYETHYLENE • Polyethylene (*see*) and oxygen combined.

OXIDIZER • A substance that causes oxygen to combine with another substance. Oxygen and hydrogen peroxide are examples of oxidizers.

OXIDIZING INGREDIENT • Hydrogen peroxide is an example that is added to hair dyes to develop the color or fix it in the hair shaft. Such ingredients often have a bleaching effect and are also disinfectants. They kill bacteria. They may damage the skin and eyes, so care should be taken to use them according to directions. *See* Oxidizer and Hydrogen Peroxide.

OXIDO REDUCTASES • Enzymes from yeast used in skin conditioners.

OXYBENZONE • Oxybenzone is an organic compound derived from benzophenone and is used in a wide spectrum of sunscreen products as a means of absorbing potentially dangerous UVA rays. It is used as a sunscreening ingredient. Sunscreens may irritate the skin and in some people cause an allergic rash. According to studies at Columbia Presbyterian Medical Center in New York City, photosensitivity (*see*) to this ingredient is increasing. The Environmental Working Group (EWG) is highlighting a study conducted by the U.S. Centers for Disease Control (CDC) alleging risks associated with oxybenzone. The organization estimates that 97 percent of Americans it tested for the study were contaminated by the ingredient, which has been linked to allergies such as hormone disruption and cell damage. The organization also says that a companion study published just a few days earlier also links the chemical to low birth weight in baby girls whose mothers are exposed to the chemical during pregnancy. However, concerns brought about by earlier scientific studies have led authorities in the EU to regulate that any sunscreen product containing a more than 5 percent dose of the ingredient should be labeled accordingly. This is because studies have shown that oxybenzone can penetrate the skin's dermal layer, where it can increase production of free radicals, leading to the production of photocarcinogens.

OXYMETHYLENE/MELAMINE COPOLYMER • Film former.

OXYQUINOLINE • 8-Hydroxyquinoline. White, crystalline powder, almost insoluble in water. Used as a fungistat and for reddish orange colors when combined with bismuth. Used internally as a disinfectant. Has caused cancer in animals both orally and when injected. The CIR Expert Panel (*see*) concluded that the available data are insufficient to support the safety of this ingredient in cosmetic products. *See* Oxyquinoline Sulfate.

OXYQUINOLINE BENZOATE • 8-Quinolinol Benzoate. The salt of benzoic acid (*see*) and oxyquinoline (*see*).

OXYQUINOLINE SULFATE • Made from phenols; composed of either white crystals or powder, almost insoluble in water and ether but soluble in alcohol, acetone, and benzene. Used as a preservative in cosmetics for its ability to prevent fungus growth and to disinfect. The CIR Expert Panel (*see*) concluded that the available data are insufficient to support the safety of this ingredient in cosmetic products. *See* Phenols for toxicity.

OXYSTEARIN • A mixture of the glycerides (*see*) of partially oxidized stearic acids (*see*) and other fatty acids (*see*). Occurs in animal fat and used chiefly in manufacture of soaps, candles, cosmetics, suppositories, pill coatings. Tan, waxy. Used as a crystallization inhibitor in cottonseed and soybean cooking. In salad oils up to 0.125 percent. Also used as a defoamer in the production of beet sugar and yeast. The Select Committee of the Federation of American Societies for Experimental Biology advising on food additives recommended further study of this additive. The final report to the FDA of the Select Committee on GRAS Substances stated in 1980 that while no evidence in the available information on it demonstrates a hazard to the public at current use levels, uncertainties exist, requiring that additional studies be conducted. The CIR (*see*) says it is safe as used in cosmetics. ASP

OYSTER SHELL EXTRACT • Shells of *Ostrea viriginca* taken from the Gulf of Mexico coast in Texas and Louisiana and from Chesapeake Bay. Used as a thickener and skin conditioner.

OZOKERITE • Ceresin. A naturally occurring, waxlike mineral; a mixture of hydrocarbons. Colorless or white when pure; horrid odor. Upon refining, it yields a hard, white, microcrystalline wax known as ceresin (*see*). Widely used as an emulsifier and thickening ingredient in lipstick and cream rouge.

OZONE • A colorless gas or dark blue liquid used as an antimicrobial ingredient in bottled water. Under the EPA Genetic Toxicology Program. Toxic effects are from inhalation.

OZONIZED CASTOR OIL • Skin conditioner.

OZONIZED JOJOBA OIL • Jojoba oil (*see*) treated with ozone. It is used in skin-conditioning creams.

OZONIZED OLIVE OIL • Skin conditioner. *See* Olive Oil and Ozone.

OZONIZED SUNFLOWER SEED OIL • Skin conditioner. *See* Ozone and Sunflower Seed Oil.

P

PABA • 4-Aminobenzoic Acid. *p*-Aminobenzoic Acid. On the Canadian Hotlist (*see*). *See* Para-Aminobenzoic Acid.

PACHYRRHIZUS EROSUS • Skin conditioner. *See* Yam.

PADIMATE A • An organic compound that is an ingredient in some sunscreens. It is derived from para-aminobenzoic acid (PABA). This aromatic chemical absorbs ultraviolet rays, thereby preventing sunburn. However, its chemical structure and behavior is similar to compounds that produce free radicals (*see*). In Europe, this chemical was withdrawn in 1989 for unstated reasons. In the United States, it was never approved for use in sunscreens.

PADIMATE O • 2-ethylhexyl 4-dimethylaminobenzoate, Escalol 507, octyldimethyl PABA. OD-PABA. An organic compound that is an ingredient in some sunscreens. It is a derivative of para-aminobenzoic acid (PABA) (*see*) formed by the condensation of 2-ethylhexanol and dimethylaminobenzoic acid. It is a yellowish oily liquid that is insoluble in water. It absorbs ultraviolet rays, thereby preventing direct DNA damage by UV-B. However, it has been reported the padimate O molecule may react with DNA and produce indirect DNA damages that are similar to those done by ionizing radiation. Therefore, padimate O is presumably a carcinogen in sunlight. This compound does not dissipate energy as fast as melanin, and therefore it is unsuitable as a sunscreen ingredient. *See* Para-Aminobenzoic Acid.

PADINA PAVONICA • A microscopic brown algae of the Dictyoataceae family that is claimed to have properties similar to those of young human skin. It is used in anti-aging skin products.

PAEONIA • Peony. Shao-yao. The root is used by herbalists as a liver tonic. Also used to treat all female "complaints," especially menstrual irregularity and abdominal pains associated with the menstrual cycle. Externally, it has been used to treat wounds and skin growths. Peony is toxic when used internally in excessive doses. Potential adverse effects from herbal use include colic, nausea, and diarrhea. It may also produce uterine contractions. Contraindicated in pregnancy.

PALM KERNEL ACID • A mixture of fatty acids from palm kernel oil (*see*). Used as an opacifier, surfactant, and emulsifier.

PALM KERNEL ALCOHOL • The mixture of fatty alcohols derived from palm kernel oil (*see*). Used as an emulsifier and stabilizer.

PALM KERNEL GLYCERIDES • A mixture of glycerides (*see*) derived from palm kernel oil (*see*).

PALM KERNEL OIL • *Elaeis guineensis.* Palm Nut. The oil from palms, particularly the African palm oil tree. White to yellowish edible fat, it resembles coconut oil more than palm oil. It is used chiefly in making soaps and ointments. On the basis of the animal and clinical data, the CIR Expert Panel (*see*) concluded that it is safe as used in cosmetic formulations.

PALM KERNELAMIDE DEA • Emulsifier and Moisturizer. A mixture of ethanolamide of the fatty acids derived from palm kernel oil (*see*). DEA residues are believed to be potential cancer-causing agents. *See* Quaternary Ammonium Compounds.

PALM KERNELAMIDE MEA • *See* Palm Kernel Oil and Quaternary Ammonium Compounds.

PALM KERNELAMIDE MIPA • *See* Quaternary Ammonium Compounds.

PALM KERNELAMIDOPROPYL BETAINE • *See* Quaternary Ammonium Compounds.

PALM OIL • *Elaesis guineensis.* Palm Butter. Palm Tallow. Oil used in baby soaps, ordinary soaps, liniments, and ointments. Obtained from the fruit or seed of the palm tree. A fatty mass with a faint violet odor. Also used to make candles and lubricants. Was teratogenic in albino rats given 3 ml daily. On the basis of the animal and clinical data, the CIR Expert Panel (*see*) concluded that it is safe as used in cosmetic formulations.

PALM OIL GLYCERIDE • *See* Palm Oil.

PALMAMIDE DEA • Antistatic ingredient. A mixture of ethanolamides of the fatty acids derived from palm oil. DEA residues are believed to be potential cancer-causing agents. *See* Palm Oil.

PALMAMIDE MEA • A mixture of ethanolamides of the fatty acids derived from palm oil (*see*). *See* Nitrosamines.

PALMAMIDE MIPA • A mixture of isopropanol amides of the fatty acids derived from palm oil (*see*). *See* Nitrosamines.

PALMAMIDOPROPYL BETAINE • *See* Palm Oil and Betaine.

PALMARIA PALMATA EXTRACT • Dulse. A natural flavoring extract from red seaweed. Used as a food condiment. GRAS

PALMAROSA OIL • Geranium Oil. The volatile oil obtained by steam distillation from a variety of partially dried grasses grown in East India and Java. Used in rose, fruit, and spice flavorings. Believed as toxic as other essential oils, causing illness after ingestion of a teaspoonful and death after ingestion of an ounce. A skin irritant. GRAS

PALMETH-2-PHOSPHATE • Surfactant and cleansing ingredient.

PALMITAMIDE DEA, MEA • *See* Palmitic Acid.

PALMITAMIDOHEXADECANEDIOL • A skin-conditioning ingredient. *See* Palm Oil and Decanoic Acid.

PALMITAMIDOPROPYL BETAINE • Widely used as an antistatic ingredient in hair conditioners. Also used as a cleansing ingredient and foam booster. *See* Palmitic Acid and Surfactants.

PALMITAMIDOPROPYLAMINE OXIDE • A hair conditioner and cleansing ingredient. *See* Palmitic Acid.

PALMITAMIDOPROPYLDIETHYLAMINE • *See* Palmitic Acid and Surfactants.

PALMITAMIDOPROPYL DIMETHYLAMINE LACTATE • *See* Quaternary Ammonium Compounds and Lactic Acid.

PALMITAMIDOPROPYL DIMETHYLAMINE PROPIONATE • *See* Quaternary Ammonium Compounds and Propionic Acid.

PALMITAMINE • The CIR Expert Panel (*see*) concluded that this ingredient is safe for use in cosmetic products.

PALMITAMINE OXIDE • Palmityl Dimethylamine Oxide. Hair conditioner. *See* Palmitic Acid and Dimethylamine.

PALMITATE • A salt of palmitic acid (*see*) used as an oil in baby oils, bath oils, eye creams, hair conditioners, and cream rouges. Occurs in palm oil, butterfat, and most other fatty oils and fats. *See* Palmitic Acid for toxicity.

PALMITIC ACID • A mixture of solid organic acids obtained from fats consisting chiefly of palmitic acid with varying amounts of stearic acid (*see*). Widely used as a texturizer in shampoos, shaving creams, and soaps. It is white or faintly yellow and has a fatty odor and taste. Palmitic acid occurs naturally in allspice, anise, calamus oil, cascarilla bark, celery seed, butter acids, coffee, tea, and many animal fats and plant oils. It forms 40 percent of cow's milk. Obtained from palm oil, Japan wax, or Chinese vegetable tallow. The CIR Expert Panel (*see*) concluded that this ingredient is safe for use in cosmetic products.

PALMITOYL CAMELLIA SINENSIS • Antioxidant. *See* Camellia Oil and Palmitic Acid.

PALMITOYL CARNITINE • A skin conditioner. *See* Palmitic Acid and Carnitine.

PALMITOYL COLLAGEN AMINO ACIDS • The condensation product of animal collagen amino acid and palmitic acid (*see both*).

PALMITOYL GLUTAMIC ACID • *See* Palmitic Acid and Glutamic Acid.

PALMITOYL GRAPE SEED EXTRACT • Antioxidant and skin protectant. *See* Palmitic Acid and Grape-Seed Oil.

PALMITOYL HYDROLYZED COLLAGEN • The condensation product of palmitic acid and hydrolyzed animal protein. The word *animal* was removed from this ingredient's name. *See* Hydrolyzed Protein.

PALMITOYL HYDROLYZED MILK PROTEIN • The condensation product of palmitic acid chloride and hydrolyzed milk protein. *See* Hydrolyzed and Milk.

PALMITOYL INULIN • Skin conditioner and emulsifier. *See* Palmitic Acid and Inulin.

PALMITOYL KERATIN AMINO ACIDS • The condensation product of palmitic acid chloride and amino acids from animal skin. *See* Keratin Amino Acids.

PALMITOYL MARE MILK • Protein from mare's milk combined with palmitic acid (*see*). Used as a skin conditioner.

PALMITOYL MYRISTYL SERINATE • Skin conditioner. *See* Palmitic Acid and Myristic Acid.

PALMITOYL OLIGOPEPTIDE • Derived from protein, it is used as a skin conditioner and cleansing ingredient.

PALMITOYL PEA AMINO ACIDS • Amino acids from peas used as a hair and skin conditioner.

PALMITOYL PG-TRIMONIUM CHLORIDE • *See* Quaternary Ammonium Compounds.

PALMITOYL QUINOA AMINO ACIDS • Used as a hair- and skin-conditioning ingredient. *See* Palmitic Acid.

PALMITOYL TETRAPEPTIDE-10 • Claimed to work topically by extending skin cells' life span. *See* Heptapeptide-6.

PALMITOYL TRIPEPTIDE-3 • PTri-3, Synthetic collagen. The effect is claimed to reverse sagging of skin caused by inflammation (glycation damage), thereby restoring skin elasticity and lifting facial contours. Marketed as a temporary alternative to cosmetic procedures. PTri-3 is often referred to as synthetic collagen, because it mimics the body's own mechanism to produce collagen. In vitro studies have shown PTri-3 to increase collagen synthesis by 119 percent. This makes it especially effective for parts of the face and body that have lost skin tissue; for example, areas with stretch marks as well as areas with crepey skin, such as the neck and upper arms. Its effect is claimed to plump out the skin from within.

PANAX GINSENG ROOT EXTRACT • Widely used in skin and hair care as well as bath preparations and toilet waters. It is also used in makeup such as eye shadow and suntan products. *See* Ginseng.

PANCREASE • *See* Pancrelipase.

PANCREATIN • Pancreatin is a mix of many different enzymes. Used in face peel products and in processing cosmetics. Should be used cautiously in people who are allergic to pork.

PANCRELIPASE • Pancrease. Viokase. Zymase. A preparation of pancreatic hormones used in the disorders of the pancreas to aid digestion. Used in processing cosmetics. May cause allergic reaction in people sensitive to pork.

PANDANUS AMARYLLISFOLIUS • A palmlike tropical tree. Extract used in fragrances, flavorings and deodorants.

PANICUM MILIACEUM • *See* Millet.

PANSY, WILD • Viola tricolor. Johnny Jump-Up. Heart's Ease. Violet. A European herb, it is grown for its large, attractive flowers. Used for colorings. The herb contains mucilaginous material that is used as a soothing lotion for boils, swellings, and skin diseases. It also contains salicylates, saponins, alkaloids, flavonoids, and tannin (*see all*).

PANTETHINE • A growth factor for *Lactobacillus bulgaricus.* Glassy, lightly yellow substance. Used in hair products such as hair sprays and moisturizing preparations.

PANTHENOL • Dexpanthenol. Vitamin B Complex Factor. Widely used in hair products and emollients, and as a supplement in foods. Employed medically to aid digestion. It is good for human tissues.

PANTHENYL ETHYL ETHER • Ethyl ether of the B vitamin panthenol (*see*).

PANTHENYL ETHYL ETHER ACETATE • The ester of acetic acid and the ethyl ether of the B vitamin panthenol (*see*).

PANTOTHENIC ACID • Vitamin B_5. A necessity in the human diet involved in the metabolism of fats and proteins. Used in hair products as a conditioner.

PANTOTHENYL TRIACETATE • *See* Panthenol.

PAPAIN • *See* Papaya.

PAPAVER • *See* Poppy Oil.

PAPAYA • *Carica papapya.* A base of organic makeup. It is a fruit grown in tropical countries. It contains an enzyme, papain, used as a meat tenderizer and medicinally to prevent adhesions. It is deactivated by cooking. Because of its protein-digesting ability, it can dissolve necrotic (dead) material. It may cause allergic reactions. It is used in cosmetics as a hair conditioner.

PAPRIKA • The finely ground pods of dried, ripe, sweet pepper. The strong, reddish orange powder is used in sausage and spice flavorings. Both paprika and paprika oleoresins are used as red coloring. Permanently listed since 1966 as a coloring.

PARA- • Prefix meaning alongside, near, or abnormal.

PARA-AMINOBENZOIC ACID • The colorless or yellowish acid found in vitamin B complex. In an alcohol and water solution plus a little light perfume, it is sold under a wide variety of names as a sunscreen lotion to prevent skin damage. It is also used as a local anesthetic in sunburn products. It is used medicinally to treat arthritis. However, it can cause allergic eczema and a sensitivity to light in susceptible people whose skin may react to sunlight by erupting with a rash, sloughing, and/or swelling. On the Canadian Hotlist (*see*).

PARA-AMINOSALICYLIC ACIDS • *See* Salicylic Acid.

PARABENS • The parabens, methyl-, propyl-, and parahydroxybenzoate, are the most commonly used preservatives in the United States. An estimated 75 to 90 percent of cosmetics use parabens, including shampoos, makeup, lotions, and deodorants. Water is the only ingredient used more frequently in cosmetics. The parabens have a broad spectrum of antimicrobial activity, were believed to be safe to use, relatively nonirritating, nonsensitizing, and nonpoisonous. They are stable over the pH (*see*) range in cosmetics and are sufficiently soluble in water to be effective in liquids. The typical paraben preservative system contains 0.2 percent methyl- and 0.1 percent propylparaben. However, in 2004, a study published in the *Journal of Applied Toxicology* reported parabens are a cause for concern. British researchers found traces of it in twenty women who had breast tumors. Parabens are believed to act like the female hormone estrogen. In high levels, estrogen can cause some women to develop breast cancer. *See* Butylparaben. Parabens received significant criticism in the European arena, particularly in France, in 2008. A campaign from a French health association focusing on the "toxic cocktail" of baby cosmetics distributed in maternity wards led to calls from the health minister for further research and even a label marking certain products as unsafe for pregnant women and young children.The European trade association jumped quickly to the defense of the ingredients, saying that only four parabens are in cosmetics on the European market and all four have been investigated and found safe by the European Commission's Scientific Committee on Consumer Products (SCCP). The number of paraben-free cosmetics is increasing because of consumer concern. Instead, ingredients such as oats, pomegranate, pineapple, and ginger are being substituted (*see all*).

PARA-DICHLOROBENZENE • 1,2-dichlorobenzene. Paracide.

PARAFFIN • Widely used in solid brilliantines, cold creams, wax depilatories, eyelash creams, and oils, eyebrow pencils, lipsticks, liquefying creams, protective creams, and mascaras; also used for extracting perfumes from flowers. Obtained from the distillate of wood, coal, petroleum, or shale oil. Colorless or white, odorless, greasy, and not digestible or absorbable in the intestines. Chlorinated paraffin waxes and hydrocarbon waxes are suspected carcinogens. Paraffin may produce purpura (a condition characterized by hemorrhage into the skin. The color is at first red, gradually darkening to purple and then fading to a brownish yellow).

PARAFFINUM LIQUIDUM • *See* Mineral Oil.

PARAFORMALDEHYDE • A white solid with the odor of formaldehyde, it is derived from it. It is used as a fungicide, to kill bacteria, and in disinfectants. It is also used in adhesives and as a waterproofing ingredient. Toxic by ingestion. *See* Formaldehyde.

PARAGUAY TEA • *See* Maté Extract.

PARA-HYDROXYBENZOIC ACID • *See* p-Hydroxybenzoic Acid.

PARA-PHENYLENE DIAMINE • PPDA. *See* Phenylenediamine.

PARESTHESIA • A sensation of numbness, prickling, or tingling.

PARETH-25–12 • A detergent. *See* C12–15 Pareth 12.

PARFUM • The EU name used to cite a product that has a fragrance added to mask a particular odor. The United States calls it "fragrance" on the label.

PARIETARIA OFFICINALIS • *See* Pellitory Extract and Spanish Pellitory Extract.

PARSLEY EXTRACT • *Petroselinum cripsum. P. sativum.* A perennial of the carrot family, it is native to Europe, especially to Sardinia, where it is believed it may have originated. It was given in a tea to colicky infants and to settle the stomachs of adults after a meal. The oil is used to induce menstruation. The crushed seeds were made into an eyewash. A tea was used for urinary infections and for insect bites and swollen glands. It is rich in vitamin C. Ancient herbalists maintained that it would help hair grow if it were rubbed into the scalp. It is a source of chlorophyll, nature's breath freshener. It also contains vitamin B, potassium, protein, apiol—an anti-inflammatory in parsley oil—and myristicin, another oil. In 1992, the FDA proposed a ban on parsley in oral menstrual drug products because it has not been shown to be safe and effective for its stated claims. *See* Parsley Oil.

PARSLEY OIL • Used as a preservative in perfume and flavoring in cosmetics, it is obtained by steam distillation of the ripe seeds of the herb. Yellow to light brown, with a harsh odor. Parsley may cause skin to break out with a rash, redden, and swell when exposed to light. It may also cause an allergic reaction in the sensitive.

PARSLEY SEED OIL • *See* Parsley Oil.

PASQUE FLOWER • *Anemone pulsatilla.* A low, perennial herb with white or purple flowers, it is used by herbalists to treat insomnia and other tension-induced conditions; it is also used to treat painful menstrual periods and painful conditions of the testes. The antibacterial effects are used by herbalists to treat skin infections and asthma.

PASSIFLORA • *See* Passionflower Extract.

PASSIONFLOWER EXTRACT • Extract of the various species of *Passiflora camata.* Indians used passionflower for swellings and sore eyes and to induce vomiting. It has been shown that an extract of the plant depresses the motor nerves of the spinal cord.

PATCHOULI OIL • Used in perfume formulations to impart a long-lasting oriental aroma in soaps and cosmetics. It is the essential oil obtained from the leaves of an East Indian shrubby mint, *Pogostemon cablin.* Yellowish to greenish brown liquid, with the pleasant fragrance of summer flowers. May produce allergic reactions.

PATHOGEN • Any microorganism causing disease.

PAULLINA CUPANA • *See* Guarana Extract.

PAULOWNIA • Chinese Emperor Tree. Skin care ingredient.

PAVONIA ODORATA • Balsam. A pubescent herb, the roots of which yield an essential oil that contains iso valeric acid, iso valeraldehyde, aromadendrene, pavonene, *a*-terpinene, azulene, and pavonenol. The roots are aromatic and possess astringent properties. Used to treat inflammations.

PAWPAW EXTRACT • Custard Apple. The extract of the fruit *Caraya papaya.* The dried and pulverized large brown seeds have been rubbed into the scalp to eradicate head lice. The fruit is rich in vitamins and minerals. If taken internally, it can cause vomiting.

PBT • Abbreviation for Persistent Bioaccumulative and Toxic or very Persistent and very Bioaccumlative (vPvB) according to European Chemicals Agency.

PCA • Pyrrolidone Carboxylic Acid. Employed in the manufacture of polyvinylpyrrolidone (*see*), which goes into hair sprays. Also a high boiling solvent in petroleum processing, and a plasticizer and coalescing ingredient for floor polishes. On the basis of the animal and clinical data, the CIR Expert Panel (*see*) concluded that it is safe as used in cosmetic formulations but should not be used in products containing nitrosating (*see*) ingredients.

PDB • Crystals made from chlorine and benzene, they have a penetrating odor, are almost insoluble in water, and are noncorrosive and nonstaining. A solvent for many organic materials, it is employed in degreasing hides and wool, metal polishes, moth repellents, general insecticides, germicides, spray deodorants, and fumigants. PDB is commonly found in room deodorizers and moth-killing products. Vapors may cause irritation to the skin, throat, and eyes, and prolonged exposure to high concentrations may cause weakness, dizziness, loss of weight, and liver damage. A well-known animal cancer-causing ingredient, the chemical can linger in the home for months or even years after use. Toxic by ingestion and inhalation, and it is irritating to mucous membranes. You can lessen your exposure to it by reading product labels and avoiding preparations that contain it (not all labels list it).

PEA EXTRACT • The extract of *Pisum sativum. See* Pea Palmitate.

PEA PALMITATE • The compound obtained by crushing peas with palmitic acid chloride. Used as a skin conditioner.

PEACH EXTRACT • *Prunus persica. See* Peach Juice Extract.

PEACH JUICE EXTRACT • The liquid obtained from the pulp of the peach, *Prunus persica*. It is used as a natural flavoring and as an emollient.

PEACH KERNEL OIL • Persic Oil. Used as an oil base in emollients, eyelash creams, and brilliantines. It is a light yellow liquid expressed from a seed. Smells like almonds. Also a flavoring in foods.

PEACH PIT POWDER • The powder obtained by grinding the pits of *Prunus persica*. It is used as an exfoliant (*see*).

PEANUT • *Arachis hypogaea*. Widely used in cosmetics as an abrasive, thickener, and skin conditioner in body and hand products, cleansing lotions, hair conditioners, and lipsticks.

PEANUT ACID • Used as a surfactant and cleansing ingredient.

PEANUT GLYCERIDES • A mixture of glycerides (*see*) derived from peanut oil (*see*).

PEANUT OIL • *Arachis* Oil. Used in the manufacture of soaps, baby preparations, hair-grooming aids, nail dryers, shampoos, and as a solvent for ointments and liniments; also in night creams and emollients. A solvent in salad oil, shortening, mayonnaise, and confections. Also used in conjunction with natural flavorings. Peanut butter is about 50 percent peanut oil suspended in peanut fibers. Greenish yellow, with a pleasant odor. Prepared by pressing shelled and skinned seeds of the peanut. It is used as a substitute for almond and olive oils in cosmetic creams, brilliantines, antiwrinkle oils, and sunburn preparations. Has been reported to be a mild irritant in soap but is considered harmless to the skin.

PEANUTAMIDE • A mixture of the ethanolamines (*see*) of the fatty acids derived from peanuts. Used as a thickener and foam booster.

PEANUTAMIDE MEA • Loramine Wax. *See* Peanut Oil.

PEANUTAMIDE MIPA • A mixture of isopropanol amides of the fatty acids derived from peanut oil (*see*).

PEAR EXTRACT • The extract of the fruit of *Pyrus communis*. Used in facial masks and bath salts, shampoos, and lip gloss.

PEARL ESSENCE • Guanine. A suspension of crystalline guanine (*see*) in nitrocellulose (*see*) and solvents. Guanine is obtained from fish scales. Used in nail polish to give it a shine. Implants of small amounts of guanine hydrochloride were lethal in mice.

PEARL POWDER • The dried powder obtained from freshwater pearls. Used to add shine to lipsticks and powders.

PEARLS • *See* Mica.

PEARLY EVERLASTING • *Anaphalis margarotacea*. An American everlasting having floccose-woolly herbage and small corymbose heads with pearly white whorls. Used in "organic" cosmetics.

PEAT • Decayed vegetable matter found in marshy or damp regions used as an anti-acne ingredient.

PECAN SHELL POWDER • From *Carya illinoinensis* shells. A coloring ingredient used in cosmetics. Employed medicinally by the American Indians. It is the nut from a hickory of the southern central United States with a rough bark and hard but brittle wood. Edible.

PECTIN • Found in roots, stems, and fruits, this soluble fiber forms an integral part of such plant structures. The richest sources of pectin are lemon and orange rind. Emulsifying ingredient used in place of various gums in toothpastes, hair-setting lotions, and protective creams. The pectins are found in roots, stems, and fruits of plants and form an integral part of such structures. They are used in cosmetics as a gelling and thickening ingredient. They are soothing and mildly acidic. Also used in foods as a "cementing ingredient" and as an antidiarrheal medication.

PED- • The Latin root means "foot," as in *pedal*. The Greek root refers to children, as in *pediatrics*.

PEG • Abbreviation for polyethylene glycol/polyethylene, used in making nonionic surfactants. The low molecular polyethylene glycols from 200 to 400 may cause hives and eczema. The higher polyethylenes are not sensitizers. *See* Surfactants and Nonionic.

PEG-4, -6, -8, -9, -10, -12, -14, -16, -18, -32, -40, -150, -200, -350 • Polymers (*see*) of ethylene oxide. Usually a waxy compound. The number refers to the liquidity; the higher the number, the harder the composition. The FDA says that solvents identifiable by PEG, polyethylene, polyethylene glycol, -eth-, or -oxynol-, may be contaminated with 1,4-dioxane, a cancer-causing agent. It can be removed by the manufacturer "without an unreasonable increase in raw material cost." Most are emulsifiers.

PEG-8 CAPRATE • The polyethylene glycol ester of capric acid. *See* Capric Acid and Polyethylene Glycol.

PEG-9 CAPRYLATE • The polyethylene glycol ester of caprylic acid (*see*).

PEG-8 CAPRYLATE/CAPRATE • The polyethylene glycol ester of a mixture of caprylic and capric acids (*see all*).

PEG-6 CAPRYLIC/CAPRIC GLYCERIDES • The ethoxylated glycerides of caprylic and capric acid derivatives. *See* Caprylic Acid, Capric Acid, and Glycerides.

PEG-3 TO -200 CASTOR OIL • Widely used in cosmetics for many applications including emollients, surfactants, skin and hair conditioning, and makeup. The polyethylene glycol derivative of castor oil (*see*). The higher the number after the listing, the more solid the compound. *See* Polyethylene Glycol.

PEG-3 TO -11 COCAMIDE • The polyethylene glycol amides of coconut acid. The higher the number, the more solid the compound. Used as emulsifiers. *See* Polyethylene Glycol and Coconut Oil.

PEG-2 TO -15 COCAMINE • The polyethylene glycol amines of coconut acid. The higher the number, the harder the compound.

PEG-5, -8 OR -15 COCOATE • The polyethylene glycol esters of coconut acid. The lower the number, the more liquid the compound. *See* Polyethylene Glycol and Coconut Oil.

PEG-2 OR -15 COCOMONIUM CHLORIDE • *See* Quaternary Ammonium Compounds.

PEG-15 COCOPOLYAMINE • The polyethylene glycol polyamine and coconut acid. *See* Polyethylene Glycol and Coconut Oil.

PEG-4 THROUGH -150 DILAURATE • The polyethylene glycol diesters of lauric acid (*see*). The higher the number, the more solid the compound. *See also* Polyethylene Glycol.

PEG-6 TO -150 DIOLEATE • The polyethylene glycol diesters of oleic acid (*see*). The lower the number, the more liquid the compound. *See* Polyethylene Glycol.

PEG-3 DIPALMITATE • The polyethylene glycol diester of palmitic acid (*see*).

PEG-2 THROUGH -175 DISTEARATE • The polyethylene glycol diesters of stearic acid. The higher the number, the more solid the compound. *See* Stearic Acid and Polyethylene Glycol.

PEG-8 OR -12 DITALLATE • The polyethylene glycol diesters of tall oil (*see*).

PEG-8 DITRIRICINOLEATE • *See* Ricinoleic Acid and Polyethylene Glycol.

PEG-22 OR -45 DODECYL GLYCOL COPOLYMERS • *See* Polyethylene Glycol.

PEG-7 OR -30 GLYCERYL COCOATE • The polyethylene glycol ethers of glyceryl cocoate. *See* Coconut Oil.

PEG-15 OR -20 GLYCERYL RICINOLEATE • The polyethylene glycol ether of glyceryl ricinoleate. The number signifies the liquidity of the compound. *See* Polyethylene Glycol and Castor Oil.

PEG-5 THROUGH -120 GLYCERYL STEARATE • *See* Polyethylene Glycol and Stearic Acid.

PEG-28 GLYCERYL TALLOWATE • *See* Tallow Glycerides and Polyethylene Glycol.

PEG-25 GLYCERYL TRIOLEATE • *See* Oleic Acid and Polyethylene Glycol.

PEG-5 THROUGH -200 HYDROGENATED CASTOR OIL • *See* Polyethylene Glycol and Castor Oil.

PEG-5 HYDROGENATED CORN GLYCERIDES • The polyethylene glycol derivative of mixed glycerides derived from hydrogenated corn oil. *See* Hydrogenation and Corn Oil.

PEG-8 HYDROGENATED FISH GLYCERIDES • The polyethylene glycol derivative of hydrogenated fish glycerides. *See* Hydrogenation and Fish Oil.

PEG-5 THROUGH -70 HYDROGENATED LANOLIN • The polyethylene glycol derivative of hydrogenated lanolin. The higher the number, the more solid the compound. *See* Polyethylene Glycol and Lanolin.

PEG-13 HYDROGENATED TALLOW AMIDE • *See* Polyethylene Glycol and Tallow.

PEG-6 THROUGH -10 ISOLAURYL THIOETHER • The polyethylene glycol ether of dodecyl mercaptan. The number signifies liquidity. *See* Polyethylene Glycol and Lauryl Alcohol.

PEG-6 OR -12 ISOSTEARATE • The polyethylene glycol ester of isostearic acid. *See* Polyethylene Glycol and Stearic Acid.

PEG-5 TO -20 LANOLATE • *See* Lanolin.

PEG-5 THROUGH -100 LANOLIN • The polyethylene glycol derivative of lanolin. The number signifies liquidity. Widely used in cosmetics. *See* Lanolin.

PEG-75 LANOLIN OIL AND WAX • *See* Lanolin.

PEG-3 TO -6 LAURAMIDE • The polyethylene glycol amide of lauric acid (*see*).

PEG-3 LAURAMINE OXIDE • *See* Lauric Acid.

PEG-LAURATE (2 THROUGH 150) • The polyethylene glycol esters of lauric acid. The number signifies liquidity. Yellow, oily liquid insoluble in water. Widely used in soaps and detergents. Emulsifier in cosmetic creams and lotions. Gives an oil-in-water emulsion. Nontoxic. May cause allergic reactions in some persons sensitive to laurates. *See* Lauric Acid.

PEG-6 METHYL ETHER • *See* Methanol.

PEG-20 METHYL GLUCOSE SESQUISTEARATE • A mixture of polyethylene glycol monoesters and diesters of methyl glucose and stearic acid (*see all*).

PEG-2 MILK SOLIDS • *See* Milk and Polyethylene Glycol.

PEG-4 OCTANOATE • The polyethylene glycol ester of caprylic acid (*see*).

PEG-2 THROUGH -9 OLEAMIDE • The polyethylene glycol amide of oleic acid (*see*). Widely used as a stabilizer and plasticizer.

PEG-2 THROUGH -30 OLEAMINE • The polyethylene glycol amine of oleic acid (*see*). Widely used in vanishing creams, soft soaps, cold creams, and many other cosmetics.

PEG-2 OLEAMONIUM CHLORIDE • *See* Quaternary Ammonium Compounds.

PEG-12, -20, OR -30 OLEATE • The polyethylene glycol ether of glyceryl oleate. *See* Polyethylene Glycol and Glycerin.

PEG-3 THROUGH -150 OLEATE • The polyethylene glycol esters of oleic acid (*see*). Widely used in cosmetic bases and shampoos. Emulsifying ingredient in creams and lotions. A dark red oil that can be dispersed in water; soluble in alcohol and miscible with cottonseed oil.

PEG-6 THROUGH -20 PALMITATE • The polyethylene glycol esters of palmitic acid (*see*).

PEG-8 PALMITOYL METHYL DIETHONIUM METHOSULFATE • *See* Quaternary Ammonium Compounds.

PEG-5 PENTAERYTHRITOL ETHER • The polyethylene glycol ether of pentaerythritol that is used as a plasticizer and synthetic lubricant. *See* Formaldehyde and Acetaldehyde.

PEG/PPG-17/6 OR 18/4 OR 23/50 OR 35/9 OR 125/30 COPOLYMERS • The copolymers produced by the interaction of ethylene oxide with propylene oxide. Used as plasticizers and bases for cosmetics. *See* Ethylene Oxide and Propylene Glycol.

PEG-8 PROPYLENE GLYCOL COCOATE • The polyethylene glycol ether of polyethylene glycol cocoate derived from coconut acid (*see*) and used as an emulsifier.

PEG-25 THROUGH -125 PROPYLENE GLYCOL STEARATE • *See* Stearic Acid.

PEG-2 OR -7 RICINOLEATE • The polyethylene glycol esters of ricinoleic acid (*see*).

PEG-8 SESQUILAURATE • The mixture of polyethylene glycol mono- and diesters of lauric acid with ethylene oxide. *See* Lauric Acid.

PEG-8 SESQUIOLEATE • The mixture of polyethylene glycol mono- and diesters of oleic acid with ethylene oxide. *See* Oleic Acid.

PEG-6, -8, -20 SORBITAN BEESWAX • The ethoxylated sorbitol derivative of beeswax with ethylene oxide. *See* Sorbitol and Beeswax.

PEG-5 OR -20 SORBITAN ISOSTEARATE • The ethoxylated sorbitol monoester of isostearic acid and ethylene oxide. *See* Sorbitol and Stearic Acid.

PEG-40 OR -75 OR -80 SORBITAN LANOLATE • The ethoxylated sorbitol derivative of lanolin and ethylene oxide of 40, 75, or 80 molecules. *See* Lanolin and Sorbitol.

PEG-3 OR -6 SORBITAN OLEATE • The ethoxylated sorbitan ester of oleic acid. *See* Oleic Acid and Sorbitan.

PEG-80 SORBITAN PALMITATE • The ethoxylated sorbitol monoester of palmitic acid (*see*).

PEG-40 SORBITAN PEROLEATE • The mixture of oleic acid esters of sorbitol. *See* Sorbitol and Oleic Acid.

PEG-3 OR -40 SORBITAN STEARATE • *See* Sorbitol and Stearic Acid.

PEG-30, -40, OR -60 SORBITAN TETRAOLEATE • *See* Oleic Acid and Sorbitol.

PEG-60 SORBITAN TETRASTEARATE • *See* Stearic Acid and Sorbitol.

PEG-2 TO -15 SOYAMINE • *See* Polyethylene Glycol and Soy Acid.

PEG-SOYA STEROLS • *See* Soybean Oil and Polyethylene Glycol.

PEG-2 THROUGH -150 STEARATE • Widely used emulsifying ingredients. On the basis of the available information the CIR Expert Panel (*see*) found it safe in the early 1980s but is considering new information to determine if the final safety assessment should be reaffirmed, amended, or have an addendum. *See* Polyethylene Glycol and Stearic Acid.

PEG-2 OR -15 STEARMONIUM CHLORIDE • *See* Quaternary Ammonium Compounds.

PEG-5 STEARYL AMMONIUM CHLORIDE • *See* Quaternary Ammonium Compounds.

PEG-12 OR -20 TALLATE • *See* Polyethylene Glycol and Tall Oil.

PEG-2 THROUGH -50 TALLOW AMINE • *See* Tallow and Polyglycerol.

PEG-3, -10, OR -15 TALLOW AMINOPROPYLAMINE • *See* Polyethylene Glycol and Tallow.

PEG-15 TALLOW POLYAMINE • *See* Tallow.

PEG-20 TALLOWATE • *See* Polyethylene Glycol and Tallow.

PEG-66 OR -200 TRIHYDROXYSTEARIN • *See* Surfactants.

PEI • Abbreviation for polyethylenimine.

PEI-7 • Polyethylenimine 7. Highly viscous liquid used as an adhesive or anchoring ingredient for cellophane and as a disinfectant for the skin. Also used in water purification.

PEI-15 THROUGH -2500 • *See* PEI-7.

PELARGONIC ACID • Nonanoic Acid. A synthetic flavoring ingredient that occurs naturally in cocoa and oil of lavender. Used in berry, fruit, nut, and spice flavorings. A strong irritant.

PELARGONIUM CAPITATUM • Fragrance ingredient. *See* Rose Geranium.

PELLIS LIPIDA • Skin fats.

PELLITORY EXTRACT • Extract of Pellitory. Parietary Extract. The extract obtained from the leaves and stem of *Parietaria officinalis*. Used as an emollient, particularly in baby creams and lotions.

PELVETIA CANALICULATA • A family of rockweed. *See* Bladder Wrack Extract.

PENGAWAR DJAMBI OIL • Oil obtained from a variety of ferns of the family Cyatheaceae. Used in emollients.

PENICILLINS • A group of beta-lactam antibiotics produced by several species of mold and/or semisynthetically. There are many kinds, and they offer a broad clinical spectrum of activity. They act by inhibiting bacterial enzymes involved in the making of cell walls. Used topically, they may cause skin rash.

PENNYROYAL EXTRACT • An extract of the flowering herb *Mentha pulegium*. Used since ancient days as a medicine, scent, flavoring, and food. Obtained from the dried flower tops and leaves, it contains tannin, which is soothing to the skin. The oil is applied externally to repel flying insects, but it must not be taken internally. Brain damage has been reported following doses of less than 1 teaspoon.

PENTA- • A prefix meaning containing five atoms or groups.

PENTADECALACTONE • Angelica Lactone. Used as a cosmetic fragrance and in berry, fruit, and liquor flavorings. It is obtained from the fruit and root of a plant grown in Europe and Asia.

PENTADECYL ALCOHOL • Pentanol. Used as an emulsifier and emollient.

PENTADESMA BUTTER • Kanya Butter. The vegetable fat extracted from the nut of *Pentadesma butyracea*. *See* Shea Butter.

PENTADIPLANDRA BRAZZEANA • Used in African folk medicine to heal wounds and as a stimulant. Used in cosmetics as a skin conditioner.

PENTADOXYNOL-200 • A surfactant and cleansing ingredient used in underarm deodorants. *See* Phenols and Polyethylene Glycol.

PENTAERYTHRITOL • Skin conditioner prepared from acetaldehyde and formaldehyde (*see both*). It is used in synthetic resins. Potential symptoms of overexposure are skin, eye, and respiratory irritation.

PENTAERYTHRITOL HYDROGENATED ROSINATE • The ester of acids derived from hydrogenated rosin (*see*) mixed with pentaerythritol (*see*).

PENTAERYTHRITYL ROSINATE • The ester of acids derived from rosin (*see*) mixed with pentaerythritol (*see*). It is used as a skin-conditioning ingredient and a thickener. The CIR Expert Panel (*see*) concluded that the data available are insufficient to support the safety of this ingredient as used in cosmetic products.

PENTAERYTHRITYL STEARATE/CAPRATE/CAPRYLATE ADIPATE • The mixed ester (*see*) of pentaerythritol and stearic, capric, caprylic, and adipic acids. Used as emulsifiers.

PENTAERYTHRITYL TETRAABIETATE • *See* Pentaerythritol and Abietic Acid.

PENTAERYTHRITYL TETRABEHENATE • The ester of pentaerythritol and behenic acid (*see both*).

PENTAERYTHRITYL TETRAOCTANOATE • *See* Caprylic Acid.

PENTAERYTHRITYL TETRAOLEATE • The ester of pentaerythritol and oleic acid (*see both*).

PENTAERYTHRITYL TETRASTEARATE AND CALCIUM STEARATE • *See* Stearic Acid.

PENTAERYTHRITYL TRIOLEATE • The ester of pentaerythritol and oleic acid (*see both*).

PENTAHYDROSQUALENE • The end product of hydrogenation (*see*) of squalene (*see*).

PENTAMETHYL-4,6-DINITROINDANE • *See* Moskene.

PENTANE • Derived from petroleum. Used as a solvent and propellant in hair sprays and shaving cream. Narcotic in high doses.

PENTANOIC ACID • Occurs naturally in apples, cocoa, coffee, oil of lavender, peaches, and strawberries. A synthetic flavoring additive used in butter, butterscotch, fruit, rum, and cheese flavorings for beverages, ice cream, ices, candy, and baked goods. Colorless, with an unpleasant odor. Usually distilled from valerian root. Some of its salts are used in medicine. A colorless, liquid organic acid that occurs in four isomeric forms and has a disagreeable odor. It occurs naturally in oils from certain marine animals and plants, and is used in flavorings, perfumes, plasticizers, and pharmaceuticals. Also used in peeling solutions for fruits and vegetables. Moderately toxic by ingestion. A corrosive irritant to skin, eyes, and mucous membranes. ASP

1-PENTANOL • Pentyl Alcohol. *n*-Amyl Alcohol. Liquid with a mild odor, slightly soluble in water. Used as a solvent. Irritating to the eyes and respiratory passages, and absorption may cause a lack of oxygen in the blood.

PENTAPEPTIDE-1 • Protein derivative used in skin conditioners.

PENTAPOTASSIUM TRIPHOSPHATE • *See* Pentasodium Pentetate.

PENTASODIUM AMINOTRIMETHYLENE PHOSPHONATE • An emulsifier. *See* Phosphoric Acid and Pentasodium Pentetate.

PENTASODIUM PENTETATE • Pentasodium Diethylenetriaminepentaacetate. Sodium Tripolyphosphate. Prepared from dehydration of mono- and disodium phosphates. An inorganic salt used as a water softener, sequestering ingredient (*see*), emulsifier, and dispersing ingredient in cosmetic cleansing creams and lotions. Moderately irritating to the skin and mucous membranes. Ingestion can cause violent purging.

PENTETIC ACID • Penthanil. Diethylenetriaminepentaacetic Acid. A chelating ingredient (*see*) to remove iron particles floating in cosmetic solutions.

PENTYL DIMETHYL PABA • The ester of pentyl alcohol and dimethyl *p* aminobenzoic acid. Used as a preservative. On the Canadian Hotlist (*see*). *See* Parabens.

PEONY • *Paeonia lactiflora.* Shao-yao. The root is used by herbalists as a liver tonic. It is also used to treat all female complaints, especially menstrual irregularity and abdominal pains associated with the menstrual cycle. Contraindicated in pregnancy. Externally, it has been used to treat wounds and skin growths. Peony is toxic when used internally in excessive doses. It is used in "organic" cosmetics.

PEPPER OIL, BLACK • A pungent oil obtained from the dried, unripe berries of the East Indian pepper plant, *Piper nigrum.* Used in flavorings. Pepper was formerly used as a carminative to break up intestinal gas and cause sweating, and as a gastric ingredient to promote gastric secretion.

PEPPERMINT • *Mentha piperita.* Brandy Mint. The oil made from the dried leaves and tops of a plant common to Asian, European, and American gardens. Peppermint is used as a flavoring in many products. In medicine, it has been used as far back as recorded history to treat indigestion and to calm spasm of the bowel. It relaxes the stomach muscles, herbalists say, and promotes burping. Modern researchers have found that peppermint contains antiulcer, anti-inflammatory, and liver bile–stimulating agents. Peppermint can also inhibit the growth of many kinds of germs. It can, however, cause allergic reactions such as hay fever and rash. In 1992, the FDA issued a notice that peppermint and peppermint spirit have not been shown to be safe and effective as claimed in OTC digestive aid products, insect bite and sting drug products, oral menstrual drug products, and in astringent.

PEPPERMINT EXTRACT • *See* Peppermint Oil.

PEPPERMINT LEAVES • *See* Peppermint Oil.

PEPPERMINT OIL • Used in toothpaste and tooth powders, eye lotions, shaving lotions, and toilet waters. It is the oil made from the dried leaves and tops of a plant common to Asian, European, and American gardens, *Mentha piperita.* Widely used as a flavoring. Can cause allergic reactions such as hay fever and skin rash.

PEPSIN • Digestive enzyme found in gastric juice that helps break down protein. Used in hair conditioners. The pepsin product used to aid digestion is obtained from the glandular layer of the fresh stomach of a hog. In 1992, the FDA proposed a ban on pepsin in oral menstrual drug products because it has not been shown to be safe and effective for its stated claims. Used as a hair- and skin-conditioning ingredient in cosmetics.

PEPTIDASES • Enzymes that cleave peptides (*see*).

PEPTIDE • Two or more amino acids chained together in head-to-tail links. Generally larger than simple amino acids or the monoamines, the largest peptides discovered thus far have forty-four amino acids. Neuropeptides signal the body's endocrine glands to balance salt and water. Opiate peptides can help control pain. The peptides work with amino acids. Peptides are really a hot subject in cosmetics, particularly in the field of products for aging skin. At this writing, another peptide compound is seeking a patent. It has the property of activating the melanogenesis and being an anti-inflammatory and acting more efficiently than other cosmetic creams for such purposes as lightening or darkening the skin.

PEPTIDE PAL-KTTKS • A patented protein, one of the newest ingredients at this writing said to counteract wrinkles. Most of the research has been done in France, and some U.S. dermatologists believe it has collagen-promoting activity. Others say that it cannot enter the skin deeply enough to have an effect.

PEPTONES • Secondary protein derivatives formed during the process of digestion— the result of the action of the gastric and pancreatic juices upon protein. In cosmetics, they are used in fermentation and to increase protein.

PERCUTANEOUS • Movement through or into the skin.

PERFLUOROCAPRYL BROMIDE • A solvent. *See* Bromides, Potassium and Sodium.

PERFLUORODECALIN • Solvent and skin-conditioning ingredient. *See* Naphthalene.

PERFLUORONONYL DIMETHICONE • A synthetic polymer (*see*) used as a skin-conditioning ingredient and occlusive. *See* Dimethicone.

PERFLUORODIMETHYLCYCLOHEXANE • A solvent. *See* Paraffin.

PERFLUOROPERHYDROPHENANTHRENE • A solvent and skin-conditioning ingredient and coloring.

PERFLUOROPOLYMETHYLISOPROPYL ETHER • A skin conditioner. *See* Fluorine Compounds and Polymer.

PERFUMES • Literally means "through smoke" because the first perfumes were incense. Thereafter, powdered flowers, leaves, wood spices, and aromatic resins were used for fragrances during religious festivals, for the home, and for the body. Some perfumes have as many as two hundred ingredients. The essential oils used for today's scents come from leaves, needles, roots, and peels of plants. Floral oils come from petals, whole flowers, gums, and resins. Animal exudates such as musk and ambergris are all used in perfumes. Isolates used in perfumes are made of individual factors in natural oils, which may also be treated chemically. Synthetic chemicals imitate natural aromas and are being used in increasing quantities today. There are four basic scents today: florals, fruits, and modern blends such as woodsy-mossy-leafy-spicy and oriental. Woodsy-mossy-leafy types have a warm aromatic scent with sandalwood, cedar wood, and balsam predominating. Orientals have subtly heavier odors. Fruity perfumes have a clean fresh fragrance. A typical basic flower perfume (rose) would include phenylethyl alcohol, 35 percent; geraniol, 48 percent; amyl cinnamaldehyde, 2 percent; benzyl acetate, 4 percent; ionone, 4 percent; eugenol, 2 percent; and terpineol, 5 percent. Perfumes are among the most frequent allergens and are left out of many hypoallergenic products. Complaints to the FDA concerning perfumes include headaches, dizziness, rash, hyperpigmentation (*see* Berloque Dermatitis), violent coughing and vomiting, skin irritation, and the explosion of the perfume container.

PERHYDROSQUALENE • *See* Squalene.

PERILLA • An Asiatic mint. Yields a dark purple coloring. Used as a skin conditioner.

PERIWINKLE EXTRACT • The extract of *Vinca minor*. *See* Myrtle.

PERLITE • Produced from natural volcanic rock and has a high surface area, high water absorption, high whiteness, and is chemically inert and lightweight, making it a good filler and extender. Absorbent, thickener, and suspending ingredient. It is also used in perfumed paper.

PERMANENT LISTING • Signifies that the FDA is convinced that a dye is safe to use as it is now employed in food, drug(s), and/or cosmetic(s). Some colorings that have been permanently listed in the past have been removed from the market because they cause cancer or unfavorable reactions.

PERMANENT WAVE NEUTRALIZER • Used to neutralize the acids that curl the hair (see Permanent Waves). May contain sodium perborate, bromates, or sodium hexylmetaphosphate (*see all*). Before 1940, bromate poisoning was rare, but when bromate was put into permanent wave neutralizers for home use, incidents became more common. Many manufacturers then substituted sodium perborate and sodium hexylmetaphosphate, a product used as a laundry detergent and in water softeners.

PERMANENT WAVES • Cold Waves. Chemicals designed to "permanently" bend or curl the hair. Once done only in beauty parlors, kits have been developed for home use. The process in both the beauty parlor and at home consists of applying a waving lotion containing thioglycolic acid, ammonia, and 93 percent water, as well as borax, ethanolamine, or sodium lauryl sulfate (*see all*). Then, after a period of time, depending upon the lotion used and the tightness of the curl desired, a neutralizer is applied. Chemicals in the neutralizer may be sodium or potassium bromate, sodium perborate, or hydrogen peroxide (see Permanent Wave Neutralizer). The thioglycolates are toxic and may cause skin irritation and low blood sugar. Among the injuries reported to the FDA were hair damage; swelling of legs and feet; eye irritations; rash in the area of the ears, neck, scalp, and forehead; and swelling of the eyelids.

PERMETHRIN • NIX. Pesticide. Used in preparations for the treatment of head lice and nits. It is used after hair has been washed with shampoo, rinsed with water, and towel dried. Potential adverse reactions include itching, burning, stinging, tingling, numbness or scalp discomfort, and mild redness or rash on the scalp. Contraindicated in patients hypersensitive to pyrethrins or chrysanthemums. Do not use on infants because their skin is more absorbent than that of children or adults.

PEROXIDE • Used in hair bleaches. It is a strong oxidant and can injure the skin and eyes. Chemists are cautioned to wear rubber gloves and goggles when handling it. May cause hair breakage and is an irritant. On the Canadian Hotlist (*see*). Canada Health says the quantity of peroxide release from an oral cosmetic must at no time cause the saliva or soft tissue of the oral cavity to exceed a concentration of 3 percent hydrogen peroxide. *See* Hydrogen Peroxide.

PERSEA GRATISSIMA • On the basis of the available information, the CIR Expert Panel (*see*) found it safe in the early 1980s but is considering new information to determine if the final safety assessment should be reaffirmed, amended, or have an addendum. *See* Avocado.

PERSIC OIL • *See* Apricot and Peach Kernel Oil.

PERSIMMON • *Diospyros kaki.* A medium-size tree that grows in the southern and eastern United States. Has a hard wood and greenish yellow or greenish white bell-shaped flowers followed by an orange to red berry that is edible. Used as a wax in cosmetics.

PERSULFATES • Ammonium. Potassium. Sodium. Salts derived from persulfuric acid, a strong oxidizer. Persulfates are excellent catalysts that speed hair color changes in hair dye. Has reportedly been linked to asthma in hairdressers. *See* Hydrogen Peroxide for toxicity.

PERUVIAN BALSAM • A dark brown, thick liquid with a pleasant, lingering odor, it is obtained in Central America near the Pacific Coast. An ingredient of topical treatments for hemorrhoids, and anti-inflammatory ointments and powders. Used in Balmex Baby Powder and Ointment, it is mildly antiseptic. May be irritating to the skin and cause contact dermatitis, and a stuffy nose. One of the most common sensitizers, it may cross-react with benzoin, benzoic acid, rosin, cinnamic acid, orange peel, and wood tars, among others. *See* Balsam Peru.

PETASITES HYBRIDUS • Butterbur. An herb that is native to temperate climates. Has a thick root and leaves that reputedly possess medicinal powers similar to coltsfoot (*see*).

PETECHIAE • Minute blood spots in the skin.

PETITGRAIN OIL • Used extensively in perfumes. It is the volatile oil obtained from the leaves, twigs, and unripe fruit of the bitter orange tree. Brownish to yellow with a bittersweet odor. Used in food flavorings. Supposedly dissolves in sweat, and under the influence of sunlight becomes an irritant. May cause allergic skin reactions.

PETROLATUM • Vaseline. Petroleum Jelly. Paraffin Jelly. Used in cold creams, emollient creams, conditioning creams, wax depilatories, eyebrow pencils, eye shadows, liquefying creams, liquid powders, nail whites, lipsticks, protective creams, baby creams, and rouge. It is a purified mixture of semisolid hydrocarbons from petroleum. Yellowish to light amber or white, semisolid unctuous mass, practically odorless and tasteless, almost insoluble in water. As a lubricant in lipsticks, it gives them a shine, and it makes creams smoother. Helps to soften and smooth the skin in the same way as any other emollient and is less expensive. The oily film helps prevent evaporation of moisture from the skin and protects the skin from irritation. However, petrolatum does cause allergic skin reactions in the hypersensitive.

PETROLEUM DISTILLATES • Hydrocarbons, Naphtha, Waxes. Condensations of a highly complex mixture of paraffinic, naphthalenic, and aromatic hydrocarbons containing some sulfur and trace amounts of nitrogen and oxygen compounds. Believed to have originated from both plant and animal sources millions of years ago. When petroleum is cracked into fractions, the gases butane, ethane, and propane, as well as naphtha, gasoline, kerosene, fuel oils, gas oil, lubricating oils, paraffin wax, and asphalt are obtained. A defoaming ingredient and a solvent for fats, oils, and detergents in cosmetics. Formerly used for bronchitis and tapeworm, and externally for arthritis and skin problems. Many petroleum products are reported to be cancer-causing ingredients. Others, presumably those used in food and cosmetics, are inert. The CIR Expert Panel (*see*) concluded that these are safe as cosmetic ingredients as currently used. *See* Kerosene for toxicity.

PEUCEDANUM GRAVEOLENS • *See* Dill.

PFAFFIA PANICULATA EXTRACT • Brazilian Ginseng. Suma. Found in the tropics, the root of this shrub is said to contain anabolic, analgesic, anticancerous, anti-inflammatory, antileukemic, antimutagenic, antiproliferative, antitumorous, aphrodisiac, estrogenic, hypocholesterolemic, immuno stimulant, nutritive, sedative, steroidal, and tonic properties. It has been used for three hundred years as an aphrodisiac by natives.

PG • Abbreviation for propylene glycol (*see*).

PG-HYDROXYETHYLCELLULOSE COCODIMONIUM • A quaternary ammonium compound (*see*) used as an antistatic ingredient in hair products. *See* Coconut Oil.

pH • The scale used to measure acidity and alkalinity. pH is the hydrogen (H) ion concentration of a solution; "p" stands for the power factor of the hydrogen ion. The pH of a solution is measured on a scale of 14. A truly neutral solution, neither acidic nor alkaline, such as water, is 7. Acid is less than 7; alkaline is more than 7. The pH of blood is 7.3; vinegar is 3.1; lemon juice is 2.3; and lye is 13. Skin and hair are naturally acidic. Soap and detergents are alkaline.

PHA • Abbreviation for polyhydroxy acids (*see*).

PHAEODACTYLUM TRICORNUTUM • Phytoplankton that has anti-inflammatory and analgesic properties according to recent studies. Used as a skin-conditioning ingredient.

PHALAENOPSIS AMABILIS EXTRACT • Used as a skin conditioner and humectant. *See* Orchid.

PHASEOLUS • Thickener. *See* Green Bean Extract and Kidney Bean Extract.

PHATIDYLCHOLINE • Fatty acids used in skin conditioners and emulsifiers. *See* Lecithin.

PHELLODENDRON • Oubaku. A family of aromatic trees of Eastern Asia that have greenish yellow flowers. Used in Eastern medicine to treat boils, carbuncles, and eczema. It is usually pounded with talc.

PHENACETIN • Acetophenetidin. Obtained from phenol and salicylic acid (*see both*). Slightly bitter, crystalline powder, used in sunscreen lotions and soothing creams. Used medicinally as an analgesic and antifever ingredient. Less toxic than acetanilid (*see*), but may cause kidney damage in prolonged and excessive internal doses.

PHENETH-6 PHOSPHATE • A surfactant (*see*). *See* Phosphorous.

PHENETHYL ACETATE • A fragrance ingredient. *See* Acetic Acid.

PHENETHYL ALCOHOL • 2-Phenylethyanol. Used as a floral scent in rose perfumes and as a preservative in cosmetics. It occurs naturally in oranges, raspberries, and tea. Used in synthetic fruit flavorings. In some studies it was found to cause birth defects in rats. It was not shown to be an irritant or sensitizer in humans. The CIR Expert Panel (*see*) concludes that it is safe as a cosmetic ingredient as currently used.

PHENETHYL DIMETHICONE • Skin conditioner. See Siloxane and Silane.

***p*-PHENETIDINE** • Hair coloring. See *p*-Aminophenol.

PHENOLPHTHALEIN • Ex-Lax. Agoral. Alophen Pills. 3,3-Bis(4-hydroxyphenyl) phthalide Correctol Laxative. Dialose. Phillips' Lax Caps. Evac-U-Gen. Feen-A-Mint. Isoplus Neutralizing Shampoo. Elasta QP Conditioning Creme Texturizing Kit For Menhair. Luster's PCJ Pretty-n-Silky No-Lye Conditioning Cream Relaxerhair relaxer. Luster's PCJ Pretty-n-Silky No-Lye Conditioning Cream Relaxer Childrens Coarsehair relaxer. Luster's PCJ Pretty-N-Silky Smooth Roots No-Lye Conditioning New Growth Relaxer Kit, Childrens Coarsehair relaxer. Luster's Curl Comb Thru Texturizer, Extra Strength Toothpaste. One or more animal studies show broad systemic effects at moderate doses (low dose studies may be unavailable for this ingredient). Suspected cancer-causing agent and may have organ system toxicity (non-reproductive). Banned in cosmetics by ASEAN, the EU, and Canada. The FDA banned it in drugs.

PHENOLIC ACID • Tannins (*see*) found in many plants, including parsley, carrots, whole grains, and berries. It has antioxidant properties, affects enzyme activity, and inhibits formation of nitrosamine, a cancer-causing agent.

PHENOLS • Carbolic Acid. Used in shaving creams and hand lotions. Obtained from coal tar. Occurs in urine and has the characteristic odor present in coal tar and wood. It is a general disinfectant and anesthetic for the skin. Ingestion of even small amounts may cause nausea, vomiting, and circulatory collapse, paralysis, convulsions, coma, and greenish urine as well as necrosis of the mouth and gastrointestinal tract. Death results from respiratory failure. Fatalities have been reported from ingestion of as little as 1.5 grams (30 grams to the ounce). Fatal poisoning can occur through skin absorption. Although there have been many poisonings from phenolic solutions, it continues to be used in commercial products. A concentration of 1 percent used to prevent itching from insect bites and sunburn, applied for several hours, caused gangrene resulting from spasm of small blood vessels under the skin. Swelling, pimples, hives, and other skin rashes following application to the skin have been widely reported. A concentration of 2 percent causes gangrene, burning, and numbness. The EU says phenol and its alkali salts used in soaps and shampoos must be listed on the label.

PHENOXYACETIC ACID • A synthetic fruit and honey flavoring agent. Also used as a fungicide to soften calluses, corns, and other hard surfaces. A mild irritant.

PHENOXYETHANOL • 2-Phenoxyethanol. Oily liquid with a faint aromatic odor and a burning taste derived from treating phenol with ethylene oxide in an alkaline medium. Widely used as a fixative for perfumes, bactericide, insect repellent, and topical antiseptic. Also used as a fragrance. It is in many cosmetics, including hair sprays, bubble baths, eye lotions, skin and body preparations, makeup, makeup removers, and shampoos. Undiluted, it is a strong eye irritant but is not irritating when diluted at 2.2 percent. Has not been found to be a skin irritant or sensitizer. The CIR Expert Panel (*see*) concluded that it is safe as a cosmetic ingredient as currently used. *See* Phenols. E

PHENOXYETHYLPARABEN • Preservative. *See* Parabens.

PHENOXYISOPROPANOL • 1-Phenoxy-2-Propanol. *See* Phenols.

PHENOXYPROPAN-2-OL • Preservative. The EU restricts it to rinse-off products only. It's prohibited in oral hygiene products.

PHENYL ACETALDEHYDE • Used in perfumes. An oily, colorless liquid with a harsh odor. Upon dilution, emits the fragrance of lilacs and hyacinths. Derived from phenethyl alcohol. Less irritating than formaldehyde (*see*), but a stronger central nervous system depressant. In addition, it sometimes produces fluid in the lungs upon ingestion. Because it is considered an irritant, it is not used in cosmetic preparations for babies.

PHENYL ANTHRANILATES • *See* Coal Tar.

PHENYL BENZOATE • Used in fragrances. *See* Benzoic Acid.

PHENYL GLYCINE • *See* Glycine.

PHENYL MERCURIC ACETATE • Preservative containing mercury and is intended for use in the area of the eye. Toxic. It is on the Canadian Hotlist (*see*). *See* Mercury Compounds.

PHENYL MERCURIC BENZOATE • It is on the Canadian Hotlist (*see*). *See* Benzoic Acid and Mercury Compounds.

PHENYL MERCURIC BORATE • Crystalline powder. Soluble in water and alcohol. Local external antiseptic. Much less toxic than most mercury compounds. It is an allergen. Banned in Canada. *See* Borates and Mercury Compounds.

PHENYL MERCURIC BROMIDE • A preservative. *See* Bromides and Mercury Compounds.

PHENYL MERCURIC CHLORIDE • A preservative. *See* Mercury Compounds.

PHENYL MERCURIC OXIDE • A preservative. It is on the Canadian Hotlist (*see*). *See also* Mercury Compounds.

PHENYL METHICONE • An emollient. *See* Silicones.

PHENYL METHYL PYRAZOLONE • A white powder made from phenylhydrazine with ethyl acetoacetate used as an intermediate in hair dyes and plastics. The EU gave manufacturers to July 2005 to submit safety information or it will propose a ban. In 2006, the EU determined it can be used safely in hair dye. *See* Resorcinol and Pyrazole.

PHENYL PELARGONATE • A liquid, insoluble in water. Used in flavors, perfumes, bactericides, and fungicides. *See* Phenols.

***o*-PHENYLPHENOL** • White, flaky crystals with a mild characteristic odor. Prepared from phenyl ether. Practically insoluble in water. An intermediate in the manufacture of cosmetic resins. Also a germicide and fungicide in cosmetics. *See* Phenols for toxicity.

N-PHENYL-*p*-PHENYLENEDIAMINE • 4-Amino Diphenylamine. White crystals, very soluble in alcohol. Used in hair dyes. Intense skin irritation and blisters reported. Similar to other compounds of the group.

N-PHENYL-*p*-PHENYLENEDIAMINE HCL • White crystals, slightly soluble in water. A constituent of hair dyes. Derived from diphenolic acid (*see*). Probably of moderate toxicity, but reports of several skin rashes from its use have been described in the literature. It is thought to be less irritating than its parent compound.

PHENYL SALICYLATE • *See* Salicylates.

PHENYL THIOGLYCOLIC ACID • *See* Thioglycolic Acid Compounds.

PHENYL TRIMETHICONE • Methyl Phenyl Polysiloxane. Silicone oil used as a skin protectant and to give it gloss. It is treated to make it water repellent. The CIR Expert Panel (*see*) concluded that it is safe as a cosmetic ingredient as currently used. *See* Silicones.

PHENYLACETIC ACID • Used as a starting material in the manufacture of perfumes and soaps. Occurs naturally in Japanese mint, oil of neroli, and black pepper. It has a honeylike odor. Also used as a synthetic flavoring for foods and in the manufacture of penicillin.

PHENYLACETONITRILE • Banned in fragrances by the United Kingdom. *See* Cyanide.

PHENYLALANINE • An amino acid (*see*) considered essential for growth in normal human beings and not synthesized by the body. It is associated with phenylketonuria (PKU), an affliction that, if not detected soon after birth, leads to mental deterioration in children. Restricting phenylalanine in diets results in improvement. Whole egg contains 5.4 percent and skim milk 5.1 percent. Used to improve penetration of emollients. The FDA has asked for further study of this amino acid as a food additive. In cosmetics, it is used in hair conditioners.

PHENYLBENZIMIDAZOLE SULFONIC ACID • PBSA. Ensulizole. An ingredient in many sunscreens was reported by Irish researchers to damage DNA when exposed to sunlight in a test tube. The University of California studied human skin samples exposed to the above UV absorbers and UV light. They found that after one hour, the chemicals had sunk below the outer layer of the skin, greatly reducing their protective power. Even more worrying, the exposed skin samples contained more reactive oxygen (ROS). ROS are free radicals that damage cells and increase the risk of skin and other cancers. Because phenylbenzimidazole sulfonic acid is water-soluble, it has the characteristic of feeling lighter on skin. As such, it is often used in sunscreen lotions or moisturizers whose aesthetic goal is a non-greasy finish. The Japanese restrict its use. *See* Ensulizole.

PHENYLDIMETHICONE • A mixture of silica gels used in tanning creams and skin care products. *See* Dimethicone.

***m*-PHENYLENE DIAMINE SULFATE** • *See* Phenylenediamine.

***p*-PHENYLENE DIAMINE SULFATE** • *See* Phenylenediamine.

PHENYLENEDIAMINE, *m*-,*o*-,*p*- • Most home and beauty parlor permanent dyes contain this chemical or a related one such as 4-nitro-*o*-phenylenediamine. Also called oxidation dyes, amino dyes, para dyes, or peroxide dyes. PPD was first introduced in 1890 for dyeing furs and feathers. It comes in about thirty shades and is used as an intermediate in coal tar dyes. May produce eczema, bronchial asthma, gastritis, skin rash, and death. Can cross-react with many other chemicals, including azo dyes used for temporary hair colorings. Can also produce photosensitization. It has reportedly caused cancer in some animal experiments and not in others. In 1979, the National Cancer Institute reported tests showing coal tar ingredients in some permanent hair dyes caused cancer when fed to laboratory rats. The Food and Drug Administration then announced it was powerless to ban the suspect hair dyes since they were exempted from such action by the 1938 Food, Drug and Cosmetic Act. The FDA tried to make manufacturers put a warning label on the hair-dye containers, but the cosmetics manufacturers successfully defeated that. The manufacturers, after the publicity, voluntarily removed a commonly used permanent hair dye—4-MMPD-4methoxy-*m*-phenylenediamine—one of six hair dyes found to cause cancer in animals. The others were 2,4-toluene diamine (used in a few permanent hair colors), 4-amino-2-nitrophenol, and 2-nitrophenylenediamine (used in many gold and reddish shade highlighters), Direct Black 38, and Direct Blue 6 (both voluntarily removed from hair dyes). Bruce Ames reported in 1978 that 150 semipermanent hair dyes he tested (see Ames Test) were mutagenic. An estimated 70 to 75 percent of the carcinogens showed up as mutagens in his test. In January 1978, NIOSH reported that a new study of beauticians and cosmetologists showed they have a higher-than-expected incidence of six kinds of cancer. That study, along with NCI's findings, led NIOSH to recommend that 2,4-diaminoanisole be treated as a human carcinogen. On April 6, 1978, the FDA issued an order that manufacturers place warnings on the labels of some permanent hair dyes that read "Warning: contains an ingredient that can penetrate your skin and has been determined to cause cancer in laboratory animals." The FDA also proposed that beauty parlors post notices urging customers to check the labels on products used in salons. The industry representatives successfully fought these suggestions and, as of this writing, no signs are posted and the labels do not carry warnings.

The FDA still has no power to ban the ingredients in hair dyes or even require manufacturers to demonstrate safety.

Not everyone agrees hair dyes are dangerous. Dr. E. Cuyler Hammond of the American Cancer Society conducted a thirteen-year test of five thousand hairdressers and a matched group of nonhairdressers and did not find any difference in the groups. However, the ACS on February 22, 1978, did issue a statement that said: "The results of studies among beauticians and women who use hair dyes have been mixed. But the regulatory agencies feel that in the absence of hard data, they must be cautious. They feel that because of the wide use by the public, even a small potential risk of cancer caused by little exposure could be associated with significant additional cancer cases. While available information does not prove or disprove that hair dyes cause cancer in humans, the ACS advises caution in the use of the substances under question until more definitive evidence is developed." A study by New York University researchers suggests that women who have used hair dye for ten years or more face an increased risk of developing breast cancer. In this study, published in the February 1979 issue of the *Journal of the National Cancer Institute,* the use of hair dye by 129 women with breast cancer was compared to 193 matched controls. In 1981, F. N. Marzulli and his colleagues at the FDA's Division of Toxicology reported skin penetration by five substances present in cosmetics. The greatest skin penetration was recorded with 2,4-toluenediamine and the least with 2,4-diaminoanisole when applied to the skin of monkeys and humans. They found 2-nitro-*p*-phenylenediamine and N-nitrosodiethanolamine showed intermediate degrees of skin penetration. Other researchers reported that hair dye containing *p*-toluenediamine sulfate (2,5-diaminotoluene) resulted in human absorption of about 0.2 percent of the material if the dye was left on for forty minutes and then rinsed off.

In 2008, a review of the evidence by a panel of the International Agency for Research on Cancer (IARC) in Lyon, France, found a "small but consistent risk of bladder cancer in male hairdressers and barbers." A second review of the evidence on personal use of hair dyes found some studies suggesting a possible association with bladder cancer and with lymphoma and leukemia. The CIR (*see*) again said that persons not sensitive to the dye may use it safely. There are 440 studies concerning the dye. Pub Med and many other regulatory and scientific groups are studying the phenylenediamine family of chemicals. *o*-Phenylamine has been banned in cosmetics by the EU. *m*-Phenylenediamine has been banned in cosmetics by the EU and Canada. *p*-Phenylamine has been restricted in cosmetics in Canada. *See also* Hair Coloring.

p-PHENYLEPHRINE HCL • Same as some nasal decongestants, it is used topically to contract blood vessels and also in eye lotions to "take the red out." Some hypersensitive individuals may experience a mild stinging sensation. Prolonged exposure to air, metal, or strong light will cause oxidation and some loss of potency. Therefore, deeply discolored solutions, although harmless, should be discarded.

PHENYLETHYL PHENYL ACETATE • A synthetic fruit and honey flavoring. *See* Coal Tar.

PHENYLMETHYLPENTANAL • A fragrance ingredient. *See* Benzene.

PHENYLPARABEN • A preservative. *See* Parabens.

PHENYLPROPANOL • Fragrance ingredient. *See* Propanol.

PHENYLPROPYLDIMETHYLSILOXYSILICATE • Film former used in hair products, as an emollient in skin conditioners. *See* Polymer.

PHEROMONE • Pheromones are chemicals secreted by humans that influence the behavior or development of others of the same species, often functioning as an attractant of the opposite sex. Pheromone has been added to fragrances for the best part of twenty years now, but ensuring that the substance remains effective once combined with a fragrance has remained a problem for many manufacturers because it is difficult to formulate. California-based Human Pheromone Sciences says it wants to build on success it has already enjoyed in the personal care area by repositioning its Natural Attraction brand based on human pheromone.

PHILADELPHUS CORONARIUS • Mock orange. Fragrance ingredient.

PHILODENDRON • The extract of powdered bark of philodendron. A popular arum houseplant, dieffenbachia or dumbcane, accounts for numerous poisonings, according to poison center reports. About 275 species occur, notably in tropical and subtropical America and in the West Indies. Species have caused dermatitis of the face, neck, hands, and arms. Some species are irritants, and some can sensitize. Since these plants trigger burning sensations, most children don't swallow them, but pets sometimes do, and the plant toxins cause swelling of the tongue and throat, which can block breathing.

PHLOROGLUCINOL • An antioxidant prepared from various acids for use in hair dyes. Consists of white crystals with a sweet taste. Discolors in the light. The aqueous solution gives a blue-violet color. The CIR Expert Panel (*see*) concluded that it cannot conclude it is safe for use in cosmetic products until the appropriate safety data have been obtained and evaluated. *See* Pyrogallol for toxicity.

PHOENIX DACTYLIFERA • Date Fruit. *See* Date.

PHONOLITE • A mineral containing iron, calcium, and sodium among other minerals. Used as an absorbent.

PHOSPHATE • A salt or ester of phosphoric acid (*see*). Used as an emulsifier, texturizer, buffering, and sequestrant in cosmetics and foods. Careful regulation of inorganic phosphates in the diet could aid lung cancer prevention and treatment, researchers have concluded from a study in mice that could call into question the high use of phosphate additives in the diet. Phosphate is an essential nutrient, however, according to Dr. Myung-Haing Cho of Seoul National University, whose work is published in the *American Journal of Respiratory and Critical Care Medicine;* the article says that phosphates are being added more commonly to processed food products and cosmetics than in the past. They are used to increase water retention and improve texture. In the 1990s, according to the article, phosphorus-containing additives contributed around 470 mg per day to the average adult diet. Now, it is estimated to have risen by as much as 1,000 mg per day.

PHOSPHATE ESTERS, ORGANIC • *See* Phosphate and Ester.

PHOSPHATE OF LIME • Calcium Diphosphate. *See* Phosphate.

PHOSPHATIDYLSERINE • Once made from cow brain, but because of Mad Cow worries, it is now made from soybeans. It has been demonstrated to speed up recovery, prevent muscle soreness, improve well-being. Consumption of phosphatidylserine may reduce the risk of cognitive dysfunction in the elderly. It is being used in anti-aging creams.

PHOSPHOLIPIDS • Phosphatides. Complex fat substances found in all living cells. Lecithin is an example. Widely used in hand creams and lotions. Phospholipids contain phosphoric acid and nitrogen and are soluble in the usual fat solvents, with the exception of acetone (*see*). They are used in moisturizers because they bind water and hold it in place.

PHOSPHORIC ACID • An acid, sequestrant, and antioxidant used in hair tonics, nail polishes, and skin fresheners. A colorless, odorless solution made from phosphate rock. Mixes with water and alcohol. Concentrated solutions are irritating to the skin.

PHOSPHORIC ANHYDRIDE • Soft, white powder absorbs moisture from the air. Derived by burning phosphorus in dry air. Used in surfactants (*see*).

PHOSPHORUS • A highly reactive, poisonous, nonmetallic element occurring naturally in phosphates, especially in apatite, and existing in three forms, white (or sometimes yellow), red, and black. An essential constituent of protoplasm, it is used in safety matches, pyrotechnics, incendiary shells, and fertilizers and to protect metal surfaces from corrosion.

PHOTODERMATITIS • Skin problems caused by exposure to light, particularly sunlight. Some prescription drugs, cosmetics, or extract from plants such as parsnips and mustard may cause the reaction in sensitive people. *See* Photosensitivity.

PHOTOSENSITIVITY • A condition in which the application or ingestion of certain chemicals, such as propylparaben (*see*), causes skin problems—including rash, hyper-pigmentation, and swelling—when the skin is exposed to sunlight. In a five-year study at Columbia Presbyterian Medical Center in New York, photosensitivity responses were most often due to fragrance ingredients (musk ambrette and 6-methyl coumarin) and sun-screen ingredients (*p*-aminobenzoic acid and esters and oxybenzone). The Columbia researchers concluded that photoallergy due to fragrances is declining, whereas reactions to sunscreen ingredients, in particular oxybenzone, are increasing.

PHOTOTOXICITY • Reaction to sunlight or ultraviolet light resulting in inflammation.

PHTHALATES • Materials are derived from the organic chemical phthalic acid (*see*). Although phthalates are used primarily as plasticizers in plastics, meaning they are used to give flexibility to rubber, plastic, or resin, they are also used in just about every major product category, such as cosmetics, construction, automotive, household, apparel, toys, packaging, and medicinal materials. Phthalates are a broad class of ingredients; each has its own benefits and toxicological profile, so each must be considered for use separately. In cosmetics, they are used as solubulizers (an agent that something is dissolved in), plas-ticizers, or denaturants (makes the product bitter to the taste). The phthalate that is most frequently used in cosmetics and personal care products is diethyl phthalate (DEP). DEP helps fragrances linger after application. Dimethyl phthalate (DMP) may also have some uses in cosmetics and personal care products. Dibutyl phthalate (DBP) is an ingredient that is claimed to be safe and effective for use in making nail polish flexible and resis-tant to chipping. However, since DBP has been banned in some countries, the use of the ingredient has been discontinued by most manufacturers. Diethylhexyl phthalate (DEHP) is no longer used in the manufacturing of cosmetic and personal care, including nail prod-ucts. Phthalates have been under scrutiny for some time now; however the picture remains unclear. World production of phthalates is estimated to be several million tons a year. Recent observations indicate some may be mutagenic, cancer-causing, and adversely affect human male sperm. The Instituto de Medicina Forense Framboyanes in Veracruz, Mexico, at this writing, is studying the effect of phthalates on sperm. DEHP, one of the most common plasticizers, and dibutyl phthalate (*see both*) are on the California potential cancer-causing agents list, and in 2004, the EU banned them in nail polish. The FDA said in 2004 that phthalates are safe for humans in the amounts to which they are exposed. The cosmetic trade group Cosmeticsinfo.org agreed. The Environmental Working Group (EWG) (*see*) called upon government agencies to inves-tigate the cumulative risks of phthalates. Although the latest round of tests, which were carried out in the fall of 2008, found that many cosmetics categories have either reduced or completely eradicated phthalates, the fragrance category still had problems with the chemical. Tests have shown that the five fragrances with the highest levels of diethyl phthalate (DEP) in 2002 still showed in 2008 more than 20,000 parts per million of the phthalate—a level that EWG deems to be potentially dangerous. A study published in the February 2008 edition of the journal *Pediatrics* suggested that the use of baby lotion, powder, and shampoo is linked to the presence of phthalates in babies. The study's researchers analyzed urine concentrations of nine different phthalate metabolites in 163 infants and concluded that the use of these baby products resulted in higher levels of phthalates in the infants. Metabolites are the substances that arise from the chemical changes that take place in living cells. Because there were serious shortcomings in this study—only one of the seven phthalate compounds reported is used in baby care products—the reported correlation between the use of infant personal care products and elevated levels of phthalates in infants some scientists found questionable. A committee of the independent National Research Council (*see*) concluded that the U.S. Environmental Protection Agency should carry out more research on the health effects of exposure to phthalates from different sources and of cumulative exposure. In addition, the EWG claims significant scientific data is now available suggesting that phthalates affect the reproductive system of humans as well as those of animals in lab tests. Although a number of consumer groups and scientists believe DEP poses a serious health risk, the Fragrance Materials Association (FMA) and the European Commission's Scientific Committee on Consumer Products (SCCP) both insist that DEP is safe for use in cosmetics at current levels. The FMA said the chemical profiles of different phthalate compounds differ significantly, which explains why DEP is considered safe in Europe while the phthalates DBP and DEHP are banned on the Continent. The National Research Council's project, launched in 2008, is funded by the EPA and will investigate the health risks posed by phthalates and the potential for conducting cumulative risk assessment. The FDA has concluded that there is no compelling evidence that DEP, as used in personal care products, poses a safety risk.

PHTHALIC ACID • A colorless crystalline organic acid prepared from naphthalene and used in the synthesis of dyes and other organic compounds. Obtained by the oxidation of various benzene derivatives, it can be isolated from the fungus *Gibberella fujikuroi*. When rapidly heated, it forms phthalic anhydride (*see*) and water. It is used chiefly in the manufacture of cosmetic esters, dyes, and nail polishes. Moderately irritating to the skin and mucous membranes. *See* Phthalates.

PHTHALIC ANHYDRIDE • Prepared from naphthalene by oxidation, it consists of lustrous white needles. It is used in the manufacture of cosmetic dyes and artificial resins. It is moderately irritating to the skin and mucous membranes. *See* Phthlates.

PHTHALIC/TRIMELLITIC/GLYCOLS COPOLYMER • *See* Phthalic Anhydride and Polymer.

PHYLLANTHUS EMBLICA • Amla. Aonla. Aola. Amalaki. Dharty. Indian Gooseberry. A medium-size deciduous tree that belongs to the plant family Euphorbiaceae. It grows in the plains and submountain on tracts all over the Indian subcontinent. Its dried fruit is used in Ayurvedic and Unani systems of medicine for various ailments like fever, liver disorder, indigestion, anemia, heart complaints, and urinary problems. It is a rich source of vitamin C that gets assimilated in the human system easily and quickly. *Phyllanthus emblica* standardized extract is used as a skin lightener for normal or hyperpigmented skin. *See* Melanin.

PHYLLOSTACHIS BAMBUSOIDES • Skin conditioner. *See* Bamboo.

PHYSALIS ALKEKENGI • *See* Cherry Pit Oil.

PHYSOSTIGMA VENENOSUM • *See* Physostigmine.

PHYSOSTIGMINE • Eserine. Antilirium. Obtained from the dried ripe seed (Calabar bean) of *Physostigma venenosum*. It is used topically to produce a contraction of the pupil and decrease pressure inside the eye in glaucoma. It is used to inhibit the destruction of acetylcholine, and its salts are banned in cosmetics by ASEAN (*see*). It is on the Canadian Hotlist (*see*).

PHYTANTRIOL • Phytantriol is an alcohol (polyol) used most often in the formulation of hair care preparations and, less often, in skin and nail preparations. An anticaking ingredient in hair and skin products used in the following product types: conditioner, mascara, shampoo, lipstick, styling gel/lotion, hair spray, foundation, other products with spf, facial moisturizer/treatment, and anti-aging products. May be toxic and irritating to the skin. The CIR Expert Panel (*see*) has listed this as top priority for review. *See* Polyols.

PHYTIC ACID • Occurs in nature in the seeds of cereal grains and is derived commercially from corn. It is used to chelate heavy metals, as a rust inhibitor, in metal cleaning, and in the treatment of hard water. Those allergic to corn may have a reaction.

PHYTOCELLTECH MALUS DOMESTICA • Uses stem cells from the stem cells of certain apples. Claims to rejuvenate skin. PhytoCellTec Malus Domestica was applied to human stem cells from umbilical cords and was found to increase the number of the stem cells in culture. Furthermore, the addition of the ingredient to umbilical cord stem cells appeared to protect the cells from environmental stress such as ultraviolet (UV) light. One of the problems with stem cells, in general, is often scientists' inability to regulate them from overproducing. If the cells keep reproducing, they may turn into a tumor.

PHYTOL • An alcohol obtained by the decomposition of chlorophyll.

PHYTOLACCA DECANDRA • *Phytolacca* spp. A tropical herb, *P. decandra,* is an extract of the roots of the pokeweed. It is considered toxic. Used for its purple coloring. On the Canadian Hotlist (*see*). The EU banned it in cosmetics. *See* Pokeweed.

PHYTONADIONE • Vitamin K (*see*).

PHYTOSOMES • A new term cosmetologists are using for the combination of liposomes (*see*) and plant extracts. They claim that the desirable substances then pass more easily through the skin. In the works are phytosomes to carry catechol, quercitrin, escin, and glycyrrhetinic acid (*see all*).

PHYTOSPHINGOSINE • A fatty alcohol used as a skin- and hair-conditioning ingredient.

PHYTOSTEROLS • Plant fatty alcohol.

PHYTOSTERYL ISOSTEARYL DIMER DILINOLEATE • A skin and hair conditioner, it is also a thickener and emollient. *See* Dilinoleic Acid.

PICEA EXCELSA • *See* Norway Spruce Extract.

PICES • Fish extract.

PICES MARINE COLLAGEN • A source of collagen from cod and pollack skin. It has a high collagen content and is almost odorless. It is claimed to be pathogen free, unlike bovine collagen, which is not always free of contaminants.

PICHI • *Fabiana imbricata.* A Peruvian shrub whose herbage yields a tonic and diuretic. It is used in "organic" cosmetics.

PICRAMIC ACID • 4, 6-Dinitro-2-Aminophenol. A red, crystalline acid obtained from phenol (*see*) and used chiefly in making azo dyes (*see*) for non-permanent hair coloring. Highly toxic material. Readily absorbed through intact skin. Vapors absorbed through respiratory tract. Produces marked increase in metabolism and temperature, profuse sweating, collapse, and death. May cause skin rash, cataracts, and weight loss. The EU gave manufacturers to July 2005 to submit safety information or the substance would be proposed for a ban. In 2007, the EU said insufficient data was presented to draw a conclusion. More data is needed. The safety of sodium picramate has been assessed by the CIR Expert Panel (*see*). The Panel evaluated the scientific data and concluded that sodium picramate was safe as a hair dye ingredient at concentrations not to exceed 0.1 percent. The EU adopted the conclusions of the agencies they had go over the scientific publications on this ingredient in 2006. The expert panels included the Scientific Committee on Consumer Products (SCCP), the Scientific Committee on Health and Environmental Risks (SCHER), and the Scientific Committee on Emerging and Newly Identified Health Risks (SCENIHR) and are made up of external experts. In addition, the

European Commission relies upon the work of the European Food Safety Authority (EFSA), the European Medicines Evaluation Agency (EMEA), the European Centre for Disease Prevention and Control (ECDC), and the European Chemicals Agency (ECHA). The SCCP is of the opinion that the information submitted is insufficient to allow a final risk assessment to be carried out. Before any further consideration, the possible genotoxic potential must be excluded. The agencies concluded the hair dye with picramic acid was safe if the level did not exceed 2 percent. However, no human tests were evaluated and its cancer-causing potential, if any, was not considered. The agencies said the hair dye is usually left on for half an hour and it is all right to repeat it each week.

PICRASMA EXCELSA • Extract of the spruce tree used as an antidandruff ingredient.

PIGMENT • Coloring.

PIGMENT BLUE 15 • The EU calls it CI 74160; the Japanese call it Ao404. Classed chemically as a phthalocyanine (copper complex) color. Used in hair dyes.

PIGMENT BLUE 15:2 • The EU calls it CI 74160; the Japanese call it Ao404. The solvent stable form of pigment blue prepared by the introduction of chlorine. Used in hair colorants. *See also* Coal Tar.

PIGMENT GREEN 7 • The EU calls it CI 74260. Classed chemically as a phthalo-cyanine (copper complex) color. Used as a hair colorant. *See* Chlorophyllin, Colors, and Coal Tar.

PIGMENT ORANGE 5 • The EU calls it CI 12075; the Japanese call it Daidai203. A monoazo color whose name can be used only when applied to batches of uncertified colors. The CTFA name for certified batches is D & C Orange No. 17 (*see*). On the Canadian Hotlist (*see*). Banned by ASEAN. *See also* Coal Tar.

PIGMENT RED 4 • The Japanese call it Aka228; the EU calls it CI 12085. It's Red 36 in the United States. A monoazo color whose name can be used only when applied to batches of uncertified color. The CTFA adopted name for certified batches is D & C Red No. 36 (*see*) used in all types of makeup except for the eye products. *See also* Coal Tar.

PIGMENT RED 5 • The EU name is CI 12490. A monoazo color (*see*). *See also* Coal Tar.

PIGMENT RED 48 • The Japanese call it Aka405; the EU calls it CI 15865. A monoazo color (*see*). *See also* Coal Tar.

PIGMENT RED 53 • The EU calls it CI 15585. The Japanese call it Aka203. A monoazo color whose name can be used only when applied to batches of uncertified color. The CTFA adopted name for certified batches is D & C Red No. 8. On the Canadian Hotlist (*see*). ASEAN bans it in cosmetics. *See also* Coal Tar.

PIGMENT RED 53:1 • The EU calls it CI 15585. The Japanese call it Aka204. The barium salt of Pigment Red 53, whose name can be applied only to uncertified batches of color. The CTFA adopted name for certified color batches is D & C Red No. 9. *See also* Coal Tar.

PIGMENT RED 57 • Red 6 for certified color, and uncertified, Pigment Red 7. A monoazo color whose name can be applied only to uncertified batches of color. The CTFA adopted name for certified batches is D & C Red No. 6. *See also* Coal Tar.

PIGMENT RED 57:1 • Name for uncertified color in the United States. Red 6 used in the EU as well as the number CI 15850. A monoazo color, it is the calcium salt of Pigment Red No. 57. The name can be applied only to batches of uncertified color. The CTFA adopted name for certified batches is D & C Red No. 7. Used in makeup polish except for around the eyes and nail. *See also* Coal Tar.

PIGMENT RED 63:1 • CI 15880 is the EU name and number. Aka220 is the Japanese name. A monoazo color whose name can be used only for batches of uncertified color.

The CTFA adopted name for certified batches is D & C Red No. 34. Used in nail polish. *See also* Coal Tar.

PIGMENT RED 64:1 • The EU name and number is CI 15800:1. Aka219 is the Japanese name. A monoazo color whose name can be applied only to uncertified batches. The CTFA adopted name for certified batches is D & C Red. No. 31. *See also* Coal Tar.

PIGMENT RED 68 • CI 15525 is the EU name and number. A monoazo color (*see*). *See also* Coal Tar.

PIGMENT RED 83 • The EU names are CI 58000 and Mordant Red 11. Alizarin. An antraquinone color. *See also* Coal Tar.

PIGMENT RED 88 • CI 73312 is the EU name. A thioindigoid color. *See also* Coal Tar.

PIGMENT RED 90:1 ALUMINUM LAKE • The EU name is CI 45380. Red 21 Lake. An insoluble pigment composed of the aluminum salt of Solvent Red 43. The CTFA name for the certified batches of this color is D & C Red No. 21 Aluminum Lake. Aluminum salt of Solvent Red 43.

PIGMENT RED 112 • EU number CI 12370. A monoazo color used in hair dyes. *See* Azo Dyes and Coal Tar.

PIGMENT RED 172 ALUMINUM LAKE • EU name, CI 45430. Japanese name AKA3. The insoluble pigment composed of the aluminum salt of Acid Red 51. The CTFA-certified name of this color is FD & C Red No. 3 Aluminum Lake. It has been prohibited in cosmetic products in the United States. Its use as a cosmetic colorant may also be restricted in other countries. *See also* Coal Tar.

PIGMENT RED 173 ALUMINUM LAKE • EU name CI 451703. An insoluble pigment composed of the aluminum salt of Basic Violet 10. The CTFA name for certified batches of this color is D & C Red No. 19 Aluminum Lake. This color has been prohibited in cosmetic products in the United States. Its use as a cosmetic colorant may also be restricted in other countries. On the Canadian Hotlist (*see*). *See* Coal Tar.

PIGMENT RED 190 • EU name CI 71140. A perylene color. Perylene has been found as a contaminant in water that is toxic to the environment. In mice, it has not been found to be carcinogenic but can be absorbed through the skin and should be avoided in cosmetics. *See also* Coal Tar.

PIGMENT VIOLET 19 • EU name CI 73900. A quinacridone color. A light-fast pigment derived from coal tar (*see*). It provides a wide range of shades, and cosmetics manufacturers are increasing its use.

PIGMENT VIOLET 23 • EU name CI 51319. A dioaxene color used in hair dye. *See also* Coal Tar.

PIGMENT YELLOW 1 • EU name CI 11680. Japanese name Ki401. A monoazo color. *See* Azo Dyes.

PIGMENT YELLOW 3 • EU name CI 11710. A monoazo color. *See* Azo Dyes and Coal Tar.

PIGMENT YELLOW 12 • Japanese name Ki205. EU name CI 21090. A diazo color. *See* Azo Dyes.

PIGMENT YELLOW 73 • EU name CI 11738. A monoazo color. *See* Azo Dyes and Coal Tar.

PIGSKIN EXTRACT • An extract of the skin of young pigs. Used in hand and hair conditioners.

PILEWORT EXTRACT • An extract of *Ranunculus ficaria,* the coarse, hairy, perennial figwort of the eastern and central United States. It was once used to treat tuberculosis.

PILOCARPINE • Used in hair tonic to stimulate the sweat glands. Derived from a tree grown in Brazil and Paraguay. Soluble in water, alcohol, and chloroform. White, water-absorbing crystals with a bitter taste. Also an antidote for atropine poisoning. Readily absorbed through the skin from the concentrations employed in hair tonics. High concentrations are known to be irritating and toxic, but no available information on toxicity in cosmetics is reported. On the Canadian Hotlist (*see*).

PILOCARPUS JABORANDI HOLMES • *See* Pilocarpine and Jaborandi. The EU has banned pilocarpine in cosmetics.

PILOCARPUS PENNATIFOLIUS • Used in shampoos and hair-grooming products. *See* Jaborandi.

PIMENTA ACRIS • Fragrance ingredient. *See* Bay Oil.

PIMENTA LEAF OIL • Jamaica Pepper. Allspice. Derived from the dried ripe fruit of the evergreen shrub grown in the West Indies and Central and South America. Used in raspberry, fruit, nut, and spice flavorings. Moderately toxic by ingestion. A severe skin irritant. GRAS

PIMENTA OFFICINALIS • Pimento. Allspice. Fragrance ingredient. Used in folk medicine to treat stomach problems, particularly gas.

PIMPINELLA ANISUM • *See* Anise.

PINE NEEDLE EXTRACT • An extract of various species of *Pinus* used to scent bath products and as a natural flavoring in pineapple, citrus, and spice flavorings. Ingestion of large amounts can cause intestinal hemorrhage.

PINE OIL • The extract from a variety of pine trees. As a pine tar it is used in hair tonics; also a solvent, disinfectant, and deodorant. As an oil from twigs and needles, it is used in pine bath-oil emulsions, bath salts, and perfumery. Irritating to the skin and mucous membranes. Bornyl acetate, a substance obtained from various pine needles, has a strong pine odor and is used in bath oils. It can cause nausea, vomiting, convulsions, and dizziness if ingested. In general, pine oil in concentrated form is an irritant to human skin and may cause allergic reactions.

PINE RESIN • Colophony. A sticky exudate used in mascara. May cause allergic reaction.

PINE TAR • A product obtained by the distillation of pinewood. A blackish brown, viscous liquid, slightly soluble in water. Used as an antiseptic in skin diseases. May be irritating to the skin.

PINE TAR OIL • Synthetic flavoring obtained from pinewood and used in licorice flavorings. Used as a solvent, disinfectant, and deodorant in cosmetics. May be irritating to the skin and mucous membranes, and large ingested doses cause central nervous system depression.

PINEAPPLE EXTRACT • *See* Pineapple Juice.

PINEAPPLE JUICE • The common juice from the tropical plant. Contains a protein-digesting and milk-clotting enzyme, bromelan (*see*). An anti-inflammatory enzyme, it is used in cosmetic treatment creams. It is also used as a texturizer.

PINECONE EXTRACT • An extract from the cones of *Pinus sylvestris*. *See* Pine Oil.

PINELLIA TERNATA • A weed that spreads easily. Used in Chinese medicine to counteract stomach problems. Used in cosmetics as a skin conditioner.

PINUS • Signifies pine, many varieties of which are used as a skin conditioner or fragrance ingredient in cosmetics. Some are also used in sunscreens.

PINUS PUMILIO OIL • Oil of Dwarf Pine Needles. Oil of Mountain Pine. *Pinus montana.* Colorless or faintly yellow liquid with a pleasant odor. Used in flavoring and perfume. Used medically as an expectorant.

PINUS SYLVESTRIS OIL • Used in antiwrinkle creams and in fragrances. *See* Pinus Pumilio Oil.

PIPER • Used in deodorants, oral care products, and skin conditioners. *See* Pepper Oil, Black.

PIPER METHYSTICUM EXTRACT • *See* Kava Kava.

PIPERIDINE • A synthetic flavoring that occurs naturally in black pepper. Has been proposed for use as a tranquilizer and muscle relaxant.

PIPERINE • Primarily found in the fruit of the pepper vine, *Piper nigrum.* The pepper vine is indigenous to the Malabar coast of India, but it is also grown in other parts of southern Asia, South America, and even Africa. Used as a fragrance. The piperine gives peppercorns their hot, biting, and very pungent taste. However, for chemical and medical use piperine is produced in the laboratory.

PIPERITONE • A synthetic flavoring ingredient that occurs naturally in Japanese mint. Used to give dentifrices a minty flavor and to give perfumes their peppermint scent.

PIPERONAL • Heliotropin. A synthetic flavoring and perfume ingredient that occurs naturally in vanilla and black pepper. White crystalline powder with a sweet floral odor. Used chiefly in perfumery. Ingestion of large amounts may cause central nervous system depression. Has been reported to cause skin rash. In lipsticks, said to produce marking of the skin. Not recommended by some cosmetic chemists because of its ability to produce skin irritation.

PIPERONYL BUTOXIDE • A-200 Pediculicide Shampoo. Lice Enz Foam. Pronto Lice Killing Shampoo. R&C Shampoo. Rid Lice Killing Shampoo. A compound derived from petroleum used in combination with pyrethrins to treat skin parasites, including lice. For external use only. Should not be inhaled or used on irritated, infected, or broken skin. Should not be used by a person sensitive to ragweed. Harmful if swallowed.

PIPSISSEWA LEAVES EXTRACT • *Chimaphila umbellata.* Love-in-Winter. Prince's Pine. King's Cure. Ground Holly. Winter Rheumatism Weed. Extracted from the leaves of an evergreen shrub, it is used in many commercial flavorings. Its leaves have been used as an astringent, diuretic, and tonic. The Cree word *pipisisikweu* means to break up—bladder stones, that is. It has properties similar to uva-ursi (*see*). Also used as a treatment for arthritis. In 1992, the FDA proposed a ban on pipsissewa in oral menstrual drug products because it had not been shown to be safe and effective as claimed.

PIROCTONE OLAMINE • Germicide in shampoos and other hair products. Used to treat dandruff. *See* Pyridium Compounds.

PISCUM LECUR • Fish liver oil.

PISTACIA LENTISCUS • Mastic gum. *See* Pistachio Nut Oil.

PISTACHIA VERA • *See* Pistachio Nut Oil.

PISTACHIO NUT OIL • *Pistacia vera.* The oil from the nut of a small tree grown in Europe, Asia Minor, and recently in the United States. Used in skin conditioners.

PISUM SATIVUM • Pea Extract. Used as a skin protectant and emollient.

PITUITARY HORMONES • Pituitrin. Used to stimulate smooth muscle contractions.

PIX • *See* Tar Oil.

PLACENTA • The afterbrith is rich with nutrients and oxygen passed to the fetus through the mammal's blood. It is rich in proteins, hormones, and vitamins. Some manufacturers reported use of extracts of both human or bovine placentas for anti-aging products. Placental proteins are used as antistatic agents and humectants, and placental fats are used as emollients. Cells, tissues, or other products of human origin are banned from use in cosmetics in the EU. Any placental extract in products purchased in the EU reportedly will be of bovine origin. *See* Placental Enzymes, Lipids, and Proteins and Placental Extract.

PLACENTAL ENZYMES, LIPIDS, AND PROTEINS • Derived from animal placenta, the vascular membrane that nourishes the fetus. Widely used in hair and skin conditioners.

PLACENTAL EXTRACT • Prepared from the placenta, the nourishing lining of the human womb that is expelled after birth. Promoted by cosmetics manufacturers as capable of removing wrinkles. The American Medical Association maintains no such evidence has been presented, nor is it likely. (Even newborn babies emerge from the womb with wrinkled skin.) On the Canadian Hotlist (*see*).

PLACENTAL PROTEIN • *See* Placental Extract.

PLANKTON EXTRACT • An extract of the marine organisms *Thalasso* plankton, a green microalgae or seaweed.

PLANT ESTROGENS • A host of estrogens (*see*) have been identified in plants. Although they are considerably less active than those in animals, chronic exposure may lead to the accumulation of levels that are active in humans.

PLANT STEROLS • Vitamin D precursors found in broccoli, cabbage, squash, and other vegetables as well as whole grains. They cause cells to differentiate.

PLANTAGO • *See* Plantain Extract.

PLANTAIN EXTRACT • The extract of various species of *Plantago major*. The starchy fruit is a staple item of diet throughout the tropics. A natural astringent and antiseptic with soothing and cooling effects on blemishes and burns.

PLAQUE • Buildup on the teeth of a film or acid-forming bacteria and material from saliva. Believed to be a main cause of gingivitis (inflamed gums), the formation of tartar, and dental cavities.

PLASTICIZERS • Chemicals added to natural and synthetic resins and rubbers to impart flexibility, workability, or distensibility without changing the chemical nature of the material. Dibutyl phthalate (*see*) is a plasticizer for nitrocellulose used in nail lacquers.

PLATINUM NANO-SIZED PARTICLES • Claim to help maintain skin's electrical balance. In very expensive creams like La Prairie. *See* Nanotechnology.

PLATYCODON GRANDIFLORUM • Balloon Flower. Kikyou. Chinese herb used as an antioxidant, antifungal, and demulcent.

PLECTRANTHUS BARBATUS • Coleus. A weed originally named from the Latin for testicles. Used as an antioxidant.

PLEUROCHRYSIS CARTERAE • Microalgae. *See* Alginates.

PLUCHEA INDICA • Skin conditioner.

PLUM EXTRACT • Extract of the fruit of the plum tree, *Prunus domestica;* the American Indians boiled the wild plum and gargled with it to cure mouth sores.

PLUMERIA • *See* Frangipani.

POA ANNUA • Annual Creeping Blue Grass. Meadow Grass. A pesty weed common in the United Kingdom. Used as a conditioner.

PODOPHYLLIN AND RESIN • *Podophyllum peltatum.* Pod-Ben. Popo-Ben. Pudofin. Mandrake. Mayapple. Verrex-C&M. An ingredient in topical medications to treat warts. Used in the treatment of benign growths, including genital and perianal warts, papillomas, and fibroids. A few hours after podophyllin is applied to a wart, the growth becomes whitened and, in one to three days, begins to disintegrate. Podophyllin can cause severe irritation of normal skin. Therefore, petrolatum is usually applied on the perimeter of the wart to keep podophyllin from touching healthy tissue. It can be toxic if too much is absorbed into the body, causing confusion, diarrhea, abdominal pain, and convulsions. The resin is poisonous and a strong purgative. Banned by the FDA, May 1992, as an ingredient in laxatives.

POGOSTEMON CABLIN • *See* Patchouli Oil.

POKEWEED • *Phytolacca americana.* Pokeroot. Coakum. Native to the southern United States and the Mediterranean area, the dried roots reduce inflammation and arthritic pains. Has antibiotic, antiviral, and anti-inflammatory properties. Among its constituents are tannin, formic acid, saponins, and alkaloids (*see all*). It is prescribed by herbalists for a variety of ailments, from swollen glands to weight loss. It is used in "organic" cosmetics. A member of the bloodberry family, it is an emetic and laxative with narcotic properties. Both berries and roots contain a dangerous drug. Some people are more sensitive to pokeweed's adverse effects than others, and fatalities have occurred. Banned in cosmetics by the EU.

POLIANTHES TUBEROSA • *See* Tuberose Oil.

POLISH REMOVER • *See* Nail Polish Remover.

POLISHING INGREDIENTS • Used in dentifrices to shine teeth. Even after removing debris and stains, teeth may still be dull. Polishing whitens and brightens teeth, and teeth that are polished are less receptive to dental plaque. Substances used to polish teeth are hydrated alumina, sodium metaphosphate, calcium phosphate, and calcium carbonate (*see all*).

POLLEN EXTRACT • An extract of flower pollen. Used as a skin conditioner.

POLOXAMER 101 THROUGH 407 • *See* Poloxamer 188. The CIR Expert Panel (*see*) has listed this as top priority for review.

POLOXAMER 188 • Poloxalene. A liquid, nonionic, surfactant polymer. If chain lengths of polyoxyethylene and polyoxypropylene are increased, the product changes from liquid to paste to solid. *See* Polymer.

POLOXAMINE 304 TO 1508 • The polyethylene, polyoxypropylene block of polymer of ethylenediamine. The numbers signify the various properties of the chemicals and whether one is to be used in food, drugs, or cosmetics. In cosmetics, it is used primarily as a surfactant (*see*).

POLY- • A prefix meaning many.

POLYACRYLAMIDE • The polymer of acrylamide monomers, it is white, solid, water soluble, and used as a thickening ingredient, suspending ingredient, and an additive to adhesives. Widely used in cosmetics including moisturizers, hair coloring, body and hand products, cold creams and cleansing lotions, makeup, and bath products. Used in tanning creams. Used in the manufacture of plastics and in nail polishes. Highly toxic and irritating to the skin. Causes central nervous system paralysis. Can be absorbed through unbroken skin. The CIR Expert Panel (*see*) concluded that it is safe as a cosmetic ingredient if used at less than 0.01 percent.

POLYACRYLAMIDOPROPYLTRIMONIUM CHLORIDE • Quaternary ammonium compound (*see*) used in hair products. *See* Acrylates.

POLYACRYLATES • Synthetic polymers used as film formers and thickeners in the manufacture of cosmetics.

POLYACRYLIC ACID • *See* Acrylic Resins.

POLYAMIDE-1 • A film former and coloring. *See* Polyacrylamide.

POLYAMINO SUGAR CONDENSATE • A skin conditioner and humectant. The condensation product of the sugars fructose, galactose, glucose, lactose, maltose, mannose, rhamnose, ribose, or xylose, with a minute amount of amino acids such as alanine, arginine, aspartic acid, glutamic acid, glycine, histidine, hydroxyproline, isoleucine, leucine, lysine, methionine, phenylalanine, proline, pyroglutamic acid, serine, threonine, tyrosine, or valine. On the basis of the available information, the CIR Expert Panel (*see*) found it safe in the early 1980s but is considering new information to determine if the final safety assessment should be reaffirmed, amended, or have an addendum. *See* Amino Acids.

POLYAMINOPROPYL BIGUANIDE • A preservative in baby products. It derived originally from a cyanide compound after undergoing several processes.

POLYBETA-ALANINE • *See* Alanine.

POLYBUTENE • Indopol. Polybutylene. A plasticizer. A polymer (*see*) of one or more butylenes obtained from petroleum oils. Used in lubricating oil, adhesives, sealing tape, cable insulation, films, and coatings. May asphyxiate. On the basis of the available information, the CIR Expert Panel (*see*) found it safe in the early 1980s but is considering new information to determine if the final safety assessment should be reaffirmed, amended, or have an addendum.

POLYCHLOROTRIFLUOROETHYLENE • Colorless, impervious to corrosive chemicals, it resists most organic solvents and heat. Nonflammable. Used as a transparent film.

POLYCYCLOPENTADIENE • A synthetic polymer (*see*) used to remove hair and to increase its thickness.

POLYDECENE • A polymerization of decylene. A colorless liquid used in flavors and fragrances.

POLYDEXTROSE • A sugar used as a bulking ingredient in skin care products.

POLYDIHYDROXYINDOLE • A phenol (*see*) used in foundations, suntan products, and mascara. *See* Phenols and Indoles.

POLYESTER-1 • A film former in hair fixatives. *See* Acrylates.

POLYETHYLACRYLATE • *See* Acrylates.

POLYETHYLENE • A polymer (*see*) of ethylene; a product of petroleum gas or dehydration of alcohol. One of a group of lightweight thermoplastics that have a good resistance to chemicals, low moisture absorption, and good insulating properties. Widely used in hand lotions, hair colorings, skin fresheners, suntan products, underarm deodorants, and makeup. No known skin toxicity, but implants of large amounts in rats caused cancer. Ingestion of large oral doses has produced kidney and liver damage.

POLYETHYLENE 6000 OR MORE • Excellent barrier to water vapor and moisture, it resists solvents and corrosive solutions. It is combustible.

POLYETHYLENE GLYCOL • PEG. Used in hair straighteners, antiperspirants, baby products, fragrances, polish removers, hair tonics, lipsticks, and protective creams. It is a binder, plasticizing ingredient, solvent, and softener widely used for cosmetic cream bases and pharmaceutical ointments. Improves resistance to moisture and oxidation.

POLYETHYLENE NAPHTHALATE • A film former. *See* Naphthas.

POLYETHYLENE TEREPHTHALATE • A synthetic polymer used as an adhesive, hair fixative, and thickener in hair coloring, foundations, indoor tanning products, leg and body paints, makeup (except eye), and nail polish and enamels. *See* Phthalates.

POLYETHYLGLUTAMATE • Film former. *See* Glutamate.

POLYGALA SENEGA • Snakeroot. *See* Senega Extract.

POLYGLUCURONIC ACID • A film former used as a humectant in conditioners. *See* Glucose.

POLYGLYCERIN-3.-4 -6 -10 • Used in conditioners and humectants. *See* Glycerin.

POLYGLYCEROL • Prepared from edible fats, oils, and esters of fatty acids. Derived from corn, cottonseed, palm, peanuts, safflower, sesame, and soybean oils, lard, and tallow. Used as an emulsifier in cosmetics. *See* Glycerol.

POLYGLYCEROL ESTER • One of several partial or complete esters of saturated and unsaturated fatty acids with a variety of derivatives of polyglycerols ranging from diglycerol to triglycerol. Used as lubricants, plasticizers, gelling ingredients, humectants, surface-active ingredients, dispersants, and emulsifiers in foods and cosmetic preparations.

POLYGLYCERYL-3 BEESWAX • Emulsifier. *See* Beeswax.

POLYGLYCERYL-10 BEHENATE/EIDOCSADIOATE • Skin conditioner and emulsifier. *See* Fish Oil and Behenic Acid.

POLYGLYCERYL-2 CAPRATE • Skin emollient and emulsifier.

POLYGLYCERYL-3 CETYL ETHER • Used in indoor tanning products. *See* Glycerol.

POLYGLYCERYL-4 COCOATE • *See* Coconut Acid and Polyglycerol.

POLYGLYCERYL-10 DECALINOLEATE • *See* Glycerin and Linoleic Acid.

POLYGLYCERYL-10 DECAOLEATE • *See* Oleic Acid and Polyglycerol.

POLYGLYCERYL-2 DIISOSTEARATE • *See* Isostearic Acid and Polyglycerol.

POLYGLYCERYL-3 DIISOSTEARATE • Widely used in makeup and moisturizers. *See* Glycerol and Isostearic Acid.

POLYGLYCERYL-6 DIOLEATE • *See* Oleic Acid and Glycerin.

POLYGLYCERYL-6 DISTEARATE • *See* Stearic Acid and Glycerin.

POLYGLYCERYL-3 HYDROXYLAURYL ETHER • *See* Lauryl Alcohol and Glycerin.

POLYGLYCERYL-4 ISOSTEARATE • Used in makeup bases and face and neck creams and lotions (excluding shaving preparations). *See* Isostearic Acid and Glycerin.

POLYGLYCERYL-2 LANOLIN ALCOHOL ETHER • *See* Lanolin Alcohol and Glycerin.

POLYGLYCERYL-LAURYL ETHER • *See* Lauryl Alcohol and Glycerin.

POLYGLYCERYL-3 OR -4 OLEATE • Oily liquid prepared by adding alcohol to coconut oil or other triglycerides with a polyglyceryl. Used in foods, drugs, and cosmetics as fat emulsifiers in conjunction with other emulsifiers to prepare creams, lotions, and other emulsion products. In addition, they may also be used as lubricants, plasticizers, gelling ingredients, and dispersants.

POLYGLYCERYL-2 OR -4 OLEYL ETHER • The ether of oleyl alcohol and glycerin (*see both*) polymer.

POLYGLYCERYL-3-PEG-2 COCOAMIDE • *See* Coconut Oil and Glycerin.

POLYGLYCERYL-2-PEG-4 STEARATE • An ether of PEG-4 stearate (*see*) and glycerin (*see*).

POLYGLYCERYL-10 PENTAOLEATE • Used in face creams. *See* Polyglyceryl and Pentanoic Acid.

POLYGLYCERYL-2-SESQUIISOSTEARATE • A mixture of esters of isostearic acid and glycerin (*see both*).

POLYGLYCERYL-2-SESQUIOLEATE • A mixture of ester of oleic acid and glycerin (*see both*).

POLYGLYCERYL SORBITOL • A condensation product of glycerin and sorbitol (*see both*).

POLYGLYCERYL-3, -4, OR -8 STEARATE • An ester of stearic acid and glycerin (*see both*).

POLYGLYCERYL-10 TETRAOLEATE • An ester of oleic acid and glycerin (*see both*).

POLYGLYCERYL-2 TETRASTEARATE • *See* Stearic Acid and Glycerin.

POLYGONATUM OFFICINALE • Solomon's Seal. Used in skin conditioners. *See* Buckwheat.

POLYGONUM • A large family of herbs. *See* Knotweed Extract.

POLYGONUM FAGOPYRUM • Skin conditioner. *See* Buckwheat.

POLYHYDROXY ACIDS • PHA. Similar to earlier alpha-hydroxy acids (AHA), which contain only one hydroxyl group. PHAs have multiple hydroxyl groups and are therefore said to be less irritating to the skin. Conventional AHAs and retinoids have been reported to cause tingling, stinging, and burning sensations in some people. PHAs may be less irritating because they are made up of larger molecules, which may penetrate the skin more slowly and thus may be gentler. Gluconolactone (*see*) is an example.

POLYHYDROXYSTEARIC ACID • A widely used suspending ingredient in cosmetics.

POLYISOBUTENE • *See* Polybutene.

POLYISOPRENE • The major component of natural rubber but also made synthetically.

POLY-L LACTIC ACID • Being studied, at this writing, as a "dermal stimulator" because it reportedly stimulates skin cells to make collagen (*see*). May require several months of application to treat wrinkles.

POLYLYSINE • A film in hair products. *See* Lysine.

POLYMER • A substance or product formed by combining many small molecules (monomers). The result is, essentially, recurring long-chain structural units that have tensile strength, elasticity, and hardness. Examples of polymers (literally, having many parts) are plastics, fibers, rubber, and human tissue.

POLYMETHACRYLAMIDE • A film former. *See* Polymer and Acrylamide.

POLYMETHYL METHACRYLATE • A widely used film former in many creams, makeup, powders, and skin care products. Also used by physicians to fill wrinkles. *See* Acrylates.

POLYMYXIN B • An antibacterial drug mainly used topically to treat infections of the skin, eyes, and ears. May cause hives, fever, and possibly fatal allergic reactions.

POLYNAPHTHALENE SULFONATE • Used as a solvent in wrinkle creams. *See* Naphthalene.

POLYOLS • Alcohol compounds that absorb moisture. They have a low molecular weight: polyols with a weight above 1,000 are solids and less toxic than those that weigh 600 or below. The latter are liquid and, although higher in toxicity, very large doses are required to kill animals. Such deaths in animals have been found to be due to kidney damage. *See* Propylene Glycol and Polyethylene Glycol as examples.

POLYOXYETHYLENE COMPOUNDS • The nonionic emulsifiers used in hand creams and lotions. Usually oily or waxy liquids.

POLYOXYMETHYLENE UREA • A bulking ingredient. The CIR Expert Panel (*see*) concluded that it is safe as a cosmetic ingredient but should not be used in aerosols. *See* Urea.

POLYOXYPROPYLENE GLYCOL • A mixture of polymers of ethylene oxide and propylene glycol (*see*) used as emollients, antistatic ingredients, and surfactants.

POLYP • Swollen or tumorous tissue that may or may not be cancerous.

POLYPERFLUOROMETHYLISOPROPYL ETHER • A skin-conditioning ingredient. *See* Polyols and Isopropyl Alchol.

POLYPHENOL • The polyphenols are compounds with antioxidant, antibacterial, and anticancer activity that are found in green tea and other foods and plants, including garlic, green tea, soybeans, cereal grains, ginger, and flaxseed. They are believed to act at both the initiation and the promotion stages of cancer development. They have been reported to interfere with tumor promotion by dampening steroid hormones. Polyphenols also act as "garbage collectors," disposing of mutagens and cancer-causing agents. Flavones (*see*) are among the best-known polyphenols. Formulations that contained methoxycinnamate, benzophenone-3, titanium dioxide, and the plant-based ingredients performed better in sunscreen in both SPF and the UVA protection, according to researchers.

POLYPOROUS UMBELLATUS • *See* Mushroom Extract.

POLYPROPYLENE • A synthetic plastic polymer with a molecular weight of 40,000 or more. Those with low molecular weight are used in gasoline additives, detergent processing, and lube oil additives as well as emulsion stabilizers. Those of higher weight are flexible. Used primarily in packaging and film forming.

POLYPROPYLENE GLYCOL • 1,2-Propanediol. A clear, colorless, viscous liquid, slightly bitter tasting, derived from propylene oxide. In cosmetics, it is the most common moisture-carrying vehicle other than water itself. It has better permeation through the skin than glycerin and is less expensive, although it has been linked to more sensitivity reactions. Absorbs moisture and acts as a solvent and a wetting ingredient. Used in liquid makeup, as a solvent for fats and oils, waxes, and resins; in cellophane, antifreeze solution, brake fluids, humectants, and preservatives. It is being reduced and replaced by safer glycols, such as butylene and polyethylene glycol.

POLYQUATERNIUM 1 THROUGH 14 • Antistatic ingredients and film formers. *See* Quaternary Ammonium Compounds.

POLYSACCHARIDES • Carbohydrates that are organic compounds consisting of carbon, hydrogen, and oxygen. The polysaccharides include starch, dextrin, glycogen, and cellulose.

POLYSILICONES • Used in lipsticks and hair products as a fixative. *See* Silicones.

POLYSORBATE-20 • A mixture of laurate esters of sorbitol and sorbitol anhydrides. It is used in facial moisturizers/treatments, anti-aging products, facial cleansers, hair color and bleaching products, foundations, body washes/cleansers, sunscreens SPF 15 and above, shampoos, styling gel/lotions, and moisturizers. The environmental working group SkinDeep says there is concern about this ingredient because: "One or more animal studies show endocrine system disruption at high doses." The CIR Expert Panel (*see*) reviewed data showing that polysorbates were not mutagens or complete carcinogens. The available data indicated that these ingredients were used in numerous preparations without clinical reports of significant adverse effects.

POLYSORBATE 40 • Widely used as an emulsifier in cosmetic creams and lotions and as a stabilizer of essential oils in water. All the polysorbates are nontoxic. The CIR Expert Panel (*see*) concluded that it is safe as a cosmetic ingredient as currently used.

POLYSORBATE 60, 80 • Both are emulsifiers that have been associated with the contaminant 1,4 dioxane, known to cause cancer in animals. The 60 is a condensate of sorbitol with stearic acid, and the 80 is a condensate of sorbitol and oleic acid (*see all*). The 60 is waxy and soluble in solvents. The 80 is a viscous liquid with a faint caramel odor and is widely used in baby lotions, cold creams, cream deodorants, antiperspirants, suntan lotions, and bath oil products. The CIR Expert Panel (*see*) concluded that these are safe as cosmetic ingredients as currently used.

POLYSORBATES 1 THROUGH 85 • These are widely used emulsifiers and stabilizers. For example, polysorbate 20 is a viscous, oily liquid derived from lauric acid. It is an emulsifier used in cosmetic creams and lotions, and a stabilizer of essential oils in water. It is used as a nonionic surfactant (*see*). Polysorbate 85 is used in tanning lotions. The polysorbate ingredients help other ingredients to dissolve in a solvent in which they would not normally dissolve. They also help to form emulsions by reducing the surface tension of the substances to be emulsified. Polysorbates are surfactants that are produced by reacting the polyol, sorbitol, with ethylene oxide. The polyoxyethylenated sorbitan is then reacted with fatty acids obtained from vegetable fats and oils such as lauric acid, palmitic acid, stearic acid, and oleic acid. Polysorbates function to disperse oil in water as opposed to water in oil. The safety of polysorbate 20, polysorbate 21, polysorbate 40, polysorbate 60, polysorbate 61, polysorbate 65, polysorbate 80, polysorbate 81, and polysorbate 85 has been assessed by the CIR Expert Panel. The panel evaluated the scientific data and concluded that polysorbates 20, 21, 40, 60, 61, 65, 80, 81, and 85 were safe as cosmetic ingredients. The Panel reviewed data showing that polysorbates were not mutagens or complete carcinogens. The available data indicated that these ingredients were used in numerous preparations without clinical reports of significant adverse effects.

POLYSTYRENE • Used in the manufacture of cosmetic resins. Colorless to yellowish oily liquid with a penetrating odor. Obtained from ethylbenzene by removing the hydrogen or by chlorination. Sparingly soluble in water; soluble in alcohol. Used in the manufacture of cosmetic resins. Used to make foam coffee cups, plates, and fast-food carry-out containers. May be irritating to the eyes and mucous membranes; in high concentrations, may be narcotic.

POLYSTYRENE LATEX • A white, plastic solid derived from petroleum and used in preparing opaque hair-waving lotions. It has outstanding moisture resistance.

POLYURETHANE • A heat-tolerating plastic produced by condensation of polyisocyanate and a hydroxyl-containing material.

POLYVINYL ACETATE • A binder, emulsion stabilizer, film former, and hair fixative. The CIR Expert Panel (*see*) concluded that it is safe as a cosmetic ingredient as currently used. *See* Polyvinylpyrrolidone.

POLYVINYL ALCOHOL • Synthetic resins used in lipstick, setting lotions, and various creams. A polymer prepared from polyvinyl acetates by replacement of the acetate groups with the hydroxyl groups. Dry, unplasticized polyvinyl alcohol powders are white to cream colored and have different viscosities. Solvent in hot and cold water, but certain ones require alcohol-water mixtures. The CIR Expert Panel (*see*) concluded that it is safe as a cosmetic ingredient as currently used.

POLYVINYL BUTYRAL • The condensation of polyvinyl alcohol and butyraldehyde (*see both*), it is a synthetic flavoring found in coffee and strawberry, and is used in the manufacture of rubber and synthetic resins and plasticizers. May be an irritant.

POLYVINYL CHLORIDE • PVC. Chloroethylene Polymer. Derived from vinyl chloride (*see*), it consists of a white powder or colorless granules that are resistant to weather, moisture, acids, fats, petroleum products, and fungus. It is widely used for everything from plumbing to raincoats. The use of PVC as a plastic wrap for food, including meats, and for human blood has alarmed some scientists. Children are at particular risk since many toys (such as chewable items) are made from PVC. Human and animal blood can extract potentially harmful chemicals from the plastic. The chemicals are added to polyvinyl chloride to make it flexible, and they migrate from the plastic into the blood and into the meats in amounts directly proportional to the length of time of storage. The result can be contamination of the blood, causing lung shock, a condition in which the patient's blood circulation to the lungs is impeded. PVC is also used in cosmetics and toiletries in containers, nail enamels, and creams. PVC has caused tumors when injected under the skin of rats in doses of 100 milligrams per kilogram of body weight.

POLYVINYL IMIDAZOLINIUM ACETATE • The polymer of vinyl imidazolinium acetate. *See* Polyvinylpyrrolidone.

POLYVINYL METHYL ETHER • *See* Polyvinyl Alcohol.

POLYVINYLPYRROLIDONE • PVP. A faintly yellow, solid, plastic resin resembling albumen. Used to give a softer set in shampoos, hair sprays, and lacquers; also a carrier in emollient creams, liquid lip rouge, and face rouge; also a clarifier in vinegar and a plasma expander in medicine. Ingestion may produce gas and fecal impaction or damage to lungs and kidneys. It may last in the system for months to a year. Strong circumstantial evidence indicates thesaurosis—foreign bodies in the lung—may be produced in susceptible individuals from concentrated exposure to PVP in hair sprays. Modest intravenous doses in rats caused them to develop tumors. The CIR Expert Panel (*see*) says based on available data, it is safe as a cosmetic ingredient.

POMADES • Almost synonymous with solid brilliantines (*see*) but of older origin. Pomades were originally made with the residual fatty material left from the enfleurage (*see*) process of extracting floral odors. Poma (apples) were used, hence giving the hairdressing its name.

POMEGRANATE • *Punica granatum.* An extract of the fruit pomegranate. Modern scientists have found that the skin of the fruit contains tannins, which from other plants have long been used in sunscreen preparations, eye lotions, and antiperspirants. In the past, it has been used to treat excessive perspiration and as a gargle for sore throats.

PONCEAU SX • A monoazo color. The name can be applied only to uncertified batches of color. The CTFA adopted name for certified batches is FD & C Red No. 4 (*see*). Widely used in all sorts of cosmetic products from perfumes to hair rinses to underarm deodorants and baby products.

PONGAMIA GLABRA • Indian Seed Oil. *Cystisus pinnatus.* An Asian evergreen used for shade. Indians have long used it to repel insects. Fats and oils used in hair and skin conditioners.

PONGAMOL • A fragrance ingredient. *See* Pongamia Glabra.

POPLAR EXTRACT • Balm of Gilead. Extract of the leaves and twigs of *Populus nigra.* In ancient times, buds were mashed to make a soothing salve to spread on sunburned areas, scalds, scratches, inflamed skin, and wounds. They were also simmered in lard for use as an ointment and for antiseptic purposes. The leaves and bark were steeped by American colonists to make a soothing tea. Supposedly relieved allergies and soothed reddened eyes.

POPPY OIL • *Papaver orientale.* A yellow to reddish oil obtained from the seeds of the poppy for use in emulsions and soaps and as a lubricant for fine machinery.

POPULUS • *See* Poplar Extract.

POPULUS NIGRA EXTRACT • The black poplar extract is used as a skin conditioner.

PORIA COCOS • A fungi used as an anticaking ingredient and emollient.

PORPHYRA UMBILICALIS • *See* Algae.

PORPHYRIDIUM CRUENTUM EXTRACT • Red Algae. Skin conditioner. *See* Algae.

PORTULACA • Portulaca is a small group of trailing annuals. *P. grandiflora,* sun plant, is a popular kind native of Brazil. Extract used as a skin conditioner and anti-aging cream. Avon, the promoter, says it "reduces the overall length, depth, and number of deep expression lines around your eyes, mouth, and forehead." Little if any scientific support has been published.

POTASSIUM • The healthy human body contains about nine grams of potassium. Most of it is found inside body cells. Potassium plays an important role in maintaining water balance and acid-base balance. It participates in the transmission of nerve impulses and in the transfer of messages from nerves to muscles. It also acts as a catalyst in carbohydrate and protein metabolism. Potassium is important for the maintenance of normal kidney function. It has a major effect on the heart and all the muscles of the body.

POTASSIUM ABIETOYL HYDROLYZED COLLAGEN • The potassium salt of the condensation product of abietic acid and hydrolyzed collagen (*see both*).

POTASSIUM ACESULFAME • Flavoring. *See* Acesulfame.

POTASSIUM ACETATE • White, crystalline, water-absorbing powder with a salt taste. Used in synthetic flavors and as a dehydrating ingredient.

POTASSIUM ACRYLATES/ACRYLAMIDE COPOLYMER • A film former. *See* Acrylamide and Acrylates.

POTASSIUM ACRYLINOLEATE • *See* Acrylinoleic Acid.

POTASSIUM ALGINATE • *See* Alginates.

POTASSIUM C12–13 ALKYL PHOSPHATE • A cleansing ingredient.

POTASSIUM ALUM • Cosmetic astringent and astringent in oral health care. *See* Alum.

POTASSIUM ALUMINUM POLYACRYLATE • A mixture of potassium and aluminum salts of polyacrylic acid used as an absorbent. *See* Acrylates.

POTASSIUM ASCORBYL TOCOPHERYL PHOSPHATE • Combination of vitamin E and vitamin C with phosphorus used as an antioxidant in moisturizers and other skin care products.

POTASSIUM ASPARTATE • The potassium salt of aspartic acid (*see*). Used as a skin conditioner.

POTASSIUM BABASSUATE • Extract of babassu (*see*) oil used as an emulsifier and cleansing ingredient.

POTASSIUM BENZOATE • A preservative. *See* Benzoic Acid.

POTASSIUM BICARBONATE • Carbonic Acid. Monopotassium Salt. Colorless, odorless, transparent crystals or powder, slightly alkaline, with a salty taste. Used as a pH adjuster in cosmetics.

POTASSIUM BINOXALATE • Potassium Acid Oxalate. Salt of Sorrel. White odorless crystals, which are poisonous, used in nail bleaches and as a stain remover.

POTASSIUM BIPHTHALATE • Phthalic Acid Potassium Acid Salt. A buffer used to affect alkalinity/acidity ratios. *See* Phthalic Acid.

POTASSIUM BORATE • Boric Acid. Potassium Salt. A crystalline salt used as an oxidizing ingredient and as a preservative in cosmetics and in flour. *See* Borates for toxicity.

POTASSIUM BROMATE • Antiseptic and astringent in toothpastes, mouthwashes, and gargles as a 3 to 5 percent solution. Colorless or white crystals. Very toxic when taken internally. Burns and skin irritation have been reported from its industrial uses. In toothpaste, it has been reported to have caused inflammation and bleeding of gums. It is a weak carcinogen in rats in oral feedings. Applied to the animal skin, it was not carcinogenic. The CIR Expert Panel (*see*) says based on available data, it is safe as a cosmetic ingredient, not to exceed 10.17 percent. It is on the Canadian Hotlist (*see*). The EU says it is not to be used in products for children under three. It also should not to be used on peeling or irritated skin.

POTASSIUM BUTYL ESTER OF PVM/MA COPOLYMER • Hair fixative.

POTASSIUM BUTYLPARABEN • Preservative. *See* Parabens.

POTASSIUM CAPRATE • A cleansing ingredient. *See* Capric Acid.

POTASSIUM CAPRYLOLYL GLUTAMATE • Amino acids used as a deodorant and cleansing ingredient.

POTASSIUM CARBONATE • Salt of Tartar. Pearl Ash. Inorganic salt of potassium. Odorless, white powder. Used in freckle lotions, liquid shampoos, vanishing creams, setting lotions, and permanent wave lotions; also in the manufacture of soap. Irritating and caustic to human skin and may cause dermatitis of the scalp, forehead, and hands.

POTASSIUM CARBOMER • Used as an emulsion stabilizer, thickener, and film former. *See* Carbomer.

POTASSIUM CARRAGEENAN • The potassium salt of carrageenan (*see*).

POTASSIUM CASEINATE • The potassium of milk proteins. *See* Casein.

POTASSIUM CASTORATE • The potassium salt of fatty acids derived from castor oil (*see*).

POTASSIUM CETYL PHOSPHATE • A mixture of esters of phosophoric acid and cetyl alcohol (*see both*).

POTASSIUM CHLORATE • Antiseptic, astringent in mouthwashes, toothpastes, and gargles as 2 to 5 percent solution. Used in bleach and freckle lotions and in permanent-wave solutions. Also used in explosives, fireworks, matches, dyeing, and in printing. May be absorbed through the skin. Irritating to the intestines and kidneys. Can cause dermatitis of the scalp, forehead, and hands. In toothpastes, reported to have caused inflammation of the gums. The salts are toxic to humans. The safety of this ingredient has not been documented and substantiated. The CIR Expert Panel (*see*) says that it cannot conclude whether potassium chlorate is safe for cosmetic products until such time that the appropriate safety data have been obtained and evaluated.

POTASSIUM CHLORIDE • Colorless or white crystals with a strong salty taste. It occurs naturally as sylvite deposits. Used in pharmaceutical and food additives as well as cosmetic ingredients. Ingestion of large doses can cause gastrointestinal irritation, purging, weakness, and circulatory collapse.

POTASSIUM CITRATE • pH adjuster. *See* Citric Acid.

POTASSIUM COCOATE • *See* Coconut Oil.

POTASSIUM COCO-HYDROLYZED PROTEIN • Hair conditioner and cleansing ingredient. On the basis of the available information, the CIR Expert Panel (*see*) found it safe in the early 1980s but is considering new information to determine if the final safety assessment should be reaffirmed, amended, or have an addendum. *See* Hydrolyzed Protein.

POTASSIUM COCOYL GLUTAMATE • Hair conditioner and cleansing ingredient. *See* Coconut Oil.

POTASSIUM COCOYL HYDROLYZED COLLAGEN • The potassium salt of the condensation product of coconut acid and hydrolyzed collagen. *See* Collagen.

POTASSIUM COCOYL HYDROLYZED POTATO, BRAN, RICE, SILK, SOY, AND WHEAT PROTEINS • Used as hair- and skin-conditioning ingredients.

POTASSIUM CORNATE • The potassium salt of fatty acids derived from corn oil. *See* Corn Oil.

POTASSIUM CYCLOCARBOXYPROPYLOLEATE • The potassium salt of cyclocarboxypropyloleate used in bath soaps and detergents.

POTASSIUM DEXTRIN OCTENYLSUCCINATE • A sugar mixed with potassium and succinic anhydride, it is used as an emulsion stabilizer and hair and skin conditioner.

POTASSIUM DIHYDROXYETHYL COCAMINE OXIDE PHOSPHATE • *See* Coconut Oil and Surfactants.

POTASSIUM DNA • The potassium salt of DNA (*see*), used in "youth creams" and other creams in which protein is included.

POTASSIUM DODECYLBENZENE SULFONATE • *See* Quaternary Ammonium Compounds.

POTASSIUM ETHYLPARABEN • *See* Parabens.

POTASSIUM FLUOROSILICATE • Oral care ingredient. *See* Potassium Fluoride and Fluorosilicate.

POTASSIUM FLUORIDE AND FLUOROSILICATE • Used in oral care products. The EU calculates at 0.15 percent when mixed with fluorine compounds. Fluorine concentration must not exceed 0.15 percent, and the EU label must say, "Contains potassium fluoride." *See* Fluoride and Silicates.

POTASSIUM GLUCOHEPTONOATE • A skin-conditioning ingredient. *See* Glucose and Heptanoic Acid.

POTASSIUM GLYCEROPHOSPHATE • Used in oral care products. *See* Phosphates.

POTASSIUM GLYCYRRHETINATE • Flavoring and skin conditioner. *See* Glycyrrhetinic Acid.

POTASSIUM GLYCOL SULFATE • *See* Polyethylene Glycol.

POTASSIUM GUAIACOL SULFONATE • *See* Quaternary Ammonium Compounds.

POTASSIUM HEMPSEEDATE • Derived from the seeds of *Cannabis sativa* used as a cleansing ingredient and emulsifier.

POTASSIUM HYALURONATE • *See* Hyaluronic Acid.

POTASSIUM HYDROGENATED COCOATE • *See* Coconut Oil and Hydrogenation.

POTASSIUM HYDROXIDE • Caustic Potash. Used as an emulsifier in hand lotions, as a cuticle softener, and as an alkali in liquid soaps, protective creams, shaving preparations, and cream rouges. It may cause irritation of the skin in cuticle removers. Extremely corrosive, and ingestion may cause violent pain, bleeding, collapse, and death. When applied to the skin of mice, moderate dosages cause tumors. May cause skin rash and burning. Concentrations above 5 percent can destroy fingernails as well. Good-quality toilet soaps do not contain more than 0.25 percent free alkali. It should be kept away from eyes, as it can cause blindness. Should be applied by professionals only, according to the EU.

POTASSIUM HYDROXYCITRATE • Skin conditioner. *See* Citric Acid.

POTASSIUM IODIDE • Potassium Salt. A dye remover and an antiseptic. Used in table salt as a source of dietary iodine. It is also in some drinking water. May cause allergic reactions.

POTASSIUM LACTATE • The salt of lactic acid (*see*) used as a buffering ingredient, exfoliant, and humectant.

POTASSIUM LAURATE • The potassium salt of lauric acid (*see*).

POTASSIUM LAURETH -4, -5, -6, -10 CARBOXYLATE • Cleansing ingredient. *See* Lauric Acid.

POTASSIUM LAURETH PHOSPHATE • Cleansing ingredient, foam booster, and solubilizing ingredient. *See* Lauryl Alcohol.

POTASSIUM LAUROYL GLUTAMATE • Amino acids used as hair conditioner.

POTASSIUM LAUROYL HYDROLYZED COLLAGEN • The potassium salt of the condensation product of lauric acid chloride and hydrolyzed collagen. *See* Hydrolyzed Collagen.

POTASSIUM LAUROYL METHYL BETA-ALANINE • Amino acid compound used as a skin conditioner.

POTASSIUM LAUROYL PCA • Skin conditioner, emulsifier, and humectant. *See* Lauric Acid.

POTASSIUM LAUROYL SARCOSINATE • Hair conditioner and cleanser. *See* Sarcosine.

POTASSIUM LAURYL SULFATE • A water softener used in shampoos. *See* Sodium Lauryl Sulfate.

POTASSIUM LINOLEATE • Used as a surfactant, emulsifying ingredient, and thickener. *See* Linoleic Acid.

POTASSIUM METABISULFITE • Potassium Pyrosulfite. White granules or powder with a sharp odor, used as an antiseptic, preservative, antioxidant, and as a developing ingredient in dyes. Also as hair waxing or straightening products. Low toxicity. Risk of eye damage. EU

POTASSIUM METHOXYCINNAMATE • Ultralight absorber used in sun protectants.

POTASSIUM METHYLPARABEN • *See* Parabens.

POTASSIUM MONOFLUOROPHOSPHATE • Oral hygiene product the EU calculates at 0.50 percent when mixed with other fluorine compounds. Fluorine concentration must not exceed 0.15 percent, and the EU label must say, "Contains potassium monofluorophosphate." *See* Fluorine.

POTASSIUM MYRISTATE • The potassium salt of myristic acid (*see*).

POTASSIUM MYRISTOYL HYDROLYZED COLLAGEN • Potassium salt of the condensation product of myristic acid chloride and hydrolyzed collagen. *See* Hydrolyzed Collagen and Myristic Acid.

POTASSIUM OCTOXYNOL-12 PHOSPHATE • The potassium salt of a mixture of esters of phosphoric acid and octoxynol (*see both*).

POTASSIUM OLEATE • Oleic Acid Potassium Salt. Used as a detergent. Yellowish or brownish soft mass. Soluble in water or alcohol.

POTASSIUM OLEOYL HYDROLYZED COLLAGEN • The potassium salt of the condensation product of oleic acid chloride and hydrolyzed collagen (*see*).

POTASSIUM PALMITATE • The potassium salt of palmitic acid (*see*).

POTASSIUM OLIVATE • *See* Olive Oil.

POTASSIUM OXIDIZED MICROCRYSTALLINE WAX • Thickener. *See* Microcrystalline Wax.

POTASSIUM PALMATE • Thickener and emulsifier. *See* Palm Oil.

POTASSIUM PALMITOYL HYDROLYZED CORN PROTEIN • Hair- and skin-conditioning ingredient and cleanser. *See* Corn.

POTASSIUM PARABEN • *See* Parabens.

POTASSIUM PCA • *See* Proline.

POTASSIUM PEANUTATE • Emulsifier. *See* Peanut Oil.

POTASSIUM PERSULFATE • Colorless, or white, odorless crystals. A powerful oxidant. Soluble in water. The solution is acid and is used in the manufacture of soaps and as a germicidal preparation for the bathroom. Aqueous solutions of 2.5 to 3 percent are not irritating to humans, but greater amounts can be very irritating. .

POTASSIUM O-PHENYLPHENATE • Preservative. *See* Phenols.

POTASSIUM PHENOXIDE • Preservative. *See* Phenols.

POTASSIUM PHOSPHATE • Monobasic, Dibasic, and Tribasic. Used as a buffering ingredient in shampoos and in cuticle removers. Colorless to white powder, also used as a yeast food in brewing industries in the production of champagne and other sparkling wines. Has been used medicinally as a urinary acidifier.

POTASSIUM POLYACRYLATE • *See* Acrylates.

POTASSIUM PROPIONATE • Preservative. *See* Propionate.

POTASSIUM PROPYLPARABEN • Preservative. *See* Parabens.

POTASSIUM RAPESEEDATE • Used as an emulsifier and thickener. *See* Rapeseed Oil.

POTASSIUM RICINOLEATE • The potassium salt of ricinoleic acid (*see*).

POTASSIUM SAFFLOWERATE • Derived from safflower oil (*see*) used as a soap.

POTASSIUM SALICYLATE • Preservative. The EU has banned it for children under three years except in shampoos. *See* Salicylates.

POTASSIUM SALTS OF FATTY ACIDS • The reaction of potassium salts on fatty acids (*see*) creates liquid soap.

POTASSIUM SILICATE • Soluble Potash Glass. Colorless or yellowish translucent to transparent glasslike particles. Used as a binder in cosmetics and in soap manufacturing. Also used as a detergent and in the glass and ceramics industries. Usually very slowly soluble in cold water.

POTASSIUM SODIUM COPPER CHLOROPHYLLIN • Chlorophyllin Copper Complex. Does not require certification. It has been permanently listed to color dentifrices that are cosmetics and is not to be used in excess of 0.1 percent in combination. *See* Chlorophyllin for toxicity.

POTASSIUM SODIUM TARTRATE • Rochelle Salt. Used in the manufacture of baking powder and in the silvering of mirrors. Translucent crystals or white, crystalline powder with cooling saline taste. Slight efflorescence in warm air. Probably used in mouthwashes, but use not identified in cosmetics.

POTASSIUM SORBATE • Sorbic Acid Potassium Salt. Used as a mold and yeast inhibitor. May cause mild irritation of the skin. On the basis of available information, the CIR Expert Panel (*see*) concluded that it is safe as presently used in cosmetic formulations.

POTASSIUM STEARATE • Stearic Acid Potassium Salt. Strongly alkaline. Used in the manufacture of soap, hand creams, emulsified fragrances, hair conditioners, lotions, and shaving creams. Acts as a defoaming ingredient. On the basis of the available information, the CIR Expert Panel (*see*) found it safe in the early 1980s but is considering new information to determine if the final safety assessment should be reaffirmed, amended, or have an addendum.

POTASSIUM STEAROYL HYDROLYZED COLLAGEN • The potassium salt of the condensation product of stearic acid chloride and hydrolyzed collagen (*see*).

POTASSIUM SULFIDE • Depilating ingredient. Toxic. Irritant. Label must read "avoid contact with eyes and keep out of reach of children." On the Canadian Hotlist (*see*). *See* Sulfides. E

POTASSIUM SULFATE • Does not occur free in nature but is combined with sodium sulfate. Colorless, or white, crystalline powder with a bitter taste. Used as a reingredient (*see*) in cosmetics and as a salt substitute. Large doses can cause severe gastrointestinal bleeding.

POTASSIUM SULFITE • *See* Sulfites.

POTASSIUM TALLATE • *See* Tall Oil.

POTASSIUM TALLOWATE • Emulsifier and moisturizer. The potassium salt of tallow acid (*see*). Has been associated with eczema (*see*).

POTASSIUM TARTRATE • Cleansing ingredient used in mouthwashes and skin care products. *See* Tartaric Acid.

POTASSIUM THIOCYANATE • An inorganic salt used in moisturizers. *See* Thiocyanate.

POTASSIUM THIOGLYCOLATE • Depilatory. *See* Thioglycolic Acid Compounds.

POTASSIUM TOLUENESULFONATE • A water-soluble powder that may be used in cosmetics as a solubilizing (*see* Solubilization) ingredient in conjunction with other detergent materials. *See* Toluene for toxicity.

POTASSIUM TRIDECETH PHOSPHATE • Cleanser.

POTASSIUM TROCLOSENE • Troclosene. Potassium. Used in solid bleaches and detergents, and as a local anti-infective ingredient.

POTASSIUM UNDECYLENATE • Fine white powder used as a bacteriostat and fungistat in cosmetics and pharmaceuticals. Toxic in high concentrations.

POTASSIUM UNDECYLENOYL CARRAGEENAN • Hair and skin conditioner. *See* Carrageenan.

POTASSIUM UNDECYLENOYL GLUTAMATE • Abrasive and hair conditioner. *See* Glutamate and Undecylenic Acid.

POTASSIUM UNDECYLENOYL HYDROLYZED COLLAGEN • *See* Hydrolyzed Protein.

POTASSIUM XYLENE SULFONATE • *See* Xylene.

POTATO EXTRACT • The extract of *Solanum tuberosum.*

POTATO STARCH • Flour prepared from potatoes, ground to a pulp, and washed of fibers. Swells in hot water to form a gel on cooling. A demulcent used in dusting powder, an emollient in dry shampoos and baby powders. With glycerin forms soothing, protective applications for eczema, skin rash, and chapped skin. May cause allergic skin reactions in the hypersensitive.

POTENTILLA • *See* Great Burnet and Tormentil.

POTENTILLA ERECTA ROOT EXTRACT • Widely used skin conditioner in shampoos and skin and hair products. *See* Tormentil.

POTERIUM OFFICINALE • *See* Great Burnet.

POULTICE • A warm mass of powdered herbs applied directly to the skin to reduce swelling.

POWDER • Face, Compact, and Dusting. Applied to the body with a puff. Usually done at the end of the makeup process. Its objective is to remove the "shine" from the face and to give a healthy subtle glow. Face powders are either loose or compacted. Talc is the principal ingredient (about 50 percent), but face powders also include about 15 percent of a clay, kaolin, and about 10 percent precipitated calcium carbonate, 10 percent zinc oxide, 10 percent zinc stearate, 5 percent magnesium carbonate (*see all*), perfume, and pigments. Also included are fractions of barium sulfate, boric acid, cetyl alcohol, titanium dioxide, rice, or cornstarch (*see all*). The absorbing, covering, and adherent properties of the face powder may be changed by varying the amounts of the ingredients or by elimination of some of them. For instance, eliminating titanium dioxide makes the powder more transparent. Various pigments are used for shades of face powder, including yellow ocher, red ocher, umber, ultramarine blue, and violet, all inorganic pigments. Organic pigments used may include D & C Red No. 7 Calcium Lake or D & C Orange No. 4 (*see both*). Problems with face powders are rare. The FDA recorded a concern with rash. Compact powder is similar to face powder but includes binders such as gums (*see*); cake makeup employs a binder such as lecithin. Also used in compact powder to make it keep its shape are glyceryl monostearate glycols or mineral oil (*see all*) and other oils. Dusting powder, usually used after a bath or shower, generally contains talc, perfumes, and zinc stearate (*see*). Toxicity concerns mechanical blocking of pores and subsequent irritation by the powders. *See* Talc and Starch for toxicity.

PPDA • Abbreviation for para-phenylenediamine. *See* Phenylenediamine.

PPG • Abbreviation for polypropylene glycol and polyoxypropylene glycol (*see both*).

PPG BUTETH-260 THROUGH -5100 • Emulsifiers. *See* Propylene Glycol.

PPG BUTETH ETHER-200 • Emulsifier. Polymer (*see*) prepared from butyl alcohol with propylene glycol (*see both*).

PPG BUTYL ETHER-300 TO -1715 • Emulsifiers. Used in many skin and hair care products. The CIR Expert Panel (*see*) has listed this as top priority for review for the whole PPG butyl ether family. May cause irritation. The CIR is concerned about the potential of absorption through the skin.

PPG-4-CETEARETH-12 • Emulsifier. *See* Cetearyl Alcohol.

PPG-10-CETEARETH-20 • *See* Cetearyl Alcohol.

PPG-4-CETETH-1 OR -5 OR -10 • *See* Cetyl Alcohol.

PPG-10-CETYL ETHER • *See* Cetyl Alcohol.

PPG-28 CETYL ETHER • *See* Cetyl Alcohol and Propylene Glycol.
PPG-30 CETYL ETHER • A liquid, nonionic, surface-active ingredient (*see*). *See* Cetyl Alcohol.
PPG-5-CETETH-10-PHOSPHATE • Used in tanning creams. *See* Cetyl Alcohol and Phosphates.
PPG-20-DECYLTETRADECETH-10 • *See* Decanoic Acid.
PPG-2 DIBENZOATE • *See* Dipropylene Glycol Dibenzoate.
PPG-24 OR -66 GLYCERETH-24 OR -12 • *See* Glycerin.
PPG-27 AND -55 GLYCERYL ETHER • *See* Glycerin and Propylene Glycol.
PPG-ISOCETYL ETHER • *See* Cetyl Alcohol.
PPG-3-ISOSTEARETH-9 • *See* Stearyl Alcohol and Propylene Glycol.
PPG-2, -5, -10, -20, -30 LANOLIN ALCOHOL ETHERS • *See* Lanolin Alcohols.
PPG-30 LANOLIN ETHER • Derived from lanolin alcohols (*see*).
PPG-5 LANOLIN WAX • An emollient. Based on the available data, the CIR Expert Panel (*see*) concludes that it is safe as used in cosmetics. *See* Lanolin and Propylene Glycol.
PPG-9 LAURATE • *See* Lauric Acid.
PPG-4 LAURETH-2, -5, -7 • Skin conditioner. *See* Lauryl Alcohol.
PPG-5-LAURETH-5 • Emollient. *See* Lauryl Alcohol.
PPG-2 METHYL ETHER • Solvent. *See* Propylene Glycol.
PPG-20-METHYL GLUCOSE ETHER • *See* Propylene Glycol and Glucose.
PPG-20-METHYL GLUCOSE ETHER DISTEARATE • *See* Propylene Glycol, Glucose, and Stearic Acid.
PPG-3-MYRETH-11 • *See* Polyethylene Glycol and Myristic Acid.
PPG-4 MYRISTYL ETHER • *See* Myristyl Alcohol.
PPG-26 OLEATE • Polyoxypropylene 2000 Monooleate. Carbowax. A solid polyethylene glycol (*see*). Each PPG is a mixture of several polymers (*see*) with various consistencies. Used as a base or carrier in hand lotions, hairdressings, and various other cosmetic lotions.
PPG-36 OLEATE • Polyoxypropylene (36) Monooleate. *See* Polypropylene and Oleic Acid.
PPG-10 OLEYL ETHER • *See* PPG-26 Oleate.
PPG-30, -50 OLEYL ETHER • *See* PPG-26 Oleate.
PPG-6-C12–18 PARETH • A mixture of synthetic alcohols. *See* Fatty Alcohols.
PPG-12-PEG-50 LANOLIN • *See* Polypropylene and Lanolin.
PPG-70 POLYGLYCERYL-10 ETHER • An alcohol used as a hair fixative. *See* Polyglycerol.
PPG-2 SALICYLATE • *See* Dipropylene Glycol Salicylate.
PPG-9-STEARETH-3 • *See* Stearyl Alcohol.
PPG-11 OR -15 STEARYL ETHER • Widely used in cosmetics as moisturizers and cleansers. *See* Polypropylene Glycol and Stearyl Alcohol.
PPG-6 TRIDECETH-8 • An alcohol used as an emollient and emulsifier. *See* Polyoxyethylene Compounds.
PPM • Parts per million.
PRASTERONE • A sterol (*see*) used as a skin conditioner.
PRECIPITATE • To separate out from solution or suspension. A deposit of solid separated out from a solution or suspension as a result of a chemical or physical change, as by the action of a reingredient (*see*).
PRECURSOR • A substance turned into another active or more mature substance by a biologic process. Beta-carotene is a precursor of vitamin A because the body can use it to make vitamin A.

PREDNISOLONE • Introduced in 1955, prednisolone is related chemically to hydrocortisone (*see*) and is used in tablet, syrup, liquid, salve, suppository, enema, and injection form. It is used to treat severe inflammation, as an immunosuppressant, and in the treatment of ulcerative colitis and proctitis. Most adverse reactions are the result of dose or length of time of administration. Contraindicated in systemic fungal infections. Prednisolone is also used in eyedrops to treat inflammation of the eyes. Potential adverse reactions for that use include increased eye pressure, thinning of the cornea, and increased susceptibility to viral and fungal eye infections.

PREDNISONE • Introduced in 1955 and related chemically to corticosteroids (*see*), prednisone is widely used to treat severe inflammation, as an immunosuppressant, and to treat acute attacks of multiple sclerosis, arthritis, and irritable bowel syndrome. Most adverse reactions are the result of dose or length of time of administration.

PREGNENOLONE ACETATE • Derived from the urine of pregnant women. Used topically as an anti-inflammatory, anti-itch ingredient. A corticosteroid.

PRENYL ACETATE • Synthetic flavoring with a fruity, pear, green taste and an aroma that is fruity, floral, and pear. Not as pungent as amyl acetate (*see*) but relatively longer lasting. Used in cosmetics, detergents, fabric softeners and soaps, and food additives. May be irritating to the skin and eyes. EAF

PRESERVATIVES • Because the presence of viable microorganisms in cosmetic products can lead to separation of emulsions, discoloration, the formation of gas and odors, and changes in the general properties, as well as possible infection for the users, a preservative must be effective against a wide range of microorganisms. It must not be toxic internally or externally. It must not alter the character of the product, and it is required to be long-lasting and inexpensive. Many kinds of yeasts, fungi, and bacteria have been identified in cosmetics, including pseudomonas, staphylococcus, and streptococcus. In many instances a product might show no visible evidence of microbial contamination and yet contain actively growing, potentially harmful germs. Esters of phydroxybenzoic acid are the most widely used preservatives.

PRESHAVING LOTIONS • *See* Shaving Lotions.

PRICKLY ASH EXTRACT • *Zanthoxylum americanum.* Toothache Tree. A native American herb, the bark and berries have been used for more than two hundred years to treat cholera, syphilis, rheumatism, gonorrhea, fevers, dysentery, neuritis, and ulcers. It has been found to contain coumarins, alkaloids (*see both*), and lignins. One of the lignins, asarinin, has been found by modern pharmaceutical researchers to have antitubercular action. The plant is a stimulant and was also used to produce perspiration. It was a popular remedy for chronic rheumatism and was used extensively in the United States for this purpose. The bark was chewed raw, or inserted into cavities, as a toothache remedy. Prickly ash bark was also used in the treatment of flatulence and diarrhea.

PRICKLY PEAR • *Opuntia tuna. See* Cactus.

PRIMROSE • *Primula vulgaris.* Easter Rose. A perennial native to Britain and Europe, it flourishes in meadows, hedges, and ditches. The name comes from the Latin word for first, *primu,* because it was the first rose of spring. Herbalists used it in a tea to treat arthritis, gout, and migraine, and as a general blood cleanser. A decoction of the root is given for catarrh, coughs, and bronchitis. It is also used to cure insomnia. It is used in "organic" cosmetics.

PRIMULA EXTRACT • The extract of various species of *Primula* taken from the rhizome and roots of the primrose or cowslip. Used as a skin-conditioning ingredient in cosmetics. In some sensitive persons, it may cause a rash.

PRISTANE • Liquid hydrocarbon obtained from shark-liver oil and from ambergris (*see both*). Used as a lubricant and anticorrosive ingredient in cosmetics.

PROANTHOCYANIDINS • *See* Anthocyanins.

PROBIOTICS • The opposite of antibiotics, certain bacteria are deliberately added to cosmetics as skin conditioners. Yogurt is an example as the product of a "friendly" bacteria. *Lactobacillus.*

PROCAINAMIDE AND ITS SALTS AND DERIVATIVES • Local anesthetic. Banned by the EU and ASEAN (*see*) in cosmetics.

PROCOLLAGEN • The precursor of collagen (*see*). Used in hair conditioners.

PROGESTERONE • A female sex hormone used in face cream for its supposed anti-wrinkle properties. There is no proven benefit to the skin, and it may be absorbed through the skin and have adverse systemic effects. The EU banned progestogens in cosmetics. *See* Hormone Creams.

PROLINAMIDOETHYL IMIDAZOLE • Used as a skin protectant. *See* Imidazole.

PROLINE • An amino acid (*see*) used as a food supplement usually isolated from wheat or gelatin. Widely used as a hair and skin conditioner in moisturizers, hair and skin preparations, and cleansing lotions. GRAS

PROPAGERMANIUM • Skin conditioner. *See* Carbomer-934, -940, -941.

PROPANE • A gas heavier than air; odorless when pure. It is used as a fuel and refrigerant. Cleared for use in a spray propellant and as an aerating ingredient for cosmetics in aerosols. May be narcotic in high doses. On the basis of the available information, the CIR Expert Panel (*see*) found it safe in the early 1980s but is considering new information to determine if the final safety assessment should be reaffirmed, amended, or have an addendum. The EU bans propane-1,2,3-trinitrate in cosmetics.

PROPANEDIOL • An alcohol used as a solvent. *See* Propylene Glycol.

PROPANOL • Another name for propyl alcohol. It is derived from propane, a flammable, gaseous paraffin hydrocarbon that occurs naturally in crude petroleum and natural gas. It is used in the manufacture of cosmetics.

PROPELLANT • A compressed gas used to expel the contents of containers in the form of aerosols. Chlorofluorocarbons were widely used because of their nonflammability. The strong possibility that they contribute to depletion of the ozone layer of the upper atmosphere has resulted in prohibition of their use for this purpose. Other propellants used are hydrocarbon gases, such as butane and propane, carbon dioxide, and nitrous oxide. The materials dispersed include shaving cream, whipping cream, and cosmetic preparations.

PROPENYL GUAETHOL • Free-flowing white powder with an odor and taste similar to vanilla but much more powerful. Used as artificial vanilla flavoring and flavor enhancer.

PROPILIS, PROPOLIS • Resinous mixture collected from tree buds by bees. Antibacterial, anti-inflammatory.

PROPIONATE • Propionic Acid, Ammonium Propionate, Calcium Propionate, Magnesium Propionate, Potassium Propionate, and Sodium Propionate prevent or retard bacterial growth. Propionic Acid is also used to control the pH of cosmetics and personal care products. Propionate is formed every day in our intestines when dietary fiber is fermented. It is subsequently absorbed into the bloodstream. It has been estimated that 5 to 10 percent of the population may have various food sensitivities or intolerance. Of this group, 30 to 40 percent may be affected by propionate, but not in isolation. Sensitivity to propionate always occurs in conjunction with sensitivity to other chemicals, either naturally occurring or added to products.

PROPIONIC ACID • Occurs naturally in apples, strawberries, tea, and violet leaves. An oily liquid with a slightly pungent, rancid odor. Can be obtained from wood pulp and waste liquor, and by fermentation. Used in perfume bases and as a mold inhibitor, antioxidant, and preservative in cosmetics. Its salts have been used as antifungal ingredients to treat skin mold. Large oral dose in rats is lethal. The Food and Drug Administration issued a notice in 1992 that propionic acid has not been shown to be safe and effective for stated claims in OTC products.

PROPIONIC ANHYDRIDE • Used in perfume oils. It has a more pungent odor than that of propionic acid (*see*).

PROPIONYL COLLAGEN AMINO ACIDS • *See* Collagen.

PROPOLIS WAX • Extracted from propolis, a resin found in beehives. *See* Beeswax.

PROPOSITION 65 • In 1986, California voters overwhelmingly approved an initiative to address growing concerns about exposures to toxic chemicals. That initiative became the Safe Drinking Water and Toxic Enforcement Act of 1986, better known by its original name, Proposition 65. It requires the governor to publish a list of chemicals that are known to the State of California to cause cancer, birth defects, or other reproductive harm. Agents that cause cancer are called carcinogens; those that cause birth defects or other reproductive harm are called reproductive toxicants. This list must be updated at least once a year. Over 550 chemicals have been listed as of April 1, 1996. Proposition 65 imposes certain controls that apply to chemicals that appear on this list. These controls are designed to protect California's drinking water sources from contamination by these chemicals, to allow California consumers to make informed choices about the products they purchase, and to enable residents or workers to take whatever action they deem appropriate to protect themselves from exposures to these harmful chemicals. Thus, Proposition 65 also provides a market-based incentive for manufacturers to remove listed chemicals from their products. The benefits of the proposition have their costs. Businesses have incurred expenses to test products, develop alternatives, reduce discharges, provide warnings, and otherwise comply with the requirements of the proposition. Recognizing that compliance with the proposition comes at a price, Cal/EPA and the Office of Environmental Health Hazard Assessment (the lead agency for Proposition 65 implementation) have worked hard to minimize any unnecessary regulatory burdens and ensure that placement of a chemical on the list is done in accordance with rigorous science in an open public process.

PROPOXYTETRAMETHYL PIPERIDINYL DIMETHICONE • Hair conditioner. *See* Silicones.

PROPYL ACETATE • Colorless liquid, soluble in water, derived from propane and acetate (*see both*). It has the odor of pears. Used in the manufacture of perfumes and as a solvent for resins. It may be irritating to the skin and mucous membranes.

PROPYL ALCOHOL • Obtained from crude fuel oil. Alcoholic and slightly overpowering odor. Occurs naturally in cognac green oil, cognac white oil, and onion oil. A synthetic fruit flavoring. Used instead of ethyl alcohol as a solvent for shellac, gums, resins, and oils; as a denaturant (*see*) for alcohol in perfumery. Not a primary irritant but, because it dissolves fat, it has a drying effect on the skin and may lead to cracking, fissuring, and infections. No adverse effects have been reported from local application as a lotion, liniment, mouthwash, gargle, or sponge bath.

PROPYL BENZOATE • Fragrance ingredient. *See* Benzoic Acid.

PROPYL GALLATE • Antioxidant and fragrance ingredient in makeup, cleansers, creams, lotions, and tanning preparations. Based on available data, the CIR Expert Panel (*see*) says it is safe as a cosmetic ingredient. Has been reported to cause allergic reactions. *See* Phenols.

PROPYL OLEATE • *See* Oleic Acid.

PROPYLAMINE • 1-Aminopropane. An alkaline base for cosmetics, it is a colorless liquid with strong ammonia odor. Miscible in water, alcohol, and ether. Strong skin irritant. May cause allergic reactions.

PROPYLENE CARBONATE • Colorless liquid used as a solvent and plasticizer. The CIR Expert Panel (*see*) says, based on available data, it is safe as a cosmetic ingredient.

PROPYLENE GLYCOL • 1, 2-Propanediol. An organic alcohol, it is one of the most widely used cosmetic ingredients. It is the most common moisture-carrying vehicle other than water itself in cosmetics. It has better permeation through the skin than glycerin and is less expensive, although it has been linked to more sensitivity reactions. Absorbs moisture and acts as a solvent and a wetting ingredient. Used in liquid makeup, foundation makeup, foundation creams, mascaras, spray deodorants, hair straighteners, liquid powders, preshave lotions, after-shave lotions, baby lotions, cold creams, emollients, antiperspirants, lipsticks, mouthwashes, stick perfumes, and suntan lotions. Propylene glycols attract water and function as moisturizers to enhance the appearance of skin by reducing flaking and restoring suppleness. Propylene glycol is also used to help stabilize formulations. Polypropylene Glycols (PPG), including PPG-9, PPG-12, PPG-15, PPG-17, PPG-20, PPG-26, PPG-30, and PPG-34, are polymers of propylene glycol and water. The number in the name represents that average number of units of propylene glycol in the compound. In 1992, the FDA proposed a ban on propylene glycol in louse-killing products because it has not been shown to be safe and effective for its stated claims. The CIR Expert Panel (*see*) says, based on available data, it is safe as a cosmetic ingredient in concentrations up to 50 percent. It has been reported to cause allergic reactions. Its use is being reduced, and it is being replaced by safer glycols such as butylene and polyethylene glycol. Propylene glycol and some other glycol compounds are used as solvents for the active ingredients in transdermal patches that are used to put medications through the skin. ASP

PROPYLENE GLYCOL ALGINATE • The propylene glycol ester of alginic acid (*see*), derived from seaweed, the most common moisture-carrying vehicle in cosmetics other than water. Used as a stabilizer and defoaming ingredient in cosmetics and food.

PROPYLENE GLYCOL CAPRYLATE • *See* Polyethylene Glycol and Capric Acid.

PROPYLENE GLYCOL DICAPRYLATE/DICAPRIATE • A gel used in emollients. The CIR Expert Panel (*see*) says, based on available data, it is safe as a cosmetic ingredient. *See* Propylene Glycol and Capric Acid.

PROPYLENE GLYCOL DICOCONATE • Mixture of propylene glycol esters of coconut fatty acids. Based on available data, the CIR Expert Panel (*see*) says it is safe as a cosmetic ingredient. *See* Propylene Glycol.

PROPYLENE GLYCOL DIOLEATE • Skin conditioner and thickener. *See* Octanoic Acid.

PROPYLENE GLYCOL DIPELARGONATE • The CIR Expert Panel (*see*) says, based on available data, it is safe as a cosmetic ingredient. Used as a skin conditioner and thickener in makeup including lipsticks and foundations, as well as in fragrances, moisturizers, and cleansers. *See* Propylene Glycol.

PROPYLENE GLYCOL LAURATE • An ester of propylene glycol and lauric acid. An emulsifying ingredient for solvents, cosmetic creams, and lotions; also a stabilizer of essential oils in water. Light orange oil, dispersible in water, soluble in alcohol and oils, but can cause allergic reactions in the hypersensitive. Based on available data, the CIR Expert Panel (*see*) says it is safe as a cosmetic ingredient.

PROPYLENE GLYCOL MYRISTATE • Used as an emollient in skin care preparations. Based on available data, the CIR Expert Panel (*see*) says it is safe as a cosmetic ingredient. *See* Propylene Glycol and Myristic Acid.

PROPYLENE GLYCOL RICINOLEATE • Ester of propylene glycol and ricinoleic acid (*see both*).

PROPYLENE GLYCOL STEARATE • Cream-colored wax. Disperses in water, soluble in hot alcohol. Widely used lubricating ingredient and emulsifier in cosmetic creams and lotions. Stabilizer of essential oils. On the basis of the available information, the CIR Expert Panel (*see*) found it safe in the early 1980s but is considering new information to determine if the final safety assessment should be reaffirmed, amended, or have an addendum.

PROPYLENE GLYCOL STEARATE SE • A widely used emulsifier. On the basis of the available information, the CIR Expert Panel (*see*) found it safe in the early 1980s but is considering new information to determine if the final safety assessment should be reaffirmed, amended, or have an addendum. *See* Propylene Glycol.

PROPYLPARABEN • Propyl *p*-Hydroxybenzoate. Developed in Europe, the esters of *p*-hydroxybenzoic acid are widely used in the cosmetic industry as preservatives and bacteria and fungus killers. They are active against a variety of organisms, are neutral, low in toxicity, slightly soluble, and active in all solutions, alkaline, neutral, or acid. Used in shampoos, baby preparations, foundation creams, beauty masks, dentifrices, eye lotions, hair-grooming aids, nail creams, and wave sets. Used medicinally to treat fungus infections. Can cause contact dermatitis. Less toxic than benzoic or salicylic acid (*see both*). *See* Parabens.

PROPYLTRIMONIUM HYDROLYZED COLLAGEN • *See* Hydrolyzed Collagen.

PROSTAGLANDINS • PGA. PGB. PGC. PGD. A group of extremely potent hormonelike substances present in many tissues. There are more than sixteen known with effects such as dilating or constricting blood vessels, stimulation of intestinal or bronchial smooth muscle, uterine stimulation, and antagonism to hormones and influencing fat metabolism. Various prostaglandins in the body can cause fever, inflammation, and headaches. Prostaglandins or drugs that affect prostaglandins are used medically to induce labor, prevent and treat peptic ulcers, control high blood pressure, in the treatment of bronchial asthma, and to induce delayed menstruation. Aspirin tends to inhibit prostaglandin production.

PROTEASE • An enzyme that breaks down protein. In 1992, the FDA issued a notice that protease had not been shown to be safe and effective as claimed in OTC digestive aid products. Used in cosmetics as a skin-conditioning ingredient.

PROTECTIVE CREAMS • Water-repellent or oil-repellent creams designed to act as barrier ingredients against irritating chemicals, including water. Some products, such as the widely used silicones, are both water- and oil-repellent. Among the chemicals used in protective creams are stearic acid, beeswax, glycerin, casein, ammonium hydroxide, zinc stearate, titanium dioxide, butyl stearate, petrolatum, polyethylene glycol, paraffin, potassium hydroxide, magnesium stearate, aluminum compounds, benzoic acid, borates, calamine, ceresin, lanolin, salicylates, sodium silicate, talc, and triethanolamine (*see all*).

PROTEIN FATTY ACID CONDENSATES • *See* Amide.

PROTEIN PAC • New name for some hair moisturizers.

PROTEINS • The chief nitrogen-containing constituents of plants and animals—the essential constituents of every living cell. They are complex but by weight contain about 50 percent carbon, about 20 percent oxygen, about 15 percent nitrogen, about 7 percent hydrogen, and some sulfur. Some also contain iron and phosphorus. Proteins are colorless, odorless, and generally tasteless. They vary in solubility. They readily undergo putrefaction, hydrolysis, and dilution with acids or alkalis. They are regarded as combinations of amino acids (*see*). Cosmetic manufacturers, particularly makers of hair products, claim that "protein enrichment" is beneficial to the hair and skin. Hair, of course, is already dead. It does consist of a type of protein, keratin (*see*), but the surface of the hair is cornified tissue that cannot be revitalized. Such products will add body to thin hair and add gloss or luster, but so will other hair conditioners (*see*). As for face creams with protein, the lubricant is more beneficial than the protein.

PRUNELLA VULGARIS • A family of herbs that yields popular fruits. Extracts used as skin conditioners.

PRUNES • A source of fiber. A plum that is dried. Fruit from a shrub related to almond, apricot, cherry, and peach.

PRUNUS AMYGDALUS, P. AMARA • *See* Almond Oil.

PRUNUS AMYGDALUS, P. DULCIS • Sweet Almond. Skin conditioner widely used in makeup, hair products, and bath products. *See* Almond Oil.

PRUNUS ARMENIACA • *See* Apricot.

PRUNUS AVIUM • *See* Sweet Cherry Extract and Oil.

PRUNUS CERASUS • Bitter Cherry. Used as an antioxidant.

PRUNUS DOMESTICA • *See* Prunes.

PRUNUS PERSICA • *See* Peach Juice Extract.

PRUNUS SEROTINA • *See* Wild Cherry Bark.

PRUNUS SPECIOSA • The EU name for cherry.

PRUNUS SPINOSA FRUIT JUICE • Blackthorn. Used as a cosmetic astringent and flavoring.

PSALLIOTA CAMPESTRIS • *See* Mushroom Extract.

PSEUDANABAENA GALEATA • Phytoplankton.

PSEUDOTSUGA • *See* Balsam.

PSIDIUM GUAJAVA • An astringent. *See* Guava.

PSORALEA EXTRACT • An extract of the fruit and seeds of *Psoralea,* a member of the pea family. One of the outstanding characteristics of this genus is its strong scent, and the resinous, dark or transparent dots which cover the leaves. The genus name *Psoralea* is based on the Greek word *psoraleos* meaning warty or scurfy, in reference to the dots or warts on the bark. Used in fragrances.

PSORALEN • Named for the Latin *psora,* meaning itch, and derived from a plant. Used in the treatment of vitiligo (lack of skin pigment), in sunscreen to increase tanning, and in perfumes. It can cause photosensitivity (*see*).

PSORIASIS • Skin disease characterized by thickened patches of inflamed red skin; sometimes accompanied by painful joint swelling and stiffness. *See* Linalool and Hydroxycitronellol.

PSYLLIUM • *Plantago psyllium.* Metamucil. Naturacil. Perdiem. Serutan Toasted Granules. Siblin. Syllact. Psyllium is a complete natural fiber, composed mostly of hemi-cellulose. It acts as a sponge, swelling as it absorbs water. It is used as a thickener and stabilizer in cosmetics.

PTEROCARPUS SANTALINUS • *See* Sandalwood Oil.

PTFE • Teflon. Used as a bulking ingredient.

PTYCHOPETALUM OLACOIDES • *See* Muira Puama Extract.

PTZ • *See* Pyrithione Zinc.

PUERARIA LOBATA • Kudzu. A woody herb that is rich in flavones that show a very similar function to estrogen. In cosmetics, it is used in breast creams, eye gels, and skin moisturizers. Kudzu root is a prized herb in Asian countries for use as a food as well as a medicine, but in the United States, it has become an invasive pest. Kudzu can grow as much as a foot a day during the summer, and sixty feet a year, prompting people to nickname it "mile-a-minute vine." It has been used as animal fodder, as soil erosion control, and in basket weaving, but it is best used in the treatment of alcoholism. In Chinese folk medicine, kudzu root tea is used to "sober up" a drunk. Kudzu is believed to be safe; however, safety in young children, pregnant and nursing women, or those with severe kidney or liver disease is not known.

PULLULAN • Starch from the yeast *Aureobasidium pullulans*. Used as a binder and film former.

PULMONARIA OFFICINALIS • *See* Lungwort.

PUMICE • Used in hand-cleansing pastes, skin-cleansing grains, toothpastes, powders, and some soaps for acne treatment. A tooth whitener in Elizabethan times. Used to rub hair from legs and as a nicotine remover paste. Light, hard, rough, porous mass of gritty, gray-colored powder of volcanic origin. Used in cosmetics for removing tough or rough skin. Pumice consists mainly of silicates (*see*) found chiefly in the Lipari Islands and in the Greek archipelago. Because of its abrasive action, daily use in dentifrices is not recommended. If used continually on dry sensitive skin, it may cause irritation. Reported to be an irritant when used with soapless detergents, but it is generally considered harmless.

PUMPKIN • *Cucurbita pepo*. A squash that is high in antioxidants and contains an enzyme with exfoliating properties. Among its ingredients are fatty oil, albumin, lecithin, and phytosterol, an alcohol, and beta-carotene (*see all*), and it is used in shampoos, conditioner, shower gels, lip glazes, enzyme peels, lotions, and soaps. Native Americans used this seed to treat problems with enlarged prostate. It has a reputation among herbalists as being a nonirritating diuretic.

PUMPKIN SEED OIL • *Cucurbita pepo* seed. The acids contained in pumpkin seed oil include palmitic, stearic, oleic, linoleic, linolenic, alpha linolenic, arachidic, and erucic (*see all*). It is high in protein, zinc, as well as polyunsaturated fats. It is made from the common pumpkin, *Cucurbita pepo* (*see*) and used in skin care products. It reputedly combats fine lines and conditions the skin. *See* Pumpkin.

PUNICA GRANATUM • *See* Pomegranate.

PURCELLINE OIL SYN • A synthetic mixture of fatty esters simulating the natural oil obtained from the preen glands of waterfowl. Used as a fixative in perfumes.

PURPLE HEATH EXTRACT • Extract of the flowers of *Erica cinerea*.

PVM/MA • Abbreviation for polyvinyl methyl ether/maleic anhydride.

PVM/MA COPOLYMER • A copolymer of methyl vinyl ether and maleic anhydride. *See* Polyvinyl Alcohols.

PVP • 1-Vinyl-2-Pyrrolidone. Abbreviation for polyvinylpyrrolidone (*see*). Widely used in the production of cosmetics such as a fixative, film former, and emulsion stabilizer.

PVP/DIMETHYLAMINOETHYL-METHYLACRYLATE COPOLYMER • A polymer prepared from vinylpryrrolidone and dimethylaminoethylmethacrylate. *See* Polyvinylpyrrolidone and Acrylates.

PVP/EICOSENE COPOLYMER • A polymer of vinylpyrrolidone and eicosine. *See* Polyvinylpyrrolidone.

PVP/ETHYL METHACRYLATE/METHACRYLIC ACID COPOLYMER • *See* Polyvinylpyrrolidone and Acrylates.

PVP/HEXADECENE COPOLYMER • Antistatic agents, binders, film formers, and viscosity controlling agents.

PVP-IODINE • Complex of polyvinylpyrrolidone and iodine (*see both*).

PVPNA COPOLYMER • A film former used in hair sprays. Based on available data, the CIR Expert Panel (*see*) says it is safe as a cosmetic ingredient. *See* Polyvinyls and Polyvinylpyrrolidone.

PVPNINYL ACETATE/ITACONIC ACID COPOLYMER • *See* Polyvinyl-pyrrolidone and Vinyl Polymers.

PYCNOGENOL • An ingredient from the French maritime pine tree, this substance is purported to be a powerful antioxidant and a blood-vessel and collagen strengthener. Used in anti-aging products. *See* Maritime Pine Extract.

PYRACANTHA FORTUNEANA FRUIT • Kiwi. Chinese Flowering Crab Apple. Skin conditioner.

PYRAZOLE • A crystalline compound used to overcome acidity of aluminum chloride in antiperspirants. Soluble in water, alcohol, ether, and benzene. A modest injection into the abdomens of mice is lethal.

PYRETHRINS • Thick esters that are the most potent insecticidal ingredients of chrysanthemum. Used in lice killing shampoos. Concerns for ingredients used in such shampoos include nerve damage, endocrine disruption, toxicity, and irritation. They may be safer than the older organophosphates (dangerous pesticides) employed, but pyrethrins must be used with great care.

PYRETHRUM • *Tanacetum cinerariifolium*. The natural insecticide obtained by extraction of chrysanthemum flowers. Can cause severe allergic dermatitis and systemic allergic reactions. Very toxic if ingested. On the Canadian Hotlist (*see*). The EU has banned *Pyrethrum album* and its galenical preparations (*see*) in cosmetics.

PYRICARBATE • Skin conditioner. *See* Carbamate.

PYRIDINE • Occurs naturally in coffee and coal tar. Disagreeable odor, sharp taste. Used as a solvent, as a denaturant for alcohol, and as a starting material in the synthesis of other compounds. Compounds that can be derived from pyridine include antihistamines and vitamins. Pyridine is obtained from bone oil or from coal tar by destructive distillation, which decomposes alkaloids that contain it. Alkaloids that contain pyridine include coniine, piperine (the alkaloid in pepper), and nicotine (present in tobacco); free pyridine is present in tobacco smoke. Used in chocolate flavorings for beverages, ice cream, ices, candy, and baked goods. Also used as a solvent for organic liquids and compounds in cosmetics. Once used to treat asthma, but may cause central nervous system depression and irritation of the skin and respiratory tract.

PYRIDIUM COMPOUNDS • A toxic, water-soluble, flammable liquid with a disagreeable odor that is obtained by distillation of bone oil or as a by-product of coal tar. Used as a modifier and preservative in shaving creams, soaps, hand creams, and lotions; also as a solvent, a denaturant in alcohol, and an industrial waterproofing ingredient. The lethal dose injected into the abdomens of rats is only 3.2 milligrams per kilogram of body weight.

PYRIDOXAL 5-PHOSPHATE • A skin conditioner. *See* vitamin B_6 and Phosphate.

PYRIDOXINE • Vitamin B_6.

PYRIDOXINE DICAPRYLATE • *See* Pyridoxine Dioctenoate.

PYRIDOXINE DILAURATE • *See* Vitamin B_6.

PYRIDOXINE DIOCTENOATE • Vitamin B_6 Hydrochloride. Texturizer. A colorless, or white, crystalline powder present in many foodstuffs. A coenzyme that helps in the metabolism of amino acids (*see*) and fats. Also soothing to skin.

PYRIDOXINE DIPALMITATE • *See* Vitamin B_6.

PYRIDOXINE GLYCYRRHETINATE • An alcohol from vitamin B_6 and glycyrrhetinic acid (*see*) used as a skin conditioner.

PYRIDOXINE HCL • *See* Vitamin B_6.

PYRIDOXINE TRIPALMITATE • Vitamin B_6 Tripalmitate. *See* Pyridoxine HCL.

PYRITHIONE ZINC • PTZ. Zinc derivative that acts as an antibacterial and antifungal ingredient for the skin. Used in shampoos. Relieves the itching and flaking associated with dandruff and with seborrheic dermatitis of the scalp.

PYROCATECHOL • Used as an antiseptic. Colorless leaflets, soluble in water; prepared by treating salicylaldehyde with hydrogen peroxide. Used in blond-type dyes as an oxidizing ingredient. It can cause eczema and systemic effects similar to phenol (*see*). Based on available data, the CIR Expert Panel (*see*) says it is unsafe for use in leave-on products and that the available data are insufficient to support the safety of pyrocatechol as used in hair dyes. On the Canadian Hotlist (*see*).

PYROGALLOL • Antiseptic hair dye for hair restorers. The first synthetic organic dye used in human hair. Discovered in 1786 and suggested for use in hair in 1845. Solution grows darker as it is exposed to air. Consists of white, odorless crystals. An aromatic alcohol of pyrogallic acid. Used medicinally as an external antimicrobial and to soothe irritated skin. Ingestion may cause severe gastrointestinal irritation, kidney and liver damage, circulatory collapse, and death. Application to extensive areas of the skin is extremely dangerous. Even with careful use, it can cause a skin rash. Its adverse effects supposedly can be reduced by adding sulfide. The CIR Expert Panel (*see*) says, based on available data, it is safe as a cosmetic ingredient. On the Canadian Hotlist (*see*). Banned in cosmetics by ASEAN.

PYROLA INCARNATA • Skin conditioner. *See* Wintergreen Oil.

PYROPHOSPHATE • Salt of Pyrophosphoric Acid. It increases the effectiveness of antioxidants in creams and ointments. In concentrated solutions it can be irritating to the skin and mucous membranes.

PYROPHYLLITE • Pencil Stone Agalmatolite. White to yellowish gray mineral consisting predominantly of anhydrous aluminum silicate (*see*) mixed with silica (*see*). Used as a coloring and opacifying ingredient. Permanently listed in 1966 for externally applied cosmetics.

PYRROLIDONE • Derived from acetylene and formaldehyde, it is used as a plasticizer, solvent, insecticide, and in special inks.

PYRUS COMMUNIS • *See* Pear Extract.

PYRUS CYDONIA • *See* Quince Seed.

PYRUS MALUS • Apple. Widely used in cosmetics. *See* Malic Acid.

PYRUS SORBUS • *See* Sorbus Extract.

PYRUVIC ACID • An important intermediate in fermentation and metabolism, it occurs naturally in coffee and when sugar is metabolized in muscle. It is isolated from cane sugar and used in flavorings and as a treatment for burns.

Q

QUARTZ • A mineral used as an abrasive. *See* Silicones.

QUASSIA AMARA • Bitter Wood. A small South American tree that has many medicinal properties according to folk medicine. It fights worms, is an astringent, soothes inflammation, and has anticancer properties. Used in cosmetics as a denaturant, skin conditioner, and tonic. Reportedly there is not enough information about this substance to judge possible adverse effects.

QUASSIN • Bitter alkaloid obtained from the wood of *Quassia amara.* Chiefly used as a denaturant for ethyl alcohol. Shavings from a plant found in Jamaica and the Caribbean islands. Used to poison flies. Toxic to humans.

QUATERNARIUM-1 THROUGH -6 • A germicide derived from lauric acid, a common constituent of vegetable fats, especially coconut oil. Positively charged with a low irritation potential, it is effective against a wide range of organisms. It is a preservative present in skin preparations. *See* Quaternarium-7.

QUATERNARIUM-7 • A surfactant and germicide derived from lauric acid (*see*). Positively charged with a low irritation potential, it is effective against a wide range of organisms.

QUATERNARIUM-8 THROUGH -14 • *See* Quaternarium-15.

QUATERNARIUM-15 • A water-soluble antimicrobial ingredient that is active against bacteria but not very active against yeast. It is a formaldehyde (*see*) releaser and is the number one cause of dermatitis from preservatives, according to the American Academy of Dermatology's Testing Tray results. It is a teratogen (*see*) in rats when administered orally but not on the skin. Conditions that favor rapid absorption from the skin, therefore, might be expected to increase the risk of birth defects. Although it is a potential sensitizer, the CIR Expert Panel (*see*) says, based on available data, it is safe as a cosmetic ingredient. It is widely used in shampoos and other hair products, face and body lotions, bath products, makeup, and cleansers as well as suntan preparations and manicuring products.

QUATERNARIUM-16 THROUGH -29 • Antistatics and surfactants. *See* Quaternarium-18.

QUATERNARIUM -18, -19, -20, -23 • Derived from cellulose (*see*), it is a film former and binding ingredient used in products to give hair a sheen.

QUARTERNARIUM-52, -53, -56, -60, -61, -63, -70, -71, -72, -73, -75, -76, -77, -78 • Antistatic ingredients and conditioners used in permanent waves and hair care products. *See* Quaternary Ammonium Compounds.

QUATERNARIUM-28 DODECYLBENZYL TRIMETHYLAMMONIUM CHLORIDE • *See* Quaternary Ammonium Compounds.

QUATERNARIUM-18 HECTORITE • Widely used in skin care, cleansing ingredients, and suntan gels. *See* Quaternary Ammonium Compounds and Hectorite.

QUATERNARY AMMONIUM COMPOUNDS • A wide variety of preservatives, surfactants, germicides, sanitizers, antiseptics, and deodorants used in cosmetics. Benzalkonium chloride (*see*) is one of the most popular. Quaternary ammonium compounds are synthetic derivatives of ammonium chloride (*see*) and are used in aerosol deodorants, after-shave lotions, antidandruff shampoos, antiperspirants, cuticle softeners, hair colorings, hair-grooming aids, hand creams, hair-waving preparations, mouthwashes, hand creams, and regular shampoos. Diluted solutions are used in medicine to sterilize the skin and mucous membranes. All the quaternary ammonium compounds can be toxic, depending upon the dose and concentration. Concentrated solutions irritate the skin and can cause necrosis of the mucous membranes. Concentrations as low as 0.1 percent are irritating to the eye and mucous membranes except benzalkonium chloride, which is well tolerated at such low concentrations. Ingestion can be fatal. *See* Quaternarium-15.

QUATERNIUM-79 HYDROLYZED COLLAGEN, -SILK, -SOY, -WHEAT, -KERATIN PROTEINS • Used as antistatic and conditioning ingredients in hair products. *See* Hydrolyzed.

QUATERNIUM-18 METHOSULFATE • Antistatic ingredient in hair products. On the basis of the available information, the CIR Expert Panel (*see*) found Quaternium-18 safe in the early 1980s but is considering new information to determine if the final safety assessment should be reaffirmed, amended, or have an addendum. *See* Quaternary Ammonium Compounds and Tallow.

QUATERNIUMS • Group of compounds used widely in cosmetics, especially in hair conditioners and shampoos. They have a variety of uses including as antistatic ingredients, antimicrobials, preservatives, surfactants, and viscosity adjusters.

QUEEN OF THE PRAIRIE • *See Filipendula rubra.*

QUEEN'S DELIGHT

QUEEN'S DELIGHT • *Stillingia sylvatica.* The root of this North American herb contains volatile oil, tannin, and resin. It is used for the treatment of chronic skin conditions such as eczema and psoriasis. It is also used by herbalists to treat bronchitis and laryngitis, especially when they are accompanied by loss of the voice. The astringent (*see*) qualities have led herbalists to use it for hemorrhoid problems.

QUERCETIN • The inner bark of a species of oak tree common in North America. Its active ingredient, isoquercitin, is used in dark brown hair-dye shades but employed mainly for dyeing artificial hairpieces. Allergic reactions have been reported.

QUERCITOL • A sweet crystalline alcohol found in acorns and oak bark and in viburnums and other plants. It is used in astringents.

QUERCITRIN • *Aesculus hippocastanum.* Yellow crystals used as a dye. Found in elder flowers. Used as an antioxidant and skin conditioner.

QUERCUS ACUTISSIMA • The EU name for sawtooth oak. Used as an astringent.

QUERCUS ALBA • The EU name for white oak bark (*see* Oak Bark Extract).

QUERCUS INFECTORIA • Oak Gall Extract. Used as an astringent. *See* Oak Bark Extract.

QUERCUS ROBUR BARK EXTRACT • English Oak. *See* Oak Bark Extract.

QUILLAJA EXTRACT • Soap Bark. Quillay Bark. Panama Bark. China Bark. The extract of the bark of *Quillaja saponaria.* The inner dried bark of a tree grown in South America. Used in fruit, root beer, and spice flavoring in foods. Used as a skin conditioner in shampoos and cleansers. Formerly used to treat bronchitis and externally as a detergent and local irritant.

QUINCE SEED • The seed of a plant, *Pyrus cydonia,* grown in southern Asia and Europe for its fatty oil. Thick jelly is produced by soaking seeds in water. Used in setting lotions, as a suspension in skin creams and lotions, as a thickening ingredient in depilatories, and as an emulsifier in fragrances, hand creams, lotions, rouges, and wave sets; medicinally as a demulcent. Has been largely replaced by cheaper substitutes. It may cause allergic reactions.

QUINIC ACID • A pH (*see*) adjuster.

QUINIDINE • An antiarrhythmic drug introduced in 1920, it is used to treat heart flutter or fibrillation. Used as a cooling and analgesic ingredient.

QUININE • The most important alkaloid of cinchona bark, which grows wild in South America. White crystalline powder, almost insoluble in water. Used as a local anesthetic, in hair tonics, and in sunscreen preparations. May cause a rash. In 1992, the FDA proposed a ban on quinine in internal analgesic products because it had not been shown to be safe and effective as claimed.

QUINOA EXTRACT • The extract of the leaves and flowers of *Chenopodium quinoa.* Natural plant extract contains a variety of amino acids used for skin hydration and softening effect. Used as toner, facial moisturizer, treatment (face), body wash, body lotion, and in shampoos.

QUINOLIN-8-OL AND BIS (8-HYDROXYQUINOLINIUM) SULFATE • Stabilizer for hydrogen peroxide in rinse-off and non-rinse-off hair care preparations. The EU limits it to 0.3 percent calculated as base.

QUINOLINE • A coal tar derivative used in the manufacture of cosmetic dyes. Also a solvent for resins. Made either by the distillation of coal tar, bones, and alkaloids or by the interaction of aniline (*see*) with acetaldehyde and formaldehyde (*see both*). *See* Coal Tar for toxicity. *See also* Colors.

QUINOLINE SALTS • A colorless, oily, very hygroscopic liquid with a disagreeable odor. Occurs in coal tar. Used in suntan preparations and perfumes as a preservative and solvent. Also a preservative for anatomical specimens.

QUINONES • Derived from benzene (*see*), used in yellow and orange to red colorings. Potent sensitizers.

R

RABBIT FAT • Rablu. Fats and oils from rabbits used as a skin conditioner.

RADISH EXTRACT • Extract of *Raphanus sativus.* The small seeds of the radish remain viable for years. Has been used as a food since ancient times. Used as a counterirritant (*see*) in herbal cosmetics.

RAFFINOSE • Sugars made from beets. Used as an emollient.

RAFFINOSE MYRISTATE • A skin-conditioning ingredient. *See* Myristic Acid and Radish Extract.

RAGWORT • The plant is a perennial and abundant in most parts of the country, on dry roadsides and waste ground and pastures, often growing in large patches and flowering in July and August. It is distributed over Europe, Siberia, and Northwest India. Used medicinally for various purposes. The leaves are used in the country for emollient poultices and yield a good green non-permanent dye. The flowers boiled in water give a fair yellow dye to wool previously impregnated with alum. The whole plant is bitter and aromatic, of an acrid sharpness, but the juice is cooling and astringent, and of use as a wash in burns, inflammations of the eye, and also in sores and cancerous ulcers—hence one of its old names, cankerwort. It is used with success in relieving rheumatism, sciatica, and gout, a poultice of the green leaves being applied to painful joints and reducing the inflammation and swelling. It makes a good gargle for ulcerated throat and mouth, and is said to take away the pain caused by the sting of bees. A decoction of the root has been reputed good for inward bruises and wounds. In some parts of the country ragwort is accredited with the power of preventing infection.

RAHNELLA/SOY PROTEIN FERMENT • Soy protein fermented by the use of the intestinal bacteria *Rahnella.* Used as a skin conditioner.

RAISIN-SEED OIL • Oil from dried grapes or berries used in lubricating creams. *See* Grape-Seed Oil.

RANSIUM DOMESTICUM • *See* Duku Extract.

RANSOU EKISU • Blue-green algae. Skin conditioner. *See* Algae.

RANUNCULUS FICARIA • *See* Pilewort Extract.

RAPE SHUSI YU • Fats and oil from the seed of *Brassica campestris* or *Brassica napus.* Used as a skin conditioner. *See* Mustard Oil and Turnip Extract.

RAPESEED ACID • A mixture of fatty acids from rapeseed, *Brassica campestris.* Used as a cleansing ingredient and in skin and hair conditioners. *See* Rapeseed Oil.

RAPESEED AMIDOPROPYL BENZYLDIMONIUM CHLORIDE • *See* Rapeseed Oil and Quaternary Ammonium Compounds.

RAPESEED AMIDOPROPYL ETHYLDIMONIUM ETHOSULFATE • *See* Rapeseed Oil and Quaternary Ammonium Compounds.

RAPESEED OIL • Brownish yellow oil from a turniplike annual herb of European origin. Widely grown as a forage crop for sheep in the United States. A distinctly unpleasant odor. Used chiefly as a lubricant, an illuminant, and in rubber substitutes; also employed in soft soaps and margarine. Can cause acnelike skin eruptions.

RAPESEED OIL UNSAPONIFIABLES • The fraction of rapeseed oil (*see*) that is not changed into a fatty alcohol when it is saponified (heated with an alkali and an acid).

RAPHANUS SATIVUS • *See* Radish Extract.

RASPBERRY JUICE • Juice from the fresh ripe fruit *Rubus idaeus,* grown in Europe, Asia, the United States, and Canada. Used as a flavoring for lipsticks, food, and medicines. It has astringent properties.

RASPBERRYKETONE GLUCOSIDE • Fragrance ingredient.

RATTLEROOT • *See* Black Cohosh.

RAUWOLFIA EXTRACT • Raudixin. Rauzide. Rauverid. Wolfina. Deserpidine. A small shrub sporting white to pink flowers, it is native to India, Indochina, Borneo, Sri Lanka, and Sumatra. Rauwolfia extracts work by blocking nerve signals that trigger constriction of blood vessels. Its medicinal properties lie in the dried root. On the Canadian Hotlist (*see*). Banned in cosmetics by the EU and ASEAN (*see*). *See* Snakeroot.

RAYON • Regenerated cellulose. Rayon is composed of man-made textile fibers of cellulose and yarn; produced from wood pulp. Its appearance is similar to silk. Used to give shine and body to face powders and in eyelash extenders in mascaras.

REACH • Abbreviation for Registration Evaluation and Authorization of Chemicals Regulation. REACH is a European Community Regulation on chemicals and their safe use. It deals with the registration, evaluation, authorization, and restriction of chemical substances. The new law entered into force on June 1, 2007. The aim of REACH is to improve the protection of human health and the environment through the better and earlier identification of the intrinsic properties of chemical substances, including cosmetic ingredients.

REBA-A • *See* Stevia Rebaudiana.

RECOMBINANT DNA • Genetic instructions artificially introduced into a cell so that the genetic and physical characteristics of the cell are altered, and the new DNA is replicated along with the natural DNA. Recombinant DNA is one technique of genetic engineering.

RECONSTRUCTED HUMAN EPIDERMIS • RHE. *See* Animal Testing for Cosmetic Safety.

RED ALGAE • A natural extract of seaweed used to carry natural spices, seasonings, and flavorings. Used in skin creams for moisturizing and soothing. *See* Alginates. GRAS

RED CLOVER • *Trifolium pratense.* Used in conditioners, moisturizers, facials, bath oils and salts, baby shampoos, hair sprays, shampoos, and soaps. It has been employed in American folk medicine for more than one hundred years to treat and prevent cancer. Also used to treat gout and as an expectorant. Used in an herbal tea for digestive disorders. Red clover has shown some estrogenic activity and has a reputation as an aphrodisiac. Some believe the enhancement of lovemaking is because of the estrogenic effect, which aids lubrication. Antibiotic tests on red clover have shown it to possess activity against several bacteria.

RED 4 • The EU name is CI 14700; the Japanese name, Aka504. Used in colognes and toilet waters, body and hand products, shampoos, moisturizers, hair conditioners, bath products, underarm deodorants, nail products, and shaving creams. *See* FD & C Red No. 4.

RED 4 LAKE • The EU name is CI 14700; the Japanese name, Aka504. *See* FD & C Red No. 4.

RED 6 • *See* D & C Red No. 6.

RED 6 LAKE • *See* D & C Red No. 6 Aluminum Lake.

RED 7 • *See* D & C Red No. 7.

RED 7 LAKE • *See* D & C Red No. 7 Aluminum Lake.

RED 17 • *See* D & C Red No. 17.

RED 21 • *See* D & C Red No. 21.

RED 21 LAKE • *See* D & C Red No. 21 Aluminum Lake.

RED 22 • *See* D & C Red No. 22.

RED 22 LAKE • *See* D & C Red No. 22.

RED 27 • *See* D & C Red No. 27.

RED 27 LAKE • *See* D & C Red No. 27 Aluminum Lake.

RED 28 • *See* D & C Red No. 28.

RED 28 LAKE • *See* D & C Red No. 28.

RED 30 • Also listed as 30 Lake, D & C Red No. 30 Lake; D & C Red 30 Aluminum and Red 30 Lake are colorants used in the formulation of blushers, lipsticks, face powders, and other makeup products, as well as bath products, cleansing products, nail polish, and enamels. The Environmental Working Group's Skin Deep says it is toxic, although it is permitted by the FDA and the EU.

RED 31 • *See* D & C Red No. 31.

RED 31 LAKE • *See* D & C Red No. 31 Calcium Lake.

RED 33 • *See* D & C Red No. 33.

RED 33 LAKE • *See* D & C Red No. 33.

RED 34 • *See* D & C Red No. 34.

RED 36 • *See* D & C Red No. 36.

RED 36 LAKE • *See* D & C Red No. 36 Lake.

RED 40 • *See* D & C Red No. 40.

RED 40 LAKE • *See* D & C Red No. 40 Aluminum Lake.

RED OIL • A commercial grade of oleic, linoleic, and stearic acids (*see all*).

RED PEPPER • Cayenne Pepper. A condiment made from the pungent fruit of the plant. Used in sausage and pepper flavorings. Also used as a stimulant in hair tonics, but may be an irritant and also cause allergic reactions.

RED PETROLATUM • A minimally refined variety of petrolatum (*see*), used as a sunscreen ingredient. May cause discoloration of the skin. E

RED RASPBERRY EXTRACT • *See* Raspberry Juice.

RED RASPBERRY LEAF EXTRACT • An extract of the leaves of the red raspberry.

RED SANDALWOOD EXTRACT • The extract of the wood of *Pterocarpus santalinus*. The use of this ingredient as a colorant in cosmetics is prohibited in the United States and may be restricted in other countries. *See* Sandalwood.

REDUCING AGENT • A substance that decreases, deoxidizes, or concentrates the volume of another substance. For instance, a reducing ingredient such as stannous chloride is used to convert a metal oxide to the metal itself. It also means a substance that adds hydrogen ingredients to another, for example, when acetaldehyde is converted to alcohol in the final step of alcoholic fermentation.

REDUCTION • The process of removing oxygen from a compound or adding hydrogen by chemical or electrochemical means. It is the reverse of oxidation.

REHMANNIA • *Radix rehmannia*. Shennong Bencao Jing. A Chinese herb used to clear heat and cool blood. The roots are dug in spring or autumn and dried in the sun. Used in skin-conditioning products.

REINGREDIENT • A chemical that reacts or participates in a reaction; a substance that is used for the detection or determination of another substance by chemical or microscopical means. The various categories of reingredients are colorimetric—to produce color—soluble compounds; fluxes—used to lower the melting point; oxidizers—used in oxidation; precipitants—to produce insoluble compounds; reducers—used in reduction (*see*); and solvents—used to dissolve water-insoluble compounds.

RELAXERS • *See* Hair Straighteners.

RENOVA • An antiwrinkle, emollient cream that contains 0.05 percent of tretinoin (*see*). The exact mechanism of Renova is unknown, but it does have an effect on skin cells. Absorption through the skin of compounds containing tretinoin varies from 1 percent to 31 percent. In a stronger version, it is used to treat acne, and that compound has been found to cause birth defects in the babies of mothers using it. Renova is used to counteract fine wrinkles and mottled skin, but it does not eliminate wrinkles, repair sun-damaged skin, reverse photoaging, or restore a more youthful or young skin cell pattern. In one study, most of the improvement in the skin occurred during the first twenty-four weeks of use. Neither the safety nor the efficacy of using Renova for more than forty-eight weeks has been established. Possible adverse reactions include skin irritation and changes in the elasticity of the skin. It should not be used if you are taking drugs that cause photosensitization, such as tetracyclines, phenothiazines, and sulfa drugs. The effect on the fetuses of animals has been equivocal. The FDA says it should not be used by pregnant women or if you are sunburned or have eczema or other chronic skin conditions. Should be applied once a day before bedtime and only enough to cover the problem areas. It should not be applied to the eyes, ears, nostrils, and mouth. *See* Tretinoin.

RESEDA LUTEOLA • Dyer's Rocket. An essential oil from the dyer's rocket, a European plant cultivated for its yellow dye.

RESINS • The brittle substance, usually translucent or transparent, formed from the hardened secretions of plants. Among the natural resins are dammar, elemi, and sandarac. Synthetic resins include polyvinyl acetate, various polyester resins, and sulfonamide resins. Resins have many uses in cosmetics. They contribute depth, gloss, flow adhesion, and water resistance. Toxicity depends upon ingredients used.

RESMETHRIN • Pesticide. *See* Pyrethrins.

RESORCINOL • A preservative, antiseptic, antifungal, astringent, and anti-itching ingredient, particularly in dandruff shampoos. Also used in hair dyes, lipsticks, and hair tonics. Also used in tanning, explosives, and the manufacture of resins. Obtained from various resins. Resorcinol's white crystals become pink on exposure to air. A sweetish taste. Irritating to the skin and mucous membranes. May cause allergic reactions, particularly of the skin. While using resorcinol, you should avoid abrasive soaps or cleansers, medicated cosmetics, preparations containing alcohol, or any other acne preparations. Since resorcinol may be absorbed through the skin, application to wounds may cause methemoglobinemia, a blood disorder, in children. The FDA issued a notice in 1992 that resorcinol has not been shown to be safe and effective for stated claims in OTC products. On the basis of the available data, the CIR Expert Panel (*see*) concluded that it is safe as a cosmetic ingredient. The EU says resorcinol must be listed on the label with the warning: "Contains resorcinol; rinse hair well after application; do not use to dye eyelashes or eyebrows; rinse eyes immediately if product comes into contact with them."

RESORCINOL ACETATE • *See* Resorcinol.

RESTHARROW EXTRACT • A European woody herb, *Onones spinosa,* with pink flowers and long, tough roots used for medicinal purposes and in emollients.

RESVERATRATE • A molecule discovered by David Sinclair, PhD of Harvard Medical School, and Leonard Guarante, PhD of the Massachusetts Institute of Technology, features significantly in Estée Lauder's new Re-Nutriv Ultimate Youth Crème. This is the newest addition to the company's anti-aging Re-Nutriv line. The molecule, Resveratrate, is able to penetrate the skin. Called the "youth molecule" by Estée Lauder, Resveratrate will be combined with South Sea pearl-micasilica, *Camelia sativa* oil, and a deep-sea organism from the Gulf of California to create Re-Nutriv Ultimate. According to *CosmeticsNews,* Elana Szyfer, senior vice president of Marketing for Estée

Lauder, said, "We would like to add new products . . . featuring this new breakthrough technology under the 'Ultimate Youth banner.'"

RESVERATROL • An antioxidant found in grapeskin and wine that is used in skin creams and as an anti-inflammatory and for skin lightening. A polyphenolic phytoalexin belonging to the group of flavanoids, it is produced by grapes and other plants in response to an infection or injury. The longer the grape juice is fermented with the grape skins the higher the resveratrol content will be. As a major constituent of red wine, resveratrol was proposed to partly account for the beneficial effects attributed to red wine in cardiovascular diseases. Resveratrol also inhibits a wide variety of biological events associated with cell proliferation and tumor progression. Resveratrol is being promoted for inclusion in emollients, patches, sunscreens, and other products intended to prevent skin cancer and other conditions associated with exposure to the sun. It is reputedly an effective anti-aging substance.

RETIN-A • A prescription drug for the treatment of acne, it is a vitamin A derivative. The medication is available in five strengths and in cream, gel, and liquid form. It has a faint medicinal odor, is greaseless, and is easily absorbed. It reportedly plumps the skin, smoothes fine wrinkles, and begins to reverse other, less visible signs of sun damage. The drug is believed to increase cell turnover, so dull surface cells are shed more quickly. It thickens the epidermis and improves texture, elasticity, and blood circulation. And it helps normalize uneven cell growth. It is not said to reduce deep wrinkles. It is expected, as of this writing, to eventually be an ingredient in over-the-counter cosmetics. The FDA began a nationwide crackdown on unlicensed manufacturers who have begun to adver-tise and distribute bogus Retin-A drugs and cosmetics. Some manufacturers are also pro-moting vitamin A in products as producing effects similar to Retin-A.

RETINAL • Skin conditioner. *See* Vitamin A and Aldehyde, Aliphatic.

RETINOIC ACID • A derivative of vitamin A. The EU has banned it and its salts in cosmetics. *See* Tretinoin and Retinoids.

RETINOIDS • Derived from retinoic acid, vitamin A, it is used to treat acne and other skin disorders. *See* Vitamin A.

RETINOL • It is on the Canadian Hotlist (*see*). *See* Vitamin A.

RETINOXYTRIMETHYLSILANE • A skin conditioner. *See* Vitamin A and Siloxanes.

RETINYL ACETATE • It is on the Canadian Hotlist (*see*). *See* Vitamin A.

RETINYL PALMITATE • The ester of vitamin A and palmitic acid, sometimes mixed with vitamin D_2 (*see all*). Widely used in makeup, skin care products, hair products, after-shave talcs, bath products, suntan gels, creams and liquids, and nail products. It was nonmutagenic in several animal species. The CIR Expert Panel (*see*) says, based on available data, it is safe as a cosmetic ingredient up to a maximum concentration of 1 percent. On the Canadian Hotlist (*see*).

RETINYL PROPIONATE • *See* Vitamin A.

RHAMNOSE • Sugar usually derived from quercetin (*see*) used as a flavoring.

RHAMNUS PURSHIANA • *See* Cascara.

RHATANY • *Krameria triandra.* The root of a shrub native to Peru that contains up to 9 percent tannin (*see*). It is a powerful astringent long used in conventional pharmacy. It is used by herbalists to treat diarrhea, hemorrhoids, and hemorrhages, or as a styptic. Rhatany is often found in herbal toothpastes and powders to treat bleeding gums.

RHE • Abbreviation for Reconstructed Human Epidermis. *See* Animal Testing for Cosmetic Safety.

RHEUM PALMATUM • *See* Rhubarb.

RHINACANTHUS COMMUNIS • A Chinese herb with antifungal properties.

RHIZOBIAN GUM • Film former and thickener derived from the bacteria *Rhizobium bacterium*. A clear, fairly recently discovered gelling gum.

RHODINOL • Used in perfumes, especially those of the rose type. Isolated from geranium or rose oils. It has the strong odor of rose and consists essentially of geraniol and citronellol (*see both*). Also used in food and beverage flavorings.

RHODIOLA SACRA • A Tibetan herb that is used in cosmetics as a skin conditioner but in Tibet to treat colds and fever.

RHODODENDRON EXTRACT • Extract of various species of rhododendron.

RHUBARB • *Rheum palmatum*. The common plant with large edible stems. It is combined with henna, black tea, and chamomile for hair dye. Its active principle is chrysophanol, which produces a desirable blond shade. It is also used to treat skin inflammation.

RHUS AROMATICA (H) (OTC) • Fragrant Sumac. Hyland's Bed Wetting Tablets. An extract of a shrub native to both temperate and warm regions. Has astringent qualities. Sumac berries contain a large amount of tannin (*see*). The root was chewed by some North American Indians to treat mouth sores.

RHUS GLABRA • *See* Sumac.

RHUS SEMIALATA EXTRACT • Chinese Sumac. *See* Sumac.

RHUS SUCCEDANEA FRUIT WAX • *See* Japan Wax.

RIBES • Astringent. *See* Currant Extract.

RIBOFLAVIN • Vitamin B_2. Lactoflavin. Formerly called vitamin G. Riboflavin is a factor in the vitamin B complex and is used in emollients. Every plant and animal cell contains a minute amount. Good sources are milk, eggs, and organ meats. It is necessary for healthy skin and respiration, protects the eyes from sensitivity to light, and is used for building and maintaining human body tissues. A deficiency leads to lesions at the corner of the mouth and to changes in the cornea.

RIBONUCLEIC ACID • *See* RNA.

RICE • *Oryza sativa*. Many cosmetic ingredients are made from rice. These include various oils and fats, rice bran oil, rice germ oil, rice bran acid, rice bran wax, and hydrogenated rice bran wax, and other extracts (*see* the following).

RICE AMINO ACIDS • A hair- and skin-conditioning ingredient from rice protein. Used as an antistatic ingredient. *See* Amino Acids.

RICE BRAN OIL • Oil expressed from the broken coat of rice grain. Used to make detergents.

RICE BRAN WAX • The wax obtained from the broken coat of rice grain.

RICE FERMENT FILTRATE • Sake. The basic process in making this ingredient is to make sugar by adding rice starch to malt microbe. Then the sugar is fermented with yeast (Moto-moromi). Next, the alcohol must be removed. The result is an ingredient used in cosmetics as an emollient.

RICE POWDER • Used in cosmetics and as a drying ingredient. May cause contact dermatitis. However, rice as a food is hypoallergenic.

RICE STARCH • Finely pulverized grains of the rice plant, *Oryza sativa,* used in baby powders, face powders, and dusting powders. A demulcent and emollient that forms a soothing, protective film when applied. It is used in the following product types: mascara, eye shadow, facial powder, foundation, shampoo, mask facial cleanser, eyeliner, anti-aging products, and facial moisturizer/treatment. May cause mechanical irritation by blocking pores and putrefying. May also cause an allergic reaction.

RICEBRANAMIDE DEA • *See* Rice Bran Oil and Ethanolamines.

RICEBRANAMIDOPROPYL HYDROXYETHYL DIMONIUM CHLORIDE • A quaternary ammonium compound (*see*) from rice bran oil.

RICINOLEAMIDE • *See* Ricinoleic Acid.

RICINOLEAMIDE DEA • Fatty acid. Antistatic ingredient foam booster, and thickness control. DEA used in deodorant sticks. *See* Ricinoleic Acid.

RICINOLEATE • Salt of ricinoleic acid found in castor oil. Used in the manufacture of soaps.

RICINOLEIC ACID • A mixture of fatty oils found in the seeds of castor beans. Castor oil contains 80 to 85 percent ricinoleic acid. The oily liquid is used in soaps, added to Turkey-red oil (*see*), and used in contraceptive jellies. Also used in cosmetics as an emollient. May cause dermatitis (*see*).

RICINOLEOAMPHOGLYCINATE • *See* Castor Oil.

RICINOLETH-40 • *See* Castor Oil.

RICINUS COMMUNIS • *See* Castor Oil. The CIR Expert Panel (*see*) has listed this as top priority for review.

RINGWORM • Tinea Corporis. A fungal (not a worm) infection, it manifests itself on the skin in round, scaly, itchy patches. Usually affects the scalp, trunk, or feet. When ringworm affects the scalp, bald patches develop. Ringworm is infectious and can be spread from a pet, such as a dog or cat, to its owner's family.

RNA • The abbreviation for ribonucleic acid. RNA is one of the molecules involved in carrying out a cell's DNA (deoxyribonucleic acid) instructions for reproduction, growth, and maturation. DNA provides the blueprint for any living organism. Used as a skin conditioner in cosmetics.

ROBINIA PSEUDACACIA • Black Locust. Used as a preservative. The tree is native to the slopes and forest margins of southern Appalachia and the Ozarks.

ROCHELLE SALT • Potassium Sodium Tartrate. Used in the manufacture of baking powder and in the silvering of mirrors. Translucent crystals or white crystalline powder with cooling saline taste. Slight efflorescence in warm air. Probably used in mouthwashes, but use not identified in cosmetics.

ROCK SALT CRYSTALS • *See* Sodium Chloride.

ROCKET EXTRACT • Extract of the leaves of *Eruca sativa*. Used in hair shampoos and in skin preparations to cut grease.

ROCKROSE • Any of several plants in the genera *Helianthemum* and *Cistus* in the family Cistaceae. They come mainly from the Mediterranean region. Used in soap making and perfumery.

ROE EXTRACT • Rosemary Oil Extract. An antioxidant from a plant. *See* Rosemary.

ROE EXTRACT • From fish eggs. Used as a conditioner, particularly for aging skin.

ROGAINE • *See* Minoxidil.

ROMAN CHAMOMILE • *See* Chamomile.

ROSA CANINA • *See* Dog Rose Extract.

ROSA CENTIFOLIA • *See* Cabbage Rose.

ROSA DAMASCENA EXTRACT • Damask Rose. Fragrance ingredient.

ROSA EGLANTERIA • Sweet Briar Rose. Fragrance ingredient.

ROSA MOSCHATA • Musk Rose. Fragrance ingredient.

ROSA MULTIFLORA • *See* Rose Extract.

ROSA ROXBURGHI • Chestnut Rose.

ROSA RUGOSA • A skin conditioner. *See* Rose Extract.

ROSA SPINOSISSIMA EXTRACT • Burnet Rose.

ROSA SPP. • *See* Rose Extract.

ROSE • *Rosa gallica*. French Rose. Red Rose. *R. officinalis* Apothecary's Rose. The use of rose petals dates back to very ancient times. Early alchemists used them for purgatives, astringents, and tonics, to treat chronic lung diseases, diarrhea, and vaginal discharges. The medicinal properties of rose petals are generally considered very mild. The buds and petals are astringent. Rosebuds are high in vitamin C, astringent tannins, and phenolic compounds.

ROSE BENGAL • A bluish red fragrant liquid taken from the rose of the Bengal region of the Asian subcontinent. Used to scent perfumes and as an edible color product to make lipstick dyes.

ROSE BULGARIAN • True Otto Oil. Attar of Roses. Rose Otto Bulgaria. One of the most widely used perfume ingredients, it is the essential oil steam-distilled from the flowers of *Rosa damascena.* The rose flowers are picked early in the morning, when they contain the maximum amount of perfume, and are distilled quickly after harvesting. Bulgaria is the main source of supply, but Russia, Turkey, Syria, and Indo-China also grow it. The liquid is pale yellow and has a warm, deep floral, slightly spicy, and extremely fragrant, red rose smell. It is used as a flavoring. Also used in mucilage and coloring. May cause allergic reactions.

ROSE EXTRACT • *Rosa damascena* or *R. multiflora.* An extract of the various species of rose, it is used in fragrances, makeup, and skin conditioners. May cause allergic reactions. GRAS

ROSE FLOWER OIL • *See* Rose Extract.

ROSE GERANIUM • Distilled from any of several South African herbs grown for their fragrant leaves. Used in perfumes and to scent toothpaste and dusting powders. May cause allergic reactions

ROSE HIPS EXTRACT • *Rosa canina.* Hipberries. An extract of the fruit of various species of wild roses, it is rich in vitamin C and is used as a natural flavoring. Widely used by organic food enthusiasts as a tonic, to ward off colds, and to ease constipation.

ROSE LEAVES EXTRACT • Derived from the leaves of a species of *Rosa.* Used in raspberry flavorings and fragrances.

ROSE OIL • Attar of Roses. Fragrant, volatile, essential oil distilled from fresh flowers. Colorless or yellow, with a strong fragrant odor and taste of roses. Used in perfumes, toilet waters, and ointments. May cause allergic reactions.

ROSE OTTO BULGARIA • *See* Rose Bulgarian.

ROSE SEED EXTRACT • Extract from the seed of *Rosa canina. See* Dog Rose Extract.

ROSE WATER • The watery solution of the odoriferous constituents of roses, made by distilling the fresh flowers with water or steam. Used as a perfume in emollients, eye lotions, and freckle lotions. May cause allergic reactions.

ROSE WATER OINTMENT • *See* Cold Cream.

ROSEMARINIC ACID • *See* Rosemary Extract.

ROSEMARY • *Rosmarinus officinalis.* Used in perfumery. The flowers and leaves of the plant are a symbol of love and loyalty. Rosemary oil is the volatile oil from the fresh flowering tops of rosemary and is used in liniments and hair tonics. Colorless to yellow, with the characteristic odor of rosemary and a warm camphorlike taste. Rosemary has the folk reputation of stimulating the growth of hair and is used in rinse water. An antioxidant, it reportedly has anti-inflammatory and antitumor properties; it supposedly is also beneficial to the skin. It is used internally as a tonic and astringent, and by herbalists as a stimulant for the nerves. Nontoxic when used externally. Irritant. May cause allergic dermatitis and photosensitivity in some people. E

ROSEMARY EXTRACT • Garden Rosemary. A flavoring and perfume from the fresh aromatic flowering tops of the evergreen shrub grown in the Mediterranean. Light blue flowers and gray-green leaves. Widely used in hair products, bubble baths, body and hand preparations, lipsticks, suntan products, perfumes, and bath soaps.

ROSEMARY OIL • The oil obtained from the flowering tops of *Rosemarinus officinalis*. *See* Rosemary.

ROSEWOOD OIL • From *Aniba rosaeodora*. Used in fragrances.

ROSIN • Colophony. Used in soaps, hair lacquers, wax depilatories, and ointments. It is also used in mascaras. It is the pale yellow residue left after distilling the volatile oil from the oleoresin obtained from various species of pine trees produced chiefly in the United States. It can cause contact dermatitis, particularly of the eyelids.

ROSIN ACRYLATE • Hair fixative. *See* Rosin and Acrylates.

ROSIN HYDROLYZED COLLAGEN • A protein used in hair and skin conditioners. *See* Rosin and Hydrolyzed.

ROSMARINIC ACID • An antioxidant. *See* Rosemary.

ROSMARINUS OFFICINALIS • *See* Rosemary.

ROUGE • One of the oldest types of makeup. Rouge is applied to the cheeks to give a rosy, healthy look. It is usually a finely divided form of ferric oxide, generally prepared by heating ferrous sulfate. Cake or compact rouge usually contains talc, kaolin, brilliant red lake (certified), zinc oxide, zinc stearate, liquid petrolatum, tragacanth, mucilage (*see all*), and perfume. Liquid rouge usually contains carmine coloring, ammonium hydroxide, glycerin (*see all*), and red coloring pigment. It may also contain polyvinylpyrrolidone or sodium carboxymethyl cellulose, glycerin, color, propylene glycol (*see all*), alcohol, perfume, and water. Rouge paste may contain carmine coloring, ammonium hydroxide, beeswax, cetyl alcohol, stearic acid, cocoa butter, and petrolatum (*see all*). Cream rouge may contain erythrosine as a coloring, stearic acid, cetyl alcohol, potassium hydroxide, glycerin, and water; or sorbitol, lanolin, mineral oil, petrolatum, a color pigment, perfume, and water; or anhydrous or emulsified carnauba wax, ozokerite, isopropyl palmitate, titanium dioxide, talc, certified colors, pigments, and perfume (*see all*). Dry rouge may contain kaolin, talc, precipitated calcium carbonate, magnesium carbonate, titanium dioxide, zinc stearate, certified colors and lakes, inorganic oxides, and perfume (*see all*). A typical formula for an emulsified rouge includes white beeswax, 12 percent; petrolatum, 24 percent; spermaceti, 8 percent; mineral oil, 22 percent; borax, 0.8 percent; water, about 30 percent; pigment, 3.1 percent; *p*-hydroxybenzoic acid, 0.1 percent; and perfume (*see all*). Rouge does not figure often in FDA complaints. In recent years there have been complaints of eye irritation and fungus.

ROYAL JELLY • Highly touted as a magic ingredient in cosmetics to restore one's skin to youthfulness. Royal jelly is the very nutritious secretion of the throat glands of the honeybee workers that is fed to the larvae in a colony, to all queen larvae, and possibly to the adult queen. It is a mixture of proteins plus about 31 percent fats, 15 percent carbohydrates, 15 percent minor growth factors, and 24 percent water and trace elements. If stored, royal jelly loses its capacity to develop queen bees.

RUBBER • Rubber, as well as rubber-based adhesives, is a common cause of contact dermatitis. The natural gum obtained from the rubber tree is not allergenic; the offenders are the chemicals added to natural rubber gum to make it a useful product. Such chemicals are accelerators, antioxidants, stabilizers, and vulcanizers, many of which can cause allergies. Two are the most frequent but certainly not the only sensitizers in rubber. They are mercaptobenzothiazole and tetramethylthiuram. Don't forget that the edge of eyelash curlers may have rubber, as well as the false eyelashes themselves. Foam rubber sponges used to apply and remove cosmetics may also cause an allergic reaction. The EU banned thiuram in cosmetics. *See* Latex.

RUBBING ALCOHOLS • Isopropyl alcohol (*see*), probably the most common rubbing alcohol, is used in astringents, skin fresheners, colognes, and perfumes. It can be irritating to the skin. Ethanol (*see*) is used in perfumes and as a solvent for oils. It also can be irritating. Rubbing alcohols are denatured with chemicals to make them poisonous so they will not be ingested as an alcoholic beverage.

RUBEFACIENTS • Help stimulate blood circulation to the scalp and the activity of the oil-secreting glands. Pilocarpine (*see*) is an example.

RUBIA TINCTORIUM • *See* Madder.

RUBUS CHINGII FRUIT EXTRACT • Chinese Raspberry. Sweet Tea. Used in folk medicine to treat urinary problems.

RUBUS DELICIOSUS • *See* Boysenberry.

RUBUS FRUTICOSUS • *See* Blackberry.

RUBUS IDAEUS • *See* Raspberry Juice.

RUBUS PARVIFOLIUS • Native Raspberry. *See* Raspberry Juice.

RUBUS STRIGOSUS • *See* Raspberry Juice.

RUBUS SUAVISSIMUL • *See* Raspberry Juice.

RUBUS VILLOSUS • *See* Blackberry.

RUE OIL • *Ruta graveolens.* A spice ingredient obtained from the fresh, aromatic, blossoming plants grown in southern Europe and the Orient. It has a fatty odor and is used in baked goods. The oil is obtained by steam distillation and is used in fragrances and in blueberry, raspberry, and other fruit flavorings. Formerly used in medicine to treat disorders and hysteria. It is on the FDA list for study of mutagenic, teratogenic, subacute, and reproductive effects. It may cause photosensitivity.

RUMEX ACETOSELLA • *See* Sorrel Extract.

RUMEX CRISPUS • *See* Curled Dock.

RUMINANT TISSUE AND TISSUE-DERIVED INGREDIENTS MATERIALS WITH SUSPECTED RISK OF INFECTIVITY • Adrenal gland, rowamyelin, basal ganglia/basal ganglion, sciatic nerve, bone marrow, sphingosine phosphatide, brain sphinogomyelin, brain extract, sphingolipid, ceramide, b-lactoside, spinal cord, ceramide dihexoside, spleen, cerebellum, suprarenal gland, cerebroside (sulfate), tetraglycosylceramide, cerebrospinal fluid, thymus gland (sweet-bread), cranial nerves, tonsil collagen (soluble), triglycosylceramide, colon, trinitrophenylaminolauroylglucocerebroside, deer fat, trinitrophenylaminolauroylgalactocerebroside, deer antler velvet, trisialoganglioside digalactosylceramide, diglycosylceramides (cytosides), disialoganglioside, dura mater elastin (source: oxen neck ligaments), eye galactocerebroside, galactosylcerebroside (sulfate ester), ganglioside, glucosylcerebroside, glycerophospholipid, glycosaminoglycan, glycosphingolipid, glycosylceramide, hypothalamus, ileum intercellular lipids (ICLs), lactocerebroside, lactosylceramide, liposomes, liver, lung, lymph nodes, monoglycosylceramide (cerebroside), monosialoganglioside, N-nervonoyl cerebroside, N-oleoyl cerebroside, N-palmitoyl cerebroside, nasal mucosa, olfactory bulb or gland, pancreas (including pancreatin), phospholipids, pineal gland, pituitary gland, and placenta. This list is not intended to identify all ruminant-derived ingredients about which the FDA and USDA have concerns. If any ruminant tissues or tissue-derived ingredients are offered for import or being used as an ingredient in cosmetics, if the ingredient is from a bovine spongiform encephalopathy (BSE) affected or at-risk country, the FDA must seek additional instructions. The British government announced on March 20, 1996, that information had been gathered about BSE in cattle that suggests a possible relationship between BSE and ten cases of a newly identified form of Creutzfeldt-Jakob disease (CJD), a similar fatal transmissible spongiform encephalopathy (TSE), in humans. To serve a mutual interest in protecting public health, the Food and Drug

Administration (FDA) believes it is prudent to reiterate concerns we have previously expressed on this issue.

BSE is an infectious neurologic disorder of cattle and is prevalent in certain parts of the world. BSE has never been diagnosed in cattle in the United States. It is believed that the rapid spread of BSE in cattle in some countries, particularly Great Britain, was caused by the feeding of certain infected cattle and sheep tissues to cattle. Although transmission of the causative agent of BSE to humans has not been definitively documented to date, inter-species transfer has been demonstrated (e.g., mice can be infected by exposure to infected bovine tissues). Developments in Great Britain raise serious questions regarding potential hazards of the use of animal tissues containing the causative agent of BSE. The FDA strongly recommends that firms manufacturing or importing cosmetic products that contain specific bovine tissues, including extracts or substances derived from such tissues, take whatever steps are necessary to assure themselves and the public that such ingredients do not come from cattle born, raised, or slaughtered in countries where BSE exists. The FDA believes that immediate and concrete steps should be taken by manufacturers to reduce the potential risk of human exposure to, or transmission of, the infectious agent which causes BSE in cattle. The list of countries where BSE is known to exist is maintained by the U.S. Department of Agriculture (USDA). They include, at the time of this writing, Northern Ireland and the Falklands, Switzerland, France, Republic of Ireland, Oman, and Portugal. A range of research projects into the exact nature of both the BSE agent and other TSE agents is ongoing. Available scientific information indicates that these agents are extremely resistant to inactivation by normal disinfection or sterilization procedures.

The cosmetic industry has historically been a user of bovine-derived raw materials. These materials include extracts of bovine organs, including brain, placenta, liver, thymus, heart, mammary gland, marrow, ovary and spleen, as well as ingredients derived from animal tissues such as glycosaminoglycans, bovine lipids, proteins, amino acids, and most recently, sphingolipids isolated from central nervous system tissue. The information that is currently available suggests that exposure of healthy, intact skin with a BSE infectious agent represents an unlikely route of infection. Nevertheless, some ingredients used in cosmetics are derived from tissues that are considered highly infectious, and, if obtained from infected animals, may contain the BSE infectious agent. The possibility of infection cannot be completely ruled out, especially if exposure occurs with abraded or damaged skin or from contact of the infectious agent with the eyes or through ingestion. Although there is still no definitive evidence that the use of bovine tissues that contain the infectious agent for BSE causes CJD in humans, the FDA is concerned that appropriate measures to eliminate the use of bovine tissues from BSE countries be instituted industrywide.

RUPTUREWORT (HERNIARIA GLABRA) • The whole plant, gathered when in flower, is astringent, very actively diuretic, and expectorant. Externally, it has been used as a poultice to speed the healing of ulcers.

RUSCOGENIN • A sterol (*see*) used as a skin-conditioning ingredient.

RUSCUS ACULEATUS • *See* Butcher's Broom.

RUTA GRAVEOLENS • *See* Rue Oil.

RUTIN • Found in many plants, especially buckwheat, tobacco, and myrtle. Used to protect blood vessels in medicines. In cosmetics, is used as a skin- and hair-conditioning ingredient and as an antioxidant.

RYE FLOUR • *Secale cereale.* The fermented grain is used as an emollient and to counteract dandruff. Used in powders.

RYOKU-CHA EKISU • Antioxidant. *See* Camellia Oil.

S

SABADILLA ALKALOIDS • Cevadilla. Caustic Barley. The dried ripe seeds of *Schoenocaulon officinale,* grown in the Andes. In 1992, the FDA proposed a ban on sabadilla in lice-killing products because it had not been shown to be safe and effective as claimed.

SABAL • *See* Saw Palmetto Extract.

SABBATIA • *See* American Centaury Extract.

SACCHARATED LIME • Produced by the action of lime upon sugar. Used as a buffer (*see*) in cosmetics and as a preservative.

SACCHARIDE HYDROLYSATE • Sugars derived from using an alkali and water on a mixture of glucose and lactose (*see*). Used as a skin conditioner. *See* Barley Extract.

SACCHARIDE ISOMERATE • *See* Saccharide Hydrolysate.

SACCHARIN • An artificial sweetener in use since 1879. It is three hundred times as sweet as natural sugar. Used as a sweetener for mouthwashes, dentifrices, and lipsticks. It sweetens dentifrices and mouthwashes in 0.05 to 1 percent concentration. It was used with cyclamates in the experiments that led to the ban on cyclamates. The FDA has proposed restricting saccharin to 15 milligrams per day for each kilogram of body weight or 1 gram per day for a 150-pound person. Now being studied by NTP (*see*) for possible delisting as a carcinogen.

SACCHAROMYCES • Yeast extracts. Used in face creams.

SACCHAROMYCES/BARLEY SEED FERMENT FILTRATE • Used as a humectant and skin conditioner. Fermented barley by the organism *Saccharomyces*. *See* Barley Extract.

SACCHAROMYCES LYSATE EXTRACT • Breakup of yeast for use as a moisturizer and humectant.

SACCHAROMYCES/SOY PROTEIN FERMENT • Fermentation of soy protein by yeast for use in skin conditioners.

SACCHARUM OFFICINARUM • Sugarcane Extract. Skin conditioner. *See* Blackstrap Powder and Sugarcane.

SAFFLOWER ACID • Fatty acids from safflower oil (*see*) used as a cleanser.

SAFFLOWER GLYCERIDE • *See* Safflower Oil.

SAFFLOWER OIL • *Carthamus tinctorius* Oil. Expressed from the seed of an Old World herb that has large bright red or orange flowers and resembles a thistle. Used in creams and lotions to soften the skin and in hair conditioners. Based on available data, the CIR Expert Panel (*see*) says it is safe as a cosmetic ingredient.

SAFFLOWERAMIDOPROPYL ETHYLDIMONIUM ETHOSULFATE • Fatty acid derived from safflower oil (*see*). Antistatic hair conditioner.

SAFFRON CROCUS EXTRACT • An extract of the flowers of *Crocus sativus*. Used in perfumery and coloring in cosmetics. It is the dried stigma of the crocus cultivated in Spain, Greece, France, and Iran. Used also in bitters, liquors, and spice flavorings. Formerly used to treat skin diseases.

SAFROLE • Found in certain natural oils such as star anise, nutmeg, and ylang-ylang. It has the odor of sassafras and root beer. Used in the manufacture of heliotropin (*see*) and inexpensive soaps and perfumes. Used as a beverage flavoring until it was banned by the FDA in 1960. The toxicity of this fragrance ingredient is being questioned by the FDA. It is an animal liver carcinogen. It has been banned as a food additive. The EU has banned it in cosmetics except for normal content in the natural essences used and provided in concentrations not to exceed 100 ppm in the finished product, 50 ppm in products for dental and oral hygiene, and provided that safrole is not present in toothpaste intended specifically for children. On the Canadian Hotlist (*see*).

SAGE EXTRACT • Used by herbalists to treat sore gums and mouth ulcers and to remove warts. The oil was used as a meat preservative.

SAGE OIL • *Salvia officinalis.* Obtained by steam distillation from the flowering tops of the plant believed by the Arabs to prevent dying. A pale yellow liquid that smells and tastes like camphor. Used to cover gray hair in some rinses and as an astringent in skin fresheners and steam baths. Supposedly has healing power.

SAGEBRUSH • *See* Sesquiterpene Lactones.

SAINT JOHN'S BEARD • *See* Locust Bean Gum.

SAINT JOHN'S WORT • *Hypericum perforatum.* Amber. Blessed. Devil's Scourge. God's Wonder Herb. Grace of God. Goatweed. Hypericum Klamath Weed. A perennial native to Britain, Europe, and Asia, it is now found throughout North America. The plant contains glycosides (sugar compounds), volatile oil, tannin, resin, and pectin (*see all*). It is used in "organic" cosmetics. It was believed to have infinite healing powers derived from the saint, the red juice representing his blood. It was used as an antivenereal. The oil is used for burns. The FDA listed Saint John's wort as an "unsafe herb" in 1977. The FDA issued a notice in 1992 that Saint John's wort has not been shown to be safe and effective as claimed in OTC digestive aid products. That does not mean, however, that it cannot be used for other purposes.

SAISIN EKISU • Asarum. An extract of the roots of *Asiasarum sieboldii* or *A. heterotropoides.* Wild Ginger. Used in bath products and deodorants. *See* Snakeroot.

SAKE • Rice wine. *See* Rice Ferment Filtrate.

SAL BUTTER • Obtained from the kernels of the sal tree, *Shorea robusta,* a tree growing wild in the jungle or forests of north, east, and central India. Sal is used locally for cooking and soap production. It is similar to cocoa butter (*see*) and is used in some similar applications. Like mango butter, it is an emollient. Used in skin and hair products, stick products, hair pomades, and dry-skin lotions.

SALACIN • A chemical derived from the bark of several species of willows and poplar trees. Aspirin and other salicylates are derived from salacin or made synthetically. Used in aromatherapy (*see*) and in astringents (*see*).

SALAD OIL • Any edible vegetable oil. Dermatologists advise rubbing salad oils or fats on the skin, particularly on babies and older persons. Vegetable oils are used in commercial baby preparations, cleansers, emollient creams, face powders, hair-grooming preparations, hypoallergenic cosmetics, lipsticks, nail creams, shampoos, shaving creams, and wave sets.

SALICARIA EXTRACT • *Lythrum salicaria.* Spiked Loosestrife. Extract of the flowering herb *L. salicaria,* which has purple or pink flowers. Used since ancient Greek times as an herb that calms nerves and soothes the skin.

SALICORNIA • Glasswort. Samphire. Pickleweed. Can provide high-quality vegetable oil per plant. Europeans perk up salads with the succulent tips of this salt marsh vegetable. Used in skin conditioners.

SALICYLAMIDE • An analgesic, fungicide, and anti-inflammatory ingredient used to soothe the skin. Gives a sensation of warmth on the tongue. In 1992, the FDA proposed a ban on the use of salicylamide to treat fever blisters and cold sores, poison ivy, poison oak, and poison sumac because it has not been shown to be safe and effective for stated claims in OTC products.

SALICYLANILIDE • Usually made from salicylic acid with aniline. Odorless leaflets, slightly soluble in water, freely soluble in alcohol. Used as a topical antifungal ingredient and in antibacterial soaps and topical preparations. In concentrated form may cause irritation of the skin and mucous membranes. When exposed to sunlight, it can cause swelling, reddening, and/or rash of the skin. Halogenated salicylanilides (those with chlorine added) are no longer permitted in cosmetics.

SALICYLATES • Amyl. Phenyl. Benzyl. Menthyl. Glyceryl. Dipropylene Glycol Esters. Salts of salicylic acid. Those who are sensitive to aspirin may also be hypersensitive to FD & C Yellow No. 5, a salicylate, and to a number of foods that naturally contain salicylate, such as almonds, apples, apple cider, apricots, blackberries, boysenberries, cherries, cloves, cucumbers, currants, gooseberries, grapes, nectarines, oil of wintergreen, oranges, peaches, pickles, plums, prunes, raisins, raspberries, strawberries, and tomatoes. The salts are used as sunburn preventatives and antiseptics.

SALICYLIC ACID • Methyl Salicylate. Occurs naturally in wintergreen leaves, sweet birch, and other plants. Synthetically prepared by heating phenol with carbon dioxide. It has a sweetish taste and is used as a preservative and antimicrobial. Used externally as an antiseptic ingredient, fungicide, and skin-sloughing ingredient. It is used as a preservative and antimicrobial at 0.1 to 0.5 percent in skin softeners, face masks, hair tonics, deodorants, dandruff preparations, protective creams, hair dye removers, and suntan lotions and oils. It is antipruritic (anti-itch). It is also used in making aspirin (*see*). It is used as a keratolytic (*see*) drug applied topically to treat acne to slough the skin. Being widely promoted at this writing in anti-aging betahydroxide products. Widely used in cleansing products, makeup, hair conditioners, bath products, and hair colorings. It is being substituted for the "alpha" in alpha-hydroxide products because it is said to be less irritating to the skin. The European Union has banned it for children under three years except in shampoos. It can be absorbed through the skin. Absorption of large amounts may cause vomiting, abdominal pain, increased respiration, acidosis, mental disturbances, and skin rashes in sensitive individuals. The Food and Drug Administration issued a notice in 1992 that salicylic acid, while useful for removing warts, is not effective as an external pain or itch reliever in insect bites and stings, poison ivy, poison sumac, and poison oak in OTC drug products. It is on the Canadian Hotlist (*see*). May cause sensitivity to sun because of the loss of the protective outer layers of skin cells. If redness, bleeding, or pain is experienced, discontinue its use.

SALICYLIDES • Any of several crystalline derivatives of salicylic acid (*see*) from which the water has been removed.

SALICYLOYL PHYTOSPHINGOSINE • Used as skin conditioner. *See* Phenols and Sphingolipids.

SALICYLYL BEESWAX • A skin conditioner. *See* Salycilates and Beeswax.

SALINE • Containing a salt. *See* Sodium Chloride.

SALIX ALBA • *See* Willow Leaf Extract.

SALIX NIGRA • *See* Willow Leaf Extract.

SALMO • *See* Salmon Egg Extract and Salmon Oil.

SALMON EGG EXTRACT • The fatty compound from salmon eggs used in cosmetic emollients.

SALMON OIL • Oil from the fish. It is used in emollients.

SALNACEDIN • Antioxidant. *See* Phenols.

SALT MINE MUD • Sediment obtained from salt mines used as an abrasive, astringent, and absorbent in cosmetic products.

SALTPETER • *See* Ammonium Nitrate.

SALVE • An unctuous adhesive composition or substance applied to wounds or sores; a healing ointment.

SALVIA HISPANICA • *See* Chia Oil.

SALVIA LAVANDULIFOLIA OIL • Fragrance Ingredient. *See* Sage Oil.

SALVIA MILTIORRHIZA EXTRACT • *See* Salvia Officinalis.

SALVIA OFFICINALIS • Sage. A member of the mint family. *Salvia officinalis* in Latin means "to save" and the Romans called it "sacred herb." Throughout history it has been used for depression, fever, respiratory infections, women's complaints, sleep inducer, diuretic, gargles, and sick room use. Widely used in cosmetics. The essential oil is anti-inflammatory, antimicrobial, antioxidant, antiseptic, antispasmodic, astringent, diuretic, hypertensive, and insecticidal. Sage was highly regarded during the Middle Ages and was used for women's complaints, nerve tonic and disorders of the kidneys and digestive system. Today the essential oil is often preferred over common sage for women's complaints, nervousness, frigidity and impotence, skin conditions, labor pain, muscle aches and tension. Chinese herbal medicine utilizes sage for women's problems. Sage is also popular in Asian medicine and cosmetics.

SALVIA SCLAREA • *See* Clary.

SAMBUCUS EXTRACT • *See* Elder Flowers.

SAND • Used as an abrasive.

SANDALWOOD • *See* Sandalwood Oil.

SANDALWOOD EXTRACT • *See* Sandalwood Oil.

SANDALWOOD OIL • Fragrance. It is the oil obtained by steam distillation from the dried ground roots and wood of the plant *Santalum album*. Has a strong, warm, persistent odor. Used in floral, fruit, honey, and ginger ale flavorings. Also used for incense and as a fumigant. May produce skin rash in the hypersensitive, especially if present in high concentrations in expensive perfumes.

SANDARAC GUM • *Callitris quadrivalvis*. Resin from a plant grown in Morocco. Used in tooth cements, varnishes, and for gloss and adhesion in nail lacquers. Also used as an incense.

SANG ZHI • Derived from the twigs of the mulberry tree, which reportedly reduces swelling.

SANGUINARIA • Bloodroot. Derived from the dried roots and rhizome of the North American herb. The resin is used to soothe the skin, and its reddish juice stanches blood when used in styptic pencils.

SANICLE • *Sanicula europaea*. A plant grown in Europe and the mountains of Africa and in the Americas. According to an old folk saying, "He who has sanicle needeth no surgeon." Since ancient times it has had a reputation for healing powers. It was used for burns and wounds. It was taken in the form of root tea for skin problems and St. Vitus's dance. Herbalists still recommend it for external use to treat skin diseases and for use in mouthwashes and gargles. A strong decoction of the leaves is used for infections.

SANICULA EUROPAEA • *See* Sanicle.

SANSHOU EKISU • Peppercorn. Prickly Ash. The fruit of *Zanthoxylum*. From a tree related to citrus trees and shrubs. It has the scent of citrus. Used as a skin conditioner. *See* Prickly Ash Extract.

SANTALUM ALBUM • *See* Sandalwood.

SANTALOL • Alcohol from sandalwood used in fragrances. *See* Sandalwood Oil.

SANTOLINA CHAMAECYPARISSUS • *See* Lavender.

SAPINDUS MUKUROSSI • *See* Soapberry Extract.

SAPONARIA EXTRACT • Soapwort. Fuller's Herb. The extract is obtained from *Saponaria officinalis,* a European and middle Asian herb that has a coarse pink or white flower and foams like soap bubbles when scratched. It is substituted for soap in shampoos.

SAPONIFICATION • The making of soap, usually by adding alkalis to fat with glycerol. To saponify is to convert to soap.

SAPONINS • Any of numerous natural or synthetic compounds derived from sugars that occur in many plants such as soapbark, soapwort, or sarsaparilla. Characterized by their ability to foam in water. Extracted from soapbark or soapwort and used chiefly as a foaming and emulsifying ingredient and detergent; also used to reduce surface tensions and to produce fine bubble lather in shaving creams, shampoos, bath oils, and dry shampoos. Yellowish to white, acrid, hygroscopic. In powder form, saponins can cause sneezing.

SARCOSINE • Found in starfish and sea urchins and also formed from caffeine. Sweetish, crystalline acids used in dentifrices as an antienzyme to prevent tooth decay. Because of excellent foaming qualities, they are also used in shampoos.

SARGASSUM • *See* Algae.

SAROTHAMNUS SCOPARIUS • *See* Broom Oil.

SARSAPARILLA EXTRACT • *Smilax aristolochiaefolia. Smilax utilis.* The dried root from tropical American plants. Used in cola, mint, root beer, sarsaparilla, wintergreen, and birch beer flavorings for beverages, ice cream, ices, candy, and baked goods. Still used for psoriasis; formerly used for the treatment of syphilis.

SASA VEITCHII • *See* Bamboo.

SASSAFRAS OIL • Used in dentifrices, perfumes, soaps, and powders to correct disagreeable odors. It is the yellow to reddish-yellow volatile oil obtained from the roots of the sassafras. It is 80 percent safrole and has the characteristic odor and taste of sassafras. Applied to insect bites and stings to relieve symptoms; also used as a topical antiseptic and to break up intestinal gas. May produce dermatitis in hypersensitive individuals.

SATUREIA HORTENSIS • *See* Savory Extract.

SAUSSUREA LAPPA • Herb of the eastern Himalayas (Kashmir) with purple florets and a fragrant root yielding an oil used in perfumery. *See* Costus.

SAVORY EXTRACT • Extract of *Satureia hortensis,* an aromatic mint known as summer or winter savory. Used as a flavoring and fragrance. A member of the mint family, savory is used for indigestion, toothache, and to soothe insect stings. Savory is also a good insect repellent.

SAW PALMETTO EXTRACT • *Serenoa repens* or *S. serrulata.* Sabal. Serenoa. A common stemless palm of southern Florida and the Indies. The fruit is used to treat debilitating and wasting conditions, prostatic enlargement, urinary tract infections, as an aphrodisiac, and for bodybuilding. The FDA does not recognize it as a drug, but in Germany it is used in OTC treatments for benign prostate enlargement. Saw palmetto contains anti-inflammatory ingredients, carotene, tannin, and estrogenic substances.

SAXIFRAGA SARMENTOSA • Rockfoil Strawberry. Begonia. Latin name derived from *saxum,* a rock, and *frangere,* to break; the plant was thought to break stones in the bladder. *See* Strawberry Extract.

SCABIOSA EXTRACT • The extract of an Old World herb, scabiosa, used to treat scabies in folk medicine.

SCCP • Three independent non-food scientific committees provide the EU Commission with the scientific advice it needs when preparing policy and proposals relating to consumer safety, public health, and the environment. The committees also draw the commission's attention to the new or emerging problems that pose an actual or potential threat. They are: the Scientific Committee on Consumer Products (SCCP), the Scientific Committee on Health and Environmental Risks (SCHER), and the Scientific Committee on Emerging and Newly Identified Health Risks (SCENIHR), and are made up of external experts. In addition, the commission relies upon the work of the European Food Safety Authority (EFSA), the European Medicines Evaluation Agency (EMEA), the European Centre for Disease Prevention and Control (ECDC), and the European

Chemicals Agency (ECHA). SCCP asks questions concerning the safety of consumer products (non-food products intended for the consumer). In particular, the committee addresses questions related to the safety and allergenic properties of cosmetic products and ingredients with respect to their impact on consumer health, toys, textiles, clothing, personal care products, domestic products such as detergents, and consumer services such as tattooing.

SCHINUS MOLLE • Brazilian Peppertree. A shrubby tree with narrow, spiky leaves, it contains many useful compounds. Used as a skin-conditioning ingredient in cosmetics. Recent scientific reports indicate extracts contain analgesic, antibacterial, antifungal, anti-inflammatory, antimicrobial, antispasmodic, antiviral, and astringent properties.

SCHIZANDRA CHINENSIS EXTRACT • An herb used by Chinese women as an aphrodisiac and youth tonic. It is a mild sedative. Also believed to increase stamina. Schizandra has been shown in modern scientific laboratories to protect against the narcotic and sedative effects of alcohol and barbiturates. It is used as a tea. Contraindicated in persons with high blood pressure, epilepsy, and increased pressure on the brain.

SCHIZONEPET TENUIFOLIA • *See* Catnip.

SCHLEICHERA TRIJUGA • Ceylon Oak. Used in hair products. *See* Shellac.

SCLAREOLIDE • Fermented Clary Sage Extract. Used as a skin conditioner. *See* Clary.

SCLEROCARYA BIRREA • Marula tree. A medium-size dioecious tree, indigenous to the woodlands of Southern Africa and the Sudano-Sahelian range of West Africa. The local populations value the yellow, aromatic, and fleshy fruits, which are eaten fresh or processed into juices and alcoholic beverages. Used as a skin conditioner in cosmetics.

SCLEROTIUM GUM • A gum produced by the bacterium *Sclerotium rolfssii*. A waxy mass of fungi and sugars used in bath gels, moisturizers, and cleansers.

SCORDININE • An ingredient in garlic used as a skin conditioner. *See* Garlic Extract.

SCROPHULARIA NODODA • *See* Figwort.

SCULLCAP • *See* Skullcap.

SCULPTURED NAILS • Methyl and polymethyl methacrylates are used to form synthetic nails. Methyl methacrylate can be highly sensitizing and polymethyl methacrylate weakly so.

SCURVY GRASS EXTRACT • The extract of the leaves and flower stalks of *Cochlearia officinalis.* The bright green leaves of this northerly herb were collected and eaten in large quantities by European seamen to prevent scurvy. The plant has the strong odor of horseradish, to which it is related.

SCUTELLARIA ROOT EXTRACT • *See* Skullcap.

SD ALCOHOLS 3-A; 23-H; 38-B; 38-F; 39-B; 39-C; 40; 40-A; 40-B; 40C146 • All ethyl alcohols denatured in accordance with government regulations. Used as thickeners, solidifiers, and liquefiers. SD 40 is one of the most popular in cosmetics. It is used as an astringent and solvent. *See* Denaturant.

SEA BUCKTHORN EXTRACT • The extract of the fruit of *Hippophae rhamnoides.* A Eurasian maritime shrub having orange-red edible berries and yielding a yellow dye. *See* Hippophae Rhamnoides.

SEA CLAY EXTRACT • A quaternary ammonium compound (*see*) made of clay from the sea used in hair and skin conditioners.

SEA ROCKET • *Cakile maritima.* Succulent herb found along the sandy shore. Used as a conditioner.

SEA SALT EXTRACT • The European market calls this maris sal. It is used in bath oils and as a skin conditioner.

SEA SILT EXTRACT • The European market calls this maris limus. The extract of marine sediments, it is used as a thickener and abrasive.

SEA URCHIN EXTRACT • Multifooted sea animals rich in the amino acid cysteine (*see*). The extract is used as a skin conditioner in cosmetics.

SEAWATER • Called maris aqua by the EU and sea mineral water or liquid by cosmetic producers. It is used as a humectant, skin conditioner, and solvent.

SEA WHIP EXTRACT • *Pseudoptero gorgia.* Gorgonian Extract. An animal with tiny, evenly distributed pores, stemps, and branches that are long and whiplike. It may be purple, red, orange, yellow, or tan. It is found attached to rocks. Its sexual reproduction is a polyp, which then reproduces asexually by budding to become the parent of a new colony. It has been found to yield a potent anti-inflammatory drug that, at this writing, is being tested as therapy for irritant contact dermatitis.

SEAWEED • A group of sea plants that yield a gelatinlike substance. *See* Algae, Carrageenan, and Kelp.

SEBACEOUS GLANDS • Oil glands that provide sebum to coat hair and the stratum corneum (*see*).

SEBACIC ACID • Decanedioic Acid. Colorless leaflets, sparingly soluble in water and soluble in alcohol. Manufactured by heating castor oil with alkalies or by distillation of oleic acid (*see*). The esters of sebacic acid are used as plasticizers in cosmetics. Also a pH adjuster.

SEBORRHEIC DERMATITIS • Skin inflammation caused by overactivity of the oil glands in the skin. Seborrheic dermatitis is a scaling disorder. Its cause is not well understood. In milder manifestations, it affects the scalp and is commonly called dandruff. In more severe cases, lesions can appear on the face and trunk. The most recent advance in the treatment of seborrheic dermatitis of the scalp is a shampoo containing the active ingredient ketoconazole, an antifungal. Recalcitrant cases may require the use of topical corticosteroids in addition to ketoconazole. Older treatments included the use of coal tar shampoos, most of which are now available over the counter, and shampoos containing selenium sulfide, also primarily OTC products. Salicylic acid solutions may help to remove scales. The EU has banned selenium in cosmetics with the exception of selenium disulfide under certain conditions.

SEBUM • The oily substance produced by the sebaceous glands (*see*).

SECALE CEREALE • *See* Rye Flour.

SECHIUM EDULE • Cho Cho. Vegetable Pear. Herbalists use it to lower high blood pressure and high cholesterol.

SEDGE ROOT • *See* Cyperus.

SEDUM ACRE • Stone Crop. Gold Moss. Flowers in spring in sunny, sandy soil. Related to houseleek (*see*). Irritating to the skin in a way similar to pepper. Contains nicotine.

SEDUM ROSEA ROOT EXTRACT • Used as an antioxidant and astringent in cosmetics.

SELENIUM ASPARTATE • The selenium salt of aspartic acid. On the Canadian Hotlist (*see*). The EU has banned selenium in cosmetics with the exception of selenium disulfide under certain conditions. *See* Aspartic Acid and Selenium Sulfide.

SELENIUM SULFIDE • Discovered in 1807 in the earth's crust, it is used in antidandruff shampoos and applied to the skin for the treatment of *Tinea versicolor* (*see*). Can severely irritate the eyes if it gets into them while the hair is being washed. May cause dryness or oiliness of hair or scalp and rarely increases normal hair loss. Occupational exposure causes pallor, nervousness, depression, garlic odor of breath, gastrointestinal disturbances, skin rash, and liver injury in experimental animals. On the Canadian Hotlist (*see*). The EU has banned selenium in cosmetics with the exception of selenium disulfide under certain conditions. Must be listed on the label with the caution to avoid contact with eyes or damaged skin.

SELF-HEAL • *Prunella vulgaris*. A perennial herb native to many countries, it was used by New England settlers to cure "female troubles" and as a tonic. Among its ingredients are volatile oils, bitter principle, and tannin (*see all*). It is used as an herbal treatment and general tonic and by herbalists as an infusion. Externally, it is used in a poultice as an antiseptic for wounds and to stop bleeding. It is also used to treat diarrhea, sore throat, and hemorrhoids.

SEMIAQUILEGIA ADOXOIDES • The root contains a number of compounds that are used in Chinese medicine to treat inflammation, swelling, and sores.

SEMPERVIVUM • Plant has irritating properties and the leaves have been found to cause skin rash. *See* Houseleek.

SENECIO • *See* Groundsel Extract.

SENEGA EXTRACT • *Polygala senega*. Snakeroot. North American Indians, particularly the Senecas, used this for snakebite. It contains saponins, mucilage, salicylic acid, and resin. Used to reduce eyelid swelling and as an emollient. It is used by herbalists as an expectorant in the treatment of bronchial asthma, to stimulate saliva, and to treat sore throats and laryngitis.

SENNA, ALEXANDRIA • Flavoring from the dried leaves of *Cassia senna* grown in India and Egypt. Has been used as a cathartic.

SENSITIVITY • Hypersensitivity. An increased reaction to a substance that may be quite harmless to nonallergic persons.

SENSITIZE • To administer or expose to an antigen provoking an immune response so that, on later exposure to that antigen, a more vigorous secondary response will occur.

SENSITIZER • An ingredient that causes an increased reaction to a substance.

SEPIA • *See* Cuttlefish Extract.

SEQUESTERING INGREDIENT • A preservative that prevents physical or chemical changes affecting color, flavor, texture, or appearance of a product. Ethylenediamine tetraacetic acid (EDTA) is an example. It prevents adverse effects of metals in shampoos.

SEQUOIA SEMPERVIRENS • Redwood. Extract of the stems of redwood used as a skin conditioner.

SEQUOIADENDRON GIGANTEA • Giant Redwood. Extract of the stems used as a skin conditioner.

SERENOA SERRULATA • *See* Saw Palmetto Extract.

SERICA • *See* Silk.

SERICIN • A protein isolated from the silkworm. Used in hair and skin conditioners.

SERINE • A nonessential amino acid (*see*), taken as a dietary supplement. It is a constituent of many proteins. *See* Proteins.

SERPENTARIA EXTRACT • Snakeroot. Snakeweed. Extracted from the roots of *Rauwolfia serpentina*, its yellow rods turn red upon drying. Used in the manufacture of resins and as a bitter tonic. Can affect heart and blood pressure when ingested.

SERUM ALBUMEN • The major protein component of blood plasma derived from bovines. Used as a moisturizing ingredient.

SERUM PROTEINS • *See* Serum Albumen.

SESAME • Seeds and Oils. *Sesamum indicum* Oil. The edible seeds of an East Indian herb that has a rosy or white flower. The seeds, which flavor bread, crackers, cakes, confectionery, and other products, yield a pale yellow oil used in the manufacture of margarine. The oil has been used as a skin softener and contains elements active against lice. It is also used in hair conditioners. May cause allergic reactions, primarily contact dermatitis. Based on available data, the CIR Expert Panel (*see*) says it is safe as a cosmetic ingredient.

SESAMIDOPROPYL BETAINE • *See* Quaternary Ammonium Compounds.

SESAMIDOPROPYL DIMETHYLAMINE • *See* Quaternary Ammonium Compounds.

SESAMIDOPROPYLAMINE OXIDE • *See* Quaternary Ammonium Compounds.

SESAMUM INDICUM SEED OIL • *See* Sesame.

SESQUITERPENE LACTONES • These compounds occur naturally in essential oils, particularly citrus oils. They have little flavor and poor water solubility, and react readily with oxygen to produce off-aroma and off-flavor notes. In recent years, more than six hundred plants have been identified as containing these substances, and more than fifty are known to cause allergic contact dermatitis. Among them are arnica, chamomile, and yarrow (*see all*).

SETTING LOTIONS • Wave-setting lotions, which women apply before rolling their hair in rollers or pins, depend on the hair-swelling ability of the water contained in them and the gum film that dries and holds the hair in place. Natural gums commonly used in such preparations are tragacanth, karaya, acacia, and quince seed, as well as sodium alginate from seaweed. Synthetic gums such as methylcellulose (*see*) are also used, but tend to flake when dry. A typical setting lotion may consist of karaya gum dissolved in ethyl alcohol and then mixed with water, glycerin, and perfume. Generally harmless but there have been some cases of scalp irritation reported to the FDA.

SHADDOCK EXTRACT • An extract of *Citrus grandis* and named for a seventeenth-century sea captain who brought the seeds back from the East Indies to Barbados. Shaddock is a very large, thick-rinded, pear-shaped citrus fruit related to and largely replaced by the grapefruit.

SHAKUYAKU • Root of the *Paeonia lactiflora* used as a skin conditioner. *See* Peony.

SHAKUYAKU EKISU • The Japanese name for peony (*see*).

SHALE EXTRACT • A fossil rock that is formed by the consolidation of mud, clay, or silt finely stratified. Contains many minerals. Used as a skin conditioner.

SHAMPOOS • Shampoos are of relatively recent origin because people used to wash their hair with soap. The original products were made of coconut oil and castile soap. In 1930, the liquid detergent shampoos were introduced, followed by the cream type, and then the liquid cream shampoos. Today, shampoos are packaged in plastic tubes or bottles, aerosol cans, jars, and glass. They have various special purposes, such as mending split ends or curing dandruff. They contain a variety of ingredients ranging from eggs to herbs. A soap shampoo today still may contain about 25 percent coconut oil, some olive oil, about 15 percent alcohol, and 50 percent glycerol and water. The soapless shampoo cream may contain 50 percent sodium lauryl sulfate, some sodium stearate (*see both*), and about 40 percent water. The liquid shampoo is the most popular today and usually contains a detergent such as triethanolamine dodecylbenzene sulfonate, ethanolamide of lauric acid (*see both*), perfume, and water. Cream shampoos may have the same ingredients as the liquid in different proportions to obtain a cream, and they usually contain lanolin. Special shampoos contain such things as dehydrated egg powder or herbs. Opacifying ingredients such as stearyl and cetyl alcohol (*see both*) may be added to the cream lotion types. Various sequestering ingredients (*see*) may be used to make the water soft to remove the film and to make the hair shinier. Various finishing ingredients, such as mineral oil and lanolin, may be added to make the hair lustrous. Water-absorbing materials such as glycerin and sorbitol (*see*) are used as conditioning ingredients; these two increase the water absorption of the hair and make it more pliable and less brittle. Preservatives such as phydroxybenzoic acid and sodium hexametaphosphate (*see*) may also be used. Ingestion of detergents can cause gastric irritation. Shampoos are among the most frequently cited products in complaints to the FDA. Reports include eye irritation; scalp irritation; tangled hair; swelling of hands, face, and arms; and split and fuzzy hair.

SHAO-YAO • *See* Peony.

SHARK-LIVER OIL • A rich source of vitamin A believed to be beneficial to the skin. A brown fatty oil obtained from the livers of the large predatory fish. Used in lubricating creams and lotions.

SHAVE GRASS • *See* Horsetail.

SHAVING CREAMS • Dry hair is hard and difficult to cut with a razor. The object of a shaving cream is to make the hair softer and easier to shave. Brushless shave creams are emulsions of oil and water, really vanishing creams rather than soaps. Not as efficient as the lathering type, they usually require that the beard (or legs) be washed with soap and water. Shaving creams, which must be applied, are soaps with small but copious bubbles known as lather. They can be applied with a brush or with an aerosol. Aerosol shaving creams produce foam. This foam is applied directly to the beard and is the most popular form used today. Some men still use the older shaving creams offered in a cake or stick. The American Medical Association recommends that men with dry or soap-sensitive skin use brushless shave creams that, because of their emollient properties, soothe the skin and do not dry it out. Men with oily skin, on the other hand, should use the lather-type cream applied by aerosol or brush. The AMA also points out that thorough washing and rinsing of the face in hot water or applying a hot wet towel for a few minutes before shaving will soften a beard.

SHAVING LOTIONS • Preshave and After-Shave. Most preshave lotions are designed to be used before shaving with an electric razor. Some are made for a regular razor and usually contain coconut oil, fatty acids, triethanolamine, alkyl arylpolyethylene glycol ether (a dispersant), water, and perfume. Preshave preparations temporarily tighten the skin to facilitate cutting the hairs. Electric razor preshave products may contain aluminum phenolsulfonate, menthol, camphor (*see all*), water, and perfume dissolved in alcohol. An oily type of preshave lotion may contain isopropyl myristate or isopropyl palmitate (*see both*), 74.5 percent alcohol, and perfume. After-shave lotions are supposed to soothe the skin, which may have been irritated by shaving. The earliest were merely substitutes for water. At the end of the nineteenth century, talcum powder appeared among men's shaving products. Then barbershop preparations such as bay rum and witch hazel came into use. By 1916, manufacturers were actively promoting men's toiletries, and today perfume is as common in men's products as it is in women's.

After-shave lotions fall into two categories: alcoholic and nonalcoholic. The most common ingredients of the alcoholic type are, in addition to alcohol, glycerin, water, certified color, and perfume. Menthol may be added to give that cool feeling to the skin. Some antiseptics such as quaternary ammonium compounds (*see*) may also be added. Alum may be used for its astringent-styptic effect; also allantoin (*see*) to promote rapid healing of razor nicks. The after-shave nonalcoholic product resembles hand lotion. In fact, hand lotion may be substituted by the consumer. Such products may be prepared from stearic acid, triethanolamine, cetyl alcohol, glycerin (*see all*), distilled water, and very small amounts of lanolin and a preservative such as *p*-hydroxybenzoic acid (*see*). Many other fats, waxes, and emulsifying ingredients may be added. Antiseptics and the soothing allantoin, as well as coloring and perfume, may be incorporated into this type of preparation. However, the best beard softener is still water. Reports of problems to the FDA include the product igniting on the face from a lighted cigarette, face irritations, burned skin and peeling, and eye irritation.

SHEA BUTTER • The natural fat obtained from the fruit of the karite tree,

Butyrosperum parkii. Also called karite butter, it is widely used in moisturizers, suntan gels and creams, cleansing products, indoor tanning preparations, hair conditioners, hair tonics, and lipsticks.

SHEA BUTTER UNSAPONIFIABLES • The fraction of shea butter that is not saponified during processing and is not turned into fatty alcohol.

SHEEP SORREL • *Rumex acetosella.* A small herb common in dry places and having a pleasant, tangy-tasting leaf. Used in "organic" cosmetics.

SHELF LIFE • Expiration Date. The amount of time for which a cosmetic product is good under normal conditions of storage and use, depending on the product's composition, packaging, preservation, and so forth. Expiration dates are, for practical purposes, rule of thumb, and a product may expire long before that date if it has not been properly stored and handled.

SHELLAC • A resinous excretion of certain insects feeding on appropriate host trees, usually in India. As processed for marketing, the lacca, which is formed by the insects, may be mixed with small amounts of arsenic trisulfide for color and with rosin. White shellac is free of arsenic. Shellac is used as a candy glaze and polish; in hair lacquer and on jewelry and accessories. It is also used as a binder in cosmetics. May cause allergic contact dermatitis. Based on available data, the CIR Expert Panel (*see*) says it is safe as a cosmetic ingredient.

SHELLAC WAX • Bleached refined shellac. *See* Shellac.

SHEPHERD'S PURSE EXTRACT • *Capsella bursapastoris.* Shepard's Skin Cream. Shepherd's Heart. A member of the mustard family. It is a white-flowered, weedy herb. Its tiny blossoms grow in the form of a cross. Pungent and bitter, it was valued for its astringent properties by early American settlers. Cotton moistened with its juice was used to stop nosebleeds. In an oil-in-water emulsion, it is used as a base for skin preparations. Among its constituents are saponins, choline, acetylcholine, and tyramine (*see all*). These preparations are used in modern medicine to stimulate neuromuscular function. The herb also reduces urinary tract irritation. It has been shown to contract the uterus and lower blood pressure. Acetylcholine and its salts are banned in cosmetics by ASEAN (*see*).

SHIELD FERN • Buckler Fern. Extract of the leaves of *Dryopteris filix-mas,* a fern that grows in Bermuda.

SHOREA ROBUSTA • *See* Damar.

SHORTENINGS • *See* Salad Oils.

SHOWER GEL • Body Shampoo. Given fancy names, but it basically has the same formulation as shampoo. However, it is usually a clear, colored gel rather than an opaque liquid.

SIDE EFFECT • An unintended but sometimes not unexpected effect of a chemical on the body, apart from the cosmetic ingredient's principal and intended action.

SIENNA • Used to color face powder. It is made from any of the various earthy substances that are brownish yellow when raw and orange-red to reddish brown when burned. They are in general darker in color and more transparent in oils than ochers. No longer authorized for use in cosmetics by the FDA.

SIGESBECKIA ORIENTALIS • Indian Weed. Hedge Mustard. St. Paul's Wort. An upright, slightly hairy annual with small, yellow, daisylike heads. Found in forested areas. Used to soothe inflammation.

SILANEDIOL SALICYLATE • Skin conditioner. *See* Salicylates.

SILANES • A foul-smelling gas that solidifies. It is used in the manufacture of silicones (*see*).

SILANETRIOL ARGINATE • Skin conditioner. *See* Arginine and Siloxane.

SILANOLS • Compounds containing hydroxyl groups bound to silicon atoms. *See* Silica.

SILICA • A white powder, slightly soluble in water, that occurs abundantly in nature and is 12 percent of all rocks. Sand is a silica. Upon drying and heating in a vacuum, hard, transparent, porous granules are formed that are used in absorbent and adsorbent material in toilet preparations, particularly skin protectant creams. Also used as a coloring ingredient. *See* Silicones.

SILICA DIMETHICONE SILYLATE • Absorbent, anticaking, antifoaming, and thickening ingredient. *See* Silica and Dimethicone.

SILICA GEL • Silicic Acid. White gelatinous substance obtained by the action of acids on sodium silicate (*see*). Odorless, tasteless, inert, white fluffy powder when dried. Insoluble in water and acids. Absorbs water readily. It is a dehumidifying and dehydrating ingredient and is widely used in cosmetics and waxes. Used in face powders, dentifrices, creams, and talcum powders as an opacifier. Soothing to skin.

SILICATES • Salts or esters derived from silicic acid (*see*). Any of numerous insoluble complex metal salts that contain silicon and oxygen that constitute the largest group of minerals, and with quartz make up the greater part of the earth's crust (as rocks, soils, and clays). *See* Silica Gel.

SILICEOUS EARTH • Purified silica (*see*) obtained by boiling with diluted acid and washing through a filter. Used in face masks.

SILICIC ACID • *See* Silica Gel.

SILICONES • Any of a large group of fluid oils, rubbers, resins, and compounds derived from silica (*see*), and which are water repellent, skin adherent, and stable over a wide range of temperatures. Sand is a silica. Used in after-shave preparations, hairwaving preparations, nail driers, hair straighteners, hand lotions, and protective creams.

SILICONE QUATERNIUM-1 THROUGH -13 • Quaternary ammonium salts used as a hair-conditioning ingredient. *See* Quaternary Ammonium Compounds.

SILK • A natural fiber secreted as a continuous filament by *Bombyx mori,* the silkworm. In the raw state, it is coated with gum that is usually removed before spinning. *See* Silk Amino Acids and Silk Powder.

SILK AMINO ACIDS • The mixture of amino acids (*see*) resulting in liquefying silk. Used in hair sprays.

SILK POWDER • Coloring ingredient in face powders and soaps obtained from the secretion of silkworms. Widely used in powders, blushers, lipsticks, mascara, foundations, hair preparations, and neck and face products. A white solid that is insoluble in water. Can cause severe allergic skin reactions.

SILKWORM EXTRACT • Bombyx. Extract obtained from crushed silkworms used as a skin conditioner.

SILOXANES • D4 and D5 found in deodorants and moisturizers may be banned in cosmetics by Canada because of environmental risks. *See* Silicones.

SILOXANETRIOL ALGINATE • Skin conditioner. *See* Siloxanes and Alginic Acid.

SILT • Sediment from inland bodies of water used as an anti-acne ingredient and cosmetic astringent.

SILVER • White metal not attacked by water or atmospheric oxygen. Used as a catalyst (*see*) and as a germicide and coloring in cosmetics such as nail polish and enamels. Pure Bioscience of San Diego partnered with Switzerland-based Ciba to help its silver-based antimicrobial ingredient in the personal care market. Ciba will market the silver dihydrogen citrate (SDC) under the trade name Ciba Tinosan SDC and claims the product's transparent and water-soluble qualities make it perfect for cosmetics formulations. The ingredient is suitable for deodorants, lotions, and liquid soaps and adds antimicrobial qualities to the product as well as improving its shelf life, according to Ciba. Pure Bioscience is positioning the ingredient as a low-toxic solution to formulators' antimicrobial needs, in an increasingly selective consumer environment. The marketers of the newer silver ingredient claim that it is "environmentally friendly," and they hope it will be accepted by the green movement (*see*). Any cosmetic containing silver and/or its salts must bear the warning to avoid contact with broken or abraded skin. Permanently listed for use in nail polish in amounts not to exceed 1 percent. Canada restricts mouthwashes to 0.04 percent or less. Silver is on the Canadian Hotlist (*see*).

SILVER BOROSILICATE • A mixture of boron (*see*), silica, sodium oxide, and silver oxide. Used as a preservative.

SILVER BROMIDE • Yellowish, odorless powder; darkens on exposure to light. Used in photography, as a topical anti-infective ingredient and astringent, and in the production of mirror finishing. May cause contact dermatitis.

SILVER FIR EXTRACT, NEEDLES AND TWIGS, OIL • *Abies alba.* The extract of the bark and needles of the silver fir tree, a small conifer. The silver fir needle is used in Europe for its medicinal properties and its fragrant scent. The essential oil is obtained by steam distillation from the needles and young twigs, fir cones, and broken-up pieces. Silver fir needle is used as an ingredient in some cough and cold remedies and rheumatic treatments and also as a fragrance component in deodorants, room sprays, disinfectants, bath preparations, soaps, and perfumes. In aromatherapy, it is used for arthritis, muscular aches, rheumatism, bronchitis, coughs, and sinusitis.

SILVER FIR OIL • *See* Silver Fir Extract.

SILVER MAGNESIUM ALUMINUM PHOSPHATE • A preservative.

SILVER NITRATE • A germicide, antiseptic, and astringent in cosmetics and a coloring ingredient in metallic hair dyes. Odorless, colorless, transparent, and poisonous. A white crystalline salt, it was used as a nineteenth-century hair dye. It darkens with exposure to light in the presence of organic matter. Silver combines readily with protein and turns brown. Disadvantages are that it may cause unpleasant off-shades and make the hair stiff. It is also adversely affected by permanent waving. On the skin, it may be caustic and irritating. If swallowed, it causes severe gastrointestinal symptoms and frequently death. The EU says it should be restricted to 4 percent and used solely for products intended for coloring eyelashes and eyebrows. Must be listed on the label along with "rinse the eyes immediately if the product comes into contact with them."

SILVER OXIDE • Germicide made from a mixture of silver nitrate (*see*) and alkali hydroxide.

SILVER SULFATE • *See* Silver Nitrate.

SILVERWEED • *Potentilla anserina.* This weed contains tannins, flavonoids, bitter principle (*see all*), and organic acids. It is an astringent used by herbalists to control the overproduction of mucus. Taken internally for hemorrhoids or used in a compress. Also used in a mouthwash for inflamed gums and mouth ulcers, and in an infusion for sore throats.

SILYBUM MARIANUM • Milk Thistle. Used as a skin conditioner. *See* Thistle.

SIMETHICONE • An antifoam compound, a silicone oil, white viscous liquid. Used as an ointment base ingredient. A topical drug vehicle and skin protectant.

SIMMONDSIA CHINENSIS • *See* Jojoba Oil.

SIN LIST • Sweden-based International Chemical Secretariat launched the Substitute It Now, or SIN, list of high-concern chemicals in 2008.

SINANOKI EKISU • *Tilia cordata.* A skin conditioner. *See* Lime.

SINE ADIPE COLOSTRUM • Nonfat colustrum. *See* Colostrum.

SINE ADIPE LAC • Nonfat dry milk.

SINGLE FLORALS • A basic type of perfume that has a definite fragrance of one flower, such as lily of the valley, carnation, or rose. This does not mean that only one note (*see* Body Note) is used. Such perfumes require skillful blending to surround the desired single floral with other notes to give it power and beauty without intruding on the single theme.

SIRAKABA EKISU • Leaves of the *Betula alba*. See Betula.

SIRAKABA JYUHI EKISU • The bark of *Betula alba*. See Betula.

SIRTUINS • Cellular enzymes are reportedly universal regulators of aging in virtually all living organisms and are a prime target for anti-aging cosmetics. They are a class of proteins found in organisms ranging from bacteria to humans. Named after the yeast gene responsible for cellular regulation in yeast, sirtuins regulate important biological pathways such as aging and stress. Regulation of metabolic processes as well as cellular defense mechanisms might ultimately be the key to a possible life-span-extending role for sirtuins in mammals. *See* Reservatrol.

SISAL • *Agave lechuguilla*. A wax and intermediate (*see*) obtained from a plant native to the Mexican desert. The dust is irritating to the respiratory tract and may cause allergic asthma. Skin toxicity unknown.

SISYMBRIUM IRIO • London Rocket. A weed that yields an aromatic oil. Used in fragrances.

SITOSTEROL • A skin conditioner. *See* Sterol.

SKATOLE • Used in perfumery as a fixative (*see*). A constituent of beetroot, feces, and coal tar. Gives a violet color when mixed with iron and sulfuric acid.

SKIN BLEACH • There are a variety of products for removing freckles, age spots (chloasma), flat moles, postinflammatory changes, and even naturally dark skin. The original bleaching creams contained ammoniated mercury (*see*), which has been banned by the FDA except for use as a preservative in eye makeup. Mercury produced some temporary lightening of the skin by causing sloughing of the outer skin, thus reducing the number of dark pigment cells near the surface. Mercury frequently caused allergic reactions and could have had adverse effects internally even though applied only to the skin. More efficient bleaching creams today use hydroquinone (*see*), which may cause some lightening of the skin in light- but not in dark-skinned blacks. After treatment is stopped, repigmentation almost always occurs. Some powerful hydroquinone products can produce blotches, allergic reactions, and other undesirable side effects. According to the American Medical Association, bleach products are useful for treating limited areas where excessive pigmentation is the result of an abnormal process. For instance, they may be of limited use in treating melasma, "the mask of pregnancy," that is, the excessive skin pigmentation fairly common in pregnant women and women taking birth control pills. The use of bleach cream is a long-term process, and often the only benefit is from the lubricating effect of the cream base, which relieves dryness of the skin. The bases of the creams and ointments are usually petrolatum, mineral oil, lanolin, or vanishing creams of the stearate type (*see all*). Active ingredients, carriers, and scents include acetic acid, alcohol, bismuth compounds, citric acid, glycerin, hydrogen peroxide, hydroquinone, monobenzone, oxalic acid, potassium carbonate, potassium chlorate, rose water, borate, sugar, benzoin, zinc oxide, and zinc peroxide (*see all*). Among problems reported to the FDA were symptoms of mercury poisoning, swelling of the face and neck, jerking of hands, skin rash, burns, and stomach distress. Mercury was banned from cosmetics in 1973 except as a preservative in eye preparations.

SKIN BRACER • There is little difference between shaving lotions (*see*) and skin bracers. A skin bracer may have a high alcohol content and may also be used as a body refresher after a bath or shower. It is made mostly of water, alcohol, and perfume. Toxicity depends upon ingredients.

SKIN CONDITIONERS • Emollients, humectants, moisturizers, protectants, and soothers.

SKIN FRESHENER • Fresheners are weaker than astringents. They are usually clear liquids designed to make the skin feel cool, tight, and refreshed. May contain about 60 percent witch hazel, about 15 percent camphorated alcohol, 24 percent alcohol, and 1 percent citric acid. May also contain arnica, bay rum, boric acid, chamomile, floral scents, glycerin, lactic acid, magnesia, menthol, lavender oil, phosphoric acid, talc, benzoin, and aluminum salts (*see all*). Depending upon the ingredients, skin fresheners may cause respiratory or allergic contact dermatitis.

SKIN LIPIDS • Mixture of fats derived from animal skin. Used in skin conditioners.

SKIN TIGHTENERS • Usually bovine serum albumin (BSA) used to make skin feel firmer. Since baby boomers may prefer to have plant-derived products, protein fractions in vegetable extracts are claimed to provide a "tightening effect."

SKULLCAP • *Scutellaria laterifolia*. Madweed. Mad Dog Scullcap. Quaker Bonnet. Huang Chi. Grown throughout the world. There are about ninety known species. It is used in cosmetics for its astringent, anti-inflammatory, antimicrobial, and antioxidant properties. Widely used during the nineteenth century to treat nervous diseases, convulsions, neuralgia, insomnia, restlessness, infertility, and even tetanus. Modern scientists have found that it stabilizes blood pressure. Skullcap tea is used as a mild tranquilizer. The sedative and antispasmodic properties led to its use in treating rabies and hence its popular name, mad dog scullcap. Cases of liver toxicity caused by the use of this herb have been reported to the Centers for Disease Control.

SLIP INGREDIENTS • Refers to ingredients that help other ingredients spread over the skin and to aid penetration into the skin. Slip ingredients also have humectant (*see*) properties. Among such ingredients are the glycols, sorbates, and glycerins.

SLIPPERY ELM BARK • *Ulmus fulva*. Bark from the North American elm. Fragrant and sticky, it contains much mucilage and powder. Used as a demulcent (*see*).

SMILAX ARISTOLOCHIAEFOLIA • Skin conditioner. *See* Sarsaparilla Extract.

SMILAX GLABRA • *See* Sarsaparilla Extract.

SMILAX UTILIS ROOT EXTRACT • *See* Sarsaparilla Extract.

SNAKE VENOM • A synthetic tripeptide protein that mimics the activity of a protein found in Wagler's pit viper venom, Walgerlin-1. A green snake, it is also called a "Temple Viper" because certain religious cults place it in their temples. Bites are not uncommon for the species; fortunately, fatalities are very rare. It has long fangs. Its venom is toxic in the blood, causing cell and tissue destruction. It is an arboreal species, and its bites often occur on the upper extremities. The cosmetic manufacturer, however, says that the protein is totally safe and has been clinically proven to reduce the size, depth, and number of wrinkles—particularly expression lines—by relaxing facial muscles. Intense Lift Concentrate, which contains Walgerlin-1, is sold in stores for $500, at this writing, and the manufacturer, Euoko, its developer, says it is more effective than leading competitive products and performs its effectiveness within a month. The Swiss muscle-relaxing tripeptide (*see* Tripeptide-1) is based on the science of the venom of the temple viper, but it is combined with a number of other peptides, vitamins, and amino acids.

SNAKEROOT • Any of numerous plants that have a reputation as remedies for snakebites. Among them, for example, senega (*Polygala senega*). The North American Indians, particularly the Senecas, used this for snakebite. It contains saponins, mucilage, salicylic acid, and resin. It is used by herbalists as an expectorant in the treatment of bronchial asthma. It also is used to stimulate saliva and to treat sore throats and laryngitis. If too much is taken, it irritates the lining of the gut and causes vomiting, according to herbalists. Various snakeroots are used in "organic" cosmetics.

SOAP • The oldest cleanser, usually a mixture of sodium salts of various fatty acids. In liquid soaps, potassium instead of sodium salts is used. Bar soaps vary in contents from brand to brand, depending on the fats or oils used. Sodium hydroxide makes a strong soap, fatty acids a mild soap. So-called neutral soaps are actually alkaline, with pH around 10 (compared to skin, which is 5 to 6.5 pH) when dissolved in water. Liquid soaps use potassium instead of sodium. Soaps are usually found in toothpastes, tooth powder, and shaving creams. Soap is usually made by the saponification of a vegetable oil with caustic soda. Hard soap consists largely of sodium oleate or sodium palmitate and is used medicinally as an antiseptic, detergent, or suppository. Many people are allergic to soaps. They may also be drying to the skin, irritate the eyes, and cause rashes, depending upon ingredients.

SOAPBERRY EXTRACT • The extract of the fruit of *Sapindus saponaria*. The berries of the tree contain as much as 37 percent saponin (*see*).

SOAPWORT • *Saponaria officinalis*. Bouncing Bet. Fuller's Herb. Sheep Weed. Bruise Wort. Saponaria. A European and middle Asian perennial herb that has a coarse pink or white flower. The name is derived from the fact that, when agitated in water, it lathers. The active principle, saponin, is a detergent. Substituted for soap in shampoos. Soapwort was prescribed by medieval Arab physicians for leprosy and other skin complaints. The leaves yield an extract that has been used to promote sweating as a remedy against rheumatism and to purify the blood.

SODIUM ACETATE • Sodium Salt of Acetic Acid. A preservative and alkalizer in cosmetics. In industrial forms, it is used in photography and dyeing processes and in foot warmers because of its heat retention ability. Medicinally it is used as an alkalizer and as a diuretic to reduce body water.

SODIUM ACETYLATED HYALURONATE • A humectant used in makeup and cleansing products. See Acetylated and Hyaluronic Acid.

SODIUM ACRYLATE/ACRYLOYLDIMETHYL TAURATE • Used as an anticaking ingredient or emulsifier and thickener. See Polymer and Acrylates.

SODIUM ACRYLATES/ACROLEIN COPOLYMER • A film former and thickener. See Acrylate

SODIUM ACRYLATES COPOLYMER • Film former and thickener. See Acrylates.

SODIUM ACRYLATE/VINYL ALCOHOL • See Polyvinyl Alcohol.

SODIUM ALGIN SULFATE • Gum used in skin conditioners and as a humectant. See Sulfuric Acid and Alginic Acid.

SODIUM ALGINATE • The sodium salt of alginic acid extracted from brown seaweed. Used as an emollient in baby lotions, hair lacquers, wave sets, and shaving creams. It acts as a stabilizer, thickener, and emulsifier.

SODIUM C12–15 ALKOXYPROPYL IMINODIPROPIONATE • The sodium salt of propionic acid (see).

SODIUM C14–17 ALKYL SEC SULFONATE • See Alcohol and Sulfonated Oils.

SODIUM C12–15 ALKYL SULFATE • See Sulfonated Oils.

SODIUM C12–18 ALKYL SULFATE • The sodium salt of the sulfate of a mixture of synthetic fatty alcohols with 12 to 18 carbons in the alkyl chain. See Sulfonated Oils.

SODIUM C16–20 ALKYL SULFATE • See Sodium C12–15 Alkyl Sulfate.

SODIUM ALLANTOIN PCA • Skin conditioner. See Allantoin.

SODIUM ALPHA-OLEFIN SULFONATES • Used in cosmetics as cleansing ingredients. The highest concentration is reportedly 16 percent in shampoos and bath and shower products. These ingredients are a mixture of sulfonate salts. Concentrations above 10 percent produced moderate eye irritation, and a concentration of 5 percent produced mild eye irritation in rabbits. In animal reproductive studies, fetal abnormalities were noted. Various studies in animals and humans showed irritation and sensitization. The CIR Expert Panel (*see*) says based on available data, these ingredients are safe up to 2 percent in leave-on products.

SODIUM ALUM • *See* Alum.

SODIUM ALUMINATE • A pH adjuster and corrosion inhibitor. *See* Aluminum Salts.

SODIUM ALUMINUM ASCORBATE • *See* Ascorbic Acid.

SODIUM ALUMINUM CHLOROHYDROXYL LACTATE • The sodium salt of lactic acid and aluminum chlorohydrate (*see both*).

SODIUM ALUMINUM LACTATE • The salt of sodium and aluminum lactate. *See* Lactic Acid.

SODIUM AMMONIUM PHOSPHATE • Transparent, odorless crystals used as an analytical reingredient.

SODIUM ASCORBYL/CHOLESTERYL PHOSPHATE • Antioxidant and skin conditioner in creams and makeup. *See* Phosphorus and Ascorbic Acid.

SODIUM ASPARTATE • The sodium salt of aspartic acid (*see*).

SODIUM BABASSUATE • Fatty acids derived from babassu (*see*). Used in cleansers.

SODIUM BEESWAX • Fatty acids derived from beeswax (*see*).

SODIUM BEHENATE • The sodium salt of behenic acid (*see*).

SODIUM BENZOATE • An antiseptic and preservative used in eye creams, vanishing creams, and toothpastes. White, odorless powder or crystals with a sweet antiseptic taste. Once used medicinally for rheumatism and tonsillitis. Now used as a preservative in margarine, codfish, and bottled soft drinks. In 1992, the FDA proposed a ban on sodium benzoate in oral menstrual drug products because it had not been shown to be safe and effective as claimed.

SODIUM BICARBONATE • Bicarbonate of Soda. Baking Soda. Used in effervescent bath salts, mouthwashes, and skin-soothing powders. It is an alkali. Its white crystals or powder are used in baking powder, as a gastric antacid, as an alkaline wash, and to treat burns. Essentially harmless to the skin, but when used on very dry skin in preparations that evaporate, it leaves an alkaline residue that may cause irritation.

SODIUM BISCHLOROPHENYL SULFAMINE • Sodium Bischlorophenyl. *See* Quaternary Ammonium Compounds.

SODIUM BISULFATE • Colorless or white crystals fused in water. Disinfectant, used in the manufacture of soaps, perfumes, foods, and pickling compounds. *See* Sodium Bisulfite.

SODIUM BISULFITE • Sodium Acid Sulfite. An inorganic salt. It is used as an antiseptic; an antifermentative in cosmetic creams, mouthwashes, bleaches, perfumes, and hair dyes; to treat parasitic skin diseases; and to remove warts. In its aqueous solution, it is an acid. Concentrated solutions are highly irritating to the skin and mucous membranes. Sodium bisulfite can cause changes in the genetic material of bacteria and is a suspected mutagen. The Select Committee on GRAS substances found it did not present a hazard at present use levels but that additional data would be needed if higher use occurred.

SODIUM BORAGEAMIDOPROPYL PG-DIMONIUM CHLORIDE PHOSPHATE • A quaternary ammonium compound (*see*) used as an antistatic ingredient.

SODIUM BORATE • Used in freckle lotions, nail whiteners, liquefying (cleansing) creams, and eye lotions as a preservative and emulsifier. Hard, odorless powder insoluble in water, it is a weak antiseptic and astringent for mucous membranes. Used also in bath salts, foot preparations, scalp lotions, permanent-wave solutions, and hair-setting lotions. Has a drying effect on the skin and may cause irritation. Continued use of a shampoo containing it will cause the hair to become dry and brittle. The FDA issued a notice in 1992 that sodium borate has not been shown to be safe and effective for stated claims in OTC products, including insect bite and sting, drug products, and in astringent (*see*) drugs. In the diet of rabbits and rats it caused growth retardation. In the diet of male rats it exerted toxic effects on the sex glands as well as infertility. On the basis of the available information, the CIR Expert Panel (*see*) found it safe in the early 1980s but is considering new information to determine if the final safety assessment should be reaffirmed, amended, or have an addendum. It is on the Canadian Hotlist (*see*). *See* Borates.

SODIUM BROMATE • Inorganic salt. Colorless, odorless crystals that liberate oxygen. Used as a solvent. Based on available data, the CIR Expert Panel (*see*) says it is safe as a cosmetic ingredient not to exceed 10.17 percent. *See* Potassium Bromate for toxicity. It is on the Canadian Hotlist (*see*).

SODIUM BUTYL ESTER OF PVM/MA COPOLYMER • A film former in hair products. *See* Polyvinyl Chloride and Acrylates.

SODIUM BUTYLOXYETHOXY ACETATE • *See* Surfactants.

SODIUM BUTYLPARABEN • A preservative. *See* Parabens.

SODIUM CAPRATE • Cleanser. *See* Capric Acid.

SODIUM CAPROAMPHOACETATE • *See* Surfactants.

SODIUM CAPROAMPHOHYDROXYPROPYLSULFONATE • *See* Quaternary Ammonium Compounds and Surfactants.

SODIUM CAPROAMPHOPROPIONATE • *See* Quaternary Ammonium Compounds and Surfactants.

SODIUM CAPRYLATE • Oil used in baby soaps, liniments, and ointments. Obtained from the fruit or seed of the palm tree. In 1992, the FDA issued a notice that sodium caprylate had not been shown to be safe and effective as claimed in OTC products. *See* Palm Oil.

SODIUM CAPRYLETH-2 CARBOXYLATE • The sodium salt of capryl alcohol. *See* Surfactants.

SODIUM CAPRYLETH-9 CARBOXYLATE • The sodium salt of capryl alcohol with carboxylic acid. *See* Surfactants.

SODIUM CAPRYLOAMPHOACETATE • *See* Surfactants.

SODIUM CAPRYLOAMPHOHYDROXYPROPYLSULFONATE • *See* Quaternary Ammonium Compounds.

SODIUM CARBOMER • An emulsion stabilizer and film former. *See* Carbomer.

SODIUM CARBONATE • Soda Ash. Small, odorless crystals or powder that occurs in nature in ores and is found in lake brines or seawater. Absorbs water from the air. Has an alkaline taste and is used as an antacid and reingredient in permanent wave solutions, soaps, mouthwashes, shampoos, foot preparations, bath salts, and vaginal douches. It is the cause of scalp, forehead, and hand rash when the hypersensitive used cosmetics containing it.

SODIUM CARBONATE PEROXIDE • *See* Sodium Carbonate.

SODIUM CARBOXYMETHYL CELLULOSE • Used in setting lotions. It is an artificial gum that dries and leaves a film on the hair. Prepared by treating alkali cellulose with sodium chloroacetate. *See* Cellulose Gums.

SODIUM CARBOXYMETHYL CHITIN • *See* Chitin.

SODIUM CARBOXYMETHYL DEXTRAN • *See* Surfactants.

SODIUM CARBOXYDECYL PEG-8 DIMETHICONE • A skin conditioner and emulsifier. *See* Siloxanes and Silanes.

SODIUM CARBOXYMETHYL STARCH • Gum derived from starch (*see*) used as a binder and thickener.

SODIUM CARBOXYMETHYL TALLOW PROPYLPROPYLAMINE • *See* Tallow.

SODIUM CARRAGEENAN • Sodium salt of carrageenan (*see*).

SODIUM CASEINATE • The soluble form of milk protein in which casein is partially neutralized with sodium hydroxide and used as a texturizer. GRAS

SODIUM CASTORATE • The sodium salt of the fatty acids derived from castor oil (*see*).

SODIUM CELLULOSE SULFATE • *See* Cellulose.

SODIUM CETEARYL SULFATE • The sodium salt of a blend of cetyl and stearyl alcohol (*see both*) and sulfuric-acid ester. A wax used as a surface-active ingredient (*see*). On the basis of the animal and clinical data, the CIR Expert Panel (*see*) concluded that it is safe as a cosmetic ingredient.

SODIUM CETETH-13 CARBOXYLATE • *See* Cetyl Alcohol.

SODIUM CETYL SULFATE • Marketed in the form of a paste. Contains alcohol, sodium sulfate (*see*), and water. A surface-active ingredient (*see*).

SODIUM CHLORIDE • Common table salt. Used as an astringent and antiseptic in mouthwashes, dentifrices, bubble baths, soap, bath salts, and eye lotions. It consists of opaque white crystals. Used topically to treat inflamed lesions. Diluted solutions are not considered irritating, but upon drying, water is drawn from the skin and may produce irritation. Salt workers have a great deal of skin rashes. Also reported to irritate the roots of the teeth when used for a long time in dentifrices.

SODIUM CHLORITE • Used as an antimicrobial in many countries and as an oxidizer and oral care ingredient. When acid is added, it forms deadly chlorine gas. *See* Sodium Chloride.

SODIUM P-CHLORO-M-CRESOL • Preservative. *See* Phenols.

SODIUM CHOLESTERYL SULFATE • Skin conditioner. *See* Cholesterol.

SODIUM CHONDROITIN SULFATE • Present in soft connective tissue, it is abundant in skin arterial walls and heart valves. Used as a hair and skin conditioner in moisturizers and body and hand products.

SODIUM CITRATE • White, odorless crystals, granules, or powder with a cool salty taste. Used as a sequestering ingredient (*see*) to remove trace metals in solutions and as an alkalizer in cosmetic products.

SODIUM COCETH SULFATE • *See* Coconut Oil.

SODIUM COCOABUTTERAMPHOACETATE • Fatty acids used in hair conditioners and cleansers. *See* Cocoa Butter.

SODIUM COCOAMINOPROPIONATE • *See* Coconut Oil.

SODIUM COCOAMPHOACETATE • Used as a hair conditioner and cleanser in hair products. *See* Coconut Oil and Surfactants.

SODIUM COCOAMPHOHYDROXYPROPYLSULFONATE • *See* Surfactants.

SODIUM COCOAMPHOPROPIONATE • *See* Surfactants.

SODIUM COCOATE • *See* Coconut Oil.

SODIUM COCOGLYCERYL ETHER SULFONATE • *See* Coconut Oil.

SODIUM COCO/HYDROGENATED TALLOW SULFATE • Surfactant (*see*) and cleansing ingredient. *See* Coconut Oil.

SODIUM COCO-HYDROLYZED COLLAGEN • The sodium salt of the condensation product of coconut acid chloride and hydrolyzed animal protein. The word *animal* was removed from the ingredient name. *See* Hydrolyzed Collagen.

SODIUM COCOMONOGLYCERIDE SULFATE • *See* Coconut Oil.

SODIUM COCOMONOGLYCERIDE SULFONATE • The fatty acids derived from coconut oil (*see*).

SODIUM COCO PG-DIMONIUM CHLORIDE PHOSPHATE • A quaternary ammonium compound (*see*). Used as an antistatic ingredient and cleanser. *See* Phosphorus.

SODIUM COCOYL COLLAGEN AMINO ACIDS • *See* Coconut Oil and Collagen.

SODIUM COCOYL GLUTAMATE • A softener. *See* Glutamate.

SODIUM COCOYL HYDROLYZED COLLAGEN • This was formerly called hydrolyzed animal protein, which it is. *See* Hydrolyzed.

SODIUM COCOYL HYDROLYZED RICE PROTEIN • Hair conditioner. *See* Coconut Oil and Rice.

SODIUM COCOYL HYDROLYZED SOY PROTEIN • Hair and skin conditioner. *See* Coconut Oil and Soybean.

SODIUM COCOYL HYDROLYZED SWEET ALMOND PROTEIN • Hair conditioner and cleanser. *See* Coconut Acids and Sweet Almond Oil and Seed Meal.

SODIUM COCOYL ISETHIONATE • The sodium salt of the coconut–fatty acid ester of isethionic acid. Used as a cleansing ingredient. On the basis of the animal and clinical data, the CIR Expert Panel (*see*) concluded that it is safe as a cosmetic ingredient up to 50 percent in rinse-off products and at 17 percent in leave-on products. *See* Coconut Oil.

SODIUM COCOYL LACTYLATE • Fatty acids used in bath soaps and detergents. *See* Coconut Acids and Lactic Acid.

SODIUM COCOYL OAT AMINO ACIDS • Hair and skin conditioner and cleanser in hair products. *See* Oat Extract.

SODIUM COCOYL SARCOSINATE • *See* Sarcosine.

SODIUM CORNAMPHOPROPIONATE • Fatty acids derived from corn used as a hair conditioning and cleansing ingredient.

SODIUM CUMENESULFONATE • A solvent. *See* Benzene and Phenols.

SODIUM CYCLAMATE • Flavoring. *See* Cyclamates.

SODIUM CYCLOPENTANE • *See* Cyclopentane.

SODIUM DECETH-2 CARBOXYLATE • *See* Polyethylene Glycol.

SODIUM DECETH SULFATE • *See* Decyl Alcohol.

SODIUM DECYLBENZENESULFONATE • Used in commercial detergents. May cause skin irritations.

SODIUM DEHYDROACETATE • Dehydroacetic Acid. A preservative; white, odorless, powdered, with an acrid taste. Used as a plasticizer, fungicide, and bacteria killer in cosmetics; also as an antienzyme ingredient in dentifrices, allegedly to prevent decay. Can cause impaired kidney function. Large doses can cause vomiting, ataxia, and confusion. There are no apparent allergic skin reactions. On the basis of the animal and clinical data, the CIR Expert Panel (*see*) concluded that it is safe as a cosmetic ingredient.

SODIUM DERMATAN SULFATE • *See* Mucopolysaccharides.

SODIUM DEXTRAN SULFATE • *See* Dextran.

SODIUM DEXTRIN OCTENYLSUCCINATE • Emollient and hair conditioner. Antistatic ingredient. *See* Dextrin.

SODIUM DIACETATE • A compound of sodium acetate and acetic acid (*see*). Used as a preservative that inhibits molds and bacteria. In 1992, the FDA proposed a ban on sodium diacetate in astringent (*see*) drug products because it had not been shown to be safe and effective as claimed.

SODIUM DICARBOXYETHYLCOCO PHOSPHOETHYL IMIDAZO-LINE • See Coconut Acids.

SODIUM DICETEARETH-10 PHOSPHATE • *See* Cetyl Alcohol.

SODIUM DICOCOYLETHYLENEDIAMINE PEG-15 SULFATE • Hair conditioner and cleanser. See Coconut Acids and Sulfuric Acid.

SODIUM DIETHYLAMINOPROPYL COASPARTAMIDE • Hair conditioner. *See* Coconut Oil and Alcohol.

SODIUM DIHYDROXYCETYL PHOSPHATE • *See* Cetyl Alcohol.

SODIUM DIHYDROXYETHYL GLYCINATE • *See* Dioctyl Sodium Sulfosuccinate.

SODIUM DILINOLEATE • Used in soaps. *See* Dilinoleic Acid.

SODIUM DIOLETH-8 PHOSPHATE • *See* Oleic Acid.

SODIUM DNA • The sodium salt of deoxyribonucleic acid. The genetic code of cells used in "youth" creams.

SODIUM DODECYLBENZENESULFONATE • A very widely used anionic detergent used in cosmetic bath products and in creams. It may irritate the skin. Will cause vomiting if swallowed. In some animal studies it caused kidney, intestinal, and liver damage when given orally. On the basis of the animal and clinical data, the CIR Expert Panel (*see*) concluded that it is safe as a cosmetic ingredient. *See* Sodium Lauryl Sulfate.

SODIUM DVB/ACRYLATES COPOLYMER • *See* Acrylates.

SODIUM EMUAMIDOPROPYL PG-DIMONIUM CHLORIDE • Fatty acids derived from emu oil (*see*) used as an antistatic and conditioning ingredient in hair products.

SODIUM ERYTHROBATE • A white, odorless powder used as an antioxidant in cosmetics.

SODIUM ETHYL ESTER OF PVM/MA COPOLYMER • Film former and hair fixative. *See* Polyvinyl Methyl Ether.

SODIUM-2-ETHYHEXYLSULFOACETATE • Light, cream-colored flakes, water soluble, good foam maker, and good in hard water. Used as a solubilizing ingredient, particularly for soapless shampoo compositions. *See* Quaternary Ammonium Compounds.

SODIUM ETHYLPARABEN • *See* Parabens.

SODIUM ETHYL-2 SULFOLAURATE • *See* Lauric Acid.

SODIUM FLUORIDE • Used in toothpastes to prevent tooth decay and as an insecticide, disinfectant, and preservative in cosmetics. Can cause nausea and vomiting when ingested and even death, depending upon the dose. Tooth enamel mottling has also been reported. The Nonprescription Drug Manufacturers Association also expressed opposition to an FDA proposal to mandate disclosure of the net fluoride content in OTC dentifrice products as a means of preventing dental fluorosis (caused by an excess intake of fluoride) in young children. The trade association insisted that there is no current scientific evidence to indicate that fluorides in dentifrices can contribute to dental fluorosis. In fluoride tablets, drops, and rinses to aid in the prevention of dental cavities. Changed from Rx to OTC. Potential adverse reactions include stomach upset, headache, weakness, and allergic reactions such as rash, eczema, and hives. Contraindicated when fluoride intake from drinking water exceeds 0.7 parts per million. Chronic toxicity can result from prolonged use of high doses. The Canadians do not permit it in dentifrices, mouthwashes, or breath drops. It is on the Canadian Hotlist (*see*). The EU calculates at 0.15 percent when mixed with other fluorine compounds. Fluorine concentration must not exceed 0.15 percent, and the EU label must say "Contains Sodium Fluouride." *See* Fluorine Compounds and Stannous Fluoride.

SODIUM FLUOROSILICATE • Oral care ingredient. The EU calculates at 0.15 percent when mixed with fluorine compounds. Fluorine concentration must not exceed 0.15 percent; the EU label must say "Contains sodium fluorosilicate." *See* Fluoride and Silicates.

SODIUM FORMATE • *See* Formic Acid.

SODIUM FUMARATE • pH adjuster. *See* Fumaric Acid.

SODIUM GLUCONATE • Made from glucose by fermentation, a white to yellowish powder, it is used in depilatories, conditioners, facial moisturizers/treatments, bar soaps, shampoos, liquid hand soaps, hair removal waxes, toothpastes, facial cleansers, and styling gels/lotions. Also used in metal cleaners, paint strippers, bottle-washing preparations, metal plating, and rust removers. One or more animal studies show broad systemic effects at high doses (low-dose studies may be unavailable for this ingredient). The FDA considers sodium gluconate GRAS for use in food as a sequestrant (*see* Sequestering Ingredient). *See* Gluconic Acid and Salts.

SODIUM GLUCURONATE • Humectant and skin conditioner. *See* Glucuronic Acid.

SODIUM GLUTAMATE • The monosodium salt of the L-form of glutamic acid. *See* Glutamic Acid.

SODIUM GLYCERETH-1 POLYPHOSPHATE • Sodium salt of a complex mixture of esters of tetraphosphoric acid with some glycerin. *See* Glycerin.

SODIUM GLYCEROTPHOSPHATE • Oral care ingredient. *See* Phosphorus and Glycerin.

SODIUM GLYCERYL OLEATE PHOSPHATE • *See* Glyceryl Monostearate.

SODIUM GUANOSINE CYCLIC MONOPHOSPHATE • Skin conditioner. *See* Phosphorus.

SODIUM HEPARIN • *See* Heparin Salts.

SODIUM HEXETH-4 CARBOXYLATE • *See* Polyethylene Glycol.

SODIUM HEXYLMETAPHOSPHATE • Graham's Salt. Used in bath salts, bubble baths, permanent-wave neutralizers, and shampoos. An emulsifier, sequestering ingredient (*see*), and texturizer. Used in foods and potable water to prevent scale formation and corrosion. Because it keeps calcium, magnesium, and iron salts in solution, it is an excellent water softener and detergent.

SODIUM HINOKITIOL • *See* Hinokitiol.

SODIUM HYALURONATE • The sodium salt of hyaluronic acid found in the umbilical cord and in the fluid between joints. It is used as a gelling ingredient and a skin conditioner in makeup, suntan products, and skin creams and lotions.

SODIUM HYALURONATE DIMETHYLSILANOL • Skin conditioner. *See* Sodium Hyaluronate and Siloxane.

SODIUM HYDROGENATED PALMATE • Cleanser. *See* Palm Kernel Acid.

SODIUM HYDROGENATED TALLOWOYL GLUTAMATE • *See* Glutamate and Tallow.

SODIUM HYDROLYZED CASEIN • Protein used as hair and skin conditioner. *See* Casein.

SODIUM HYDROSULFATE • A bacterial inhibitor and antifermentative.

SODIUM HYDROSULFITE • *See* Sulfites.

SODIUM HYDROXIDE • Caustic Soda. Soda Lye. An alkali and emulsifier in liquid face powders, soaps, shampoos, cuticle removers, hair straighteners, shaving soaps, and creams. White or nearly white pellets, flakes, or sticks. Readily absorbs water. Also a modifier for food starch, a glazing ingredient for pretzels, and a peeling ingredient for tubers and fruits. The FDA banned use of more than 10 percent in household liquid drain cleaners. If too much alkali is used, dermatitis of the scalp may occur. Its ingestion causes vomiting, prostration, and collapse. Inhalation causes lung damage. Keep away from eyes. Can cause blindness. Should be applied by professionals only, according to the EU.

SODIUM HYDROXYMETHANE SULFONATE • Sodium Formaldehyde Bisulfite. *See* Formaldehyde.

SODIUM HYDROXYMETHYL GLYCINATE • *See* Glycine.

SODIUM HYPOCHLORITE • Made by the addition of chlorine to sodium hydroxide, it is used for bleaching paper pulp and textiles, in water purification, in fungicides, as a swimming pool disinfectant, in laundry products, and as a germicide. Liquid household bleaches are approximately 5 percent sodium hypochlorite solutions. It is also an antiseptic for wounds.

SODIUM IODATE • Used in dusting powder and to soothe the skin. White, crystalline powder. Antiseptic, particularly to the mucous membranes. The safety of this ingredient has not been documented and substantiated according to the CIR Expert Panel (*see*), and the Panel cannot conclude whether sodium is safe in cosmetics.

SODIUM IODIDE • White, odorless, water-absorbing crystals. Slowly becomes brown on exposure to air. *See* Sodium Iodate.

SODIUM C8–16 ISOALKYLSUCCINYL LACTOGLOBULIN SULFONATE • Protein derived from milk used as a skin-conditioning ingredient in face powders.

SODIUM C4–12 OLEFIN/MALEIC ACID COPOLYMER • Kao Soap. The sodium salt of a polymer synthesized from C4–12 olefins and maleic anhydride (*see*). Used as a demulcent.

SODIUM C14–16 OLEFIN SULFONATE • Widely used in bath products, hair colorings, and cleansers. *See* Sulfonated Oils.

SODIUM ISETHIONATE • *See* Sodium Hydroxide.

SODIUM ISOBUTYLPARABEN • Preservative. *See* Parabens.

SODIUM ISOOCTYLENE/MA COPOLYMER • *See* Maleic Acid and Polymer.

SODIUM ISOPROPYLPARABEN • Preservative. *See* Parabens.

SODIUM ISOSTEARATE • Cleanser. *See* Stearic Acid.

SODIUM ISOSTEARETH-6 CARBOXYLATE • *See* Isostearic Acid.

SODIUM ISOSTEAROAMPHOACETATE • *See* Surfactants.

SODIUM ISOSTEAROAMPHOPROPIONATE • *See* Quaternary Ammonium Compounds.

SODIUM ISOSTEROYL LACTYLATE • The sodium salt of isostearic acid and lactyl lactate. *See* Stearic Acid and Lactic Acid.

SODIUM LACTATE • Plasticizer substitute for glycerin. Colorless, thick, odorless liquid miscible with water, alcohol, and glycerin. Widely used as a buffer, humectant, and exfoliant in moisturizers and other skin and hair products. Solution is neutral. *See* Lactic Acid.

SODIUM LACTATE METHYLSILANOL • *See* Silanols.

SODIUM LANETH SULFATE • *See* Lanolin.

SODIUM LANOLATE • *See* Lanolin.

SODIUM LARDATE • Fatty acids derived from lard used as emulsifiers and surfactants.

SODIUM LAURAMIDO DIACETATE • Surfactant. *See* Sodium Diacetate.

SODIUM LAURAMINOPROPIONATE • *See* Propionic Acid.

SODIUM LAURATE • *See* Sodium Lauryl Sulfate.

SODIUM LAURETH-4 CARBOXYLATE • *See* Polyethylene Glycol and Lauric Acid.

SODIUM LAURETH-5 CARBOXYLATE • *See* Polyoxyethylene Compounds and Lauric Acid.

SODIUM LAURETH-4 PHOSPHATE • Widely used emulsifier and cleanser used in shampoos, bath soaps, cleansing products, bubble baths, body and hand products, makeup, and baby shampoos. *See* Sodium Lauryl Sulfate.

SODIUM LAURETH SULFATE • The sodium salt of sulfated ethoxylated lauryl alcohol, widely used as a water softener and in baby and other nonirritating shampoos as a wetting and cleansing ingredient. Has caused eye and skin irritation in experimental animals and in some human test subjects. The irritant effects are similar to those produced by other detergents and are affected by concentration. On the basis of the available information, the CIR Expert Panel (*see*) found it safe in the early 1980s but is considering new information to determine if the final safety assessment should be reaffirmed, amended, or have an addendum. *See also* Surfactants.

SODIUM LAURETH-5, -7, AND -12 SULFATES • The 12 is widely used in cosmetics including bath products, hair coloring, and makeup as well as baby shampoos. *See* Sodium Laureth Sulfate and Polyethylene Glycol.

SODIUM LAURIMINODIPROPIONATE • Antistatic agent and surfactant. *See* Quaternary Ammonium Compounds.

SODIUM LAUROAMPHOACETATE • *See* Surfactants.

SODIUM LAUROAMPHOHYDROXYPROPYLSULFONATE • *See* Surfactants.

SODIUM LAUROAMPHO PG-ACETATE PHOSPHATE • *See* Surfactants.

SODIUM LAUROAMPHOPROPIONATE • The safety of this ingredient has not been documented and substantiated according to the CIR Expert Panel (*see*), which said it cannot conclude whether it is safe in cosmetics. *See* Quaternary Ammonium Compounds.

SODIUM LAUROYL ASPARTATE • Hair conditioner and cleanser. *See* Lauric Acid and Aspartic Acid.

SODIUM LAUROYL COLLAGEN AMINO ACIDS • Formerly called sodium lauroyl animal collagen amino acids, but the name was changed to remove the word *animal*. *See* Collagen and Amino Acid.

SODIUM LAUROYL GLUTAMATE • A softener and hair conditioner. *See* Glutamate.

SODIUM LAUROYL HYDROLYZED COLLAGEN • The salt of the condensation product of lauric acid and hydrolyzed collagen used as a hair and skin conditioner. *See* Hydrolyzed Collagen.

SODIUM LAUROYL HYDROLYZED SILK • Hair and skin conditioner. *See* Lauric Acid and Hydrolyzed Silk.

SODIUM LAUROYL ISETHIONATE • Sodium Lauryl Isethionate. It is a mild synthetic soap. *See* Surfactants.

SODIUM LAUROYL LACTYLATE • *See* Lauric Acid.

SODIUM LAUROYL METHYLAMINOPROPIONATE • *See* Lauric Acid.

SODIUM LAUROYL SARCOSINATE • Widely used in shampoos, bath products, foundation, and cleanser. *See* Sarcosine.

SODIUM LAUROYL TAURATE • *See* Surfactants.

SODIUM LAUROYLISETHIONATE • *See* Sodium Lauryl Sulfate.

SODIUM LAURYL BENZENE SULFONATE • *See* Sodium Lauryl Sulfate.

SODIUM LAURYL SULFATE • A detergent, wetting ingredient, and emulsifier widely used in bubble baths, emollient creams, cream depilatories, hand lotions, cold permanent waves, soapless shampoos, and toothpastes. Prepared by sulfation of lauryl alcohol followed by neutralization with sodium carbonate. It emulsifies fats. May cause drying of the skin because of its degreasing ability, and it is an irritant to the skin. Has been associated with eczema (*see*). On the basis of the available information, the CIR Expert Panel (*see*) found it safe in the early 1980s but is considering new information to determine if the final safety assessment should be reaffirmed, amended, or have an addendum.

SODIUM LAURYL SULFOACETATE • *See* Sodium Lauryl Sulfate.

SODIUM LIGNOSULFONATE • The sodium salt of polysulfonated lignin derived from wood. It is used as a dispersing ingredient. A tan, free-flowing powder, it is also used as an emulsifier, stabilizer, and cleaning ingredient.

SODIUM MAGNESIUM SILICATES • *See* Silicates.

SODIUM MALATE • Skin conditioner and humectant. In anti-aging products. *See* Malic Acid.

SODIUM MANNOSE PHOSPHATE • A skin conditioner made from a sugar. *See* Mannose.

SODIUM MANNURONATE METHYLSILANOL • *See* Silanols.

SODIUM MA/VINYL ALCOHOL COPOLYMER • A film former. *See* Maleic Acid and Vinyl Polymers.

SODIUM/MEA LAURETH-2 SULFOSUCCINATE • Emulsifier. *See* Surfactants.

SODIUM METABISULFITE • An inorganic salt. A bacterial inhibitor and antioxidant in cosmetics, including hair products, cleansers, bath preparations, underarm deodorants, and moisturizers. Used as an antifermentative in sugar, and a preservative for fruits and vegetables. *See* Bisulfites.

SODIUM METABORATE • *See* Boric Acid.

SODIUM METAPHOSPHATE • Graham's Salt. Used in dental polishing ingredients, detergents, water softeners, sequestrants, emulsifiers, food additives, and textile laundering. *See* Sodium Hexylmetaphosphate.

SODIUM METASILICATE • An alkali usually prepared from sand and soda ash. Used in detergents. Caustic substance, corrosive to the skin, harmful if swallowed, and cause of severe eye irritations. Preserves eggs in egg shampoos.

SODIUM METHYL COCOYL TAURATE • Cleanser in shampoos, bath soaps, coloring, and other hair products. *See* Ox Bile and Coconut Oil.

SODIUM METHYL LAUROYL TAURATE • *See* Surfactants.

SODIUM METHYL OLEOYL TAURATE • *See* Ox Bile.

SODIUM METHYL PALMITOYL TAURATE • *See* Surfactants.

SODIUM METHYL STEAROYL TAURATE • *See* Taurine.

SODIUM METHYL-2 SULFOLAURATE • *See* Lauric Acid.

SODIUM METHYLNAPHTHALENE SULFONATE • *See* Sulfonated Oils.

SODIUM n-METHYL-n-OLEYL TAURATE • *See* Ox Bile.

SODIUM METHYLESCULETIN ACETATE • Oral care ingredient. *See* Phenols.

SODIUM METHYLPARABEN • *See* Parabens.

SODIUM MONOFLUOROPHOSPHATE • Used in toothpaste to prevent cavities in the United States but not permitted in dentifrices, mouthwashes, or breath drops in Canada. It is on the Canadian Hotlist (*see*). *See* Sodium Fluoride.

SODIUM MONOUNDECYLENAMIDO MEA-SULFOSUCCINATE • *See* Dioctyl Sodium Sulfosuccinate and Sulfonated Oils.

SODIUM MYRETH SULFATE • A cleansing and emulsifying ingredient. Data indicating that a shampoo containing 7 percent and 20 percent dilution of this ingredient induced mild to moderate eye irritation in some animal studies. On the basis of animal and clinical data, the CIR Expert Panel (*see*) concludes that it is safe as a cosmetic ingredient in the present practices of use and concentration. *See* Myristyl Alcohol.

SODIUM MYRISTATE • *See* Myristic Acid.

SODIUM MYRISTOAMPHOACETATE • Hair conditioner. *See* Surfactants.

SODIUM MYRISTOL GLUTAMATE • *See* Glutamic Acid.

SODIUM MYRISTOYL HYDROLYZED COLLAGEN • *See* Hydrolyzed Collagen and Myristic Acid.

SODIUM MYRISTOYL ISETHIONATE • *See* Myristic Acid.

SODIUM MYRISTOYL SARCOSINATE • *See* Sarcosine.

SODIUM MYRISTYL SULFATE • *See* Myristyl Alcohol.

SODIUM NAPHTHALENESULFONATE • Surfactant. *See* Naphthalene and Sulfonated Oils.

SODIUM NAPHTHOL SULFONATE • Absorbent. *See* Phenols and Sulfonic Acids.

SODIUM NITRATE • Chile Saltpeter. Chile Niter. Used in oral care products and emollients. Occurs as a mineral found in the mountains of Chile. In 1992, the FDA proposed a ban on sodium nitrate in oral menstrual drug products because it had not been shown to be safe and effective as claimed. Sodium salt of nitric acid. *See* Nitrates.

SODIUM NITRITE • *See* Nitrite.

SODIUM *m*-NITROBENZENESULFONATE • Viscosity controlling agent. The CIR Expert Panel (*see*) concludes that the data available are insufficient to support the safety of this ingredient as used in cosmetics. *See* Benzene and Phenols.

SODIUM 5-NITROGUAIACOLATE • Coloring. *See* Guaiacol.

SODIUM NONOXYNOL-6 PHOSPHATE OR -9 PHOSPHATE • A complex mixture of esters of phosphoric acid and nonoxynol (*see both*).

SODIUM NONOXYNOL-1 OR -4 SULFATE • *See* Sulfonated Oils.

SODIUM OCTOXYNOL-2-, -9 SULFATE • Cleanser. *See* Polyethylene Glycol and Octanoic Acid.

SODIUM OCTYL SULFATE • *See* Sulfonated Oils.

SODIUM OLEAMIDOPROPYL PG-DIMONIUM CHLORIDE PHOSPHATE • Antistatic ingredient and hair conditioner. *See* Quaternary Ammonium Compounds.

SODIUM OLEATE • Sodium salt of oleic acid. White powder, fatty odor, alkaline. Used in soaps.

SODIUM OLEOAMPHOACETATE • Hair-conditioning and cleansing ingredient. *See* Quaternary Ammonium Compounds.

SODIUM OLEOAMPHOHYDROXYPROPYLSULFONATE • *See* Quaternary Ammonium Compounds.

SODIUM OLEOAMPHOPROPIONATE • *See* Quaternary Ammonium Compounds.

SODIUM OLEANOLATE • Skin conditioner. *See* Oleic Acid.

SODIUM OLEOYL HYDROLYZED COLLAGEN • Formerly called sodium oleoyl hydrolyzed animal protein. *See* Proteins and Hydrolyzed.

SODIUM OLEOYL ISETHIONATE • *See* Sulfonated Oils.

SODIUM OLETH-7 OR -8 PHOSPHATE • The sodium salts of the phosphate esters of oleth used in mild detergents such as baby shampoos.

SODIUM OLETH SULFATE • *See* Polyethylene Glycol and Oleyl Alcohol.

SODIUM OLEYL SULFATE • Widely used in cosmetics as a cleansing ingredient including in foundations, cleansing lotions, makeup, bath products, hair colorings, nail products, and moisturizers. *See* Surfactants.

SODIUM OLIVATE • Fatty acids from olives used as cleansers and emulsifiers.

SODIUM OXALATE • Sodium Salt of Oxalic Acid. White, odorless, crystalline powder used as an intermediate (*see*), in hair dyes, and as a texturizer. Corrosion inhibitor. Toxic when ingested and may be irritating to the skin.

SODIUM OXYNOL-2 ETHANE SULFONATE • *See* Sulfonated Oils.

SODIUM PALM GLYCERIDE SULFONATE • Fatty acids from palm oil (*see*) used as a cleansing ingredient.

SODIUM PALM KERNELATE • *See* Palm Kernel Acids.

SODIUM PALMITATE • Used in soap and bath products and moisturizers. Sodium salt of palmitic acid (*see*).

SODIUM PALMITOYL CHONDROITIN SULFATE • Hair and skin conditioners. *See* Palmitic Acid and Sodium Chondroitin Sulfate.

SODIUM PALMITOYL HYDROLYZED COLLAGEN • Hair and skin conditioner. *See* Hydrolyzed Collagen.

SODIUM PALMITOYL PROLINE • Skin conditioner. *See* Amino Acids.

SODIUM PALMOYL GLUTAMATE • Cleansing ingredient. *See* Amino Acids and Glutamate.

SODIUM PANTETHEINE SULFONATE • Skin conditioner. *See* Sulfonic Acid.

SODIUM PANTOTHENATE • Hair conditioner. *See* Pantothenic Acid.

SODIUM PARABEN • Preservative. *See* Parabens.

SODIUM C11–15 PARETH-7 CARBOXYLATE • The sodium salt of C1115 pareth. Used as a gelling ingredient. *See* Alkanolamines.

SODIUM C12–15 PARETH-7 CARBOXYLATE • The sodium salt of C1215 pareth-7 carboxylic acid. Used as a gelling ingredient.

SODIUM C12–13 PARETH SULFATE • The sodium salt of sulfated polyethylene glycol ether of a mixture of synthetic alcohols. *See* Polyethylene Glycol.

SODIUM C12–15 PARETH-6 CARBOXYLATE • The sodium salt of the organic acid. *See* Alkanolamines.

SODIUM C12–15 PARETH SULFATE • A mixture of fatty alcohols. *See* Sulfated Oil and Polyethylene Glycol.

SODIUM PARETH-15–7 OR 25–7 CARBOXYLATE • *See* Fatty Alcohols.

SODIUM PARETH-23 OR -25 SULFATE • *See* Fatty Alcohols.

SODIUM PCA • A naturally occurring component of human skin that is believed to be in part responsible for its moisture-binding capacity. It is highly water absorbing and at high humidity dissolves in its own water hydration. Application of this compound to the skin as a humectant (*see*) is claimed to increase softness. On the basis of the animal and clinical data, the CIR Expert Panel (*see*) concluded that it is safe as used in cosmetic formulations but should not be used in cosmetics containing nitrosating (*see*) ingredients.

SODIUM PCA METHYSILANOL • *See* Sodium PCA.

SODIUM PEANUTAMPHOACETATE • Hair conditioner from peanut oil (*see*).

SODIUM PEANUTATE • Fatty acids derived from peanut oil used as an emulsifier and cleanser. *See* Peanut Oil.

SODIUM PEG-6 COCAMIDE CARBOXYLATE • *See* Coconut Oil.

SODIUM PEG-8 COCAMIDE CARBOXYLATE • *See* Coconut Oil.

SODIUM PEG-3 LAURAMIDE CARBOXYLATE • *See* Lauric Acid.

SODIUM PERBORATE • White crystals soluble in water, used as a reingredient (*see*), antiseptic, deodorant, bleach, and in dentifrices as a tooth whitener; also in foot baths and detergents. Ulcerations of the mouth have been reported in its use in dentifrices. Strong solutions that are very alkaline are irritating if permitted on the skin. It is on the Canadian Hotlist (*see*) and is not permitted in mouthwash, dentifrices, or "other" purposes that involve long-term use in the oral cavity. May be used as a tooth-bleaching agent if safety data is submitted.

SODIUM PERCARBONATE • Stable, crystalline powder derived from sodium carbonate and hydrogen peroxide (*see both*). Used as a denture cleaner and mild antiseptic. Toxic by ingestion. *See* Peroxide.

SODIUM PEROXIDE • A strong oxidizing ingredient and irritant. Used to purify water and germicidal soaps.

SODIUM PERSULFATE • Oxidizing ingredient that promotes emulsion used in hair-waving solution. An inorganic salt; a crystalline powder that decomposes in moisture and warmth. Can cause allergic reactions in the hypersensitive. The CIR Expert Panel (*see*) concludes there is not enough information about this ingredient to "support safety" in cosmetics.

SODIUM PHENATE • *See* Phenols.

SODIUM PHENOLSULFONATE • *See* Phenols.

SODIUM PHENOXIDE • *See* Phenols.

SODIUM *o*-PHENYL PHENATE • Antiseptic, germicide, fungicide, and preservative used in cosmetic creams and lotions. Yellow flakes or powder with a slight soap odor. Soluble in water, alcohol, and acetone. A skin irritant. Regarded as more effective than phenol (*see*) and cresol (*see*) because it has greater germ-killing power, may be used in smaller concentrations, and is less irritating to the skin, although it is often considered toxic by some cosmetic companies for use in products.

SODIUM PHOSPHONO-PYRIDOXYLIDENERHODANINE • Antioxidant. *See* Phosphorus Compounds.

SODIUM PHOSPHATE • Buffer and effervescent used in manufacture of nail enamels and detergents. White, crystalline or granular powder, stable in air. Without water, it can be irritating to the skin but has no known skin toxicity.

SODIUM PHTHALATE STEARYL AMIDE • *See* Quaternary Ammonium Compounds.

SODIUM PHYTATE • Oral care ingredient. *See* Phytic Acid.

SODIUM PICRAMATE • Sodium Salt of Picramic Acid. A hair colorant. It is a mutagen and a mild sensitizer in animal studies. It may be a mild sensitizer in humans. It is used in hair dyes at concentrations of 0.1 percent to 1 percent. On the basis of the available animal data, the CIR Expert Panel (*see*) concluded that it is safe as a cosmetic ingredient at concentrations not to exceed 0.1 percent. *See* Picramic Acid.

SODIUM POLYACRYLATE • Film former, thickener, and hair fixative. *See* Acrylic Resins.

SODIUM POLYACRYLATE STARCH • *See* Starch and Acrylates.

SODIUM POLYDIMETHYLGLYCINOPHENOLSULFONATE • *See* Sulfonated Oils.

SODIUM POLYGLUTAMATE • *See* Glutamic Acid.

SODIUM POLYMETHACRYLATE • *See* Acrylates.

SODIUM POLYNAPHTHALENE SULFONATE • *See* Sulfonated Oils.

SODIUM POLYSTYRENE SULFONATE • It is on the Canadian Hotlist (*see*). *See* Polystyrene.

SODIUM POTASSIUM ALUMINUM SILICATE • Thickener. *See* Silicates.

SODIUM PROPIONATE • Colorless, or transparent, odorless crystals that gather water in moist air. Used as a preservative in cosmetics and foodstuffs to prevent mold and fungus. It has been used to treat fungal infections of the skin but can cause allergic reactions. The Food and Drug Administration issued a notice in 1992 that sodium propionate has not been shown to be safe and effective for stated claims in OTC products.

SODIUM PROPOLY PPG-2 ACETATE • Surfactant and cleanser. *See* Acetic Acid.

SODIUM PROPYLPARABEN • *See* Parabens.

SODIUM PYRITHIONE • Sodium salt of pyrithione zinc derivative. Used as a fungicide and bacteria killer. Used in dandruff shampoos to control dandruff and as an antibacterial in soaps and detergents. On the Canadian Hotlist (*see*).

SODIUM PYROPHOSPHATE PEROXIDE • White powder, water soluble, used as a denture cleanser, in dentifrices and household laundry detergents, and as an antiseptic. *See* Hydrogen Peroxide.

SODIUM PYRUVATE • Skin conditioner. *See* Propionic Acid.

SODIUM RAPESEEDATE • Fatty acids derived from rapeseed oil (*see*) used in cleaners and emulsifiers.

SODIUM RIBOFLAVIN PHOSPHATE • Skin conditioner. B vitamin containing sodium phosphate (*see*).

SODIUM RIBONUCLEIC ACID • SRNA. Skin conditioner. Used in makeup and skin care preparations. The basic instructions in the cell that tell it how to behave. Since it is believed that the RNA in the cell may make mistakes as we age, it is added to some anti-aging creams.

SODIUM RICINOLEATE • The sodium salt of ricinoleic acid (*see*).

SODIUM RICINOLEOAMPHOACETATE • *See* Quaternary Ammonium Compounds.

SODIUM RNA • *See* Sodium Ribonucleic Acid.

SODIUM ROSINATE • Derived from rosin (*see*), used as a cleanser and thickener.

SODIUM SACCHARIN • An artificial sweetener in dentifrices, mouthwashes, and lipsticks. In use since 1879. Pound for pound, it is three hundred times as sweet as natural sugar but leaves a bitter aftertaste.

SODIUM SAFFLOWERATE • Derived from safflower oil (*see*), it is used as a cleanser.

SODIUM SALICYLATE • A white, odorless, crystalline powder used in shaving creams and in sunscreen lotions. Becomes pinkish upon long exposure to light; also used to lower fever and kill pain in animals. Mild antiseptic analgesic and preservative. May cause nasal allergy. The European Union has banned it for children under three years except in shampoos. *See* Salicylates.

SODIUM SARCOSINATE • The sodium salt of sarcosine. *See* Sarcosine.

SODIUM SCYMNOL SULFATE • Used as a skin conditioner. *See* Sterol.

SODIUM SESQUICARBONATE • White crystals, flakes, or powder produced from sodium carbonate. Soluble in water. Used as an alkalizer in bath salts, shampoos, tooth powders, and soaps. Irritating to the skin and mucous membranes. May cause allergic reaction in the hypersensitive.

SODIUM SHALE OIL SULFONATE • Preservative. *See* Shale Extract and Sulfonated Oils.

SODIUM SILICATE • Water Glass. An anticaking ingredient preserving eggs, detergents in soaps, depilatories, and protective creams. Strongly alkaline. As a topical antiseptic can be irritating and caustic to the skin and mucous membranes. If swallowed, it causes vomiting and diarrhea.

SODIUM SILICOALUMINATE • *See* Silicates.

SODIUM SOAP • *See* Sodium Stearate.

SODIUM SORBATE • A preservative used in cheeses alone or in combination with potassium sorbate or sorbic acid (*see both*). It is also used in fruit butter, artificially sweetened fruit jelly, presersves, jams, and margarines. Also migrates from packaging into food. GRAS In 1984 in the journal *Food Chemistry,* researchers reported that sodium sorbate is a genotoxicity (*see*) agent, although its potency seems to be weak, and that sorbic acid and potassium sorbate are less genotoxic than the sodium salt. ASP

SODIUM SOY HYDROLYZED COLLAGEN • Formerly called hydrolyzed animal protein, but the *animal* name was removed. The sodium salt of the condensation product of soya acid chloride and hydrolyzed animal protein. *See* Collagen.

SODIUM STANNATE • An inorganic salt. White or colorless crystals. Absorbs water from air. Used in hair dyes and permanent waves.

SODIUM STARCH OCTENYLSUCCINATE • *See* Cornstarch.

SODIUM STEARATE • 92.82 percent stearic acid (*see*). Made by action of caustic soda on animal or vegetable oils. A fatty acid widely used in deodorant sticks, stick perfumes, toothpastes, soapless shampoos, and shaving lather. A white powder with a soapy feel and a slight tallowlike odor. Slowly soluble in cold water or cold alcohol. Also a waterlike odor. Also a waterproofing ingredient and has been used to treat skin diseases and in suppositories. One of the least allergy-causing of the sodium salts of fatty acids. Nonirritating to the skin. On the basis of the available information, the CIR Expert Panel (*see*) found it safe in the early 1980s but is considering new information to determine if the final safety assessment should be reaffirmed, amended, or have an addendum. E

SODIUM STEARETH-4 PHOSPHATE • *See* Surfactants.

SODIUM STEAROAMPHOACETATE • *See* Sodium Stearate.

SODIUM STEAROAMPHOHYDROXYPROPYLSULFONATE • A surfactant used in hair conditioners and foam boosters. *See* Stearic and Sulfonic Acids.

SODIUM STEAROMAMPHOPROPIONATE • *See* Quaternary Ammonium Compounds.

SODIUM STEAROYL CASEIN • Hair conditioner and cleanser. *See* Casein.

SODIUM STEAROYL CHONDROITIN SULFATE • Hair and skin conditioner. *See* Sodium Chondroitin.

SODIUM STEAROYL DNA • Skin conditioner. *See* DNA.

SODIUM STEAROYL GLUTAMATE • Hair- and skin-conditioning ingredient. *See* Glutamate.

SODIUM STEAROYL HYALURONATE • Skin conditioner. *See* Hyaluronic Acid.

SODIUM STEAROYL HYDROLYZED COLLAGEN • *See* Hydrolyzed Collagen.

SODIUM STEAROYL LACTALBUMIN • Stearic acid and milk albumin (*see both*) used as skin and hair conditioners.

SODIUM STEAROYL LACTYLATE • *See* Lactic Acid.

SODIUM STEAROXY PG-HYDROXYETHYLCELLULOSE SULFONATE • Gum used as a thickener. *See* Hydroxyethylcellulose.

SODIUM STEAROYL HYDROLYZED CORN PROTEIN • *See* Corn and Hydrolyzed.

SODIUM STEAROYL HYDROLYZED SILK • *See* Hydrolyzed Silk.

SODIUM STEAROYL HYDROLYZED SOY PROTEIN • Hair conditioner. *See* Soy.

SODIUM STEARYL DIMETHYL GLYCINE • Emulsifier. *See* Amino Acids.

SODIUM STEARYL SULFATE • *See* Surfactants.

SODIUM STEARYL PHTHALAMATE • Emulsifying ingredient. *See* Benzoic Acid.

SODIUM STYRENE/ACRYLATES/DIVINYLBENZENE COPOLYMER • An opacifier. *See* Styrene, Benzene, and Acrylates.

SODIUM STYRENE/ACRYLATES/PEG-10 DIMALEATE COPOLYMER • An opacifier. *See* Styrene and Acrylates.

SODIUM STYRENE/PEG-10 MALEATE/NONOXYNOL-10 MALEATE/ ACRYLATES COPOLYMER • Opacifier. *See* Styrene and Acrylates.

SODIUM SUCCINOYL GELATIN • Skin conditioner. *See* Gelatin.

SODIUM SUCROSE OCTASULFATE • Skin conditioner. *See* Sucrose.

SODIUM SULFANILATE • The sodium salt of sulfanilic acid (*see*). Used as a hair coloring.

SODIUM SULFATE • Salt Cake. Occurs in nature as the minerals mirabilite and thenardite. Used chiefly in the manufacture of dyes, soaps, and detergents. Also as a chewing gum base and, used medicinally, to reduce body water. It is a reingredient (*see*) and a precipitant; mildly saline in taste. Usually harmless when applied in toilet preparations. May prove irritating in concentrated solutions if applied to the skin, permitted to dry, and then remain. May also enhance the irritant action of certain detergents. Based on the available data, the CIR Expert Panel (*see*) concluded it is safe as used in rinse-off formulations, and safe up to 1 percent in leave-on formulations.

SODIUM SULFIDE • Depilatory. Toxic. Irritating. The label must carry a warning to avoid contact with the eyes and to keep out of reach of children.

SODIUM SULFITE • An antiseptic, preservative, and antioxidant used in hair dyes. It has been used medicinally as a topical antifungal ingredient. It is also used as a bacterial inhibitor in wine brewing and distilled beverage industries. Also an antifermentative in the sugar and syrup industries and an antibrowning ingredient in cut fruits. Products containing sulfites may release sulfur dioxide. If this is inhaled by people who suffer from asthma, it can trigger an asthmatic attack. Sulfites are known to cause stomach irritation, nausea, diarrhea, skin rash, and swelling in sulfite-sensitive people.

SODIUM SULFONATE • A bubble bath, clarifying ingredient, and a dispersing ingredient used to make shampoos clear. *See* Sulfonated Oils.

SODIUM SUNFLOWERAMIDOPROPYL PG-DIMONIUM CHLORIDE PHOSPHATE • Antistatic ingredient in hair conditioners. *See* Quaternary Ammonium Compounds.

SODIUM SURFACTIN • Fatty acids from the fermentation of *Bacillus subtilis*, a soil bacteria. Used as an emulsifier.

SODIUM TALLAMPHOPROPIONATE • *See* Quaternary Ammonium Compounds.

SODIUM TALLATE • Cleanser and emulsifier from tall oil (*see*).

SODIUM TALLOW SULFATE • A defoamer, emollient, intermediate (*see*), and surface-active ingredient. A mixture of sodium alkyl sulfates. *See* Tallow.

SODIUM TALLOWAMPHOACETATE • *See* Tallow and Acetic Acid.

SODIUM TALLOWAMPHOPROPIONATE • *See* Tallow and Sodium.

SODIUM TALLOWATE • The sodium salt of tallow (*see*). Used in soaps and detergents. Has been associated with eczema.

SODIUM TAURINE COCOYL METHYLTAURATE • Cleanser and emulsifier from taurine and coconut oil (*see both*).

SODIUM/TEA-LAUROYL COLLAGEN AMINO ACIDS • *See* Collagen and Lauric Acid.

SODIUM/TEA-LAUROYL HYDROLYZED COLLAGEN • Formerly had "animal protein" in its name. It is still a mixture of sodium and triethanolamine salts of the condensation product of undecylenic acid chloride and hydrolyzed animal protein. *See* Hydrolyzed Protein.

SODIUM/TEA-LAUROYL HYDROLYZED KERATIN • *See* Hydrolyzed Keratin and Lauric Acid.

SODIUM/TEA-LAUROYL KERATIN AMINO ACIDS • *See* Keratin and Amino Acids.

SODIUM/TEA-UNDECYLENOYL HYDROLYZED COLLAGEN • Formerly had "animal protein" in the name. It is still a mixture of sodium and triethanolamine salts of the condensation product of undecylenic acid chloride and hydrolyzed animal protein. *See* Animal Collagen.

SODIUM THIOGLYCOLATE • Depilatory. The sodium salt of mercaptoacetic acid. *See* Thioglycolic Acid Compounds.

SODIUM TOCOPHERYL PHOSPHATE • Antioxidant. *See* Vitamin E.

SODIUM TOLUENESULFONATE • Methylbenzenesulfonic Acid. Sodium Salt. An aromatic compound that is used as a solvent. *See* Benzene.

SODIUM TREHALOSE SULFATE • Skin conditioner. *See* Carboyhdrates.

SODIUM TRIDECETH-3, -6, -7, -12 CARBOXYLATE • The sodium salt of tridecyl alcohol and carboxylic acid. *See* Tridecyl Alcohol.

SODIUM TRIDECETH SULFATE • Widely used sodium salt of sulfated ethoxylated tridecyl alcohol. Used as an emulsifier. *See* Tridecyl Alcohol and Alkyl Sulfates.

SODIUM TRIDECYL SULFATE • Cleanser used in cold creams and baby shampoos. *See* Sulfonated Oils.

SODIUM TRIDECYLBENZENE SULFONATE • A mixture of alkyl benzene sulfonates used as a synthetic detergent. *See* Sodium Dodecylbenzenesulfonated Oil.

SODIUM TRIMETAPHOSPHATE • *See* Sodium Metaphosphate.

SODIUM TRIPOLYPHOSPHATE • STPP. Used in bubble baths and as a texturizer in soaps, it is a crystalline salt, moderately irritating to the skin and mucous membranes. Ingestion can cause violent purging. *See* Sodium Phosphate.

SODIUM UNDECYLENATE • Preservative. A sodium salt of undecylenic acid. Occurs in sweat. A topical fungicide. Liquid or crystals with a sweaty odor prepared from castor oil.

SODIUM UNDECYLENOAMPHOACETATE • *See* Quaternary Ammonium Compounds.

SODIUM UNDECYLENOAMPHOPROPIONATE • *See* Quaternary Ammonium Compounds.

SODIUM UROCANATE • The sodium salt of urocanic acid. *See* Histidine.

SODIUM URSOLATE • Skin conditioner. *See* Ursolic Acid.

SODIUM USNATE • Germicide. *See* Usnic Acid.

SODIUM XYLENESULFONATE • Used as a solubilizer. An isolate from wood and coal tar. *See* Xylene.

SODIUM ZINC CETYL PHOSPHATE • Colorant. *See* Zinc and Phosphate.

SOLANUM DULCAMARA • *See* Dulcamara Extract.

SOLANUM LYCOCARPUM • *See* Lycopodium.

SOLANUM LYCOPERISCUM • Tomato extract.

SOLANUM MELONGENA • *See* Eggplant.

SOLANUM MURICATUM EXTRACT • *See* Potato Extract.

SOLANUM NIGRUM • Black Nightshade. In homeopathic and Indian medicine it is used for "rejuvenating," to soothe the eyes and inflammation as well as skin diseases. On the Canadian Hotlist (*see*). The EU has banned *Solanum nigrum* and its galenical preparations in cosmetics.

SOLANUM TUBEROSUM • *See* Potato Extract.

SOLAR ELASTOSIS • Degeneration and loosening of collagen (*see*) under the skin, frequently resulting from exposure to sunlight over a period of years.

SOLIDAGO ODORA • *See* Goldenrod.

SOLOMON'S SEAL • *Polygonatum officinale.* A perennial herb, the root was formerly used for its emetic properties and externally for bruises near the eyes, as well as for treatment of tumors, wounds, poxes, warts, and pimples. It was thought to help mend broken bones. In sixteenth-century Italy, it was used in a wash believed to maintain healthy skin. The roots contain allantoin (*see*), used today as an anti-inflammatory and healing ingredient.

SOLUBILITY • The degree to which a chemical can dissolve in a solvent, forming a solution.

SOLUBILIZATION • The process of dissolving in water such substances as fats and liquids that are not readily soluble under standard conditions by the action of a detergent or similar ingredient. Technically, a solubilized product is clear because the particle size of an emulsion is so small that light is not bounced off the particle. Solubilization is used in colognes and clear lotions. Sodium sulfonates (*see*) are common solubilizing ingredients.

SOLUBILIZED VAT BLUE 5 • A vat dye in the form of a soluble sodium salt of a sulfuric acid monoester. Vat dyes are more expensive than ordinary dyes and are used in pastels. *See* Vat Dyes for toxicity.

SOLUBILIZED VAT DYES • Sodium salts of vat dyes. They are comparatively expensive but give excellent penetration and fastness. *See* Vat Dyes.

SOLUBLE COLLAGEN • The protein source derived from the connective tissue of young animals. It is widely used in skin and hair conditioners. Formerly had "animal" in the name. *See* Solubilization and Collagen.

SOLUBLE PROTEOGLYCAN • Softened protein with a high sugar content.

SOLUM DIATOMEAE • *See* Diatomaceous Earth.

SOLUM FULLONUM • *See* Fuller's Earth.

SOLVENT • A liquid capable of dissolving or dispensing one or more substances. Methyl ethyl ketone is an example of a solvent.

SOLVENT BLACK 3 • EU name CI 26150. A diazo color. *See* Solvent Dye.

SOLVENT BLUE 35 • EU name CI 61554. Classed chemically as an anthraquinone (*see*) color. On the Canadian Hotlist (*see*). *See* Solvent Dye.

SOLVENT DYE • Generally insoluble in water, but dissolves in varying degrees in different organic media in liquid, molten, and solid forms. These include alcohols, oils, fats, and waxes. The use of a solvent dye depends upon fastness to light and adequate solubility, in powders, resins, and plastic. Can be irritating to the skin.

SOLVENT GREEN 3 • EU name CI 61565. An anthraquinone (*see*) color. The name can be used only when applied to uncertified batches of this color. The CTFA adopted name for certified (*see*) batches is D & C Green No. 6 (*see*).

SOLVENT GREEN 7 • EU name CI 59040. A pyrene color, the name can be used only for batches of uncertified color. The CTFA adopted name for certified (*see*) batches is D & C Green No. 8 (*see*). Pyrene is a cancer-causing ingredient.

SOLVENT ORANGE 1 • EU name CI 11920. A monoazo (*see*) dye.

SOLVENT RED 1 • EU name CI 12150. A monoazo (*see*) dye. *See also* Solvent Dye.

SOLVENT RED 3 • EU name CI 12010. A monoazo color (*see*). *See also* Solvent Dye.

SOLVENT RED 23 • EU name CI 26100. Japanese name Aka225. A diazo (*see*) color. The name can be used only for uncertified batches of this color. The CTFA adopted name for certified (*see*) batches is D & C Red No. 17 (*see*).

SOLVENT RED 24 • Calico Oil Red. EU name CI 26105 (banned by the EU). Japanese name Aka501. A diazo (*see*) color. On the Canadian Hotlist (*see*). *See also* Solvent Dye.

SOLVENT RED 43 • EU name CI 45380. Japanese name Aka223. A fluoran color. The sodium salt of this is Acid Red 87. The Solvent Red 43 name can be used only when applied to uncertified batches of color. The CTFA adopted name for certified (*see*) batches is D & C Red No. 21.

SOLVENT RED 48 • EU name CI 45410. Japanese names Aka104(1), Aka218, or Aka231. A fluoran color. The sodium salt is Acid Red 92. The name Solvent Red 48 can be used only for uncertified batches. The CTFA adopted name for certified (*see*) batches is D & C Red No. 27.

SOLVENT RED 49:1 • Japanese name Aka215. A xanthene (*see*) color. It is the stearic acid salt of Basic Violet 10. The name Solvent Red 49:1 can be applied only to batches of uncertified color. The CTFA adopted name for certified (*see*) batches is D & C Red No. 37 (*see*). The use of this color certified as D & C Red No. 37 has been banned in the United States in cosmetic products. Its use in cosmetics in other countries may also be restricted. On the Canadian Hotlist (*see*).

SOLVENT RED 72 • Orange Red 5. EU name CI 45370. Japanese name Daidai201. A fluoran color. The name can be applied only to uncertified batches. The CTFA adopted name for certified (*see*) batches is D & C Orange No. 5 (*see*).

SOLVENT RED 73 • Orange 10. EU name CI 45425. Japanese name Daidai206 or Daidai207. A fluoran color. The sodium salt is Acid Red 95. The name Solvent Red 73 can be applied only to uncertified batches of color. The CTFA adopted name for certified (*see*) batches is D & C Orange No. 10 (*see*).

SOLVENT VIOLET 13 • EU name CI 60725. Japanese name Murasaki 201. An anthraquinone color. The name is applied only to uncertified batches of this color. The CTFA adopted name for certified (*see*) batches is D & C Violet No. 2 (*see*).

SOLVENT YELLOW 13 • A quinoline color. The name can be applied only to uncertified batches of this color. The CTFA adopted name for certified (*see*) batches is D & C Yellow No. 11 (*see*).

SOLVENT YELLOW 18 • Food Yellow 12. A monoazo color (*see*).

SOLVENT YELLOW 29 • EU name CI 21230. A diazo (*see*) color.

SOLVENT YELLOW 33 • EU name CI 47000. Japanese name Ki204. A quinoline (*see*) color. The CTFA-certified (*see*) name for this color is D & C Yellow No. 11.

SOLVENT YELLOW 44 • EU name CI 56200. Disperse Yellow. An aniline (*see*) color.

SOLVENT YELLOW 85 • A coal tar color. Not listed by the EU or Japanese.

SOLVENT YELLOW 172 • A coumarin (*see*) color not listed by the EU or Japanese.

SOMAT-, SOMATO- • Prefixes pertaining to the body.

SONCHUS OLERACEUS • Milk Thistle. An annual herb with yellow semiflorets, it blossoms in spring and summer and can be found growing by the roadside or in fields all over China. It is eaten in salads in China as well as used in medicine. It reportedly has immunity aids. *See* Thistle.

SOPHORA ANGUSTIFOLIA ROOT EXTRACT • Minor source of kushen, an ancient Chinese medicine. Both sophora and its alkaloids are effective for treating urticaria, acute eczema, pudendal eczema, and other types of dermatitis. One of the alkaloids, aloprene, was shown to be a potent inhibitor of swelling induced by many ingredients.

SOPHORA JAPONICA • Pagoda Tree. Scholar Tree. The United States Agricultural Research Service renamed the tree *Styphnolobium* instead of *Sophora.* Has antibacterial properties.

SORBATE • A salt of Sorbic Acid. A material that has been or is capable of being taken up by another substance by either absorption or adsorption.

SORBETH-6 • *See* Sorbitol

SORBETH-20, -30, -40 • *See* Sorbitol.

SORBETH-6 HEXASTEARATE • *See* Sorbitol and Stearic Acid.

SORBIC ACID • A white, free-flowing powder obtained from the berries of the mountain ash. Also made from chemicals in the factory. Used in cosmetics as a preservative and humectant. A mold and yeast inhibitor. Used as a replacement for glycerin in emulsions, ointments, embalming fluids, mouthwashes, dental creams, and various cosmetic creams. A binder for toilet preparations and plasticizers. Produces a velvetlike feel when rubbed on skin. Sticky in large amounts. May cause skin irritation in susceptible people. On the basis of available information, the CIR Expert Panel (*see*) concluded that it is safe as presently used in cosmetic formulations.

SORBITAN • A compound from sorbitol that has the water removed.

SORBITAN CAPRYLATE • An emulsifier. *See* Sorbitan and Caprylic Acid.

SORBITAN COCOATE • An emulsifier. *See* Sorbitan and Coconut Oil.

SORBITAN DIISOSTEARATE • An emulsifier. The diester of isostearic acid (*see*) and hexitol.

SORBITAN DIOLEATE • An emulsifier. The diester of oleic acid and hexitol anhydrides derived from sorbitol. *See* Sorbitan Fatty Acid Esters.

SORBITAN DISTEARATE • An emulsifier. *See* Stearic Acid and Sorbitol.

SORBITAN FATTY ACID ESTERS • Mixture of fatty acids (*see*), esters of sorbitol (*see*), and sorbitol with the water removed. Widely used in the cosmetics industry as an emulsifier and stabilizer. Also used to prevent irritation from other cosmetic ingredients.

SORBITAN ISOSTEARATE • An emulsifier. *See* Sorbitan Fatty Acid Esters.

SORBITAN LAURATE • An emulsifier in cosmetic creams and lotions; a stabilizer of essential oils in water. *See* Lauric Acid.

SORBITAN OLEATE • Sorbitan Monooleate. An emulsifying ingredient, defoaming ingredient, and plasticizer. *See* Oleic Acid.

SORBITAN OLIVATE • *See* Sorbitan and Olive Oil.

SORBITAN PALMITATE • Derived from sorbitol (*see*). An emulsifier in cosmetic creams and lotions, a solubilizer of essential oils in water. On the basis of available information, the CIR Expert panel (*see*) concluded that it is safe as presently used in cosmetic formulations.

SORBITAN SESQUIISOSTEARATE • *See* Sorbitol and Isostearic Acid.

SORBITAN SESQUIOLEATE • A widely used emulsifier. *See* Sorbitol and Oleic Acid.

SORBITAN SESQUISTEARATE • *See* Sorbitan Stearate.

SORBITAN STEARATE • Sorbitan Monostearate. An emulsifier in cosmetic creams and lotions, a solubilizer of essential oils in water. Used in antiperspirants, deodorants, cake makeup, hand creams, hair tonics, rouge, and suntan creams. Manufactured by reacting edible commercial stearic acid with sorbitol (*see both*). On the basis of available information, the CIR Expert Panel (*see*) concludes that it is safe as presently used in cosmetic formulations.

SORBITAN TRIISOSTEARATE • On the basis of available information, the CIR Expert Panel (*see*) concluded that it is safe as presently used in cosmetic formulations. *See* Stearic Acid.

SORBITAN TRIOLEATE • On the basis of available information, the CIR Expert Panel (*see*) concluded that it is safe as presently used in cosmetic formulations. *See* Sorbitol.

SORBITAN TRISTEARATE • An emulsifier and alternate for sorbitan stearate (*see*). On the basis of available information, the CIR Expert Panel (*see*) concluded that it is safe as presently used in cosmetic formulations.

SORBITOL • A humectant. Gives a velvety feel to skin. Used as a replacement for glycerin in emulsions, ointments, embalming fluid, mouthwashes, dental creams, and various cosmetic creams. A binder for toilet preparations and a plasticizer and a flavoring ingredient. Also used in hair sprays, beauty masks, cuticle removers, foundation cake makeup, hand lotions, liquid powders, dentifrices, after-shave lotions, deodorants, antiperspirants, shampoos, and rouge. First found in the ripe berries of the mountain ash; it also occurs in other berries (except grapes), and in cherries, plums, pears, apples, seaweed, and algae. Consists of white hygroscopic powder, flakes, or granules with a sweet taste. It is a texturizing ingredient and a sequestrant. Also used in antifreeze, in foods as a sugar substitute, in writing inks to ensure a smooth flow from the point of the pen, and to increase the absorption of vitamins in pharmaceutical preparations. Medicinally used to reduce body water and for intravenous feedings, if taken externally. However, if ingested in excess, it can cause diarrhea and gastrointestinal disturbances; it may also alter the absorption of other drugs, making them less effective or more toxic.

SORBITYL ACETATE • Made from sorbitol and acetic acid (*see both*).

SORBITYL FURFURAL • Antioxidant made from sorbitol and furfural (*see both*).

SORBITYL SILANEDIOL • Humectant made from sorbitol and siloxanes (*see both*).

SORBUS EXTRACT • Service Tree Extract. The extract of *Sorbus domestica.* An extract that was used by the American Indians to make a wash for eyes that were sore and blurred from the sun, as from climbing and hiking, and from dust.

SORREL EXTRACT • *Rumex acetosella.* An extract of the various species of *Rumex.* The Europeans imported this to the Americas, and the Indians adopted it. Originally the root was used as a laxative and as a mild astringent. It was also used for scabs on the skin and as a dentifrice. It was widely used by American medical circles to treat skin diseases.

SOUHAKUHI EKISU • The root bark extract of *Morus alba,* white mulberry. Has many uses in folk medicine such as treating tumors, as an astringent, to treat bug bites and wounds, and to soothe a sore throat. It does have many compounds that are biologically active, such as sugars, nicotinic acid, and vitamin A. Used as a skin conditioner in cosmetics.

SOUR DOCK (H) • A weed with coarse leaves that is a member of the sorrel family and contains a sour juice. Used by herbalists to treat wounds and sore throats.

SOUTHERNWOOD • *Artemisia abrotanum.* Native to southern Europe and widely grown in English gardens, it belongs to the Compositae family. Pliny thought it had aphrodisiac qualities when placed under a mattress. It reputedly made hair grow on bald heads. Used in herbal teas as a sedative. It is also used by herbalists to bring on delayed menstruation, from which it got the nickname "lad's love." It is also used to remove threadworms in children. It is used in "organic" cosmetics.

SOY • Protein extracts of soy beans and soy milk, including isoflavones such as genistein and daidzein, are becoming increasingly used in anti-aging cosmetics. The proteins have been reported to have anticancer, antipigmentary, and antioxidant properties, at least in mouse skin. Genistein and daidzein, which are hormonelike ingredients, appear to increase hyaluronic acid (*see*). Another soy protein derivative, Bowman-Birk proteinase inhibitor, has been reported to protect against sun damage to the skin.

SOY ACID • A mixture of the fatty acids derived from soybean oil (*see*).

SOY AMINO ACIDS • Used in hair and skin conditioners. *See* Soy and Amino Acids.

SOY FLOUR • *See* Soybean Oil.

SOY GERM EXTRACT • Formerly called soy extract. *See* Soybean Oil.

SOY STEROL • *See* Soybean Oil.

SOY STEROL ACETATE • *See* Soybean Oil and Acetate.

SOYA HYDROXYETHYL IMIDAZOLINE • *See* Ethylenediamine and Urea.

SOYAETHYL MORPHOLINIUM ETHOSULFATE • *See* Soy and Sulfated Oil.

SOYAMIDE DEA • Fatty acids derived from soybeans used as a thickener and foam booster in shampoos and other hair products. *See* Soybean.

SOYAMIDOPROPYL BENZYLDIMONIUM CHLORIDE • *See* Quaternary Ammonium Compounds.

SOYAMIDOPROPYL DIMETHYLAMINE • *See* Amide.

SOYAMIDOPROPYL ETHYLDIMONIUM ETHOSULFATE • *See* Quaternary Ammonium Compounds.

SOYAMINE • Antistatic ingredient used in hair products. *See* Soybean Oil.

SOYAMINOPROPYLAMINE • *See* Quaternary Ammonium Compounds.

SOYATRIMONIUM CHLORIDE • Soya Trimethyl Ammonium Chloride. *See* Ammonium Chloride and Soybean Oil.

SOYBEAN • An erect, bushy, hairy legume, *Glycine max,* native to Asia and extensively cultivated in China, Japan, and elsewhere. Its seeds contain glycerides of linoleic, oleic, linolenic, and palmitic acids. *See* Soybean Oil.

SOYBEAN FLOUR • Used as a thickener.

SOYBEAN OIL • Extracted from the seeds of plants grown in eastern Asia, especially Manchuria, and the midwestern United States. Used in the manufacture of soaps, shampoos, and bath oils. Pale yellow to brownish yellow. Also used in the manufacture of margarine. Soybean flour contains practically no starch and is widely used in dietetic foods. May cause allergic reactions, including hair damage and acnelike pimples.

SOYBEAN OIL UNSAPONIFIABLES • The fraction of soybean oil that is not saponified (turned into fatty alcohol) in the refining of soybean oil fatty acids.

SOYBEAN PALMITATE • Used as a skin conditioner. *See* Palmitic Acid and Soybean.

SOYOU EKISU • Shiso. An extract of the leaves and twigs of *Perilla ocimoides,* an Asiatic mint, used in cosmetics as a fragrance additive and as a skin conditioner.

SOYTRIMONIUM CHLORIDE • Antistatic ingredient. *See* Quaternary Ammonium Compounds.

SPANISH MOSS • *Tillandsia usneodides.* Black Moss. Long Moss. Old Man's Beard. A plant that forms tufts of hairlike grayish green strands upon the trunks and branches of many trees in the southern United States and West Indies. Used in "organic" cosmetics.

SPANISH PELLITORY EXTRACT • Extract of the root of *Anacyclus pyrethrum.* Used as an insecticidal ingredient.

SPARTIUM JUNCEUM • Spanish Broom. Fragrance ingredient. In its medicinal properties, Spanish broom closely resembles the common broom, but it is from five to six times more active. The symptoms produced by overdoses are vomiting and purging, with renal irritation. The flowers yield a yellow dye.

SPEARMINT OIL • *Mentha viridis.* Used in perfumes, perfumed cosmetics, and toothpaste. It is the essential volatile oil obtained by steam distillation from the fresh aboveground parts of the flowering plant grown in the United States, Europe, and Asia. It is colorless, yellow or yellow-green, with the characteristic taste and odor of spearmint. Also used as a flavoring ingredient in food. May cause allergic reactions such as skin rash.

SPEEDWELL • Used in shampoos. It is an herb, a common, hairy perennial grown in Europe, with pale blue or lilac flowers. It has a reputation among herbalists of inducing sweating and restoring healthy body functions; also as a treatment for hemorrhages, and a medication for skin diseases. Used as an astringent.

SPELT • The popularity of spelt has rocketed in recent years, leading to a 130 percent increase in European product launches containing the ancient grain over the past three years. Spelt has been used in foods since about 8000 B.C. In line with the growing trend for natural cosmetics, spelt grain is appearing in an increasing number of skin and hair care products being launched across Europe. Although the number of beauty products being launched with the ingredient is still tiny, it is growing in popularity, particularly among organic product producers. Because of its structure, spelt is naturally pest resistant and therefore ideal for chemical-free production. The grain's popularity has reached such heights that people are even slathering spelt germ oil on their skin and hair. One UK spa has a whole treatment therapy on it. It is expensive for a wheat-free cosmetic and treatment. The full treatment and a bottle of spelt germ oil reportedly costs hundreds of dollars. For those allergic to wheat, however, it may be worth it.

SPENT GRAIN WAX • *Hordeum vulgare.* The ingredient made from the extraction of the residual dry grains obtained from the malting process in beer production. Used as an emollient and anti-inflammatory in cosmetics.

SPERGULARIA RUBRA • Sandspurry. Sabline roughe. *Tissa rubra. Birda rubra.* An herb common in Britain in sandy, gravelly heaths near the sea. Flowers all summer. Long used in bladder disease. Soothing to mucous membranes.

SPERMACETI • Cetyl Palmitate. Used as a base for ointments and creams, and as an emollient in cleansing creams. Also in shampoos, cold creams, and other creams to improve their gloss and increase their viscosity. Derived as a wax from the head of the sperm whale. Generally nontoxic but may become rancid and cause irritations.

SPERMINE • Found widely in living tissues along with spermidine. It was originally isolated from semen. Used as a skin-conditioning ingredient.

SPF • Sun Protectant Factor. A rating scale indicating how much time you can expose your skin to the sun before you will burn when using a particular sunscreen.

SPHAGNUM SQUARROSUM • Peat Moss. Skin conditioner.

SPHINGANINE • An unusual fat that accumulates when animals are exposed to a fumonisin, a harmful mold on corn. It is found concentrated in mammalian skin and may serve as a natural antifungal barrier, preventing infection by harmful fungi. In cosmetics, it is used as a skin and hair conditioner.

SPHINGOLIPIDS • A group of fats that yield aminoglycols. *See* Glycols.

SPHINGOMONAS FERMENT EXTRACT • A bacteria that can break up compounds.

SPICY BOUQUETS • One of the basic perfume types, they derive their characteristics from spice-giving ingredients, such as cinnamon, clove, vanilla, and ginger, but they may also be characterized by spiciness inherent in the flower notes of the perfume composition.

SPIKE LAVENDER OIL • French Lavender. Used in perfumes. A pale yellow, stable oil obtained from a flower grown in the Mediterranean region. A lavenderlike odor.

Used in cologne and toilet water; blended with lavender oil, soaps, and varnishes. Used also for fumigating, to keep moths from clothes, and in food and beverage flavorings.

SPIKENARD • *Aralia racemosa.* Nard. American herb of the ginseng family used for skin ailments such as acne, rash, and general skin problems. Also used for coughs, colds, and other chest problems.

SPILANTHES ACMELLA • Toothache Plant. Brazilian Cress. Chewing on the leaves used to treat toothache. It is also said to be effective against bacteria. No reported toxicity.

SPINACEA OLERACEA • *See* Spinach Extract.

SPINACH EXTRACT • An extract of the leaves of spinach, *Spinacea oleracea.* Powdered spinach leaf. Used to add green color to some soaps. Also used in masks and other cosmetics. May cause allergic skin reaction in the sensitive.

SPINAL CORD EXTRACT • The extract obtained from animal spinal cords.

SPINAL LIPID EXTRACT • The extract of fats from animal spinal cords.

SPIRAEA EXTRACT • Queen Meadow. An extract from the flowers of *Spiraea ulmaria.* Contains an oil similar to wintergreen (*see*). The roots are rich in tannic acid (*see*).

SPIRAEA ULMARIA EXTRACT • Used as a skin conditioner. *See* Spiraea Extract.

SPIRLODELA • *Herba spirodelae.* Fuping. Duckweed. Oriental herb used to promote sweating and relieve itching and swelling.

SPIRONOLACTONE. • Aldactone. Is used to treat many different disorders, from high blood pressure to fluid retention. Although the U.S. Food and Drug Administration doesn't recognize spironolactone as an acne treatment, it is often prescribed off-label to treat hormonally influenced breakouts. Spironolactone is used as an acne treatment for women only. Banned in UK cosmetics.

SPIRULINA EXTRACT • An extract of spirula, a many-chambered shell coiled in flat spirals. Occurs in most tropical seas. Humectant (*see*) used in hair and skin conditioners.

SPLEEN EXTRACT • The extract of bovine spleen used in "youth" cream.

SPONDIAS AMARA • Wu Feng. Tonic Plums. Extract of a tree that is used to treat oily skin.

SPONGE • The dried ground skeleton of the freshwater sponge *Spongia fluviatilis. S. tosta.* Named for the Greek word *spongos,* for "fungus," sponges are elastic porous masses of horny fibers that form the skeletons of marine animals of the lower species. *S. tosta* is a genus of subtropical sponges that are commercially important. They absorb water. Homeopathic medicines use sponge as a remedy for coughs and dry mucus. Sold to consumers to apply cosmetics and to help get rid of dead skin cells by scrubbing the face.

SPOTTED DOGFISH SKIN EXTRACT • Nurse Hound. An extract of the skin of *Scyliorhinus manicula,* a spotted fish. Used in anti-aging products.

SPOTTED HEMLOCK ROOT EXTRACT • An extract of the roots of *Conium maculatum. See* Hemlock Oil.

SPRAY DEODORANT • With antiperspirant action. Usually contains aluminum phenolsulfonate, 10 percent; propylene glycol, 5 percent; alcohol, 85 percent; and perfume. May seriously irritate the eyes, especially if you wear contact lenses. Dispenses by aerosols (*see*). Caution is advised, especially since aerosol is a highly efficient way of delivering materials to the lungs. It is an unnecessary and potentially harmful product. *See* Deodorants.

SPRUCE NEEDLES, TWIGS, and OIL • Colorless to light yellow, pleasant-smelling oil obtained from the needles and twigs of various spruces and hemlocks. Used chiefly in scenting soaps and cosmetics but also used as a flavoring. *See* Hemlock Oil. ASP

SPRUCE OIL • *See* Spruce Needles, Twigs, and Oil.

SQUALENE • Obtained from shark-liver oil. Occurs in smaller amounts in olive oil, wheat germ oil, and rice bran oil. It has a faint agreeable odor and is tasteless and miscible with vegetable and mineral oils, organic solvents, and fatty substances. Also found in human sebum. Insoluble in water. A lubricant and perfume fixative. A bactericide, an intermediate (*see*) in hair dyes, and used in surface-active ingredients. On the basis of the available information, the CIR Expert Panel (*see*) found it safe in the early 1980s but is considering new information to determine if the final safety assessment should be reaffirmed, amended, or have an addendum.

SQUALI LECUR • *See* Shark-liver Oil.

STAB • FDA abbreviation for stabilizer.

STABILIZER • A substance added to a product to give it body and to maintain a desired texture—for instance, the stabilizer alginic acid, which is added to cosmetics.

STACHYS OFFICINALIS • Wood Betony. Lousewort. A common herb of eastern North America and the British Isles, it has been used for centuries to treat diarrhea, and as an astringent, and sedative and dream repressant. Also is reputedly good for chronic headache. In cosmetics, it is used as an astringent and fragrance. Tincture of betony is used in the treatment of allergic rhinitis and hay fever.

STANNIC CHLORIDE • Tin Tetrachloride. A thin, colorless, fuming caustic liquid, soluble in water, used as a mordant (*see*) in metallic hair dye and as a reingredient (*see*) in perfumes and soaps. May be highly irritating to the eyes and mucous membranes.

STANNOUS CHLORIDE • Tin Dichloride. An antioxidant, soluble in water, and a powerful reducing ingredient, particularly in the manufacture of dyes. May be irritating to the skin and mucous membranes.

STANNOUS FLUORIDE • Tin Difluoride. Fluoristan. Prepared by dissolving tin in hydrofluoric acid. Used in dentifrices as a decay preventative in the United States but not permitted in dentifrices, mouthwashes, or breath drops in Canada. It is on the Canadian Hotlist (*see*). The EU calculates at 0.15 percent when mixed with fluorine compounds. Fluorine concentration must not exceed 0.15 percent, and the EU label must say "Contains stannous fluoride." *See* Fluoride.

STANNOUS PYROPHOSPHATE • Salt of Tin. It is poorly absorbed from the gastrointestinal tract. Used as an oral care ingredient. *See* Phosphate.

STAPHYLOCOCCI • Spherical bacteria that tend to grow in clumps like bunches of grapes. They are common inhabitants of the skin and of nasal passages. Some strains cause little trouble but some, called "resistant staph," tend to proliferate and are difficult to treat. *Staphylococcus aureus* is the most virulent type and is a frequent cause of boils, sties, abscesses, bone marrow infection, and pneumonia.

STAR ANISE • *Illicium verum.* Chinese Anise. Yellow-Flowered Starry Aniseed Tree. A small tree grown in Asia and North America, the fruit has been employed in Chinese medicine for centuries, particularly to cure arthritis. The seeds and oil have stimulant, carminative, diuretic, and digestive properties. Star anise also is used to soothe inflamed mucous membranes of the nasal passages. The fruit is used today in herbal teas. In China, the seeds are used to treat toothache, and the essential oil is given to children with colic. In scientific experiments, alcoholic extracts of the fruit were effective against gram-positive and gram-negative bacteria and fungi. Star anise contains a high level of anethole, which can produce hives, scaling, and blisters when applied directly to the skin.

STAR OF BETHLEHEM • *See Ornithogallum Umbellatum.*

STARCH • Acid Modified. Pregelatinized and Unmodified. Starch is stored by plants and is taken from wheat, potatoes, rice, corn, beans, and many other vegetable foods. Insoluble in cold water or alcohol but soluble in boiling water. Comparatively resistant to naturally occurring enzymes, and for this reason processors modify starch to make it more digestible. Used in dusting powders, dentifrices, hair colorings, rouge, dry shampoos, baby powders, emollients, and bath salts. Soothing to the skin and used to treat rashes. Used internally as a gruel in diarrhea. Allergic reaction to starch in toilet goods includes stuffy nose and other symptoms due to inhalation. Absorbs moisture and swells, causing blocking and distension of the pores leading to mechanical irritation. Particles remain in pores and putrefy, accelerated by sweat.

STARCH ACETATE • Hair- and skin-conditioning ingredient. *See* Acetic Acid and Starch.

STARCH/ACRYLATES/ACRYLAMIDE COPOLYMER • A film former and thickener. *See* Acrylamide and Starch.

STARCH DIETHYLAMINOETHYL ETHER • *See* Starch.

STARCH HYDROXYPROPYLTRIMONIUM CHLORIDE • An antistatic ingredient in hair products. *See* Quaternary Ammonium Compounds.

STARCH TALLOW • Fatty acids derived from tallow (*see*) used as an emollient.

STATUS COSMETICUS • A term used to describe patients intolerant of all cosmetics.

STEAPYRIUM CHLORIDE • A quaternary ammonium compound (*see*) used as an antistatic ingredient in hair products.

STEARALKONIUM BENTONITE • *See* Quaternary Ammonium Compounds.

STEARALKONIUM CHLORIDE • Improves the ability to comb the hair and adds shine. It is used in concentrations of less than 0.1 percent to 5 percent. On the basis of the available information, the CIR Expert Panel (*see*) found it safe in the early 1980s but is considering new information to determine if the final safety assessment should be reaffirmed, amended, or have an addendum. *See* Quaternary Ammonium Compounds.

STEARALKONIUM HECTORITE • Used in a wide variety of cosmetics as a suspending ingredient. Based upon the available data, the CIR Expert Panel (*see*) concluded that it is safe for use in cosmetics. *See* Quaternary Ammonium Compounds.

STEARAMIDE • An emulsifier. Colorless leaflets, insoluble in water. *See* Stearic Acid.

STEARAMIDE DEA • Stearic Acid Diethanolamine. *See* Stearamide.

STEARAMIDE DIBA STEARATE • An emulsifier. *See* Stearamide.

STEARAMIDE MEA STEARATE • *See* Stearamide.

STEARAMIDE MIPA • *See* Stearamide.

STEARAMIDE OXIDE • A hair conditioner. *See* Stearamide.

STEARAMIDOETHYL DIETHANOLAMIDE • *See* Diethanolamine.

STEARAMIDOETHYL DIETHYLAMINE • *See* Quaternary Ammonium Compounds.

STEARAMIDOETHYL ETHANOLAMINE • *See* Ethanolamines.

STEARAMIDOPROPYL BETAINE • *See* Quaternary Ammonium Compounds.

STEARAMIDOPROPYL CETEARYL DIMONIUM TOYSYLATE • *See* Quaternary Ammonium Compounds.

STEARAMIDOPROPYL DIMETHYLAMINE • *See* Dimethylamine.

STEARAMIDOPROPYL DIMETHYLAMINE LACTATE • *See* Quaternary Ammonium Compounds.

STEARAMIDOPROPYL DIMETHYLAMINE STEARATE • *See* Quaternary Ammonium Compounds.

STEARAMIDOPROPYL MORPHOLINE • *See* Quaternary Ammonium Compounds.

STEARAMIDOPROPYL MORPHOLINE LACTATE • *See* Quaternary Ammonium Compounds.

STEARAMIDOPROPYL PYRROLIDONYLMETHYL DIMONIUM CHLORIDE • *See* Quaternary Ammonium Compounds.

STEARAMIDOPROPYL TRIMONIUM METHOSULFATE • *See* Quaternary Ammonium Compounds.

STEARAMIDOPROPYLALKONIUM CHLORIDE • *See* Quaternary Ammonium Compounds.

STEARAMIDOPROPYLAMINE OXIDE • *See* Quaternary Ammonium Compounds.

STEARAMINE OXIDE • Used in hair products as a foam builder, a thickener, a stabilizer, and a conditioner as well as an antistatic ingredient. On the basis of the available information, the CIR Expert Panel (*see*) concluded that it is safe as a cosmetic ingredient for rinse-off products, but for leave-on products it should be limited to 5 percent. *See* Stearic Acid.

STEARATES • *See* Stearic Acid.

STEARDIMONIUM HYDROXYPROPYL HYDROLYZED COLLAGEN • An antistatic ingredient in hair products and a skin-conditioning ingredient. *See* Quaternary Ammonium Compounds.

STEARDIMONIUM HYDROXPROPYL HYDROLYZED SILK, OR SOY OR VEGETABLE OR WHEAT PROTEINS • Used as antistatic ingredients in hair products. *See* Quaternary Ammonium Compounds.

STEARDIMONIUM HYDROXYPROPYL PANTHENYL PEG-7 DIMETHICONE CHLORIDE • Used to make hair easier to comb. *See* Phosphorus and Silanes.

STEARETH-2 • A polyoxyethylene (*see*) ether of fatty alcohol. The oily liquid is used as a surfactant (*see*) and emulsifier (*see*). Widely used in hand and body products, cleansing lotions, tanning products, baby lotions, powders, and makeup. On the basis of available information, the CIR Expert Panel (*see*) concluded that it is safe as presently used in cosmetic formulations.

STEARETH-3, -4, -6, -10, -11, -13, -15, -16, -20, -21, -25, -27, -30, -40, -50, -100 • The polyethylene glycol ethers of stearyl alcohol. The number indicates the degree of liquidity; the higher, the more solid. Surfactants and emulsifying ingredients. *See* Steareth-2.

STEARETH-10 ALLYL ETHER/ACRYLATES COPOLYMER • *See* Acrylates.

STEARETH-5 STEARATE • *See* Stearic Acid.

STEARIC ACID • Widely used in deodorants and antiperspirants, liquid powders, foundation creams, hand creams, hand lotions, liquefying creams, hair straighteners, protective creams, shaving creams, and soap. Occurs naturally in butter acids, tallow, cascarilla bark, and other animal fats and oils. A white, waxy, natural fatty acid, it is the major ingredient used in making bar soap and lubricants. A large percentage of all cosmetic creams on the market contain it. It gives pearliness to hand creams. It is also used as a softener in chewing gum base, for suppositories, and as a food flavoring. It is a possible sensitizer for allergic people. The CIR Expert Panel (*see*) concluded that this ingredient is safe for use in cosmetic products. Vegans are really careful about this one since they consider that it often comes from animal fats from pigs and cows, etc. *See* Fatty Acids.

STEARIC HYDRAZIDE • Used in cosmetic products at concentrations of use of less than 1 percent. Hydrazides and their salts are prohibited for use in cosmetic products by the European Economic Community. The safety of stearic hydrazide has not been documented and substantiated. The CIR Expert Panel (*see*) cannot conclude that this ingredient is safe for use in cosmetic products until the appropriate safety data have been obtained and evaluated. *See* Stearic Acid and Hydrazine.

STEARMIDOETHYL DIETHYLAMINE • *See* Stearic Acid and Diethylamine.

STEAROAMPHOACETATE • *See* Quaternary Ammonium Compounds.

STEAROAMPHOCARBOXYGLYCINATE • *See* Surfactants.

STEAROAMPHODIACETATE • *See* Quaternary Ammonium Compounds.

STEAROAMPHOHYDROXYPROPYLSULFONATE • *See* Quaternary Ammonium Compounds.

STEAROAMPHOPROPIONATE • *See* Stearic Acid and Propionic Acid.

STEARONE • Derived from stearic acid. It is insoluble in water and is used as an antiblocking ingredient. *See* Stearic Acid.

STEAROXY DIMETHICONE • *See* Stearic Acid and Dimethicone.

STEAROXYTRIMETHYLSILANE • *See* Stearic Acid and Silicones.

STEAROYL GLUTAMIC ACID • A hair- and skin-conditioning ingredient. *See* Glutamic Acid.

STEAROYL LACTYLIC ACID • *See* Stearic Acid and Lactic Acid.

STEAROYL SARCOSINE • *See* Sarcosine.

STEARTRIMONIUM CHLORIDE • The CIR Expert Panel (*see*) concludes, on the basis of animal studies, this ingredient is safe for use in rinse-off products, and for use at concentrations of up to 0.25 percent in leave-on products. *See* Quaternary Ammonium Compounds.

STEARTRIMONIUM HYDROLYZED ANIMAL PROTEIN • *See* Quaternary Ammonium Compounds.

STEARYL ACETATE • The ester of stearyl alcohol and acetic acid (*see both*).

STEARYL ALCOHOL • Stenol. A mixture of solid alcohols prepared from sperm whale oil. Unctuous, white flakes, insoluble in water, soluble in alcohol and ether. Can be prepared from sperm whale oil. A substitute for cetyl alcohol (*see*) to obtain a firmer product at ordinary temperatures. Used in pharmaceuticals, cosmetic creams, for emulsions, as an antifoam ingredient, and a lubricant; also in depilatories, hair rinses, and shampoos. Has reportedly caused allergic reactions.

STEARYL BEHENATE • Ester of stearyl alcohol and behenic acid (*see both*).

STEARYL BETAINE • *See* Surfactants and Stearic Acid.

STEARYL CAPRYLATE • Ester of stearyl alcohol and citric acid (*see both*).

STEARYL CITRATE • The ester of stearyl alcohol and citric acid (*see both*).

STEARYL DIMETHICONE • A synthetic wax. *See* Silicones.

STEARYL ERUCAMIDE • *See* Quaternary Ammonium Compounds.

STEARYL ERUCATE • *See* Stearyl Alcohol and Erucic Acid.

STEARYL GLUCOSIDE • A wetting ingredient that lowers water's surface tension, permitting it to spread out and penetrate more easily. Widely used surfactant in hair dyes and shampoos. *See* Lauryl Alcohol.

STEARYL GLYCYRRHETINATE • The ester of stearyl alcohol and glycyrrhetinic acid (*see both*).

STEARYL HEPTANOATE • The ester of stearyl alcohol and heptanoic acid. Used as a wax and in skin emollients. On the basis of available information, the CIR Expert Panel (*see*) concluded that it is safe as presently used in cosmetic formulations. *See* Stearyl Alcohol and Heptanoic Acid.

STEARYL HYDROXYETHYL IMIDAZOLINE • *See* Quaternary Ammonium Compounds.

STEARYL LACTATE • An emulsifier that occurs in tallow and other animal fats as well as vegetable oils.

STEARYL OCTANOATE • The ester of stearyl alcohol and 2-ethylhexanoic acid. *See* Stearyl Alcohol.

STEARYL STEARATE • The ester of stearyl alcohol and stearic acid (*see both*).

STEARYL STEAROYL STEARATE • *See* Stearyl Alcohol.

STEARYLDIMETHYLAMINE • *See* Stearyl Alcohol.

STEARYLDIMONIUM HYDROXYPROPYL HYDROLYZED CASEIN • *See* Quaternary Ammonium Compounds.

STEARYLDIMONIUM HYDROXYPROPYL HYDROLYZED COLLAGEN • The quaternary ammonium chloride. *See* Hydrolyzed Collagen.

STEARYLDIMONIUM HYDROXYPROPYL HYDROLYZED KERATIN • *See* Quaternary Ammonium Compounds and Hydrolyzed Keratin.

STEARYLDIMONIUM HYDROXYPROPYL HYDROLYZED SILK • *See* Quaternary Ammonium Compounds and Silk.

STEARYLDIMONIUM HYDROXYPROPYL HYDROLYZED VEGETABLE PROTEIN • *See* Quaternary Ammonium Compounds and Hydrolyzed Vegetable Protein.

STEARYLDIMONIUM HYDROXYPROPYL HYDROLYZED WHEAT PROTEIN • *See* Quaternary Ammonium Compounds and Wheat Germ.

STEARYLTRIMONIUM HYDROXYETHYL HYDROLYZED COLLAGEN • *See* Hydrolyzed Collagen.

STEARYLTRIMONIUM METHOSULFATE • *See* Quaternary Ammonium Compounds.

STELLARIA MEDIA • *See* Chickweed.

STEPHANIA • Used by Chinese and other herbalists as analgesic, antipyretic, anti-inflammatory, antitumor, antibacterial, antihypertensive, diuretic. It is promoted as an herb for arthritic and rheumatic conditions caused by wind, damp, and coldness; it can also be used for heat, depending on the other herbs with which it is combined. Also said to be useful for the treatment of generalized swelling, swollen glands, and deficient mother's milk. The FDA has warned against its use as a dietary supplement because serious side effects have been reported and it has been banned in at least one country.

STERCULIA URENS GUM • *See* Gum Karaya.

STEROL • Any class of solid complex alcohols from animals and plants. Cholesterol is a sterol and is used in hand creams. Sterols are lubricants in baby preparations, emollient creams and lotions, emulsified fragrances, hair conditioners, hand creams, and hand lotions.

STEVIA REBAUDIANA • Rebiana, Reb A. Truvia. Sweetleaf. Candy leaf. Flavoring ingredient equal in sweetness to sugar. Extract of the leaves of a Paraguayan plant claimed to have antibacterial, antifungal, anti-inflammatory, antimicrobial, antiviral, antiyeast, cardiotonic, diuretic, hypoglycemic, hypotensive, tonic, and vasodilator effects. However, in animal experiments it was found to be toxic to pregnant rodents and to affect the kidneys. The FDA has given the long-awaited green light for Reb A, the sweetener made from the stevia leaf, to be used in food and beverages, opening the floodgates for new product launches. The FDA has concluded that it has no objection to rebiana (Reb A), at 95 percent purity or above, having GRAS status as a general purpose sweetener for food, drink, and eventually for cosmetics.

STEVIOSIDE • Derived from *Stevia rebaudiana*, a South American plant. The plant leaves have been used for centuries to sweeten bitter beverages and to make tea in the plant's native Paraguay. Since the 1970s stevioside has been used as a sweetener in Japan. In 1999, the Joint Expert Committee on Food Additives of the World Health Organization (JECFA) and the Scientific Committee for Food of the European Union reviewed stevioside and determined that on the basis of the scientific data currently available, stevioside is not acceptable as a sweetener. Stevioside is allowed in food for sweetening purposes in Japan, South Korea, and Brazil. Used in the United States in the 1980s, banned in 1991, and then allowed in as a dietary supplement, not a food additive. *See* Stevia Rebaudiana.

STIFFENING INGREDIENT • An ingredient to add body to shaving soaps and creams. Many of the gums, such as karaya and carrageenan (*see*), are used for this purpose.

STILLINGIA • Chinese Tallow Tree. Queen's Root. Yaw Root. Dried roots of a southeastern U.S. plant. An acrid resin; fixed and volatile oils. Used as a drying oil in cosmetics. Formerly used medicinally to induce vomiting.

STIPA TENACISSIMA • Esparto grass. Porcupine Grass. From the family of Gramineae. It is used as a cosmetic wax. The grass has been found to cause asthma.

ST. JOHN'S WORT • *See* Saint John's Wort.

STOMACH EXTRACT • Extract of bovine stomachs, it is used as a humectant in skin conditioners.

STONEROOT • *Collinsonia canadensis.* Horse Balm. Used for its constituents of resin, saponin, and tannic acid (*see all*). An erect, smooth perennial; a strong scented herb of eastern North America with pointed leaves. It produces a chocolate-colored powder with a peculiar odor and bitter astringent taste. Soluble in alcohol. *See* Collinsonia Canadensis.

STORAX • Styrax. Sweet Oriental Gum. Used in perfumes. It is the resin obtained from the bark of an Asiatic tree. Grayish brown, fragrant semiliquid, containing styrene and cinnamic acid (*see both*). Also used in food and beverage flavorings. Moderately toxic when ingested. Can cause urinary problems when absorbed through the skin. Can cause skin irritation, welts, and discomfort when applied topically. A common allergen.

STPP • *See* Sodium Tripolyphosphate.

STRAMONIUM • *Datura stramonium.* Thorn Apple. Jimsonweed. Stinkweed. Used in antiperspirants for its antiperspirant properties. Obtained from the dried leaves and flowering tops of a plant grown in Europe, Asia, and the United States. Leaves contain 0.25 to 0.45 percent alkaloids consisting of atropine, hyoscyamine, and scopolamone. It is used medicinally to treat intestinal spasms, asthma, and Parkinson's disease. The EU has banned it in cosmetics.

STRATUM CORNEUM • The outermost, horny cell layer of your skin, which serves to retain body water and prevent the entry of chemical irritants.

STRAWBERRY EXTRACT • *See* Strawberry Juice.

STRAWBERRY JUICE • *Fragaria chiloensis. F. vesca.* Strawberry was said to stop bleeding, slow excessive menstruation, and cure gout. Externally, it was used as a lotion for eczema and to prevent wrinkles. A concoction of the root and herb is said to be good for ulcers and liver disorders. In 1992, the FDA issued a notice that strawberry had not been shown to be safe and effective as claimed in OTC digestive aid products. Fresh, ripe strawberries are reputed to contain ingredients that soften and nourish the skin. Widely used in natural cosmetics today. No scientific evidence of benefit or harm.

STRAWFLOWER EXTRACT • The extract of *Helichrysum italicum,* grown for its bright yellow, strawlike flowers. Used in coloring.

STREPTOCOCCUSTHERMOPHILUS/MILK FERMENT LYSATE • The fermentation of milk with *Streptococcus thermophilus* with subsequent removal of the microorganism's cells. Used as a skin conditioner.

STREPTOMYCIN • Sulfate. An antibiotic active against streptococcal infections. May cause skin reactions.

STRIVECTIN • A cream promoted to combat stretch marks and then to combat wrinkles. Deionized water, C12–15 alkyl benzoate, sesame oil, caprylic/capric triglyceride, sweet almond oil, cetearyl olivate, sorbitan olivate, striadril complex (see product details for ingredients list), glycerin, PPG-12/SMDI copolymer, glyceryl stearate and PEG-100 stearate, cocoa butter, stearic acid, shea butter, tocopheryl acetate, mango butter, peppermint oil, methylparaben, xanthan gum, propylparaben, triethanolamine, butylene glycol, disodium EDTA, retinyl palmitate, tetrahexyldecyl ascorbate (*see* entries as appropriate).

STRONTIUM • Strontium is an alkaline earth metal that gives off radiation used to treat cancer. Strontium hydroxide is used as a pH adjuster. Strontium chloride is used as an oral care and skin-conditioning ingredient, and strontium nitrate is also used as an oral care ingredient and skin conditioner. Strontium peroxide is a white, odorless, and tasteless powder derived by passing oxygen over hot strontium. Used as a bleaching ingredient and antiseptic. It is highly flammable and explosive. Strontium sulfide and strontium thioglycolate are used as depilating ingredients. A number of its salts are toxic. May cause skin rash, irritation, and hair breakage. On the Canadian Hotlist (*see*).

STRONTIUM ACETATE HEMIHYDRATE • Used in toothpaste. See Strontium Chloride Hexahydrate.

STRONTIUM CHLORIDE HEXAHYDRATE • Used in toothpaste and shampoo and face care products. Restricted to 3.5 percent when mixed with other permitted strontium products, and total strontium content must not exceed 3.5 percent. In shampoo, it must not exceed 2.10 percent. The label must list it and caution that it should not be frequently used by children.

STRONTIUM DIOXIDE • Bleaching ingredient. Harmful by skin contact and damaging to the eyes. It is restricted to professional use only. See Strontium.

STRONTIUM HYDROXIDE • Used chiefly in making soaps and greases in cosmetics. pH regulator in depilatory products. Colorless, water-absorbing crystals or white powder. Absorbs carbon dioxide from the air. Very alkaline in solution. Irritating when applied to the skin. See Strontium.

STRONTIUM LACTATE, STRONTIUM NITRATE, STRONTIUM POLY-CARBOXYLATE • All are banned in cosmetics by ASEAN. See Strontium.

STRONTIUM PEROXIDE • Used in rinse-off hair care preparation. Should be used only by professionals. See Strontium.

STRYCHNINE • A powerful poison from the seeds of *Strychnos nux-vomica*. It is toxic by ingestion and inhalation. Produces an intense green mascara, and some women use it as an astringent. On the Canadian Hotlist (*see*).

STRYCHNOS • The seed of *Strychnos nux-vomica,* a tree that abounds on the Malabar and Coromandel coasts of the East Indies. From this seed the deadly poisons known as strychnine and brucine are obtained. The seeds are sometimes called Quaker buttons. On the Canadian Hotlist (*see*). Banned in cosmetics by the EU. See Strychnine.

STYPTIC • An agent that reduces or stops external bleeding. Among the herbs that are used for this purpose are raspberry and yellow dock.

STYPTIC PENCIL • A cylindrical stick composed of potassium aluminum sulfate, glycerin, and talc. It has an astringent effect, tending to contract or bind. Designed to check blood flow, primarily from razor nicks. May sting but has no known toxicity.

STYRAX • *See* Storax.

STYRENE • Obtained from ethylbenzene by taking out the hydrogen. Colorless to yellowish, oily liquid with a penetrating odor. Used in the manufacture of cosmetic resins and in plastics. May be irritating to the eyes and mucous membranes, and in high concentrations, it is narcotic.

STYRENE/ACRYLAMIDE COPOLYMER • An opacifier. *See* Acrylates.

STYRENE/ACRYLATE COPOLYMER • An opacifier. *See* Acrylates.

STYRENE/ACRYLATE/AMMONIUM METHACRYLATE COPOLYMER • Polymer (*see*) of styrene and a monomer of acrylic acid, methacrylic acid, or one of their esters. Used in liquid eyeliners. *See* Styrene and Acrylates.

STYRENE/ACRYLIC ACID COPOLYMER • *See* Styrene and Acrylates.

STYRENE/MA COPOLYMER • *See* Styrene and Maleic Acid.

STYRENE/VP COPOLYMER • Prepared from vinyl pyrrolidone and styrene monomers, it is used in liquid eyeliners as a carrier for color. *See* Styrene and Polyvinylpyrrolidone.

SUBCUTANEOUS • Under the skin.

SUBTILISIN • An enzyme obtained by fermentation of the bacterias *Bacillus subtilis* or *B. liceniformis*. Used as a skin conditioner. This enzyme is also used in detergents.

SUCCINIC ACID • Butanedioc acid. Occurs in fossils, fungi, lichens, etc. Prepared from acetic acid (*see*). Odorless; very acid taste. The acid is used as a plant-growth retardant. Used as a germicide and mouthwash, and in perfumes and lacquers; also used as a buffer and neutralizing ingredient. Has been employed medicinally as a laxative. Large amounts injected under the skin of frogs kills them.

SUCCINIC ANHYDRIDE • A starch modifier. *See* Succinic Acid.

SUCCINOGLYCAN • A sugar produced by the fermentation of *Agrobacterium tumefaciens*. Used as a skin conditioner.

SUCROSE • Sugar. Cane Sugar. Saccharose. A sweetening ingredient and food, a starting ingredient in fermentation production, a preservative and antioxidant in the pharmacy, a demulcent, and a substitute for glycerin (*see*). Workers who handle raw sugar often develop rashes and other skin problems. When it oxidizes with sweat, sugar draws water from the skin and causes chapping and cracking. Infections, erosions, and fissures around the nails can occur.

SUCROSE ACETATE ISOBUTYRATE • A denaturant for rubbing alcohols (*see both*) and used as a plasticizer for nail products and eye makeup.

SUCROSE BENZOATE • *See* Benzoic Acid.

SUCROSE BENZOATE/SUCROSE ACETATE ISOBUTYRATE/BUTYL BENZYL PHTHALATE COPOLYMER • The condensation polymer of sucrose benzoate, sucrose acetate isobutyrate, and butyl benzyl phthalate monomers. Used as a film former.

SUCROSE BENZOATE/SUCROSE ACETATE ISOBUTYRATE/BUTYL BENZYL PHTHALATE/METHACRYLATE COPOLYMER • The condensation product of sucrose benzoate, sucrose acetate isobutyrate, butyl benzyl phthalate, and methyl methacrylate monomers. Used as a film former. *See* Acrylates.

SUCROSE COCOATE • *See* Coconut Acids and Sucrose.

SUCROSE DILAURATE • *See* Lauric Acid.

SUCROSE DISTEARATE • A mixture of sucrose and lauric acid (*see both*).

SUCROSE LAURATE • A mixture of sucrose and lauric acid (*see both*).

SUCROSE MYRISTATE • Emulsifier. May promote acne. *See* Myristic Acid and Sucrose.

SUCROSE OCTAACETATE • A preparation from sucrose (*see*). A synthetic flavoring. Used in adhesives and nail lacquers; a denaturant for alcohol.

SUCROSE OLEATE • *See* Oleic Acid and Sucrose.

SUCROSE PALMITATE • *See* Palmitic Acid and Sucrose.

SUCROSE POLYLAURATE • *See* Lauric Acid and Sucrose.

SUCROSE POLYOLEATE • *See* Oleic Acid and Sucrose.

SUCROSE POLYSTEARATE • *See* Stearic Acid and Sucrose.

SUCROSE RICINOLEATE • *See* Ricinoleic Acid and Sucrose.

SUCROSE STEARATE • A mixture of sucrose and stearic acid (*see both*).

SUCROSE TETRASTEARATE TRIACETATE • *See* Stearic Acid and Sucrose.

SUCROSE TRIBEHENATE • *See* Behenic Acid and Sucrose.

SUCROSE TRISTEARATE • *See* Stearic Acid and Sucrose.

SUDAN III • Oil Red. Oil Scarlet. Solvent Red 23. A reddish brown powder used in coloring for waxes, oils, stains, dyes, and resins. May cause contact dermatitis (*see*).

SUGAR • *See* Sucrose.

SUGAR MAPLE • *Acer saccharinum* Extract. Used as a flavoring and skin conditioner.

SUGARCANE • *Saccharum officinarum.* Used as a flavoring and skin conditioner.

SUIKAZURA EKISU • *See* Honeysuckle.

SULFAMIC ACID • A cleansing ingredient in cosmetics and used in the manufacture of hair dyes and lakes (*see*). A strong, white, crystalline acid used chiefly as a weed killer, in cleaning metals, and as a flameproofing and softening ingredient. Moderately irritating to the skin and mucous membranes.

SULFANILIC ACID • Grayish white crystals made from aniline and sulfuric acid (*see both*). Used in dyes and medicines as an antibacterial.

SULFATED CASTOR OIL • *See* Sulfated Oil and Castor Oil.

SULFATED GLYCERYL OLEATE • Produced by adding sulfuric acid to glyceryl oleate. *See* Sulfated Oil and Glyceryl Oleate.

SULFATED OIL • Sulphated Oil. A compound to which a salt of sulfuric acid has been added to help control the acid-alkali balance.

SULFATED OLIVE OIL • *See* Sulfated Oil and Olive Oil.

SULFATED PEANUT OIL • *See* Sulfated Oil and Peanut Oil.

SULFATES • Sulphates. A salt or ester of sulfuric acid (*see*). Used in detergents and shampoos. May cause an allergic reaction to those sensitive to sulfur.

SULFIDES • Inorganic sulfur compounds that occur free or in combination with minerals. They are salts of a weak acid and are used as hair-dissolving ingredients in depilatories. They are skin irritants and may cause hair breakage. On the Canadian Hotlist (*see*).

SULFITES • Sodium, Potassium, and Ammonium. In organic compounds, sulfites can be added to cosmetics as preservatives. Sulfites can cause serious and even fatal reactions in persons sensitive to them. Such adverse responses include acute asthma attacks, loss of consciousness, anaphylactic shock, diarrhea, and nausea occurring soon after ingesting sulfiting ingredients. There have been seventeen deaths that the FDA has determined were "probably or possibly" associated with sulfites in foods. The Scientific Committee on Cosmetics and Non-Food Products (SCCNFP) of the European Union meeting in Brussels 2003 concluded that inorganic sulfites and bisulfites do not pose a health risk when used in cosmetic products at concentrations up to 0.67 percent in oxidative hair dye products, up to 6.7 percent in hair-waving/straightening products, up to 0.45

percent in self-tanning products for the face, and up to 0.40 percent in self-tanning products for the body. The FDA requires sulfites must be declared on the labels of wine and packaged foods sold in supermarkets when they are added in excess of 10 parts per million. Despite reports of severe or even fatal reactions to sulfites, there are six sulfiting ingredients currently listed as GRAS chemical preservatives. They are sulfur dioxide, sodium sulfite (*see*), sodium bisulfate (*see*) and potassium bisulfite, and sodium and potassium metabisulfite (*see*).

SULFONAMIDE FORMALDEHYDE • A solvent in nail polish and the most frequent cause of nail polish dermatitis, which generally affects the neck.

SULFONAMIDE RESINS • Sulfanilamide. The use of sulfonamides dates back to 1934, when the dye prontosil was shown to cure certain infections caused by bacteria. Sulfonamides are bacteria killers and are used to inhibit germ growth in cosmetics. They are also used to contribute depth, gloss, flow adhesion, and water resistance to films in nail lacquers. They may cause allergic reactions. On the Canadian Hotlist (*see*).

SULFONATED OILS • Sulfated. Prepared by reacting oils with sulfuric acid. Used in soapless shampoos and hair sprays as an emulsifier and wetting ingredient. Shampoos containing sulfonated oils were first manufactured in 1880 and were effective in hard or soft water. Sulfonated oils strip color from both natural and colored hair and can bring out streaks. Sulfated castor oil has been used to remove all types of dye. Applied to hair and heated, it is used as a hair treatment. Sulfonated oils are used in hair tonics that remain on the hair as hairdressings. May cause drying of the skin.

SULFONIC ACIDS • Strong organic acids used in detergents, dyes, and resins. Unlike ordinary soaps, they do not leave a scum.

SULFOSUCCINIC ACID • From sulfur and succinic acid. Used as a surfactant (*see*) and a solubilizing ingredient.

SULFUR • Aveeno Cleansing Bar. Clearasil Adult. Brimstone. Buf-Bar. Fostex Regular Strength. Fostex. Fostril. Liquimat. Lotio Alsulfa. Meted 2. Acnomel Cream. Sastid. Sebucare. Sebulex Antiseborrheic Treatment Shampoo. Sebutone Cream Shampoo. Pernox. Sulfacet R. Sulpho-Lac Acne Maximum Strength Meted. An element that occurs in the earth's crust in the free state and in combination. A mild topical antibacterial and antifungal agent used in preparations for acne and dandruff. Also a stimulant to healing when used on rash. May cause irritation of the skin. In 1992, the FDA issued a notice that sulfur had not been shown to be safe and effective as claimed in OTC products, including those for treatment of poison ivy, poison sumac, and poison oak, and sulfur (sublimed) in products to kill lice. Sulfur was also placed on the banned list for diaper rash, fever blister, and cold sore drug products because it had not been shown to be safe and effective as claimed. In homeopathic medicines, it is used to ease burning pains, eruptions, sensations, discharges, and offensive odors. It is also used for shortness of breath.

SULFUR TAR COMPLEX • Product obtained from the distillation of wood of various species of fir and treated with sulfur. Used in treatment shampoos and skin problems.

SULFURATED LIME • Used to treat acne, scabies, and other skin disorders. Avoid using abrasive soaps or cleansers, alcohol containing preparations, and other topical acne preparations while using sulfurated lime. May cause skin irritation.

SULFURIC ACID • Sulphuric Acid. Sul-Ac. Oil of Bitriol. A clear, colorless, odorless, oily acid used to modify starch and to regulate acid-alkalinity. It is very corrosive and produces severe burns on contact with the skin and other body tissues. Inhalation of the vapors can cause serious lung damage. Diluted sulfuric acid has been used to stimulate appetite and to combat overalkaline stomach juices. It is used as a topical caustic in cosmetic products. If ingested undiluted, it can be fatal. Homeopaths used it to treat anemia, bruises, diarrhea, exhaustion, hot flashes, and thrush. The final report to the FDA of the Select Committee on GRAS Substances stated in 1980 that it should continue its GRAS status with no limitations other than good manufacturing practices. The FDA data bank, PAFA, has fully up-to-date toxicology information available on this food additive.

SULFURIZED JOJOBA OIL • A mixture of sulfur and jojoba oil (*see both*).

SULFURIZED HYDROLYZED CORN PROTEIN • Protein from the reaction of sulfur with hydrolyzed corn protein (*see*) used as a hair conditioner.

SULPH • *See* Sulfur.

SULPHUR • *See* Sulfur.

SUMA • *Pfaffia paniculata*. Para Todo. Brazilian Ginseng. The South American version of ginseng (*see*). Has been referred to as "Para Todo," meaning "for all things," by Brazilian Indian tribes who first discovered the medicinal uses of the herb. In North America, it has been used to treat exhaustion resulting from viruses such as Epstein-Barr and Chronic Fatigue Syndrome. Among its constituents are saponins and germanium (*see both*). A tonic to increase energy.

SUMAC • *Rhus glabra*. Sumach. Sweet Sumach. A number of members of this genus possess poisonous properties. *Rhus* is found growing wild in all parts of the United States. The bark and fruit are astringent. Sumac berries are used as a gargle in decoction form for the chest pain angina. The decoction also is gargled for throat irritation and to help asthmatics breathe easier. The high tannin (*see*) content in the berries explains why it was used to treat diarrhea. The root was chewed by some North American Indians for mouth sores.

SUNBURN LOTION • Includes Creams and Sprays. Serious sunburn requires medical attention, and the use of oils, including butter, is not recommended. However, there are a number of soothing lotions, creams, and sprays for mild sunburn on the market. A common formula includes mineral oil, 10 percent; lanolin, 2.5 percent; propylene glycol, 2.5 percent; triethanolamine, 5.0 percent (*see all*); and water, distilled, 80 percent.

SUNFLOWER • *Helianthus annuus*. Indian Sunflower. Lady Eleven O'Clock. Marigold of Peru. Introduced into the United States from Mexico and Peru, the seeds are used in medicine as a diuretic and a soothing tonic for coughs. Used today as a dietary supplement. High in vitamin E. Used in skin conditioners, cleansers, emulsifiers, surfactants, and thickeners.

SUNFLOWER SEED EXTRACT • An extract of the seed of *Helianthus annuus*. Used in skin creams.

SUNFLOWER SEED OIL • Widely used in many cosmetic products including bath products, makeup, cleansing products, depilatories, hair conditioners, shampoos, other hair care products, skin care products, and suntan products. The Food and Drug Administration (FDA) includes sunflower seed oil and its triglycerides or fatty acids on its list of indirect food additives. These ingredients may be used as components of resinous and polymeric coatings having incidental contact with food. The addition of hydrogen atoms to sunflower seed oil results in hydrogenated sunflower seed oil. Sunflower seed glyceride is a mixture of mono-, di-, and triglycerides derived from sunflower seed oil. Sunflower seed acid is a mixture of fatty acids derived from sunflower seed oil.

SUNFLOWER SEED OIL GLYCERIDE • *See* Sunflower Seed Oil and Glycerides.

SUNSCREEN PREPARATIONS • A product that includes the term "sunscreen" in its labeling or in any other way represents or suggests that it is intended to prevent, cure, treat, or mitigate disease or to affect a structure or function of the body comes within the definition of a drug by FDA regulations. Sunscreen active ingredients affect the structure or function of the body by absorbing, reflecting, or scattering the harmful, burning rays of the sun, thereby altering your body's response to solar radiation. These ingredients also help to prevent diseases such as sunburn and may reduce the chance of premature skin aging, skin cancer, and other harmful effects due to the sun when used in conjunction with limiting sun exposure and wearing protective clothing. If you see the term "sunscreen" or similar sun protection terminology in the labeling of a product, do you expect the product to protect you in some way from the harmful effects of the sun, irrespective of other labeling statements? Consequently, the use of the term "sunscreen" or similar sun protection terminology in a product's labeling generally causes the product to be subject to regulation as a drug. However, sunscreen ingredients may also be used in some products for nontherapeutic, nonphysiologic uses (e.g., as a color additive or to protect the color of the product). If your cosmetic product contains a sunscreen ingredient and uses the term "sunscreen" or similar sun protection terminology anywhere in its labeling, the term must be qualified by describing the cosmetic benefit provided by the sunscreen ingredient. Preparations to prevent painful sunburn that encourage a change in pigmentation (a tan) have a large market. Suntan creams (emulsions) may contain *p*-aminobenzoic acid, mineral oil, sorbitan stearate, poloxamers (*see all*), and 62 percent water. A suntan ointment may contain petrolatum, stearyl alcohol, mineral oil, sesame oil, and calcium stearate (*see all*). A suntan lotion may contain methyl anthranilate, propylene glycol, ricinoleate, glycerin (*see all*), and about 65 percent alcohol and 10 percent water. A suntan oil may contain salicylates, about 40 percent sesame oil (*see both*), and 55 percent mineral oil. Sunscreen preparations may also contain alcohol, *p*-aminobenzoic acid and derivatives, benzyl salicylate, cinnamic acid derivatives, and coumarin (*see all*). A common suntan oil formula includes 2-ethyl hexyl salicylate, 5 percent; sesame oil, 40 percent; mineral oil, about 55 percent; perfume; color; and an antioxidant.

Complaints to the FDA concerning sunscreen preparations include rash, blisters, burns, yellowed skin, and even death. The newer brands of sunscreens available protect against UVA rays of the sun, which tan, and UVB rays, which burn. They are called broad-spectrum sunscreens, and they list the UVA blocker, oxybenzone, among their ingredients. It has become common practice to add sunscreening ingredients to cosmetics to protect against the adverse effects of ultraviolet rays. In a study done at Case Western Reserve University, Cleveland, Ohio, it was shown that cosmetic preparations containing sunscreening ingredients are protective against the sun's rays and should therefore be encouraged. Regular use of sunscreens over the years may reduce your chance of skin damage, some types of skin cancer, and other harmful effects due to the sun. Epidemiologists believe the rising toll of melanoma (*see*) may well be attributed to the desire to acquire tans at a time when UVA radiation is growing more destructive because of thinning of the ozone layer. Sunscreens are considered over-the-counter drugs in the United States but cosmetics in the European Union. The United States uses sun protection factor (SPF) measured according to standard FDA protocol, while the European Union does not have mandatory methods for assessing SPF. The following is a concensus of manufacturers and dermatologists:

- Apply sunscreen thirty minutes before sun exposure to all uncovered skin except the eyelids.

- Make sure it is a "broad spectrum" product that protects against both UVA and UVB rays.

- Use at least an SPF (sun protection factor) of 15, but if you are fair skinned, increase your protection to an SPF of 25 or more. The SPF number is based on the multiplication of the time it would take you to first turn slightly red from the sun. That is, if your skin begins to turn pink after ten minutes, a product with SPF of 15 would theoretically keep you from sunburning for 150 minutes under ultraviolet radiation. Recognize, however, that SPF 30 does not give twice the protection of SPF 15. SPF 15 absorbs 93 percent of the sunburning rays, and SPF 30 absorbs 97 percent.

- Choose a sunscreen that says it is "noncomedogenic" (doesn't cause blackheads).
- Make sure it is "waterproof" if you lap swim or play tennis or golf, or other outdoor activity that involves water or a lot of sweating.
- Reapply your sunscreen about every two hours when outdoors.
- Wear a sunscreen all year around because you can get casual sun exposure during any season. Many don't wear sunscreen in the winter because they feel it's impossible for the skin to be sun damaged in the cold weather. In fact, UVA rays reflect off snow and levels increase at higher elevations, which is where you find ski resorts and mountain climbers.

If you are allergic to sunscreen chemicals—and many people are—try zinc oxide cream, which is a sunblock (an opaque substance that physically blocks the sun's rays).

In 1999 and 2003, there were warnings that wearing sunscreen may make you more vulnerable to skin cancer. A study, published in the *U.S. Journal of the National Cancer Institute,* said that people who wore higher-factor sunscreens tended to stay out much longer, because they felt protected from the risk of sunburn. A British biochemist has suggested that the cocktail of chemicals involved in sunscreens could be converted into free radicals (*see*) , which could cause cell damage and lead to cancer. Caution: There has been concern for a long time about lathering your skin with chemicals that may be in sunscreens. The trend in the newest medical literature tends to recommend sun protective clothing rather than or in addition to sunscreens. There are sunscreens currently being developed that contain new active ingredients that are said to be more protective against UVA rays and may soon be available in the United States. New formulations are also being developed to address special environments and seasonal-related issues. Stay tuned as the final verdict on sunscreens' benefits and disadvantages is not in at this writing.

SUNSET YELLOW • EU name CI 15985. Japanese name Ki5. A monoazo color, Sunset Yellow can be used only when applied to batches of uncertified color. The CTFA adopted name for certified (*see*) batches is FD & C Yellow No. 6 (*see*).

SUNSET YELLOW ALUMINUM LAKE • EU name CI 15985. Japanese name Ki5. Uncertified it is called Yellow 6 Lake.

SUNTAN PREPARATIONS • There are "tanning pills" manufactured as capsules intended for ingestion. These products usually contain beta-carotene and/or canthaxanthin (*see*). They act by entering the bloodstream and are partially deposited in skin tissue, giving the skin a tanlike color. Neither beta-carotene nor canthaxanthin is approved for this use, and tanning pill products containing these color additives are considered adulterated. "Suntan accelerators" are considered drugs. *See* Sunscreen Preparations.

SUNTANNING PRODUCTS • The FDA requires a warning statement for suntanning cosmetic products containing no sunscreen ingredients (21 CFR 740.19). The warning statement must read as follows: "Warning—This product does not contain a sunscreen and does not protect against sunburn. Repeated exposure of unprotected skin while tanning may increase the risk of skin aging, skin cancer, and other harmful effects to the skin, even if you do not burn."

SUPERCHAR • *See* Activated Charcoal.

SUPEROXIDE DISMUTASE • A copper-containing protein enzyme that decomposes oxygen.

SURFACE-ACTIVE INGREDIENT • Any compound that reduces surface tension when dissolved in solution. There are three types: detergents, wetting ingredients, and emulsifiers (*see all*).

SURFACTANTS • These are wetting ingredients. They lower water's surface tension, permitting it to spread out and penetrate more easily. These surface-active ingredients are classified by whether or not they ionize in solution and by the nature of their electrical charges. There are four major categories—anionic, nonionic, cationic, and amphoteric. Anionic surfactants, which carry a negative charge, have excellent cleaning properties. They are stain and dirt removers in household detergent powders and liquids and in toilet soaps. Nonionic surfactants have no electrical charge. Since they are resistant to hard water and dissolve in oil and grease, they are especially effective in spray-on oven cleaners. Cationic surfactants have a positive charge. These are primarily ammonia derivatives and are antistatic and sanitizing ingredients used as friction reducers in hair rinses and fabric softeners. Amphoteric surfactants may be either negatively charged or positively charged, depending on the activity or alkalinity of the water. They are used for cosmetics where mildness is important, such as in shampoos and lotions.

SURMA • A lead-based eye cosmetic used by Chinese women. Medical personnel are campaigning to inform the women about the danger of the cosmetic.

SUS • Pigskin extract.

SUTILAINS • Enzymes obtained from the bacteria *Bacillus subtillis.*

SVHC • Abbreviation for Substances of Very High Concern according to the European Chemicals Agency.

SWEET ALMOND OIL • *Prunus amygdalus. P. dulcis.* Used in perfumes and in the manufacture of fine soaps and emollients. Expressed from the seeds of a plant. Colorless or pale yellow, oily liquid, almost odorless, with a bland taste. Insoluble in water. On the basis of the available information, the CIR Expert Panel (*see*) found it safe in the early 1980s. In 2002, as part of the scheduled reevaluation of ingredients, the CIR Expert Panel considered available new data and reaffirmed the above conclusion. *See* Bitter Almond Oil.

SWEET BAY OIL • Used in perfumes. It is the yellow-green volatile oil from the leaves of the laurel.

SWEET BIRCH • *See* Methyl Salicylate.

SWEET CHERRY EXTRACT and OIL • *Prunus avium.* A tall pyramidlike Eurasian tree with reddish-brown bark, white flowers, and fruits that are often small and bitter in the wild but have been cultivated into sweet-flavored cherries. The extract is used in flavorings and in "organic" cosmetics. The oil is used as a skin-conditioning ingredient.

SWEET CLOVER EXTRACT • The extract of various species of *Melilotus,* grown for hay and soil improvement. It contains coumarin (*see*) and is used as a scent to disguise bad odors.

SWEET FLAG • *See* Calamus Root Extract.

SWEET GRASS EXTRACT • The extract of *Hierochloe borealis.* Any of various grasses of sweet flavor or odor such as manna grass or holy grass.

SWEET MARJORAM OIL • *Origanum majorana.* Pot Marjoram. Used in perfumery and hair preparations. The natural extract of the flowers and leaves of two varieties of the fragrant marjoram. Also a food flavoring.

SWEET VIOLET EXTRACT • The extract of the flowers of *Viola odorata* of Eurasia and North Africa, which is the source of many of the commercially developed violets. Used in perfumery.

SWEET WOODRUFF • *See* Woodruff.

SWERTIA EXTRACT • The extract of flowers, leaves, and stems of various species of swertia. A small genus of herbs found in the western United States. Has a thick, bitter-tasting root and dull-colored flowers. Used as a wax and in hair-grooming aids as well as in skin conditioners.

SWIFTLET NEST EXTRACT • An extract from the nest of swiftlets used as a skin conditioner. The nests are used for bird's nest soup popular in Chinese restaurants.

SYLVIC ACID • *See* Abietic Acid.

SYMPATHETIC NERVOUS SYSTEM • One of the major divisions of the autonomic nervous system; it regulates involuntary muscle action such as the beating of the heart and breathing. The sympathetic nerves that leave the brain and spinal cord, pass through the nerve cell clusters (ganglia), and are distributed to the heart, lungs, intestines, blood vessels, and sweat glands. In general, sympathetic nerves dilate the pupils, constrict small blood vessels, and increase heart rate. They are the nerves that prepare us for fight or flight. The other part of the autonomic system, parasympathetic nerves, slows things down after you stop exercising or the danger has passed. The system also involves circulating substances produced by the adrenal gland.

SYMPHYTUM OFFICIALE • *See* Comfrey.

SYMTRIOL • A new preservative at this writing. It contains 1,2-octanediol and 1,2-hexanediol, which are both moisturizers that also have antimicrobial properties and can therefore help reduce the amount of preservative required in a formulation. Added to the patent-pending blend is methylbenzyl alcohol, which is a "nature-identical" compound used in fragrances. It is often added to cosmetics and perfumes for its floral scent, although formulators using SymTriol may, if desired, mask the scent with other fragrances. Methylbenzyl alcohol also has antifungal effects. Its manufacturer, Symrise, claims that it complements the antimicrobial properties of the 1,2-alkanediol blend and is going to be marketed to formulators who wish to reduce preservatives such as parabens and formaldehyde in cosmetics.

SYNECHOCOCCUS/MANGANESE FERMENT • An extract of a fermentation product of the bacteria *Synechococcus* with manganese ions. Used as a skin conditioner.

SYNERGISTIC EFFECT • A substance that coordinates action with another substance.

SYNSEPALUM DULCIFICUM • Miracle Fruit. Berries are eaten fresh. Africans sometimes use the fruits to improve the taste of stale food. Fruits are being investigated as a possible source for a natural food sweetener. Used in cosmetics as a skin conditioner.

SYNTHETIC • Made entirely of artificial means and not found in nature. They usually are compounded from chemicals derived from crude oil, coal tar, or minerals.

SYNTHETIC BEESWAX • A mixture of alcohol esters.

SYNTHETIC CANDELILLA WAX • *See* Swertia Extract and Candelilla Wax.

SYNTHETIC CARNAUBA • *See* Carnauba Wax.

SYNTHETIC HECTORITE • *See* Hectorite.

SYNTHETIC JAPAN WAX • *See* Japan Wax.

SYNTHETIC JASMINE • *See* Cinnamic Aldehyde.

SYNTHETIC SPERMACETI • Widely used substitutes for spermaceti (*see*).

SYNTHETIC WAX • A hydrocarbon wax derived from various oils.

SYRINGA VULGARIS • *See* Lilac.

SYSTEMIC • Having a generalized effect; causing physical or chemical changes throughout the body.

T

TABEBUIA • Lapacho. Pau D'arco. *Tabecuia heptaphylla* or *T. impetiginosa.* The inner bark of a tree in the forests of Brazil, it was used by Brazilian Indians for the treatment of cancer. Used as a skin conditioner and humectant in cosmetics. Contains quinones and lapachol. It also is used to treat fungal and parasitic infections, and to aid digestion. Also reportedly lowers blood sugar. It is now being studied in Brazil to treat cancers, including leukemia.

TAED • Tetraacetylethylenediamine is a bleaching activator that is mainly used in detergents and additives for laundry washing and dishwashing. Very low toxicity.

TAGETES • Meal, Extract, and Oil. The meal is the dried, ground flower petals of the Aztec marigold, a strong-scented, tropical American herb, mixed with no more than 0.3 percent ethoxyquin, an herbicide and antioxidant. The extract is taken from tagetes petals. Both the meal and the extract are used to enhance the yellow color of chicken skin and eggs. The oil is extracted from the Aztec flower and used in fruit flavorings and in cosmetics as a skin conditioner.

TAIMU YU • Essential oil from the herb *Thymus serpillum* or *T. vulgarus.* Used as a fragrance ingredient and skin conditioner. *See* Thyme.

TAISOU EKISU • Chinese date extract of *Ziziphus jujuba,* which can be eaten hard and ripe, when it tastes like an apple, or it can be left on the tree to dry naturally, when it tastes like a date. It is used as a skin conditioner.

TALC • French Chalk. The main ingredient of baby and bath powders, face powders, eye shadows, liquid powders, protective creams, dry rouges, face masks, foundation cake makeups, skin fresheners, foot powders, and face creams. Gives a slippery sensation to powders and creams. Talc is finely powdered native magnesium silicate, a mineral. It usually has small amounts of other powders such as boric acid or zinc oxide added as a coloring ingredient. Prolonged inhalation can cause lung problems because it is similar in chemical composition to asbestos, a known lung irritant and cancer-causing ingredient. The EU says the label must read "Keep powder away from children's nose and mouth."

TALCUM POWDER • Talc-based powders have been linked to ovarian cancer. In Boston's Brigham and Women's Hospital, of 215 women with ovarian cancer, 32 had used talcum powder on their genitals and sanitary napkins. Talc easily works its way up the reproductive tract. Eventually, a few particles reach the ovary and may set the stage for cancer. All factors considered in the study, the risk of ovarian cancer was raised to 3.28 times greater for women who use talc than for women who don't. Daniel Cramer, M.D., the obstetrician-gynecologist who wrote of the findings in the journal *Cancer,* said further studies are needed before doctors could recommend that women should not use talc but said that he himself advises patients to use other products such as cornstarch-based powders or creams. Talcum powder has been reported to cause coughing, vomiting, or even pneumonia when it is used carelessly and inhaled by babies. The EU says the label must read "Keep powder away from children's nose and mouth." *See* Talc.

TALL OIL • Liquid Rosin. A by-product of the pine wood pulp industry and used to scent shampoos, soaps, varnishes, and fruit sprays. *Tall* is Swedish for "pine." Dark brown liquid; acrid odor. A fungicide and cutting oil. It may be a mild irritant and sensitizer. On the basis of available information, the CIR Expert Panel (*see*) concluded that it is safe as presently used in cosmetic formulations.

TALL OIL ACID • A mixture of rosin (*see*) and fatty acids recovered from tall oil (*see*). Used as a surfactant and cleansing ingredient.

TALL OIL BENZYL HYDROXYETHYL IMIDAZOLINIUM CHLORIDE • *See* Quaternary Ammonium Compounds and Tall Oil.

TALL OIL GLYCERIDES • A mixture of glycerides derived from tall oil. *See* Glycerides and Tall Oil.

TALL OIL HYDROXYETHYL IMIDAZOLINE • *See* Tall Oil and Imidazoline.

TALL OIL STEROL • *See* Phytosterols.

TALLAMIDE DEA • Antistatic and viscosity adjuster. DEA residues are cancer suspects. *See* Tall Oil.

TALLAMPHOPROPIONATE • *See* Tall Oil.

TALLOL • *See* Tall Oil.

TALLOW • The fat from the fatty tissue of bovine cattle and sheep in North America. Used in shaving creams, lipsticks, shampoos, and soaps. White, almost tasteless when pure, and generally harder than grease. May cause eczema and blackheads. On the basis of available information, the CIR Expert Panel (*see*) concluded that it is safe as presently used in cosmetic formulations. Tallow derivative means any chemical obtained through initial hydrolysis, saponification, or transesterification of tallow; chemical conversion of material obtained by hydrolysis, saponification, or transesterification may be applied to obtain the desired product. The UK does not prohibit the supply of a cosmetic product that contains any tallow derivative as long as the relevant method set out was used in the manufacture of that derivative and the manufacturer of the derivative has certified that that method was used in its manufacture.

TALLOW ACID • *See* Tallow.

TALLOW ALCOHOL • Fatty alcohol from tallow (*see*) used as an emulsifier and thickener.

TALLOW AMIDE • *See* Tallow.

TALLOW AMIDE DEA AND MEA • *See* Tallow.

TALLOW AMINE • *See* Tallow.

TALLOW AMINE OXIDE • *See* Tallow.

TALLOW DIHYDROXYETHYL BETAINE • An antistatic ingredient, a hair and skin conditioner, a thickener, and a cleanser. *See* Tallow and Quaternary Ammonium Compounds.

TALLOW GLYCERIDES • A mixture of triglycerides (fats) derived from tallow.

TALLOW HYDROXYETHYL IMIDAZOLINE • *See* Tallow and Imidazoline.

TALLOW IMIDAZOLINE • *See* Tallow.

TALLOW TRIMONIUM CHLORIDE • Tallow. Trimethyl Ammonium Chloride. *See* Quaternary Ammonium Compounds.

TALLOWALKONIUM CHLORIDE • *See* Tallow and Quaternary Ammonium Compounds.

TALLOWAMIDOPROPYL BETAINE • *See* Quaternary Ammonium Compounds.

TALLOWAMIDOPROPYL HYDROXYSULTAINE • *See* Quaternary Ammonium Compounds.

TALLOWAMIDOPROPYLAMINE OXIDE • *See* Tallow.

TALLOWAMINOPROPYLAMINE • *See* Quaternary Ammonium Compounds.

TALLOWAMPHOACETATE • *See* Quaternary Ammonium Compounds.

TALLOWETH-6 • *See* Tallow.

TAMARIND EXTRACT • The extract of *Tamarindus indica,* a large tropical tree grown in the East Indies and Africa. Preserved in sugar or syrup, it is used as a natural fruit flavoring. The pulp contains about 10 percent tartaric acid (*see*).

TAMARINDUS INDICA • *See* Tamarind Extract.

TAMARIX CHINENSIS • Salt Cedar. Extract of the leaves and flowers *Tamarix chinensis,* used as a skin conditioner and humectant. In humid weather, salt is secreted in droplets on the twigs of this shrub.

TAMPER-RESISTANT PACKAGING • Each manufacturer and packer who packages a cosmetic liquid oral hygiene product or vaginal product for retail sale shall package the product in a tamper-resistant package, if this product is accessible to the public while held for sale. A tamper-resistant package is one having an indicator or barrier to entry that, if breached or missing, can reasonably be expected to provide visible evidence to consumers that tampering has occurred. To reduce the likelihood of substitution of a tamper-resistant feature after tampering, the indicator or barrier to entry is required to be distinctive by design (e.g., an aerosol product container) or by the use of an identifying characteristic (e.g., a pattern, name, registered trademark, logo, or picture). For purposes of this entry, the term "distinctive by design" means the packaging cannot be duplicated with commonly available materials or through commonly available processes. The term "aerosol product" means a product that depends upon the power of a liquified or compressed gas to expel the contents from the container. A tamper-resistant package may involve an immediate-container and closure system or secondary-container or carton system or any combination of systems intended to provide a visual indication of package integrity. The tamper-resistant feature shall be designed to and shall remain intact when handled in a reasonable manner during manufacture, distribution, and retail display.

TANACETUM CINERARIIFOLIUM • *See* Pyrethrins.

TANAKURA CLAY • Native clay obtained from the Tanakura area in Japan. It is used as an absorbent and thickener.

TANGERINE OIL • *Citrus tangerina.* The oil obtained by expression from the peels of the ripe fruit from several related tangerine species. Reddish orange, with a pleasant orange aroma. Used in blueberry, mandarin, orange, tangerine, and other fruit flavorings. Used in "organic" cosmetics. A skin irritant. GRAS

TANG KUEI EXTRACT • The extract of the roots of *Angelica sinensis. See* Dong Quai.

TANNIC ACID • Used in sunscreen preparations, eye lotions, and antiperspirants. It occurs in the bark and fruit of many plants, notably in the bark of the oak and sumac, and in cherry, coffee, and tea. Used medicinally as a mild astringent, and when applied it may turn the skin brown. Also used in food flavorings. Tea contains tannic acid, and this explains its folk use as an eye lotion. Excessive use in creams or lotions by hypersensitive persons may lead to irritation, blistering, and increased pigmentation. Low toxicity orally, but large doses may cause gastric distress. The FDA issued a notice in 1992 that tannic acid has not been shown to be safe and effective as claimed in OTC digestive aid products, fever blister treatment products, and products to treat poison ivy, poison oak, and poison sumac. A mild temporary stinging sensation may be experienced with this use. Tannic acid in astringents, drugs, diaper rash products, fever blister preparations, and cold sore drugs were also on the list. It may still be used for other purposes.

TANNIN • Any of a broad group of plant-derived phenolic compounds characterized by their ability to precipitate proteins. Some are beneficial and some are toxic, depending upon their source. Tannins in herbs are astringents (*see*). They are soothing to the skin and mucous membranes. They can bind to the tissues of the intestines and reduce diarrhea and internal bleeding. Herbalists use them to treat burns and for wound healing. *See* Tannic Acid.

TANSY • *Tanacetum vulgare*. Bitter Buttons. Parsley Fern. A native of Greece, tansy is widespread in the United States in gardens and along highways. During the fifteenth century, it was used in a tea for gas, children's colic, and abdominal cramps, gout, and even for the plague. It was used for centuries by young girls in tea to alleviate slow and painful menstruation. It was considered a laxative, a gentle stimulant to digestion, and even a sedative. The plant is still listed in the United States Pharmacopeia chiefly for its use as a tea to avert colds and externally for use on bruises, tumors, and inflammations. If too much of tansy is taken, it can result in vomiting, convulsions, and death.

TAPIOCA STARCH • Used as a thickener.

TARAKTOGENOS KURZII • *See* Chaulmoogra Oil.

TARAXUM OFFICINALE • *See* Dandelion Leaf and Root.

TARCHONANTHUS CAMPHORATUS • Camphor Bush. Small tree named from the Greek meaning "funeral." Used in folk medicine to treat sinus problems and headache, it is also used in massaging to treat stiffness. In cosmetics, it is used as a fragrance.

TAR OIL • The volatile oil distilled from wood tar, generally from the family Pinaceae. Used externally to treat skin diseases, the principal toxic ingredients are phenols and naphthalenes. Toxicity estimates are hard to make because even the U.S. Pharmacopeia does not specify the phenol content of official preparations. However, if ingested, it is estimated that one ounce would kill. *See* Pine Tar Oil, which is a rectified tar oil used as a licorice flavoring.

TARO • *Colocasia esculenta*. Elephant's Ear. Dasheen. A starchy root grown throughout the tropics for its edible starch. It has to be peeled to remove its poisonous outer covering. Used to make the Hawaiian dish poi. Used in "organic" cosmetics.

TARRAGON • *Artemisia dracunculus*. Used in perfumery to improve the note (*see*) of chypre-type perfumes (*see*). Derived from the dried leaves of a small European perennial, wormwood. Pale yellow oil grown for its pungent aroma. Also used in making pickles and vinegar.

TARS • An antiseptic, deodorant, and bug killer. Any of the various dark brown or black bituminous, usually odorous, viscous liquids or semiliquids obtained by the destructive distillation of wood, coal, peat, shale, and other organic materials. Used in hair tonics and shampoos and as a licorice food flavoring. May cause allergic reactions.

TARTARIC ACID • Effervescent acid used in bath salts, denture powders, nail bleaches, hair-grooming aids, hair rinses, depilatories, and hair coloring. Widely distributed in nature in many fruits but usually obtained as a by-product of winemaking. Consists of colorless or translucent crystals or a white, fine-to-granular, crystalline powder that is odorless and has an acid taste. In strong solutions it may be mildly irritating to the skin.

TARTRAZINE • FD & C Yellow No. 5. Bright orange-yellow powder used in foods, drugs, and cosmetics and as a dye for wool and silk. Those allergic to aspirin are often allergic to tartrazine. Allergies have been reported in persons eating sweet corn, soft drinks, and cheese crackers—all colored with Yellow No. 5. It is derived from coal tar. The British and the EU Parliament want to ban this color because it reportedly exacerbates hyperactive behavior in children. Tartrazine (E102) is a yellow color used in a range of foods including soft drinks, sweets, and sauces. Studies have shown that eating foods or drinks containing tartrazine can cause nettle rash (urticaria), dermatitis (an allergic skin condition), asthma, or rhinitis (runny nose) in a very small number of people. The use of tartrazine has decreased in recent years. ASP. E

TAURINE • An amino acid found in almost every tissue of the body and is especially high in human milk. Most infant soy-protein formulas are now supplemented with taurine. Taurine is almost absent from vegetarian diets. It is believed necessary for healthy eyes, and it is an antioxidant. It is also used as a nutritional supplement in feed for growing chicks. Some researchers theorize irregular heartbeat is characteristic of lack of blood to the heart and may be partly due to loss of intracellular taurine. Much like magnesium, taurine affects membrane excitability by normalizing potassium flux in and out of the heart muscle cells. Supplementation may prevent digitalis-induced arrhythmias.

TAXUS CUSPIDATA • Japanese Yew.

TBS • *See* Tribromosalan.

TBHQ • *See* Tertiary Butylhydroquinone TCC • *See* Triclocarban.

TDI OXIDIZED MICROCRYSTALLINE WAX • Microcrystalline wax (*see*) that has been treated with toluene (*see*). Used as a thickener.

TEA- • The abbreviation for triethanolamine.

TEA • The leaves, leaf buds, and internodes of plants having leaves and fragrant white flowers, prepared and cured to make an aromatic beverage. Cultivated principally in China, Japan, Ceylon, and other Asian countries. Tea is a mold stimulant, and its tonic properties are due to the alkaloid caffeine; tannic acid (*see*) makes it astringent. Used by natural cosmeticians to reduce puffiness around the eyes. A cotton or gauze pad is dampened with a weak solution of tea and placed on the eyelids. One then lies down for five to ten minutes.

TEA EXTRACT • Now being studied for anti-aging properties. Has been reported to inhibit absorption of UV radiation. *See* Chinese Tea Extract.

TEA SORBATE • *See* Triethanolamine and Sorbic Acid.

TEA TREE OIL • Essential oil from the leaves of an Australian tree, *Melaleuca alternifolia.* Used as a germicide in cosmetics. Eleven to thirteen times as powerful as carbolic acid. Penetrates the skin quickly and accelerates the healing of skin disorders.

TEA-ABIETOYL HYDROLYZED COLLAGEN • The salt of the condensation product of abietic acid chloride and hydrolyzed animal protein. The word *animal* was taken out of this ingredient's name. Used as a skin conditioner. *See* Hydrolyzed Protein.

TEA-ACRYLATES/ACRYLONITROGENS COPOLYMER • *See* Acrylates.

TEA-ALGINATE • Salt of alginic acid (*see*) used as an emulsifier and thickener.

TEA-C12–15 ALKYL SULFATE • *See* Triethanolamine, Alcohol, and Sulfates.

TEA-CANOLATE • A cleanser and emulsifier derived from canola oil (*see*).

TEA-COCOATE • The triethanolamine (*see*) soap derived from coconut fatty acids (*see*).

TEA-COCOYL ALANINATE • Hair-conditioning ingredient. *See* Allantoin and Coconut Oil.

TEA-COCOYL GLUTAMATE • Softener. *See* Coconut Acids and Glutamic Acid.

TEA-COCOYL HYDROLYZED COLLAGEN • Can cause sensitivity. *See* Hydrolyzed Collagen, Animal Protein Derivative, and Anionic Surfactants.

TEA-COCOYL HYDROLYZED SOY PROTEIN • Hair conditioner. Can cause sensitivity. *See* Coconut Oil and Soy.

TEA-COCOYL SARCOSINATE • *See* Cocoyl Sarcosine.

TEA-DEXTRIN OCTENYLSUCCINATE • An emulsifier, humectant, emollient, and hair conditioner. *See* Dextrin.

TEA-DODECYLBENZENESULFONATE • *See* Sulfonated Oils.

TEA-EDTA • *See* Ethylenediamine Tetraacetic Acid.

TEA-HYDROCHLORIDE • The salt of hydrochloric acid (*see*).

TEA-HYDROGENATED TALLOWOYL GLUTAMATE • A softener. *See* Glutamate.

TEA-HYDRIODIDE • *See* Iodide.

TEA-ISOSTEARATE • *See* Triethanolamine and Isostearic Acid.

TEA-LACTATE • *See* Triethanolamine and Lactic Acid.

TEA-LANETH-5 SULFATE • *See* Surfactants.

TEA-LAURAMINOPROPIONATE • *See* Quaternary Ammonium Compounds.

TEA-LAURETH SULFATE • *See* Anionic Surfactants.

TEA-LAUROYL COLLAGEN AMINO ACIDS • Protein enhancer for cosmetic creams. *See* Hydrolyzed Protein.

TEA-LAUROYL GLUTAMATE • A softener. *See* Glutamate.

TEA-LAUROYL KERATIN AMINO ACIDS • *See* Keratin Amino Acids.

TEA-LAUROYL LACTYLATE • *See* Lauric Acid and Triethanolamine.

TEA-LAUROYL SARCOSINATE • *See* Sarcosine.

TEA-LAURYL BENZENE SULFONATE • *See* Surfactants.

TEA-LAURYL SULFATE • Widely used cleansing ingredient and emulsifier. Used in hair products, bath preparations, body and hand preparations, and mud packs. Concentrations greater than 10.5 percent may cause irritation, especially if allowed to remain in contact with the skin for significant periods of time. On the basis of the available information, the CIR Expert Panel (*see*) found it safe in the early 1980s but is considering new information to determine if the final safety assessment should be reaffirmed, amended, or have an addendum. *See* Sodium Lauryl Sulfate.

TEA-MYRISTAMINOPROPIONATE • *See* Surfactants.

TEA-MYRISTATE • Emulsifier and surfactant. May promote acne. *See* Myristic Acid and Surfactants. E

TEA-MYRISTOL HYDROLYZED COLLAGEN • *See* Animal Protein and Surfactants.

TEA-OLEAMIDO PEG-2 SULFOSUCCINATE • Triethanolamine and succinic acid (*see both*).

TEA-OLEATE • Triethanolamine Oleate. *See* Oleic Acid and Ethanolamines.

TEA-OLEOYL HYDROGENATED COLLAGEN • The hydrolyzed collagen is the salt of the condensation product of oleic acid and collagen.

TEA-OLEOYL SARCOSINATE • *See* Oleic Acid and Sarcosine.

TEA-PALM KERNEL SARCOSINATE • *See* Palm Kernel Oil and Sarcosine.

TEA-PALMITATE • Emulsifier and surfactant. May cause contact dermatitis. *See* Palmitic Acid.

TEA-C12–13 PARETH-3 SULFATE • Emulsifier. *See* Triethanolamine and Sulfates.

TEA-PCA • *See* Ethanolamines.

TEA-PEG-3 COCOAMIDE SULFATE • *See* Surfactants.

TEA-SALICYLATE • *See* Salicylic Acid and Triethanolamine.

TEA-STEARATE • Emulsifier and surfactant. Widely used in makeup and moisturizers. May cause sensitivity. *See* Triethanolamine and Stearic Acid.

TEA-SULFATE • *See* Triethanolamine and Sulfuric Acid.

TEA-TALLATE • *See* Fatty Acids and Tall Oil.

TEA-TRIDECYLBENZENESULFONATE • *See* Surfactants.

TEA-UNDECYLENOYL HYDROLYZED COLLAGEN • *See* Hydrolyzed Protein.

TECOMA CURIALIS EXTRACT • *See* Lapacho Extract.

TELANGIECTASIS • The dilation of groups of small blood vessels, appearing as fine lines on the skin.

TELFAIRIA PEDATA OIL • Oyster Nut Oil. From a perennial grown in Central and East Africa. It is drought tolerant and can grow at elevations up to 2,000 m. The nuts are relished by people in Tanzania and are normally planted directly in the drip line of existing trees. The species existence in cultivation in Meru (Kenya), Kabale (Uganda), Mauritius. Malawi is given by some authors. The seed is rich in fats and minerals, is part of the traditional food of breastfeeding mothers, and is now primarily eaten by children. The nuts are sold by vendors in Tanzanian markets. Used as an emollient and cover-up in cosmetics. Used as a gel for African hair.

TEMPORARY TATTOOS • Those applied to the skin with a moistened wad of cotton, which fade several days after application. Many contain color additives approved for cosmetic use on the skin. However, the FDA has received reports of allergic reactions to some temporary tattoos. An import alert is in effect for several foreign-made temporary tattoos. According to Consumer Safety Officer Allen Halper of the FDA's Office of Cosmetics and Colors, the temporary tattoos subject to the import alert are not allowed into the United States because they don't have the required ingredient declaration on the label or they contain colors not permitted for use in cosmetics applied to the skin. Henna (*see*), a coloring made from a plant, is approved only for use as a hair dye, not for direct application to the skin, as in the body-decorating process known as mehndi. This unapproved use of a color additive makes these products adulterated and therefore illegal. An import alert is in effect for henna intended for use on the skin. The FDA has received reports of injuries to the skin from products marketed as henna. Since henna typically produces a brown, orange-brown, or reddish-brown tint, other ingredients must be added to produce other colors, such as those marketed as "black henna" and "blue henna." So-called black henna may contain the coal tar color *p*-phenylenediamine (*see*), also known as PPD. This ingredient may cause allergic reactions in some individuals. The only legal use of PPD in cosmetics is as a hair dye. It is not approved for direct application to the skin. Even brown shades of products marketed as henna may contain other ingredients intended to make them darker or make the stain last longer. In addition to color additives, these skin-decorating products may contain other ingredients, such as solvents. Cosmetics including temporary skin-staining products that are sold on a retail basis to consumers must have their ingredients listed on the label. Without such an ingredient declaration, they are considered misbranded and are illegal in interstate commerce. The FDA requires the ingredient declaration under the authority of the Fair Packaging and Labeling Act (FPLA). Because the FPLA does not apply to cosmetic samples and products used exclusively by professionals—for example, for application at a salon, or a booth at a fair or boardwalk—the requirement for an ingredient declaration does not apply to these products.

TEN-K • *See* Potassium Chloride.

TEPHROSIA PURPUREA • Skin conditioner. The plant is used as a digestive, diuretic, and antitussive in Ayurvedic (Indian) medicine. It has undergone clinical trials in viral hepatitis and is claimed to improve liver function. The roots have weak insecticidal action. In the commonly used doses no adverse reactions are reported.

TERATOGENIC • From the Greek *terat* (monster) and Latin *genesis* (origin): the origin or cause of a monster—or defective—fetus.

TEREBINTH • *See* Turpentine Tree.

TEREPHTHALIC ACID/ISOPHTHALIC ACID/SODIUM ISOPHTHALIC ACID SULFONATE/GLYCOL COPOLYMER • Synthetic hair fixative. *See* Phthalic Acid and Sulfonates.

TEREPHTHALYLIDENE DICAMPHOR SULFONIC ACID • Ecamsule. It is an organic compound that absorbs ultraviolet (UV) light. The FDA approved it for OTC sunscreen as has the European Commission. Based on their review, the EU concluded that use of this ingredient in cosmetic products as a UV light absorber at a maximum concentration of 10 percent would not pose a health hazard. They also concluded that this ingredient could be used in combination with any other listed UV absorber up to the 10 percent concentration level.

TERMINALIA CATAPPA • Belongs to a large family of tropical trees and shrubs. *See* Almond Oil.

TERPENELESS OILS • An essential oil from which the terpene components have been removed by extraction and fractionation, either alone or in combination. The terpeneless grades are more highly concentrated than the original oil. Removal of the terpenes is necessary to inhibit spoilage, particularly of oils derived from citrus. *See* Terpenes.

TERPENES • A class of unsaturated hydrocarbons occurring in most essential oils and plant resins. Among terpene derivatives are camphor and menthol (*see both*). Some terpenes are used as antiseptics.

TERPINEOL • A colorless, viscous liquid with a lilaclike odor, insoluble in mineral oil and slightly soluble in water. It is primarily used as a flavoring ingredient but is also employed as a denaturant to make alcohol undrinkable. It has been used as an antiseptic. It can be a sensitizer.

TERPINYL ACETATE • Colorless liquid, odor suggestive of bergamot and lavender. Slightly soluble in water and glycerol. Derived by heating terpineol with acetic acid (*see both*). Used as a perfume and flavoring ingredient.

TERPINYL FORMATE • Formic Acid. A synthetic fruit-flavoring ingredient. *See* Turpentine for toxicity.

TERPINYL PROPIONATE • A synthetic fruit-flavoring ingredient, colorless with a lavender odor. Derived by heating terpineol with propionic acid (*see both*). Used as a synthetic fruit-flavoring ingredient for beverages, ice cream, ices, candy, and baked goods. *See* Turpentine for toxicity.

TERSA-TAR • *See* Coal Tar.

TERTIARY BUTYLHYDROQUINONE • TBHQ. This antioxidant was put on the market after years of pressure by food manufacturers to get it approved. It contains the petroleum-derived butane and is used either alone or in combination with the preservative-antioxidant butylatedhydroxyanisole (BHA) and/or butylated hydroxytoluene (BHT). Application to the skin may cause allergic reactions. On the Canadian Hotlist (*see*).

TESLAC • Neither an anabolic nor androgenic steroid. It is considered a sex hormone that is a relative of testosterone and was developed for women for medical purposes. Teslac is widely used in the steroid community as probably the most effective anti-estrogen. When combined with Proviron, Teslac is almost certain to completely prevent estrogen conversion and its associated problems. It is also reputed to stimulate the body's natural production of testosterone. Testolactone is the chemical name of the active ingredient in Teslac. Teslac is a registered trademark of E.R. Squibb & Sons, Inc. in the United States and/or other countries.

TESTICULAR CANCER • Tumors in the testicles, which account for the majority of solid malignancies in males under thirty years of age.

TESTICULAR EXTRACT • Extract of bovine testicular tissue.

TESTICULAR HYDROLYSATE • The testicular hydrolysate of animal testicular tissue. Used in skin creams.

TESTOSTERONE • The male hormone. Women have some of it too. The FDA maintains "cosmetics" containing hormones are drugs. Manufacturers, however, are using substitutes, such as wild yam, that produce diosgenin, a precursor to natural progesterone, though not actual progesterone and dihydro-testosterone (DHT), a by-product of testosterone. Potential adverse reactions to the hormone testosterone in women include acne, edema, oily skin, weight gain, hairiness, hoarseness, clitoral enlargement, changes in libido, flushing, sweating, and vaginitis with itching. In both sexes, edema, gastroenteritis, nausea, vomiting, diarrhea, constipation, change in appetite, bladder irritability, jaundice, liver toxicity, and high levels of calcium can occur. Presumably, the substitute testosterones are so weak that they probably have no effect but results are still uncertain. Testosterone is in some male skin creams. China has asked for a ban on testosterone in cosmetics.

TESTRED • *See* Methyltestosterone.

TETRAACETYLPHYTOSPHINGOSINE • Hair and skin conditioner. *See* Acetic Acid and Phytosphingosine.

TETRAAMINOPYRIMIDINE SULFATE • The EU gave manufacturers to July 2005 to submit safety information or the substance will be proposed for a ban. A hair coloring. It is being used to test irritation instead of the Draize test (*see*). *See* Coal Tar.

TETRABORATES • Bath products. Should not be used in products for children under three years. In hair-waving products for adults, should be rinsed well, according to the EU.

TETRABROMOFLUORESCEIN • Eosine Yellow. A red color with a yellowish or brownish tinge prepared by adding bromine fluorescein (*see*). Used to make lipstick indelible and to color nail polish. It may cause photosensitivity (*see*) and has caused inflamed lips and respiratory and gastrointestinal symptoms. Tetrabromofluorescein is also used to dye wool, silk, and paper. The EU bans bromine in cosmetics.

TETRABUTYOXYPROPYL TRISILOXANE • An emollient. *See* Silicones.

TETRACAINE • Pontocaine. Pontocaine Eye. A local anesthetic used by doctors who apply permanent "makeup"—tattooing for the lips and around the eyes. Potential adverse reactions include skin reactions and swelling. On the Canadian Hotlist (*see*). The EU and ASEAN (*see*) have banned it in cosmetics.

TETRACHLOROETHYLENE • Perchloroethylene. A colorless, nonflammable liquid with a pleasant odor, made from acetylene and chlorine. Used as a solvent in cosmetics. Narcotic in high doses. Has a drying action on the skin and can lead to adverse skin reactions. On the Canadian Hotlist (*see*). The EU banned it in cosmetics.

TETRADECENE • An emollient. *See* Decanoic Acid.

TETRADECYLEICOSANOIC ACID • Emulsifier and thickener. *See* Decanoic Acid.

TETRADECYLEICOSANOL • Emollient. *See* Myristic Acid and Arachadonic Acid.

TETRADECYLEICOSYL STEARATE • Skin conditioner. *See* Stearic Acid and Myristic Acid.

TETRADECYLOCTADECANOIC ACID • Emulsifier. *See* Decanoic Acid.

TETRADECYLOCTADECANOL • *See* Octanoic Acid and Alcohol.

TETRADECYLOCTADECYL BEHENATE • Emulsifier and emollient. *See* Behenamide.

TETRADECYLOCTADECYL MYRISTATE • Emulsifier, opacifier, and skin conditioner. *See* Myristic Acid.

TETRADECYLOCTADECYL • Stearate. Emulsifier, skin conditioner, opacifier. *See* Stearic Acid.

TETRADIBUTYL PENTAERITHRITYL HYDROXYHYDROCINNAMATE • Antioxidant. *See* Cinnimate and Phenols.

TETRAETHYLTHIURAM DISULFIDE • Thiram. An agricultural chemical found to be a degerming ingredient when incorporated in soap. A disinfectant, insecticide, fungicide, and bacteria killer. May cause irritation of nose, throat, and skin. Can cause allergic skin reactions. The EU banned thiuram in cosmetics.

TETRAGLYCOSYLCERAMIDE • Derives from the covering of nerve tissue of animals. Used in skin creams and moisturizers. Producers claim ceramide-containing compositions have a high capacity for recovering diminished water-retaining properties of preheated or damaged skin. Furthermore, they maintain that the ceramide-containing compositions protect the skin against irritation.

TETRAHEXYLDECYL ASCORBATE • Antioxidant and skin conditioner. *See* Ascorbic Acid.

TETRAHYDROBISDEMTHOXYDIFERULOYMETHANE • Antioxidant and oral care ingredient. *See* Curcumin and Phenols.

TETRAHYDROCURCUMINOIDS • Curcuminoids from turmeric (*see*) without the yellow color, providing antioxidant protection and skin-lightening effects.

TETRAHYDROFURAN • Solvent derived from furan for natural and synthetic resins, particularly vinyls, protective coatings, adhesives, and printing inks. Toxic by ingestion.

TETRAHYDROFURFURYL ACETATE • *See* Furfural.

TETRAHYDROFURFURYL ALCOHOL • A liquid that absorbs water and is flammable in air. A solvent for cosmetic fats, waxes, and resins. Mixes with water, ether, and acetone. Mildly irritating to the skin and mucous membranes. *See* Furfural.

TETRAHYDROGERANYL HYDROXYL STEARATE • *See* Stearic Acid and Hydroxylation.

TETRAHYDRO-6-NITROQUINOXALINE • Hair coloring. *See* Coal Tar.

TETRAHYDROPIPERINE • Skin conditioner. *See* Piperine.

TETRAHYDROXYPROPYL ETHYLENEDIAMINE • Clear, colorless, thick liquid, a component of the bacteria-killing substance in sugarcane. It is strongly alkaline and is used as a solvent and preservative. It may be irritating to the skin and mucous membranes and may cause skin sensitization.

TETRAMETHRIN • Preservative. *See* Pyrethrins.

TETRAMETHYL AMMONIUM CHLORIDE • *See* Quaternary Ammonium Compounds.

TETRAMETHYL CYCLOPENTENE BUTENOL • A fragrance ingredient.

TETRAMETHYL DECYNEDIOL • *See* Fatty Alcohols.

TETRAMETHYL TETRAPHENYL TRISILOXANE • Skin conditioner. *See* Siloxanes.

TETRAPEPTIDE-1 • Combination of the amino acids leucine, praline, threonine, and valine used as a skin conditioner.

TETRAPOTASSIUM PYROPHOSPHATE • TKPP. A sequestering, clarifying, and buffering ingredient for shampoos. Produced by molecular dehydration of dibasic sodium phosphate. Insoluble in alcohol. A water softener in bath preparations.

TETRASELMIS SUECICA • Extract of a sea plankton. *See* Algae.

TETRASODIUM DICARBOXYETHYLSTEARYL SULFOSUCCINANATE • *See* Surfactants.

TETRASODIUM EDTA • Sodium Edetate. Powdered sodium salt that reacts with metals. A sequestering ingredient and chelating ingredient (*see both*) used in cosmetic solutions. Widely used in baby products, colognes, bath products, eye makeup, fragrance, hair coloring, powder and sprays, cuticle softeners, and indoor tanning preparations. Can deplete the body of calcium if taken internally. *See* Ethylenediamine Tetraacetic Acid.

TETRASODIUM ETIDRONATE • *See* Tetrasodium EDTA.

TETRASODIUM PYROPHOSPHATE • TSPP. A buffering and chelating ingredient (*see both*). Also used in dentifrices, hair colorings, permanent waves, cleansers, and face and neck products. *See* Sodium Pyrophosphate Peroxide.

TETRAHYDROZOLINE AND ITS SALTS • Used to take the red out of the eyes in eye drops and as a nasal decongestant. Among the more serious adverse effects are irritation to mucosa, rebound nasal congestion, and effects associated with systemic absorption, including sedation, alterations in cardiovascular functions, and hypertension. Banned in cosmetics by ASEAN and the EU.

TEUCRIUM CANADENSE • Creeping Germander. *See* Germander Extract.

TEUCRIUM SCORODONIA • *See* Germander Extract.

TEXTURIZER • A chemical used to improve the texture of various cosmetics. For instance, in creams that tend to become lumpy, calcium chloride (*see*) is added to keep them smooth.

THALASSOTHERAPY • *Thalassa* is Greek for sea. It is usually a spa treatment that uses seawater and seaweed to "oxygenate, tone, moisturize, and revitalize the body and the skin." The theory is that seawater contains at least sixty different minerals and trace elements, most of which are essential to the human organism. These include iodine, iron, copper, zinc, manganese, strontium, molybdenum, boron, and a vast range of vitamins, trace elements, minerals, and plankton. These natural elements can be found in seaweed at concentrations of 50,000 to 100,000 times the quantities found in seawater. *See* Ascophyllum Nodosum.

THAUMATOCOCCUS DANIELLII • Thaumatin. A mixture of intensely sweet-tasting proteins extracted from the fruit of a West African plant, *Thaumatococcus daniellii*. It has about 2,000 to 3,000 times the sweetness of sugar. It does contain calories. The fruits of the plant have been used for centuries by the West Africans as a source of sweetness. It is also sold in Japan. Because of problems with stability, taste profile, and compatibility, thaumatin is used primarily as a flavor enhancer, at levels below the sweet-taste threshold. It is awaiting approval in the United States.

THEANINE • An amino acid used as an emollient. *See* Amino Acids.

THENOYL METHIONATE • An amino acid compound used to treat hair.

THEOBROMA CACAO • *See* Theobroma Oil.

THEOBROMA GRANDIFLORUM • Cupuaçu Tree. Native in the southeast of Pará, Brazil, the fruit pulp is used for the production of juice, ice cream, yogurts, and other fresh products. Closely related to the cocoa tree, which makes it sometimes a cocoa substitute. Used in cosmetics as a skin-conditioning ingredient.

THEOBROMA OIL • Cacao Butter. Cocoa Butter. Yellowish white solid with chocolatelike taste and odor derived from the cacao bean. Widely used in confections, suppositories, pharmaceuticals, soaps, and cosmetics. Also used as a skin protectant but may cause allergic reactions in the sensitive.

THEOBROMINE • The alkaloid found in cocoa, kola nuts, tea, and chocolate products, closely related to caffeine. It is used as a diuretic, smooth muscle relaxant, heart stimulant, and blood-vessel dilator in medications. In cosmetics, it is used as a skin conditioner. The EU bans bromine in cosmetics. *See* Theobroma Oil.

THEOPHYLLINE • A white powder, soluble in water. Occurs in tea. It is used in cosmetics as a skin conditioner. It is a smooth muscle relaxant, heart stimulant, and diuretic (reduces body water). It can cause nausea and vomiting if ingested. The toxic dose in man is only 2.9 milligrams per kilogram of body weight. It is on the Canadian Hotlist (*see*).

THEVETIA NERIFOLIA JUSS • On the Canadian Hotlist (*see*). The EU banned it in cosmetics. *See* Oleander.

THIABENDAZOLE • A mold retardant. Moderately toxic by ingestion.

THIAMINE • Vitamin B_1. Essential nutrient for calcium metabolism and also involved in nerve function.

THIAMINE DIPHOSPHATE • Most abundant form of thiamine in animal tissue. *See* Thiamine.

THIANTHOL • Ingredient claimed to aid the promotion of skin support membrane. It is used to make artificial skin. *See* Niacin.

THICKENERS • Substances to add body to lotions and creams. Those usually employed include such natural gums as sodium alginate and pectins.

THIGH CREAMS • Many of these creams said to slim and counteract cellulite (*see*) on thighs contain aminophylline (*see*), an approved prescription drug used in the treatment of asthma. Since some individuals suffer from allergic reactions to ethylenediamine, a component of aminophylline, the FDA is concerned about the use of this ingredient in cosmetics. Drugs, unlike cosmetics, alter the structure or function of the body and are subject to an intensive review and approval process by the FDA before their release to the public. Thigh creams may more appropriately be classified as drugs under the Food, Drug, and Cosmetic Act since removal or reduction of cellulite affects the "structure or function" of the body.

THIMEROSAL • Mercurochrome. The metallo-organic compound also called merthielate. Used as a bacteriostat and fungistat in eye preparations. May cause allergic reaction from either the mercury or the salicylates in the compound. It is on the Canadian Hotlist (*see*).

THIO- • Prefix used to indicate sulfur in a compound usually as a substitute for oxygen.

2,2´-THIOBIS (4-CHLOROPHENOL) • *See* Phenols.

THIOCTIC ACID • Antioxidant. *See* Valeric Acid.

THIOCYANATE • Colorless or white crystals derived from cyanide. Used in animal feed to stimulate growth.

THIODIGLYCOL • *See* Thioglycolic Acid Compounds.

THIODIGLYCOLAMIDE • *See* Quaternary Ammonium Compounds.

THIODIPROPIONIC ACID • An acid freely soluble in hot water, alcohol, and acetone. Used as an antioxidant in general food use. Used also for soap products and polymers (*see*) of ethylene. GRAS

THIOGLYCERIN • A depilatory and hair-waving or hair-straightening ingredient. *See* Thioglycolic Acid Compounds and Glycerin.

THIOGLYCEROL • Used in soothing skin lotions. Prepared by heating glycerin (*see*) and alcohol. Yellowish, very viscous liquid, with a slight sulfur odor. Used to promote wound healing.

THIOGLYCOLATE • A salt or ester of thioglycolic acid; frequently used in bacterial media to reduce their oxygen content so as to create favorable conditions for the growth of bacteria.

THIOGLYCOLIC ACID COMPOUNDS • Thioglycollic Acid. Prepared by the action of sodium sulfohydrate on sodium chloroacetate. A liquid with a strong unpleasant odor; mixes with water and alcohol. The ammonium and sodium salts are used in permanent wave solutions and as a hair straightener. The EU recommends it be applied by professionals. The calcium salts are used in depilatories, hair-waving solutions, and lotions. Thioglycolates can cause hair breakage, skin irritations, severe allergic reactions, and pustular reactions. On the Canadian Hotlist (*see*). Canadians limit it to 5 percent in depilatories.

THIOINDIGOID DYE • *See* Vat Dyes and Indigo.

THIOKOL • One of the first synthetic elastomers (*see*), it is used in face masks and nail enamels and in the manufacture of rubbers and resins.

THIOLACTIC ACID • Used in depilatories and hair-waving preparations. *See* Thioglycolic Acid Compounds.

THIOLANEDIOL • An antibacterial. *See* Phenols.

THIOMALIC ACID • *See* Malic Acid.

THIOMORPHOLINONE • *See* Morpholine.

THIONYL CHLORIDE • Pale yellow or red liquid with suffocating odor. Used in pesticides and plastics. Strong irritant to the skin.

THIOSALICYLIC ACID • Sulfur yellow flakes, slightly soluble in hot water. Used in the manufacture of cosmetic dyes.

THIOSINAMINE • Thios. Made from mustard oil, alcohol, and ammonia, it is used by homeopaths to treat scars.

THIOTAURINE • An antioxidant. *See* Taurine.

THIOUREA • White, lustrous crystals with a bitter taste made by heating ammonium thiocyanate. Used in hair preparations, and as a mold inhibitor. A carcinogen. May not be used in food products. Skin irritant. Allergenic. On the Canadian Hotlist (*see*). The EU banned it in cosmetics with one exception, its use in hair straighteners.

THIOXANTHINE • *See* Xanthene.

THISTLE • *Carduus marianus. Cnicus benedictus. Sonchus oleraceus.* Sow Thistle. Holy Thistle. Several thistles were used as medicinal herbs, including holy thistle. Holy thistle is a native of Greece and Italy and is an annual. Sow thistle, a vile-smelling weed, appeared in English medicine in 1387 and was mentioned frequently since then as a tonic. It is used in "organic" cosmetics. Cotton thistle extract can help repair and restructure damaged skin, claims the French ingredients supplier Gattefossé. The ingredient, named Gatuline Skin-Repair Bio, is designed for use in anti-aging products and sunburn treatments, as well as products designed to help skin damaged by cosmetic treatments such as dermabrasion and peels.

THIURAM • On the Canadian Hotlist (*see*). The EU banned it in cosmetics. *See* Tetraethylthiuram Disulfide.

THREONINE • An essential amino acid (*see*); the last to be discovered (1935). Prevents the buildup of fat in the liver. Occurs in whole eggs, skim milk, casein, and gelatin. Used in hair and skin conditioners.

THUJA OCCIDENTALIS • *See* White Cedar Leaf Oil.

THUJA OIL • *Thuja occidentalis.* Northern White Cedar. Cedar Leaf Oil. The twigs of this evergreen contain volatile oils, glycosides, flavonoids, mucilage, and tannin (*see all*). Thuja's main action is due to its stimulating volatile oil. It is used by herbalists as an expectorant, a stimulant to smooth muscles, a diuretic, and an astringent. Has a marked antifungal effect and is used externally for ringworm. Also used to treat psoriasis and urinary incontinence due to loss of muscle tone. Thuja preparations are toxic when ingested in large amounts. They can cause miscarriage, a drop in blood pressure, spasms, coma, and even death. The oil is contraindicated in pregnancy, or in persons with gastrointestinal inflammation, liver, or kidney dysfunction. *See* White Cedar Leaf Oil.

THUJOPSIS DOLABRATA • A Japanese tree that contains a compound that is antifungal. It is used as a skin-conditioning ingredient in cosmetics.

THUNDER GOD VINE • *Tripterygium wilfordii.* Lei Gong Tang. The Chinese have been using the root medicinally for centuries to treat arthritis, systemic lupus erythematosus, chronic hepatitis, and a variety of skin disorders.

THURFYLNICOTINATE HCL • Skin conditioner. *See* Nicotinic Acid.

THYME • *Thymus vulgaris.* Used to flavor toothpastes and mouthwashes, and to scent perfumes, after-shave lotions, and soap. It is a seasoning from the dried leaves and flowering tops of the wild, creeping thyme grown in Eurasia and throughout the United States. May cause contact dermatitis and hay fever.

THYMINE • Skin conditioner. A derivative of nucleic acids (*see*). Originally derived from the thymus glands of animals.

THYMOL • Used in mouthwashes and to scent perfumes, after-shave lotions, and soap. Obtained from the essential oil of lavender, origanum oil, and other volatile oils. It destroys mold and is a topical antifungal ingredient with a pleasant aromatic odor. It is omitted from hypoallergenic cosmetics because it can cause allergic reactions. GRAS. ASP

THYMUS CITRIODORUS • Lemon Thyme. *See* Thyme.

THYMUS EXTRACT • The extract of animal thymus gland, an organ in the chest that helps to activate the body's defenses against infections. Used in skin creams.

THYMUS HYDROXYLATE • The hydrolysate of animal thymus derived by acid, enzyme, or other method of hydrolysis. *See* Thymus Extract.

THYMUS SERPILLUM • Taimu Yu. Wild Thyme. Used as a moisturizer. *See* Thyme.

THYMUS VULGARIS • Skin-conditioning ingredient in many cosmetics. *See* Thymus Serpillum.

THYMUS ZYGIS OIL • Fragrance ingredient. *See* Thyme.

THYROID HORMONE • The thyroid gland is an endocrine (meaning ductless) gland, which secretes its hormones directly into the bloodstream. It is located in the lower front part of the neck just in front of the trachea. The thyroid gland needs iodine to make thyroid hormones. These hormones influence many bodily functions, such as physical growth and development, metabolism, puberty, organ function, fertility, and body temperature. These functions depend on two of the most important hormones released from the thyroid gland, triiodothyronine (T3) and thyroxine (T4).

THYROPROPIC ACID AND ITS SALTS • A relative of thyroid hormone with a slightly different structure. Banned by the UK and ASEAN (*see*) in cosmetics. *See* Thyroid Hormone.

THYROTHRICINE • An antibacterial substance produced by the growth of *Bacillus brevis Dubos* (Fam. Bacteriaceae), used in mouthwash. Banned in cosmetics by ASEAN (*see*), the UK, and the EU, and it is on the Canadian Hotlist (*see*).

TIARE FLOWER • The flower obtained from *Gardenia tahitensis. See* Gardenia.

TILIA AMERICANA • *See* Basswood Extract.

TILIA CORDATA OIL AND WATER • A skin conditioner used in many cleansing creams and lotions as well as skin fresheners, eye makeup preparations, and bath products. *See* Linden Extract.

TILIA PLATYPHYLLOS • *See* Linden Extract.

TILIA TOMENTOSA • *See* Linden Extract.

TILIA VULGARIS • *See* Linden Extract.

TILLANDSIA USNEODIDES • *See* Spanish Moss.

TIMONACIC • Skin conditioner. Prepared from the amino acid cysteine and formaldehyde. Used in medicine to protect the liver.

TIN CHLORIDE • *See* Stannous Chloride.

TIN OXIDE • A coloring ingredient and an abrasive in cosmetics. A brownish black powder insoluble in water.

TINCTURE • A solution in alcohol of the flavors derived from plants obtained by mashing or boiling.

TINEA CRURIS • *See* Jock Itch.
TINCTURE OF BENZOIN • *See* Benzoin.
TINEA PEDIS • *See* Athlete's Foot.
TINEA VERSICOLOR • An eruption of tan or brown patches on the skin of the trunk, often appearing white in contrast with tan skin after exposure to the summer sun.
TINOSAN • Swiss ingredient manufacturer Ciba says at this writing, it is readying its Tinosan SDC antimicrobial for the European market and should have it approved by mid-2009 for use as a preservative. Tinosan SDC has been developed around a water-soluble silver citrate complex that helps kill a wide range of potentially harmful microorganisms. Clinical trials conducted by the company have shown that the ingredient has broad-spectrum activity covering gram-positive and gram-negative bacteria, which includes strains such as *Staphylococcus aureus, Escherichia coli,* and *Pseudomonas aeruginosa,* together with yeasts and molds. It is said to be ideal for a variety of hair and skin care applications, including liquid soaps, clear gels, shampoos, and skin care products such as cleansers, face creams, and body care lines.
TINOSORB • Methylene-bisbenzotriazolyltetramethylbutylphenol. Reduces transmission of excessive UVA and UVB radiation through fabrics to the skin. A panel including Congressman Nita Lowey and Ciba Corporation has called on the FDA to speed up approval of UV filters and tighten up regulations on sunscreens, an effort organized by Citizens for Sun Protection. Lowey accused the FDA of failing to approve "highly effective sunscreen ingredients" that she claimed were available in every other country except the United States. Tinsorb, which is under consideration before the FDA, is described by the company as a "photostable, broad spectrum UV filter that provides protection against UV rays." A petition sent to the FDA and signed by all the panelists, sponsored in part by Ciba, drew particular attention to the need for filters that provide excellent protection against UVA rays and appealed to the regulator to act immediately to approve such ingredients. Tinsorb may also be an ingredient in skin-lightening products.
TIOXOLONE • Prepared from resorcinol (*see*). Used in dandruff shampoo.
TIPA • The abbreviation for triisopropanolamine.
TIPA-LAURETH SULFATE • *See* Surfactants.
TIPA-LAURYL SULFATE • *See* Surfactants.
TIPA-STEARATE • *See* Stearic Acid.
TISANE • An infusion of dried leaves or flowers that is used as a beverage or a mild medicine.
TITANIUM DIOXIDE • The greatest covering and tinting power of any white pigment used in bath powders, nail whites, depilatories, eyeliners, white eye shadows, antiperspirants, face powders, protective creams, liquid powders, lipsticks, hand lotions, and nail polish. Occurs naturally in three different crystal forms. Used chiefly as a white pigment and as an opacifier; also a white pigment for candy, gum, and marking ink. In high concentrations the dust may cause lung damage. Permanently listed for general cosmetic coloring in 1973.
TITANIUM HYDROXIDE • Thickener and opacifier. *See* Titanium Dioxide.
TITANIUM OXYNITRIDE • An abrasive and antistatic hair product ingredient, it is formed by the reaction of titanium dioxide (*see*) and ammonia gas.
TITANIUM SALICYLATE • A preservative. *See* Salicylates.
TOAD FLAX • *Linaria vulgaris.* Yellow Toad Flax. Snap Dragon. Butter and Eggs. Ramsted. A woody herb native to Europe and introduced in North America and Great Britain, it is valued for both external and internal use. It is employed to treat hemorrhoids and skin diseases. The flowers are sometimes mixed with vegetable oils to make a lini-

ment. Taken internally, an infusion of the leaves has been used by herbalists to eliminate kidney stones. Toad flax is reportedly both diuretic and cathartic.

TOBACCO EXTRACT • Extract of Nicotiana tabacum (*see*).

TOCOCYSTEAMIDE • Antioxidant. *See* Tocopherol.

TOCOPHERETH 5–18 • Antioxidants. *See* Tocopherol.

TOCOPHEROL • Vitamin E. Widely used antioxidant in baby preparations, deodorants, and hair-grooming aids. Obtained by the vacuum distillation of edible vegetable oils. Used as a dietary supplement and as an antioxidant for essential oils and fats. Helps form normal red blood cells, muscle, and other tissues. Protects fat in the body's tissues from abnormal breakdown. Experimental evidence shows vitamin E may protect the heart and blood vessels and retard aging. May cause a skin rash.

TOCOPHERSOLAN • Antioxidant. *See* Tocopherol.

TOCOPHERYL ACETATE • Antioxidant and skin conditioner widely used in makeup, moisturizers, bath products, hairsprays, indoor tanning preparations, and cleansers. *See* Tocopherol.

TOCOPHERYL GLUCOSIDE • Vitamin E and glucose. *See* Tocopherol.

TOCOPHERYL LINOLEATE • Vitamin E and linoleic acid (*see both*).

TOCOPHERYL NICOTINATE • Antioxidant and skin conditioner used in hand products, foundations, and hair products. A combination of vitamin E and vitamin B_1. *See* Tocopherol and Nicotinic Acid.

TOCOPHERYL SUCCINATE • Vitamin E Succinate. Obtained by the distillation of edible vegetable oils and used as a dietary supplement and as an antioxidant for fats and oils.

TOCOQUINONE • Antioxidant. *See* Tocopherol.

TOCOTRIENOLS • Oral care ingredient and skin conditioner. *See* Tocopherol.

TOILET SOAP • A mild, mostly pure soap made from fatty materials of high quality, usually by milling and molding to form cakes. Usually contains an emollient (*see*), perfume, color, and stabilizer with preservatives. More pleasant to use and less drying to the skin.

TOILET WATER • The scent is similar to that of perfume, but it does not last as long and is not as strong or as expensive. Usually made by adding a large amount of alcohol to the perfume formula. In Europe, it is called "lotion"—8 ounces of perfume oil per gallon as compared to 20 to 24 ounces per gallon for perfumes. Considered moderately toxic if swallowed. Skin reactions depend upon ingredients.

TOLBUTAMIDE • Orinase. In a class of drugs called sulfonylureas. Oral antidiabetic. It causes functioning beta cells in the pancreas to release insulin, leading to a drop in blood sugar levels; used to treat type II diabetes mellitus. According to the United Kingdom, must not form part of the composition of cosmetic products.

TOLERANCE • The ability to live with an allergen.

TOLNAFTATE • *See* Naphthalene.

TOLU BALSAM • Extract and Gum. Extract from the Peruvian or Indian plant. Contains cinnamic acid and benzoic acid (*see both*). Used in flavorings. Mildly antiseptic and may be mildly irritating to the skin.

TOLUENE • Antioxidant and solvent. Used in nail polish up to 50 percent. Obtained from petroleum or by distilling Tolu balsam. Used chiefly as a solvent. Resembles benzene but is less volatile, flammable, or toxic. May cause mild anemia if ingested and is narcotic in high concentrations. It can cause liver damage and is irritating to the skin and respiratory tract. While halogenated hydrocarbons like toluene are assumed responsible for health risks, long-term effects of low-level exposure to them have been found in at least twenty cities where toluene is present in the drinking water. On the basis of available information, the CIR Expert Panel (*see*) concluded that it is safe as presently used in cosmetic formulations. *See* Toluene Sulfonamide/Formaldehyde Resin.

TOLUENE-2, 5-DIAMINE • Hair coloring. The EU now allows 10 percent in hair dyes. The compound has been banned in Germany, Sweden, and France. On the Canadian Hotlist (*see*). *See* Toluene and Coal Tar.

TOLUENE-3, 4-DIAMINE • An intermediate chemical in the manufacture of polyurethanes; dyes for textiles, fur, and leather, varnishes, pigments, and hair dyes. In a National Cancer Institute study, it caused liver cancer when fed to rats and mice, as well as breast cancer in female rats. In tests, a closely related compound, 2,4-toluenediamine, had the greatest absorption through the scalp of the hair dyes tested. *See* Phenylenediamine.

TOLUENE-2, 5-DIAMINE SULFATE • Hair coloring.

TOLUENE SULFONAMIDE/FORMALDEHYDE RESIN • TSAFr. It is used as a "nail strengthener" or hardener, and to improve adhesion and gloss. There is supposed to be no free formaldehyde in this widely used formula. Large cosmetics manufacturers stopped producing nail hardeners with free formaldehyde in the 1960s because of the frequent adverse reactions reported. This compound is a strong sensitizer while in the liquid state but not when solidified; therefore, if it doesn't touch the skin while being applied, even a person sensitive to the ingredients may not have a reaction. Those allergic to this common ingredient of nail polishes almost always have allergic reactions on the eyelids, the sides of the neck, and around the mouth and almost never on the hands. On the basis of available information, the CIR Expert Panel (*see*) concluded that it is safe as presently used in cosmetic formulations.

TOLUENE SULFONIC ACID • Surfactant. *See* Toluene.

TOLUIDINES, THEIR ISOMERS, SALTS AND HALOGENATED AND SULPHONATED DERIVATIVES • Coal tar colors. Banned in cosmetics by the EU and ASEAN (*see*). Toluidine Red was formerly D & C Red No. 571 and is also known as Toluidine Scarlet 1207.

p-**TOLYL ACETATE** • *p*-Cresyl Acetate. A synthetic butter, caramel, fruit, honey, nut, and spice flavoring for cosmetics and beverages, ice cream, ices, candy, baked goods, chewing gum, and gelatin.

TOLYLALDEHYDE • Colorless liquid from benzene. Used in perfumes and flavorings. *See* Tolu Balsam.

o-**TOLYL BIGUANIDE** • Antioxidant used in bath products. *See* Toluene.

TOMATO EXTRACT • Tomatine. Extract from the fruit of the tomato, *Solanum esculentum.* Used as a fungicide and as a precipitating ingredient.

TOMATO OIL • *Solanum lycopersicum.* Oil from tomatoes used as a skin-conditioning ingredient.

TONER • In cosmetics, an organic pigment that is used at full strength. For example, D & C Red No. 7 (*see*).

TONKA • Tonka Bean. Coumarouna Bean. Black, brownish seeds with a wrinkled surface and brittle, shiny, or fatty skins. A vanillalike odor and a bitter taste. Used in the production of natural coumarin (*see*), flavoring extracts, and toilet powders.

TOOTHPASTE • *See* Dentifrices.

TOP COAT • Same ingredients as in base coat (*see*) so as to give the nail enamel a greater gloss and to help prevent chipping.

TOP NOTE • The first impression of a fragrance upon the sense of smell. The most volatile part of the perfume. It is one of the most important factors in the success of the perfume, but does not persist after the first sniff.

TOPAZ • A mineral containing mostly aluminum and silicate (*see both*) used as an abrasive.

TOPICAL • Used to describe the application of a drug directly to the external site on the body where it is intended to have its effect.

TOPICAL STARCH • Stored by plants, it is taken from grains of wheat, potatoes, rice, and many other vegetables. In 1992, the FDA proposed a ban on topical starch in astringent (*see*) drug products, and in fever blister and cold sore products because it had not been shown to be safe and effective as claimed.

TORMENTIL • *Potentilla procumbens. P. tormentilla.* Septfoil. Hippocrates used it for skin problems. The earliest citation of this plant in England appeared in 1387 recommending it for toothaches. Tormentil is a powerful astringent. Through the years it came to be used for piles, fevers, canker sores, and to relieve pain. It is used by herbalists as a gargle for sore throats and sore mouths. Supposedly a piece of cloth soaked in a decoction of it covering a wart will cause the growth to turn black and fall off. The same decoction is recommended for sores and ulcers. A fluid extract of the root is used by herbalists to stop bleeding of the gums and of cuts. The root contains more tannin (*see*) than oak bark.

TORREYA CALIFORNICA • *See* Nutmeg.

TOSYLAMIDE/EPOXY RESIN • A widely used resin in nail polish and other manicuring preparations. *See* Acrylates.

TOSYLAMIDE/FORMALDEHYDE RESIN • Film former, plasticizer used in nail polish and enamels, base coats and undercoats. *See* Formaldehyde and Toluene.

TOSYLCHLORAMIDE SODIUM • The EU says it should not be used above 0.2 percent concentration.

TOTAROL • Antioxidant and deodorant used in oral care products. Totarol is a naturally occurring plant extract with antibacterial and antioxidant properties. The most abundant source of totarol is the heartwood of New Zealand's totara tree. Totarol is advertised as effective against acne and tooth decay bacteria and is reportedly active against penicillin- and methicillin-resistant strains of *Staphylococcus aureus.* Totarol is in cosmetic formulations, soaps, toothpastes, skin cleansers, and disinfectants. The producers claim it is a nonprimary irritant and nonprimary sensitizer to the human skin.

TOUCH-ME-NOT • *See* Impatiens.

TOUGARASI EKISU • *See* Capsicum.

TOUHI EKISU • *See* Bitter Orange Oil.

TOUKI • Used as an abrasive and skin conditioner. *See* Angelica.

TOUNIN EKISU • Skin conditioner. *See* Peach Kernel Oil.

TOURMALINE • A compound of silicate, boron, and aluminum containing varying amounts of iron, magnesium, manganese, calcium, sodium, potassium, lithium, and fluorine. Thickener.

TOXICITY • The capacity of a substance to dangerously impair body functions or to damage body tissue.

TOXICOKINETICS • Essentially the study of how a substance gets into the body and what happens to it in the body. The relationship between the systemic exposure of a compound and its toxicity. It is used primarily for establishing relationships between exposures in toxicology experiments in animals and the corresponding exposures in humans.

TRACHEA HYDROLYSATE • The use of an enzyme or some other method to remove the water from animal tracheas. Used as a cartilage ingredient.

TRAGACANTH • *See* Gum Tragacanth.

TRAILING ARBUTUS EXTRACT • The extract of the leaves of *Epigaea repens.* *See* Arbutus Extract.

TRANEXAMIC ACID • Decreases external blood loss. Used as a cosmetic astringent and skin conditioner.

TRANSDERMAL • A drug delivery system consisting of an adhesive patch containing a medication that diffuses through the skin and acts systemically in the body. Examples include nicotine-containing patches to help people stop smoking, and nitroglycerin-containing patches to treat and prevent angina (chest pain) attacks.

TRANSGENIC ANIMAL, PLANT, OR CROP • An animal, plant, or crop in which the hereditary DNA (*see*) has been altered through genetic engineering by adding DNA from a source other than its parent.

TRANSLUCENT POWDER • Because it contains more titanium dioxide (*see*) than other face powders, translucent makeups are actually more opaque. But other than that, they contain the same ingredients.

TRAVELER'S JOY • *Clematis vitalba*. Old Man's Beard. A woody vine native to Europe and imported to North America, it is used in homeopathic medicine to treat genitourinary tract ailments and skin diseases. Herbalists use it to relieve migraine attack. The plant is toxic and may cause skin irritation.

TREMELLA FUCIFORMIS • Skin conditioner and humectant. *See* Mushroom Extract.

TREE MOSS • *Climacium*. Lichen that grows on trees. Used in fragrances and flavors. The EU says it must be listed on leave-on and rinse-off products.

TREHALOSE • Flavoring. A sugar that yields glucose (*see*) on hydrolysis, and this is obtained from trehala, ergot of rye, and many fungi in which it is stored.

TRETHOCANIC ACID • Exfoliating ingredient. Used in anti-aging products. Can cause sensitivity to sunlight. Discontinue use if bleeding and pain are experienced.

TRETINOIN • Vitamin A Retinoic Acid. Retin-A. A prescription cream, gel, or solution introduced in 1973 to treat severe acne and fine wrinkles from sun-damaged skin. Clinically, according to researchers at Emory University Medical School, Atlanta, Georgia, patients experience decreased wrinkling, improved texture, and pinkening of sallow skin. However, the changes induced by topical tretinoin extend beyond a cosmetic. Microscopic, ultrastructural, and biochemical alterations, the researchers say, indicate that topical tretinoin is a significant medical therapy and requires medical supervision. Potential adverse reactions include a feeling of warmth, slight stinging, local redness, peeling, chapping, swelling, blistering, crusting, and temporary increase or decrease in pigmentation and acne. Contact with eyes and mouth should be avoided. Topical preparations containing sulfur, resorcinol, or salicylic acid increase risk of skin irritation and should not be used with tretinoin. Contraindicated in hypersensitivity to any tretinoin components. Should be used with caution in eczema. Increased sensitivity to wind and cold may occur. No medicated cosmetics should be used. On the Canadian Hotlist (*see*). The EU and ASEAN (*see*) have banned it in cosmetics.

TRIACETIN • Glyceryl Triacetate. Primarily a solvent for hair dyes. Also a fixative in perfume and used in toothpaste. A colorless, somewhat oily liquid with a slight fatty odor and a bitter taste. Obtained from adding acetate to glycerin (*see both*). In 1992, the FDA issued a notice that triacetin had not been shown to be safe and effective as claimed in OTC products.

TRIALKANOLAMINES • Used in non-rinse-off products at a concentration restricted to 2.5 percent. *See* Fatty Acid Dialkanolamides.

2,5,6-TRIAMINO-4-PYRIMIDINOL SULFATE • A hair coloring.

TRIARACHIDIN • Made from glycerin and arachidic acid (*see both*), it is used as a skin-conditioning ingredient and thickener.

TRIBEHENIN • Glyceryl Tribehenate. Skin conditioner in makeup, cleansers, moisturizers, deodorants, and suntan products. *See* Behenic Acid and Glycerin.

TRIBEHENIN PEG-20 ESTERS • Derived from glycerin, it is used as a skin conditioner, emollient, and emulsifier. *See* Glycerin.

TRIBENZOIN • Skin conditioner. *See* Glycerin.

TRIBENZOYL TRIRICINOLEIN • Used as a hair and skin conditioner and emollient. *See* Glycerin and Benzoic Acid.

TRIBROMOSALAN • TBS. 3,4′,5-Tribromosalicylanilide. Used in medicated cosmetics; an antiseptic and fungicide. Salicylanilide is an antifungal compound used to treat ringworm. TBS is contained in the most popular soaps to kill skin bacteria. Used as a germicide, frequently replacing hexachlorophene (*see*). Prohibited in cosmetics by the FDA in 2000 because it may cause allergic reaction when skin is exposed to the sun. On the Canadian Hotlist (*see*). The EU has banned it.

3,4′,5-TRIBROMOSALICYLANILIDE • Produces a powerful and prolonged photosensitizing effect. The EU says this substance should therefore be prohibited in cosmetic products. *See* Tribromosalan.

TRIBULUS TERRESTRIS • Plant that grows in many tropical and moderate areas of the world. Many different cultures have used it for a number of conditions. For example, the Greeks used *Tribulus terrestris* as a diuretic and a mood-enhancer. Indians used it as a diuretic, antiseptic, and anti-inflammatory. The Chinese used it for a variety of liver, kidney, and cardiovascular diseases. The people of Bulgaria used *Tribulus terrestris* as a sex enhancer and to treat infertility. Used in anti-aging cosmetics today because of its alleged hormonelike action.

TRIBUTYL CITRATE • Used as a plasticizer and solvent. The triester of butyl alcohol and citric acid (*see both*), it is a pale yellow, odorless liquid used as a plasticizer, antifoam ingredient, and solvent for nitrocellulose. Low toxicity.

TRI (BUTYLCRESYL) BUTANE • Used as a stabilizer. *See* Phenols.

TRICALCIUM PHOSPHATE • The calcium salt of phosphate (*see*). A polishing ingredient in dentifrices; also an anticaking ingredient in table salt and vanilla powder, and a dietary supplement. *See* Calcium Phosphate.

TRI-C12–13 • Alkyl Citrate. A combination of alcohol and citric acid (*see both*), it is used as an emollient.

TRICAPRIN • *See* Decanoic Acid.

TRICAPRYLIN • A fragrance ingredient and skin conditioner used in lipsticks, foundations, moisturizer, and hand and body lotions and creams. *See* Caprylic Acid and Glycerin.

TRICAPRYLYL CITRATE • Made from capryl alcohol and citric acid, it is a skin conditioner. *See* Capric Acid and Citric Acid.

TRICETEARETH-4 OR -5 PHOSPHATE • An emulsifier. *See* Phosphoric Acid and Surfactants.

TRICETETHS • Emulsifiers. *See* Cetearyl Alcohol.

TRICETYL PHOSPHATE • A wax. *See* Phosphoric Acid and Cetyl Alcohol.

TRICETYLMONIUM CHLORIDE • *See* Quaternary Ammonium Compounds.

TRICHLOROACETIC ACID • Topical preparation containing salicylic acid; used to treat warts. On the Canadian Hotlist (*see*). Banned by the UK and ASEAN (*see*) in cosmetics.

TRICHLOROETHANE • Used in cosmetics as a solvent and degreasing ingredient. Nonflammable liquid. Insoluble in water and absorbs some water. Less toxic than carbon tetrachloride, which is used in fire extinguishers. Trichloroethane solutions are irritating to the eyes and mucous membranes, and in high concentrations they can be narcotic. Can be absorbed through the skin. Inhalation and ingestion produce serious symptoms, ranging from vomiting to death. The CIR Expert Panel (*see*) has listed this as top priority for review.

TRICHODESMA ZEYLANICUM OIL • Wild Borage. English Camel Bush. Skin conditioner. From eastern tropical Africa to India, Ceylon, western Malaysia, and Australia, apparently introduced and naturalizing elsewhere. Is toxic to cattle.

TRICHOSANTHES KIRILOWII • Snake Gourd. Chinese Cucumber. It reportedly helps stimulate the production of body fluids, thus relieving dryness. It is said to disperse phlegm, remove pus, and expel toxic matter and is anti-inflammatory and can act as a natural antibiotic, expectorant, and laxative; and it can be used for abscesses, boils, and hemorrhoids.

TRICLOCARBAN • Trichlorocarbanilide. TCC. Widely used bacteria killer and antiseptic in soaps, medicated cosmetics, deodorants, and cleansing creams. Prepared from aniline (*see*). In May 1983, it was revealed that tests for this soap ingredient were falsified and that rat deaths were not reported. The reasons for the deaths were not confirmed. Reports in the scientific literature in 2001 suggest that use of antibacterials such as this may cause resistant germs.

TRICLOSAN • A broad-spectrum antibacterial ingredient, active primarily against some types of bacteria, that is the target of controversy at this writing. It is used in deodorant soaps, vaginal deodorant sprays, and other cosmetic products as well as in drugs and household products. Its deodorant properties are due to the inhibition of bacterial growth. Can cause allergic contact dermatitis, particularly when used in products for the feet. The EPA registers it as a pesticide, giving it high scores as a risk to both human health and the environment. The U.S. Pharmacopeia recently proposed a new monograph for the specific testing of triclosan. It is a chlorinated aromatic, similar in molecular structure and chemical formula to some of the toxic chemicals—dioxins, PCBs, and Agent Orange. It is on the Canadian Hotlist (*see*). Canadians limit it to a concentration of 0.3 percent or less. The latest research into the antibacterial ingredient triclosan brings fresh evidence that it can have a significant impact on thyroid function and the onset of puberty in male rats. The Swiss company that makes it, Ciba, claims triclosan is effective at very low concentration levels and therefore the amount used to produce results in consumer products is hundreds of times lower than doses showing effects in animals. The team at Ciba is eager to emphasize that in most personal care products the dosing level of triclosan is normally at 0.1 percent to 0.2 percent. Furthermore, Ciba maintains that through testing on different animals and human volunteers, the company has evidence refuting allegations that concurrent use of several personal care products containing triclosan can lead to accumulated levels of the substance that can be potentially dangerous. Furthermore, blood concentrations appear to decrease once triclosan is no longer used by a person.

Criticism of the use of this antimicrobial ingredient in cosmetics and personal care products is coming from Europe and America. In 2008, a number of public health and environment groups banded together to lobby against all nonmedical uses of triclosan and triclocarban. The lobby groups claimed scientific studies have linked the chemical to endocrine system disruption, cancer, and increased skin sensitization, in addition to noting its ability to persist in aquatic environments. Industry again supported the use of this ingredient, stating there is no conclusive evidence to suggest it is harmful to humans as well as pointing out that it can play an invaluable role in protecting against potentially pathogenic organisms. The promotion to frequently "wash your hands" is a result of the promotion of antibacterial products containing triclosan. Experiments suggest the ingredient can be toxic to laboratory rats, but the company argues that the levels used in personal care products are much smaller than those used in the study. Ciba says even the cumulative effect of using multiple triclosan-containing products as part of a beauty regimen will lead to blood triclosan levels 200–300 times smaller than those shown to have an effect in the animal study. Researchers at the University of North Carolina State University, however, say that a study they conducted on rats showed a dramatic decrease in the thyroid hormone thyroxine following exposure to increasing concentrations of triclosan. The study used newly weaned rats that were fed quantities of triclosan in doses of 0, 3, 30, 100, 200, or 300 mg/kg of body weight over a 31-day period. The purpose of the experiment was to determine what effect triclosan has on thyroid hormone levels as a means of gauging how this might impact the onset of puberty. The researchers found that at doses of up to 3 mg there was no detectable difference in thyroid activity. However, at 30 mg, thyroxine levels decreased by 47 percent, and at 300 mg, activity decreased by 81 percent. As thyroxine is a crucial chemical in the development of puberty and a functioning metabolism in males, the researchers suggest that the impact of triclosan may consequently lead to a variety of health-related issues both before and after birth. Hypothyroid (low thyroid) can lead to a variety of serious conditions such as obesity, infertility, and even neurological problems—conditions that are related to the all-important influence thyroxine has on the metabolism.

The research findings reaffirm a growing body of scientific evidence underlining the potential toxicity of triclosan, a danger that is exacerbated by the fact that it is used in a wide number of personal care products, including toothpaste, soap, and deodorant. Although regulatory authorities all over the world dictate that formulators use doses of triclosan at levels deemed not to pose a risk to human health, some industry experts believe that concurrent use of multiple personal care products might lead to a cumulative exposure that could pose a greater danger. In 2008, the international NGO (*see*) ChemSec released a list of 267 chemical substances that included triclosan, for which it feels companies should be searching for alternatives.

TRICONTANYL PVP • *See* Polyvinylpyrrolidone.

TRICRESYL PHOSPHATE • TCP. A plasticizer in nail polishes and a strengthener in lubricants. Colorless or pale yellow liquid. Can cause paralysis many days after exposure. For instance, in 1960, approximately ten thousand Moroccans became ill after ingesting cooking oil adulterated with turbojet engine oil containing 3 percent TCP. Can be absorbed through the skin and mucous membranes, causing poisoning. Persons sensitive to the plasticizer in eyeglass frames may develop a skin rash from tricresyl. Toxic dose in man is only 6 milligrams per kilogram of body weight. On the Canadian Hotlist (*see*).

TRIDECETH-2, -3, -5, -7, -9, -10, -12, -15, -20, -50 • The number signifies the viscosity. *See* Polyethylene Glycols.

TRIDECETH-4, -7, OR -19 CARBOXYLIC ACID • A surfactant (*see*). *See also* Polyoxyethylene and Carboxylic Acid.

TRIDECETH-3 OR -6 PHOSPHATE • The number signifies viscosity. *See* Phosphoric Acid and Polyethylene Glycol.

TRIDECYL ALCOHOL • Derived from tridecane, a paraffin hydrocarbon obtained from petroleum. Used as an emulsifier in cosmetic creams, lotions, and lipsticks.

TRIDECYL BEHENATE • A skin-conditioning ingredient. *See* Behenic Acid.

TRIDECYL COCOATE • A skin-conditioning ingredient. *See* Coconut Oil.

TRIDECYL ERUCATE • Skin conditioner. *See* Erucic Acid and Tridecyl Alcohol.

TRIDECYL ETHYLHEXANOATE • An emollient. *See* Octanoic Acid.

TRIDECYL ISONONANOATE • Emollient. Used in lipsticks and tanning products. The CIR Expert Panel (*see*) concluded it was safe in 2008.

TRIDECYL LAURATE • Skin conditioner. *See* Dodecanoic Acid and Lauric Acid.

TRIDECYL MYRISTATE • Skin conditioner. May promote acne. *See* Myristic Acid and Tridecyl Alcohol.

TRIDECYL NEOPENTANOATE • Emollient used in moisturizers and face powders. *See* Neopentyl Alcohol and Tridecyl Alcohol.

TRIDECYL SALICYLATE • *See* Salicylates.

TRIDECYL STEARATE • *See* Stearic Acid.

TRIDECYL STEAROYL STEARATE • *See* Stearic Acid.

TRIDECYL TRIMELLITATE • *See* Trimellitic Acid.

TRIDECYLBENZENE SULFONIC ACID • *See* Sulfonamide Resins and Surfactants.

TRIDETH-3 • *See* Tridecyl Alcohol.

TRIDETH-6, -10, -12 • *See* Tridecyl Alcohol.

TRIERUCIN • Made from glycerin and erucic acid (*see both*). Used as a skin-conditioning ingredient and also used as a thickener.

TRIETHANOLAMINE • A coating ingredient for fresh fruit and vegetables and widely used in surfactants (*see*) and as a dispersing ingredient and detergent in hand and body lotions, shaving creams, soaps, shampoos, and bath powders. Its principal toxic effect in animals has been attributed to overalkalinity. Gross pathology has been found in the gastrointestinal tract in fatally poisoned guinea pigs. It is an irritant. It has been found, in tests in Italy at the University of Bologna, to be the most frequent sensitizer among the common emulsifiers used in cosmetics. On the basis of available information, the CIR Expert Panel (*see*) concluded that it is safe as presently used in cosmetic formulation but in products intended for prolonged contact with the skin, the concentration should not exceed 5 percent and be used only in rinse-off products. Should not be used with nitrosating ingredients (*see* Nitrosamines).

TRIETHANOLAMINE DODECYLBENZENE SULFONATE • Linear. Made from ethylene oxide and used in bubble baths and soapless shampoos. May be mildly irritating to the skin. *See* Ethanolamines.

TRIETHANOLAMINE-*d*-1–2-PYRROLIDONE-5-CARBOXYMETHYLATE • Triethanolamine. A colorless liquid, soluble in water, and used as a soap base and oil emulsifier. *See* Triethanolamine Stearate.

TRIETHANOLAMINE STEARATE • Made from ethylene oxide. Used in brilliantines, cleansing creams, foundation creams, hair lacquers, liquid makeups, fragrances, liquid powders, mascara, protective creams, baby preparations, shaving creams and lathers, and preshave lotions. A moisture absorber, viscous, used in making emulsions. Cream colored, turns brown on exposure to air. May be irritating to the skin and mucous membranes, but less so than many other amines (*see*).

TRIETHANOLAMINE TRISODIUM PHOSPHATE • Made from ethylene oxide and used in cuticle softeners. May be mildly irritating to the skin. *See* Ethanolamines.

TRIETHONIUM HYDROLYZED COLLAGEN ETHOSULFATE • *See* Hydrolyzed Animal Protein and Quaternary Ammonium Compounds.

TRIETHYL CITRATE • Citric Acid. Ethyl Citrate. Plasticizer in nail polish. Odorless, practically colorless, bitter; also used in dried egg as a sequestering ingredient (*see*) and to prevent rancidity.

TRIETHYLENE GLYCOL • Used in stick perfume. Prepared from ethylene oxide and ethylene glycol (*see both*). Used as a solvent. *See* Polyethylene Glycol for toxicity. The CIR Expert Panel (*see*) has listed this as top priority for review.

TRIETHYLENE GLYCOL HYDROGENATED ROSINATE • Derived from triethylene glycol (*see*) and rosin (*see*). Used as a skin conditioner and thickener.

TRIETHYLHEXANOIN • Fragrance used in hair and skin products as well as lipsticks and face powders. Derived from hexanoic acid and glycerin (*see both*).

TRIFLUOROMETHYL C1–4 ALKYL DIMETHICONE • *See* Silicones.

TRIFLUOROPROPYL CYCLOPENTASILOXANE • Hair and skin conditioner. *See* Siloxane and Fluoride.

TRIFOLIUM PRATENSE • *See* Clover.

TRIGLYCERETH-7 CITRATE • Humectant and skin conditioner from citric acid and glycerin.

TRIGONELLA FOENUM-GRAECUM • *See* Fenugreek Seed.

TRIHEPTANOIN • Skin conditioner and thickener. *See* Heptanoic Acid.

TRIHEPTYLUNDECANOIN • Skin conditioner and thickener. *See* Glycerin and Undecanoic Acid.

TRIHEXYLDECYL CITRATE • Skin conditioner and opacifier. *See* Citric Acid.

1,2,4-TRIHYDROXYBENZENE • Hair coloring. *See* Coal Tar.

TRIHYDROXYBENZENE • *See* Benzene.

TRIHYDROXY STEARIN • Isolated from cork and used as a thickener.

TRIHYDROXYMETHOXYSTEARIN • Used as a skin conditioner, a solvent, and a thickener in cosmetic formulations at concentrations up to 5 percent. On the basis of available information, the CIR Expert Panel (*see*) concluded that it is safe as presently used in cosmetic formulations. *See* Stearic Acid.

TRIHYDROXYPALMITAMIDOHYDROXYPROPYL MYRISTATE • Skin conditioner. *See* Palmitic and Myristic Acids.

TRIHYDROXYSTEARIN • Skin conditioner and thickener used in makeup, lipsticks, and skin care products. *See* Octanoic Acid.

TRIISOCETYL CITRATE • *See* Citric Acid.

TRIISOCETYL STEARATE • Made from citric acid and isocetyl alcohol (*see both*). Used as a skin-conditioning ingredient. On the basis of the available animal and human data, the CIR Expert Panel (*see*) concludes that this ingredient is safe as used in cosmetics.

TRIISODECYL TRIMELLITATE • Skin conditioner, lip gloss, lipstick, anti-aging creams, and lip plumper. *See* Tridecyl Alcohol.

TRIISOPALMITIN • A skin-conditioning ingredient made from palmitic acid and glycerin (*see both*).

TRIISONONANOIN • *See* Glycerin and Nonanoic Acid.

TRIISOPROPANOLAMINE • A white crystalline solid. A mild base used as an emulsifying ingredient.

TRIISOPROPYL CITRATE • Emollient. *See* Citric Acid.

TRIISOPROPYL TRILINOLEATE • *See* Isopropyl Alcohol and Trilinoleic Acid.

TRIISOSTEARIN • *See* Glycerin and Isostearic Acid.

TRIISOSTEARIN PEG-6 ESTERS • Emollient and emulsifier. *See* Isostearic Acid and Polyethylene Glycol.

TRIISOSTEARYL CITRATE • Skin conditioner in face powders. *See* Citric Acid.

TRIISOSTEARYL TRILINOLEATE • *See* Isostearyl Alcohol and Trilinoleic Acid.

TRILACTIN • Skin conditioner. *See* Lactic Acid and Glycerin.

TRILANETH-4 PHOSPHATE • *See* Lanolin Alcohols.

TRILAURIN • Widely used in makeup, body and hand preparations, and bath products. *See* Lauric Acid.

TRILAURYL CITRATE • *See* Lauryl Alcohol and Citric Acid.

TRILAURYL PHOSPHATE • Skin conditioner and plasticizer. *See* Phosphoric Acid.

TRILAURYLAMINE • *See* Lauryl Alcohol.

TRILINOLEIC ACID • Trimer Acid. *See* Linoleic Acid.

TRILINOLEIN • The triester of glycerin and linoleic acid (*see both*).

TRIMAGNESIUM PHOSPHATE • Magnesium Phosphate. Tribasic. Occurs in nature as the mineral bobierite. A white, crystalline powder, it absorbs water and is used in cosmetics as an alkali.

TRIMELLITIC ACID • Colorless crystals from coal used in the manufacture of plastics, dyes, adhesives, and polymers.

TRIMETHYLHEXANOL • *See* Hexanol.

TRIMETHYLOLPROPANE TRICAPRYLATE/TRICAPRATE • *See* Caprylic Acid.

TRIMETHYLOLPROPANE TRIETHYLHEXANOATE • Skin conditioner used in lipsticks and foundations. *See* Hexanoic Acid.

TRIMETHYLOLPROPANE TRIISOSTEARATE • *See* Propane and Isostearic Acid.

TRIMETHYLOLPROPANE TRILAURATE • Skin conditioner. *See* Dodecanoic Acid.

TRIMETHYLOLPROPANE TRIOCTANOATE • *See* Propane and Octanoic Acid.

TRIMETHYLPENTANEDIOLISOPHTHALIC ACID/TRIMELLITIC ANHYDRIDE COPOLYMER • *See* Copolymer.

TRIMETHYLSILOXYSILICATE • *See* Silicates.

TRIMETHYLSILYLAMODIMETHICONE • *See* Silicones.

TRIMETHYLSILYL TRIMETHYLSILOXY SALICYLATE • Skin conditioner. *See* Siloxane and Salicylates.

TRIMYRISTIN • Glyceryl Trimyristate. Solid triglyceride of myristic acid that occurs in many vegetable fats and oils, particularly in coconut oil and nutmeg butter. Used as an emollient in cold creams and for shampoos.

TRIOCTANOATE • *See* Octanoic Acid.

TRIOCTANOIN • *See* Octanoic Acid and Glycerin.

TRIOCTYLDODECYL BORATE • Preservative. *See* Borates.

TRIOCTYLDODECYL CITRATE • *See* Citric Acid.

TRIOLEIN • Glyceryl Trioleate. From the Palestine olive and one of the chief constituents of nondrying oils and fats used in cosmetics as a skin conditioner and thickener in creams and oils.

TRIOLETH-8 PHOSPHATE • Derived from phosphoric acid and oleyl alcohol (*see both*).

TRIOLEYL PHOSPHATE • Used as an emulsifier. *See* Oleyl Alcohol.

TRIPABA PANTHENOL • *See* Panthenol and PABA.

TRIPALMITIN • Used as a skin conditioner and thickener. Occurs in fats and is prepared from glycerol and palmitic acid (*see both*). *See* Palmitic Acid for toxicity.

TRIPALMITOLEIN • Skin conditioner. *See* Oleic Acid and Palmitic Acid.

TRIPEPTIDE-1 • Synthetic protein used as a skin conditioner. *See* Amino Acids.

TRIPHENYL PHOSPHATE • A noncombustible substitute for camphor in celluloid. Colorless; insoluble in water. Stable, fireproof, and used as a plasticizer in nail polish. Causes paralysis if ingested and skin rash in hypersensitive people. Inhalation of only 3.5 milligrams per kilogram of body weight is toxic to humans.

TRIPHENYL TRIMETHICONE • Antifoaming ingredient and skin conditioner. *See* Silicones.

TRIPHENYLMETHANE GROUP • Tritan. Certified dyes made from the reduction (*see*) of carbon tetrachloride and benzene with aluminum chloride. Very soluble in water, affected by light and alkalis. Among the triphenylmethane group are FD & C Blue No. 1 and FD & C Green Nos. 1, 2, and 3. *See* Colors for toxicity.

TRIPOLYPHOSPHATE • A buffering ingredient in shampoos. A phosphorus salt. Used to soften water, as an emulsifier, and as a dispersing ingredient. May cause esophageal stricture if swallowed. Moderately irritating to the skin and mucous membranes. Ingestion can cause violent vomiting.

TRIPOTASSIUM EDTA • *See* EDTA Salts.

TRIPROPYLAMINE • Clear liquid, ammonia-like odor used in dyes, agrochemicals, pharmaceuticals, rubber and plastic additive industries, cosmetics and catalysts (zeolite). Toxic if inhaled or swallowed. Corrosive. Severe skin irritant. FAO/WHO last evaluated this flavoring additive in 2005. The committee determined the ADI "as conditional" but pointed out there was no safety concern at current levels of intake when used as a flavoring agent. The evaluation is conditional because the estimated daily intake is based on the anticipated annual volume of production. The conclusion of the safety evaluation of this substance will be revoked if use levels or poundage data are not provided before the end of 2007. As of this writing, no action has been taken. EAF

TRIPROPYLENE GLYCOL CITRATE • *See* Propylene Glycol.

TRIRICINOLEIN • Made from glycerin and ricinoleic acid (*see both*), it is used as a skin-conditioning ingredient and a thickener. The ester of glycerin and sebacic acid (*see both*).

TRISEBACIN • Skin conditioner and thickener.

TRIS-ETHOXYDIGLOCOL PHOSPHATE • Skin conditioner and humectant. *See* Phosphorus.

TRIS (HYDROXYMETHYL) NITROMETHANE • Crystals from ethyl acetate and benzene (*see both*). Soluble in alcohol. Inhibits bacterial growth in water systems, cutting oils, nonprotein glues, and sizings. Irritating to the skin and mucous membranes. May release formaldehyde (*see*).

TRIS (NONYLPHENYL) PHOSPHITE • *See* Phenols.

TRISILOXANE • Skin conditioner and antifoaming ingredient. *See* Siloxanes.

TRISODIUM EDTA • *See* Tetrasodium EDTA.

TRISODIUM GLYCYRRHIZATE • Flavoring and skin conditioner. *See* Glycyrrhizic Acid.

TRISODIUM HEDTA • Mineral-suspending ingredients. *See* Sequestering Ingredient.

TRISODIUM HYDROXY EDTA • *See* Tetrasodium EDTA.

TRISODIUM HYDROXYETHYL ETHLENEDIAMINETRIACETATE • *See* Tetrasodium EDTA.

TRISODIUM INOSITOL TRIPHOSPHATE • Skin conditioner. *See* Inositol and Phosphorus.

TRISODIUM LAUROAMPHO PG-ACETATE PHOSPHATE CHLORIDE • *See* Quaternary Ammonium Compounds.

TRISODIUM NTA • *See* Sequestering Ingredient.

TRISODIUM PHOSPHATE • Obtained from phosphate rock. Highly alkaline. Used in shampoos, cuticle softeners, bubble baths, and bath salts for its water-softening and cleaning actions. Phosphorus was formerly used to treat rickets and degenerative disorders and is now used as a mineral supplement for foods; also in incendiary bombs and tracer bullets. Can cause skin irritation from alkalinity.

TRIS-OLEOYLTROMETHAMINE ETHAN SULFATE • Skin conditioner. *See* Oleic Acid.

TRISTEARIN • Present in many animal and vegetable fats, especially hard ones like tallow and cocoa butter, it is used in surfactants, quaternary ammonium compounds, and emollients.

TRISTEARYL CITRATE • The triester of stearyl alcohol and citric acid (*see both*).

TRISTEARYL PG-PHOSPHATE DIMONIUM CHLORIDE • *See* Quaternary Ammonium Compounds.

TRITICUM VULAGRE (WHEAT) BRAN LIPIDS • *See* Wheat Germ.

TRIUNDECANOIN • *See* Glycerin and Undecanoic Acid.

TROMETHAMINE • Made by the reduction (*see*) of nitro compounds, it is a crystalline mass used in the manufacture of surface-active ingredients (*see*). Used as an emulsifier and fragrance in cosmetic creams and lotions, mineral oil, and paraffin wax emulsions. Used medicinally to correct an overabundance of acid in the body.

TROMETHAMINE ACRYLATES/ACRYLONITROGENS COPOLYMER • *See* Acrylates.

TROMETHAMINE MAGNESIUM ALUMINUM SILICATE • *See* Silicates.

TROPAEOLUM MAJUS • *See* Indian Cress Extract.

TROPIC ACID • An exfoliant. *See* Beta Hydroxy Acids.

TROXERUTIN • Skin conditioner. A derivative of the natural bioflavonoid rutin (*see*) extracted from *Sophora japonica* (Japanese pagoda tree). Common usage is mainly in the treatment of varicose veins and hemorrhoids. Troxerutin may also act to improve capillary function, reduce capillary fragility, and reduce abnormal leakage. Applications also exist for reducing the occurrence of night cramps and other circulatory problems.

TRUE FIXATIVE • This holds back the evaporation of other materials. Benzoin is an example. *See* Fixative.

TRUVIA • *See* Stevia.

TRYPTOPHAN • Hair conditioner. Although it is sold over the counter, it is not believed to be completely harmless and has been suspected of being a co-carcinogen (*see*) and affecting the liver when taken in high doses. In cosmetics, it is used to increase the protein content of creams and lotions. A tremendous amount of research is now in progress with this amino acid (*see*). First isolated in milk in 1901, it is now being studied as a means to calm hyperactive children, induce sleep, and fight depression and pain. The FDA called for further study of this additive. ASP

TSAFr • Abbreviation for toluene sulfonamide/formaldehyde resin (*see*).

TUAMINOHEPTANE AND ITS ISOMERS AND SALTS • A nasal decongestant. A vasoconstrictor. Banned in cosmetics by the EU and ASEAN (*see*), and it is on the Canadian Hotlist (*see*).

TUBER MELANOSPORUM • Truffle Oil. Skin conditioner and humectant. A gourmet mushroom collected only in winter.

TUBEROSE OIL • *Polianthes tuberosa.* Derived from a Mexican bulbous herb commonly cultivated for its spike of fragrant, white, single or double flowers that resemble small lilies. Tuberose oil is used in perfumes. Can cause allergic reactions. GRAS. EAF

TULIPA KAUFMANNIANA • Skin conditioner. Soon after its discovery on the Central Asian mountain slopes, the Kaufmann's tulip was introduced to Europe. In 1872, the Dutch company Van Tubergen bought the first species and started the wide-scale selling of the bulb. The tulip was described in 1877 by Eduard Regel of the St. Petersburg

Botanic Garden. The tulip was named after Konstantin Kaufmann, the governor of Tashkent at that time.

TUMERIC • *See* Turmeric.

TUNA EXTRACT • The extract of the fish species *Thunnus. See* Fish Oil.

TURKEY-RED OIL • One of the first surface-active ingredients (*see*). Used in shampoos. Contains sulfated castor oil. It has been used to obtain bright, clear colors in dyeing fabrics. *See* Sulfonated Oils.

TURMERIC • Tumeric. Derived from an East Indian herb, *Curcuma longa*. An aromatic, pepperlike, but somewhat bitter, taste. The cleaned, boiled, sun-dried, pulverized root is used in coconut, ginger ale, and curry flavorings. The oleoresin (*see*) is obtained by extraction of one or more of the solvents acetone, ethyl alcohol, ethylene dichloride (*see all*), and others. It is used in spice flavorings. Both turmeric and its oleoresin have been permanently listed as yellow colorings since 1966. Turmeric has medicinal properties and is used for several applications including hair care, sunscreen, and anti-acne.

TURMERIC OIL • Curcuma Longa. Curcuma Longa Roots. Obtained by steam distillation or solvent extraction of the powdered rhizome of species of the genus *Curcuma* (Family: Zingiberaceae). Of these species, *Curcuma longa* is the most well known.

TURNERA DIFFUSA • *See* Damiana Leaves.

TURNIP EXTRACT • The extract of *Brassica rapa*. Biennial herbs with thick root. Has a hairy skin.

TURPENTINE • Any of the various resins obtained from coniferous trees. A yellowish, viscous exudate with a characteristic smell, it is a natural solvent composed of pine oils, camphenes, and terpenes. It is used as an external analgesic, fragrance ingredient, and thinner. The volatile components of turpentine, pinene, and carene may be hazardous to the lungs. Turpentine is readily absorbed through the skin. Irritating to the skin and mucous membranes and can cause allergic reactions. In addition, it is a central nervous system depressant. Death is usually due to respiratory failure. As little as 15 milliliters has killed children.

TURPENTINE GUM • A solvent in hair lotions, waxes, and perfume soaps and used to soothe skin. It is the oleoresin from a species of pines. Also a food flavoring. Readily absorbed through the skin. Irritating to the skin and mucous membranes. In addition to being a local skin irritant, it can cause allergic reactions.

TURPENTINE TREE • *Pistacia terebinthus. Pinus taeda.* Terebinth. White Turpentine. Spirits of Turpentine. The term turpentine refers to vegetable juices, liquids, or gums containing the essential oil generally procured from various species of pine; other trees, such as the European larch, also yield turpentine. *P. terebinthus* is a small tree native to Greece. The common American, or white, turpentine, which is listed as terebintha in the U.S. Pharmacopeia, is from *P. taeda*. The oil or "spirit" is a local irritant, and somewhat antiseptic. Turpentine baths, arranged so that vapors were not inhaled, were given to patients with chronic arthritis. Applied topically as a liniment or ointment, it is used by herbalists to treat arthritis and nerve pain. It was also used topically to treat and promote the healing of burns, and to heal parasitic skin diseases. Terebene, which is derived from oil of turpentine, is used orally or by inhalation as an antiseptic and expectorant. In 1992, the FDA proposed a ban for the use of turpentine oil to treat fever blisters and cold sores, in insect bite and sting drug products, and in those to treat poison ivy, poison sumac, and poison oak because it had not been shown to be safe and effective as claimed in these OTC products.

TURTLE OIL • The oil of *tartaruchus*, used in emollients. At one time there was a great deal of hype about the antiwrinkle benefits of this ingredient but, as pointed out, it never did much for a turtle's skin.

Powders with a cornstarch base may be preferred over those with a talc base. Avoid inhaling and contact with the eyes or other mucous membranes. Should not be applied on blistered, raw, or oozing skin or over deep or puncture wounds. Patients with impaired circulation, including diabetics, should consult a physician before using.

UNDECYLENOYL COLLAGEN AMINO ACIDS • The treatment of animal collagen with acid to obtain amino acids. Used as a protein additive.

UNDECYLENOYL GLYCINE • Hair conditioner and cleanser. *See* Glycine and Undecylenic Acid.

UNDECYLENOYL HYDROLYZED COLLAGEN • A hair and skin conditioner. *See* Undecylenic Acid and Hydrolyzed Collagen.

UNDECYLENOYL INULIN • Emollient and emulsifier. *See* Undecylenic Acid and Inulin.

UNDECYLENOYL PEG-5 PARABEN • Preservative. *See* Parabens and Polyethylene Glycol.

UNDECYLENOYL WHEAT AMINO ACIDS • Hair conditioner and cleanser. *See* Undecylenic Acid and Wheat.

UNDECYLENOYL XANTHAN GUM • Emulsifier and hair conditioner. *See* Xanthan Gum and Undecylenic Acid.

UNDECYLENYL ALCOHOL • Colorless liquid with a citrus odor. Used in perfumes. It is combustible but has a low toxicity.

UNDECYLIC ACID • *See* Undecylenic Acid.

UNDECYLPENTADECANOL • Used as a skin conditioner. *See* Fatty Alcohols.

UNIPERTAN • A tanning accelerator made of collagen, tyrosine, and riboflavin, all of which are derived from animals. But there is a vegetarian version of this suntanning compound.

UNSAPONIFIABLE OLIVE OIL • The oil fraction that is not broken down in the refining of olive fatty acids. *See* Olive Oil.

UNSAPONIFIABLE RAPESEED OIL • The oil that is not broken down in the refining of rapeseed oil fatty acids. *See* Rapeseed Oil.

UNSAPONIFIABLE SHEA BUTTER • The fraction of shea butter that is not broken down during processing. *See* Shea Butter.

UNSAPONIFIABLE SOYBEAN OIL • The fraction of soybean oil that is not broken down in the refining recovery of soybean oil fatty acids. *See* Soybean Oil.

URACIL • Skin conditioner. It occurs in combined form in many important biological molecules, including RNA and several coenzymes active in carbohydrate metabolism. Used in cancer chemotherapy.

UREA • Carbamide. A product of protein metabolism excreted from human urine. Used in yeast food and wine production up to two pounds per gallon. It is used to "brown" baked goods such as pretzels and consists of colorless or white, odorless crystals that have a cool salty taste. An antiseptic and deodorizer used in liquid antiperspirants, ammoniated dentifrices, roll-on deodorants, mouthwashes, hair colorings, hand creams, lotions, and shampoos. Medicinally, urea is used as a topical antiseptic and as a diuretic to reduce body water. Its largest use, however, is as a fertilizer, and only a small part of its production goes into the manufacture of other urea products. The final report to the FDA of the Select Committee on GRAS Substances stated in 1980 that it should continue its GRAS status with no limitations other than good manufacturing practices. On the Canadian Hotlist (*see*). Permitted in concentrations equal to or less than 10 percent in Canada.

UREA-D-GLUCURONIC ACID • A humectant. *See* Glucuronic Acid.

UREA-FORMALDEHYDE RESIN • UFFI. A large class of resins, the mixture of urea and formaldehyde (*see both*), were the first colored plastics made. The adverse health effects of UFFI are hotly debated. People exposed to UFFI in buildings report shortness of breath, headache, stuffy nose, irritated eyes, cough, frequent "colds," rash, fatigue, sore throat, and vomiting. *See* Formaldehyde.

UREA PEROXIDE • When used in over-the-counter drugs, the established name for this ingredient is carbamide peroxide. A strong oxidizing ingredient, it is used for softening wax. It is on the Canadian Hotlist (*see*) and in that country it is not permitted in dentifrices, mouthwashes, or "other" purposes that involve long-term use in the oral cavity. May be used as a tooth-bleaching agent if safety data submitted and concentration limited to 3 percent and labeled for use for no more than fourteen days unless under the supervision of a dentist.

UREASE • An enzyme that hydrolyzes urea (*see*) to ammonium carbonate (*see*).

URETHANE • A known carcinogen for several species of animals, and, as such, must be viewed as a potential carcinogen for humans as well. The degree of risk to humans, though, is not known. The FDA says scientific data are simply too limited to assess the risk posed by low levels of the chemical in alcoholic beverages. Concern in this country over urethane (also called ethyl carbamate) began in November 1985 with news reports that Canadian authorities had detected the chemical in certain wines and distilled spirits. It is used in hair products as a film former and thickener. On the Canadian Hotlist (*see*). *See also* Polyurethane.

URIC ACID • White, odorless, tasteless crystals. It forms the end product of nitrogen metabolism of birds and scaly reptiles. It is present in small amounts in human urine. Used as a skin conditioner. *See* Allantoin.

UROCANIC ACID • 3-Imidazol-4-ylacrylic acid. Skin conditioner and sunscreen. Prepared from histidine (*see*). The CIR Expert Panel (*see*) says there is insufficient data to conclude that this ingredient is "safe for use in cosmetics." Because of this, sunscreens containing urocanic acid should not be used by consumers when trying to minimize the potential of increased sun sensitivity due to alpha-hydroxy acid (AHA) use. The safety of this ingredient has not been documented and substantiated. On the Canadian Hotlist (*see*). Banned in cosmetics by ASEAN (*see*).

URSOLIC ACID • Fragrance ingredient and skin conditioner that naturally occurs in a large number of vegetarian foods, medicinal herbs, and other plants. For a long time, it was considered to be pharmacologically inactive. Thus, ursolic acid and its alkali salts (e.g., potassium or sodium ursolates) were exclusively used as emulsifying agents in pharmaceutical, cosmetic, and food preparations. It has now been found to be medicinally active both topically and internally. Its anti-inflammatory, antitumor (skin cancer), and antimicrobial properties are being used in some cosmetics. Its overall toxicity (both chronic and acute) is low. It is reportedly not a primary irritant or sensitizer and has been termed "dermatologically innocuous."

URTICA DIOICA • *See* Nettles.

URTICA URENS • Stinging Nettles. Used to treat insect bites and stings, burns and scalds, heavy or prolonged menstruation, leucorrhoea, hives, eczema, itchy blotches, ill effects of eating shellfish, sore throat, rheumatism, gout, gravel, vertigo, diminished secretion of milk.

USNEA BARBATA • *See* Lichen Extract.

USNIC ACID • Antibacterial compound found in lichens. Pale yellow, slightly soluble in water.

UVA-URSI • *Arctostaphylos uva-ursi.* Bearberry. An astringent used to treat bladder problems, it is believed that its action is due to the high concentration of the antiseptic arbutin. Contains a natural hydroquinone (a bleaching agent used in skin preparations) sugar complex that is used to help fade hyperpigmentation spots on the skin by interfering with melanin (see) synthesis. Crude extracts of uva-ursi reportedly possess some anticancer property. In 1992, the FDA proposed a ban on uva-ursi in oral menstrual drug products because it had not been shown to be safe and effective for its stated claims.

V

VA • Abbreviation for vinyl acetate (see).

VA/BUTYL MALEATE/ISOBORNYL ACRYLATE COPOLYMER • Film former in hair products. The copolymer of vinyl acetate, butyl maleate, and isobornyl acrylate monomers. See Vinyl Polymers.

VA/CA COPOLYMER • Binder, hair fixative, and emulsifier. An epidemiological study of hairdressers, who would inhale more VA/CA than the average person, did not show lung problems. On the basis of the available information, the CIR Expert Panel (see) found it safe in the early 1980s but is considering new information to determine if the final safety assessment should be reaffirmed, amended, or have an addendum. See Vinyl Acetate.

VACCINIUM ANGUSTIFOLIUM • See Bilberry Extract.

VACCINIUM MACROCARPON • See Cranberry.

VACCINIUM MYRTILLUS • Skin conditioner. See Bilberry Extract.

VACCINIUM VITIS-IDAEA • Lingonberry. Mountain Cranberry. Koemomo. Cowberry. Used as a flavoring and as a cough and throat soother by Alaskan Indians. Used as an antioxidant, skin conditioner, and humectant in cosmetics.

VA/CROTONATES COPOLYMER • Aerosol fixative in hair sprays. A polymer of vinyl acetate and one or more monomers consisting of crotonic acid or any of its simple esters. *Croton tiglium* oil is banned in cosmetics by the EU. See Vinyl Polymers and Crotonic Acid.

VA/CROTONATES/METHACRYLOXYBENZOPHENONE-1 COPOLYMER • Synthetic polymer used as a hair fixative and ultraviolet light absorber. See Benzophenones 1–12 and Vinyl Acetate.

VA/DBM COPOLYMER • Film former for hair products. See Vinyl Acetate and Malic Acid.

VAGINAL DEODORANTS • Formerly called "Feminine Hygiene Sprays." Introduced in 1966, vaginal deodorant sprays have grown very popular. Marketed as mists or powders in aerosol sprays and widely advertised as products to keep women feeling "feminine," they are designed to prevent "feminine odor" and to give that "clean feeling." Classified as cosmetics, these deodorants did not need clearance for the ingredients. Reports to the FDA of irritations and other problems from the sprays within the last two years include bladder infections, burning, itching, swelling, rash, boils in the vaginal area, and blood in the urine. Physicians recommend soap and water as more beneficial than the sprays, and that concentrating chemicals, including perfumes, in one area is not wise because of the possibility of allergic reactions and irritations. Ingredients in vaginal deodorants include emollients such as glycerides, myristate, polyoxyethylene derivatives, perfumes, and propellants. Some sprays, in addition, contain an antibacterial. The allergic and skin reactions may not only occur in the women who use these products but also in their male partners who are exposed to the ingredients during sexual relations. Among some of the problem spray ingredients identified were benzalkonium chloride, chlorhexidine, isopropyl myristate, and perfume. The FDA says such products are misbranded unless the labeling bears explicit warnings and directions for safe use (when applicable). Additionally, these products may be considered misbranded if the labeling contains the word *hygiene* or a similar word. If the product is represented to have a medical usefulness, it may be considered a drug and would be misbranded. Most vaginal deodorants are similar to shampoos containing sodium lauryl sulfate (*see*), which can cause irritation. Other ingredients, such as alcohol and other antimicrobials (*see*), can also cause irritation.

VALERIA INDICA • Skin conditioner. *See* Damar.

VALERIAN • The extract of *Valeriana officinalis*. A perennial native to Europe and the United States, it was reputed to be a love potion. Used in massage oils today and in aromatherapy. The herb has been widely studied in Europe and Russia, and the major constituents, the valepotriate, have been reported to have marked sedative, anticonvulsive, blood pressure–lowering, and tranquilizing effects. It has been used for centuries to treat panic attacks. In Germany, valerian preparations have been used for more than a decade to treat childhood behavioral disorders, supposedly without the side effects experienced with pharmaceuticals for that purpose. It has been reported that it also helps concentration and energy. Prolonged use of valerian may result in side effects such as irregular heartbeat, headaches, uneasiness, nervousness, and insomnia. Very large doses may cause paralysis. *See* Valeric Acid.

VALERIANA CELTICA • Found in Alpine pastures. *See* Valerian.

VALERIANA FAURIEI • Skin conditioner. *See* Valerian.

VALERIANA OFFICINALIS • *See* Valerian.

VALERIANA WALLICHII • *See* Valerian.

VALERIC ACID • Used in the manufacture of perfumes. Occurs naturally in apples, cocoa, coffee, oil of lavender, peaches, and strawberries. Colorless, with an unpleasant odor. Usually distilled from the roots of valerian (*see*). It is used also as a synthetic flavoring, and some of its salts are used in medicine.

VALINE • An essential amino acid (*see*). Occurs in the largest quantities in fibrous protein. It is indispensable for growth and nitrogen balance. Used in suntan lotions, and hair and skin conditioners. Nontoxic in cosmetics, but the FDA has asked for further study of this ingredient as a food additive.

VANCIDE FP • *See* Captan.

VANILLA EXTRACT • Used in perfumes and flavorings. Extracted from the full-grown unripe fruit of the vanilla plant of Mexico and the West Indies.

VANILLA PLANIFOLIA EXTRACT • *See* Vanilla Extract.

VANILLA TAHITENSIS • Used in hair conditioners and shampoos. *See* Vanilla Extract.

VANILLIN • Used in perfumes. Occurs naturally in vanilla and potato parings but is an artificial flavoring and scent made synthetically from eugenol (*see*); also from the waste of the wood pulp industry. One part vanillin equals 400 parts vanilla pods. The lethal dose in mice is 3 grams (30 grams to the ounce) per kilogram of body weight. A skin irritant that produces a burning sensation and eczema. May also cause pigmentation of the skin.

VANILLYL BUTYL ETHER • Hair and skin conditioner. *See* Phenols.

VANISHING CREAM • An emollient cream that creates the feeling of vanishing when rubbed on the skin. *See* Emollients.

VASELINE • Petroleum Jelly. Petrolatum. Paraffin Jelly. Used in cold creams, emollient creams, conditioning creams, wax depilatories, eyebrow pencils, eye shadows, liquefying creams, liquid powders, nail whites, lipsticks, protective creams, baby creams, and rouge. While usually soothing to the skin, it may cause allergic reactions, particularly in creams and hairdressings, because it is a derivative of petroleum.

VASOCONSTRICTION • A decrease in the diameter of a blood vessel.

VASOCONSTRICTOR • A substance that causes a narrowing of the blood vessels. Cold, stress, nicotine, and certain drugs such as ergotamine are vasoconstrictors.

VAT DYES • Water-soluble aromatic organic compounds. They dissolve in water when vatted with an alkaline solution of the reducing agent (*see*) sodium hydrosulfite. Good fastness. Considered low in toxicity.

VAT RED 1 • EU name CI 73360; Japanese name Aka226. An indigoid color. The certified name of this color is D & C Red No. 30. *See* Vat Dyes.

VA/VINYL BUTYL BENZOATE CROTONATES COPOLYMER • A polymer of vinyl acetate, vinyl *t*-butylbenzoate, and one or more monomers of crotonic acid or one of its simple esters. Film former in hair products. *Croton tiglium* is banned in cosmetics by the EU. *See* Vinyl Polymers.

VA/VINYL CROTINATES/VINYL NEODECANOATE • Used in hair sprays. *See* Vinyl Polymers and Decanoic Acid.

VEGETABLE GLYCERIDES PHOSPHATE • A skin conditioner. *See* Vegetable Oils.

VEGETABLE GLYCERIN • Products made of plants such as avocado instead of animal-derived glycerin (*see*).

VEGETABLE GUMS • Includes derivatives from quince seed, karaya, acacia, tragacanth, Irish moss, guar, sodium alginate, potassium alginate, ammonium alginate, and propylene glycol alginate. All are subject to deterioration and always need a preservative. The gums function as liquid emulsions; that is, they thicken cosmetic products and make them cream. No known toxicity. May cause allergic reactions in hypersensitive persons.

VEGETABLE OILS • Peanut, sesame, olive, and cottonseed oil obtained from plants and used in baby preparations, cleansing creams, emollient creams, face powders, hair-grooming aids, hypoallergenic cosmetics, lipsticks, nail creams, shampoos, shaving creams, and wave sets.

VELVET EXTRACT • *Cervus elaphus.* Elk. Wapiti. Red Deer. Extract of the antler "velvet" is associated with anti-aging, immune support, mood disorders, blood enrichment, chronic joint pain of osteoarthritis, the side effects of chemotherapy, bone and muscle growth, joint restoration, healthy sexual function in men and women, and increased energy levels. Used in cosmetics as a skin conditioner and humectant.

VERATALDEHYDE • Derived from petroleum. Has the odor of vanilla beans. Used in perfumery.

VERATRUM • Veratrine is a poisonous alkaloid obtained from the root helebore (*Veratrum*) and from sabadilla seeds as a white crystalline powder, having an acrid, burning taste. It is sometimes used externally, as in ointments, in the local treatment of neuralgia and rheumatism. Called also veratria, and veratrina. On the Canadian Hotlist (*see*). Banned in cosmetics by the EU.

VERBASCUM THAPSUS • *See* Mullein Extract.

VERBENA OFFICINALIS EXTRACT • Has a characteristic odor; insoluble in water. Used as a perfume ingredient. The flower water is used as a skin conditioner. Not permitted in fragrances by the UK. *See* Terpenes.

VERONICA EXTRACT • Extract of the flowering herb veronica, a small herb of wide distribution that has pink or white flowers. Used in perfumery and skin conditioners. *See* Speedwell.

VETIVER OIL • Vetiverol. Khus-Khus. Stable, brown to reddish brown oil from the roots of a fragrant grass. Used in soaps and perfumes, it has an aromatic to harsh, woodsy odor.

VETIVER RECTIFIED • Perfume ingredient. *See* Vetiver Oil.

VETIVEROL • *See* Vetiver Oil.

VETIVERYL ACETATE • *See* Vetiver Oil.

VIBURNUM EXTRACT • Haw Bark. Black Extract. Extract of the fruit of a hawthorn shrub or tree. Used in fragrances and in butter, caramel, cola, maple, and walnut flavorings for beverages. Has been used as a uterine antispasmodic.

VIBURNUM PRUNIFOLIUM POWDER • *See* Viburnum Extract.

VICIA FABA • *See* Faba Bean Extract.

VIGNA RADIATA • Mung bean. Best known in the United States as the bean used for production of bean sprouts. The mung bean is commonly known in Asia as the green gram. Other common names include golden gram, moong, and chop suey bean. Contains an enzyme that processes protein. Used as a skin conditioner.

VINCA MAJOR • *See* Periwinkle Extract.

VINEGAR • Used for hundreds of years to remove lime soap after shampooing. It is a solvent for cosmetic oils and resins. Vinegar is about 4 to 6 percent acetic acid. Acetic acid occurs naturally in apples, cheese, grapes, milk, and other foods, but it may cause an allergic reaction in those allergic to corn.

VINYL ACETATE • Used as film former. Vapors in high concentration may be narcotic; animal experiments show low toxicity.

VINYL BROMIDE • A flame retardant. A cancer-causing ingredient.

VINYL CAPROLACTAM/PVP/DIMETHYLAMINOETHYL METHACRYLATE COPOLYMER • *See* Vinyl Polymers.

VINYL CHLORIDE • Banned in aerosol cans for hair sprays and deodorants in 1974. It is a proven cause of liver cancer in workers who work with the compound. On the Canadian Hotlist (*see*). Banned in cosmetics by the EU and the FDA.

VINYL DIMETHICONE • *See* Dimethicone and Vinyl Acetate.

VINYL POLYMERS • Includes resins used in false nails and nail lacquer preparations. A major class of polymer (*see*) material widely used in plastics, synthetic fibers, and surface coatings. Such materials are derived from the polymerization of vinyl groups, which include vinyl acetate and vinyl chloride. Vinyls are made from the reaction between acetylene and certain compounds such as alcohol, phenol, and amines. Inhalation of 300 parts per million is toxic in man.

VINYL PYRROLIDONE • *See* Polyvinylpyrrolidone.

VINYLDIMETHICONE • *See* Silicones and Vinyl Polymers.

VIOLA ODORATA • Sweet Violet. Skin conditioner. Medicinal and edible, the flowers and leaves of viola are made into a syrup used in alternative medicine mainly for respiratory ailments. Flowers are also edible and used as food additives, for instance in salad, made into jelly, and candied for decoration. New research has detected the presence of a glycoside of salicylic acid (natural aspirin), which substantiates its use for centuries as a medicinal remedy for headache, body pains, and as a sedative.

VIOLA TRICOLOR • *See* Pansy, Wild.

VIOLET EXTRACT • Flowers and Leaves. Green liquid with typical odor of violet. It is taken from the plant widely grown in the United States. Used in perfumes, face powders, and for coloring inorganic pigments. May produce skin rash in the allergic. *See* Viola Odorata.

VIOLET 2 • EU name CI 60725. Japanese name Murasaki 201. An anthraquinone (*see*) color. *See* Coal Tar.

VISCOSITY • Thickness or resistance to flow or alteration of shape. Ingredients are added to cosmetics to make them thinner or thicker. Shampoo contains mostly water so thickeners are added to improve pouring properties. Lipsticks are made with light oils or fatty alcohols that soften the wax.

VISCUM ALBUM • *See* Mistletoe.

VISNAGA VERA EXTRACT • Used as a skin conditioner promoted as useful to counteract cellulite (*see*). A plant related to celery (*see*) and may cause an allergic reaction.

VITAMIN A • A yellow, viscous liquid insoluble in water. Used in lubricating creams and oils for its alleged skin-healing properties. Can be absorbed through the skin. Its absence from the diet leads to a loss in weight, retarded growth, and eye diseases. Too high a level can cause the skin to turn yellow and can cause birth defects and pressure on the brain. *See also* Retinoids and Retin-A.

VITAMIN B$_6$ • Pyridoxine hydrochloride. A colorless or white crystalline powder added to evaporated milk base in infant foods. Present in many foodstuffs. Especially good sources are yeast, liver, and cereals. A coenzyme that helps in the metabolism of amino acids (*see*) and fat. Permits normal red blood cell formation. The final report to the FDA of the Select Committee on GRAS Substances stated in 1980 that it should continue its GRAS status with no limitations other than good manufacturing practices. The FDA is doing a toxicology search on this additive.

VITAMIN C • *See* Ascorbic Acid.

VITAMIN D$_2$ • Calciferol. A pale yellow, oily liquid, odorless, tasteless, and insoluble in water. Used for its alleged skin-healing properties in lubricating creams and lotions. The absence of vitamin D in the food of young animals can lead to rickets, a bone-affecting condition. It is soluble in fats and fat solvents and is present in animal fats. Absorbed through the skin, its value in cosmetics has not been proven. The final report to the FDA of the Select Committee on GRAS Substances stated in 1980 that there is no evidence in the available information that it is a hazard to the public when used as it is now, and it should continue its GRAS status with limitations on amounts that can be added to food. Dermatologists recommend vitamin D supplements. The American Academy of Dermatology (AAD) is backing efforts to encourage increased consumption of vitamin D through food and dietary supplements. In a position statement on vitamin D at this writing, the academy stressed the importance of obtaining adequate levels of the vitamin without overexposure to cancer-causing UV radiation from sunlight or tanning machines. "Vitamin D is essential for optimal health, and the medical literature supports safe ways to get it—a healthy diet which incorporates foods naturally rich in vitamin D, vitamin D-fortified foods and beverages, and vitamin D supplements," said dermatologist C. William Hanke, MD, president of AAD. "And, according to the medical literature, unprotected exposure to UV radiation from sunlight (natural) or indoor tanning devices (artificial) is not safe. Individuals who intentionally expose themselves to UV radiation for vitamin D are putting their health at risk for developing skin cancer." AAD said it supports the recommended daily intake levels provided in guidelines from the Institute of Medicine (IOM) and is urging physicians to do the same.

VITAMIN E • *See* Tocopherol.

VITAMIN E ACETATE • *See* Tocopherol.

VITAMIN E SUCCINATE • *See* Tocopherol.

VITAMIN K • Recommended daily allowance for adults has not been established, but the safety and adequate daily dietary intake level is listed at 0.07 to 0.14 mg. It is necessary for blood clotting. Current research seems to indicate it helps maintain bone mass in the elderly and prevents osteoporosis.

VITAVERIA ZIZANOIDES • *See* Vetiver Oil.

VITEX AGNUS CASTUS • Chaste Tree Berry. Used as an astringent and anti-aging ingredient. Chasteberry has been used since ancient times as a female remedy. One of its properties was to reduce sexual desire, and it is recorded that Roman wives whose husbands were abroad with the legions spread the aromatic leaves on their couches for this purpose. It became known as the chasteberry tree. During the Middle Ages, chasteberry's supposed effect on sexual desire led to it becoming a food spice at monasteries, where it was called "monk's pepper" or "cloister pepper." In tradition, it was also known as an important European remedy for controlling and regulating the female reproductive system. Recent investigations show the presence of compounds that are able to adjust the production of female hormones. It is said to contain a progesterone-like compound. The EU banned progestogens in cosmetics.

VITEX TRIFOLIA • Vervain. *See* Vitex Agnus Castus.

VITILIGO • Leukoderma. Irregular white patches of skin, sometimes streaks of white or gray hair due to lack of pigment. Usually, there is a family tendency to develop this condition. The white patches are most noticeable when surrounded by deeply tanned skin. It is not a systemic but merely a cosmetic condition.

VITIS VINEFERA • *See* Grape Leaf Extract.

VITREOSCILLA FERMENT • An extract of the bacterial culture derived from the bacteria *Vitreoscilla*. Used as a skin conditioner.

VITULUS • Calf blood or calf skin extract. Used in emollients.

VOANDZEIA SUBTERRANEA • Ground Nut. Skin conditioner. The entire plant is similar to the common peanut. Carried to America by slaves, it has never become as popular as the peanut, which has a higher level of protein. Seeds contain 14–24 percent protein and about 60 percent carbohydrate. The protein is reported to be higher in the essential amino acid methionine than other grain legumes. Bambara groundnuts contain 6–12 percent oil, which is less than half the amount found in peanuts.

VOLCANIC ASH • Abrasive, absorbent, and bulking ingredient.

VOLATILE OILS • Volatility in oils is the tendency to give off vapors, usually at room temperature. The volatile oils in plants such as peppermint or rose produce the aroma. The volatile oils in plants stimulate the tissue with which they come into contact, whether they are inhaled, ingested, or placed on the skin. They can relax or stimulate, irritate or soothe, depending upon their source and concentration.

VP/ACRYLATES/LAURYL METHACRYLATE COPOLYMER • Hair fixative. *See* Acrylates Copolymer.

VP/DIMETHYLAMINOETHYLMETHACRYLATE COPOLYMER • Hair fixative in hair-grooming products and mascara. *See* Acrylates Copolymer.

VP/EICOSENE COPOLYMER • Film former and thickener in suntan products, makeup, and moisturizers. *See* Arachidic Acid and Polyvinylpyrrolidone.

VP/VA COPOLYMER • Binder, film former, and hair fixative in hair-grooming products, and makeup including eyeliner and mascara. *See* Vinyl Acetate and Vinyl Pyrrolidone.

W

WALNUT EXTRACT • *Juglans nigra.* An extract of the husk of the nut of *Juglans* species, used in walnut flavorings and for brown coloring. The fruit is used by herbalists to promote strength and weight gain and to treat skin diseases, including eczema, herpes, and psoriasis.

WALNUT LEAVES • Used in hair products for "split ends." *See* Walnut Extract.

WALNUT OIL • *See* Walnut Extract.

WALNUT SHELL POWDER • The ground shell of English walnuts, *Juglans regia*. *See* Walnut Extract.

WALTHERIA INDICA • Sleepy Morning. Ualoa. Small shrublike weed with aromatic flowers. Mixed with ferulic acid (*see*) to lighten age spots. The plant is believed to have tannins and combats bacteria and viruses.

WASABIA JAPONICA • Japanese Horseradish. Preservative. Has been reported to have antifungal and antibacterial effects and to aid metabolism of B_1.

WATER • Aqua. The major constituent of all living matter and the ingredient used most in the cosmetic industry. Because of this fact, the industry fought labeling that required listing ingredients in descending order since water would be first most of the time. However, listing in descending order is now required. It is important that water used in cosmetics be sterile to avoid contamination of the product. Manufacturers may also have to soften water in some areas because of the high mineral content that may affect the texture and appearance of the finished product.

WATER CHESTNUT EXTRACT • The extract of the seeds of *Eleocharis dulcis*, which has an edible nutlike fruit. *See* Cyperus.

WATER LILY • *Nymphaea alba*. Water Rose. Cultivated in pools, this beautiful and romantic flower was used in folk medicine to depress sexual function. Externally, white and yellow water lilies were used to treat various skin disorders such as boils, inflammations, tumors, and ulcers.

WATERCRESS EXTRACT • Extract obtained from *Nasturtium officinalis*, a water-loving plant. Used in emollients for oily skin.

WATERMELON • *Citrullus vulgaris*. Succulent fruit of the gourd family, native to tropical Africa, and under cultivation on every continent. The sweet, juicy fruit may be red, white, or yellow. Used in "organic" cosmetics.

WAVE SET • *See* Setting Lotions.

WAXES • Obtained from insects, animals, and plants. Waxes have a wide application in the manufacture of cosmetics. Beeswax, for instance, is a substance secreted by the bee's special glands on the underside of its abdomen. The wax is glossy and hard but plastic when warm. Insoluble in water but partially soluble in boiling alcohol. Used in hair-grooming preparations, hair straighteners, as an epilatory (hair pull) to remove unwanted hair, and as the traditional stiffening ingredient (*see*) in lipsticks. Wax esters such as lanolin or spermaceti (*see both*) differ from fats in being less greasy, harder, and more brittle. Waxes are generally safe for the skin but may cause allergic reactions in the hypersensitive, depending upon the source of the wax.

WAXING • A method of hair removal for large areas of skin such as the legs and forearms. Melted or cold wax tapes are placed over the hairs, which then become caught in the wax as it hardens. The hair roots are not usually killed, and the hair reappears in a few weeks or so. Some claim that after several treatments, the hair doesn't reappear or is nearly unnoticeable.

WELAN GUM • Emulsifier and thickener. Produced by the fermentation of sugars.

WETTING INGREDIENTS • Any of numerous water-soluble ingredients that promote spreading of a liquid on a surface or penetration into a material such as skin. It lowers surface tension for better contact and absorption.

WHEAT AMINO ACIDS • Emulsifier used in hair and skin conditioners. *See* Wheat Germ and Amino Acids.

WHEAT BRAN • The broken coat of *Triticum aestivum*. *See* Wheat Germ and Wheat Bran Lipids.

WHEAT BRAN LIPIDS • An extract of the coat of wheat. *See* Wheat Germ.

WHEAT FLOUR • Milled from the kernels of wheat, *Triticum aestivum*. Used as an abrasive and thickener. *See* Wheat Starch.

WHEAT GERM • *Triticum vulgare*. The golden germ of the wheat is high in vitamin E. It is used by organic cosmeticians to make a face mask to counteract dry skin. Here is the formula: Crush 1/4 cup wheat germ plus 1 tablespoon sesame seeds with a mortar and pestle or with the back of a spoon. Add 2 tablespoons of fresh olive oil and mix well. Spread on face and neck. Leave on for 10 minutes. Remove with lukewarm water. Then rinse with cold water. Apply a rinse of chilled witch hazel (*see*). In low concentrations, it has not been found to cause sensitization. On the basis of available information, the CIR Expert Panel (*see*) concluded that it is safe as presently used in cosmetic formulations. *See* Tocopherol.

WHEAT GERM ACID • An emollient ingredient. On the basis of the available information, the CIR Expert Panel (*see*) found it safe in the early 1980s but is considering new information to determine if the final safety assessment should be reaffirmed, amended, or have an addendum.

WHEAT GERM EXTRACT • Widely used extract of wheat germ used in anti-aging and other emollients. *See* Tocopherol.

WHEAT GERM GLYCERIDES • Used in emollients. On the basis of the available information, the CIR Expert Panel (*see*) found it safe in the early 1980s but is considering new information to determine if the final safety assessment should be reaffirmed, amended, or have an addendum. *See* Tocopherol and Glycerides.

WHEAT GERM OIL • *Triticum vulgare*. Used in hair conditioners, emollients, and solvents. On the basis of available information, the CIR Expert Panel (*see*) concluded that it is safe as presently used in cosmetic formulations. *See* Tocopherol.

WHEAT GERM OIL UNSAPONIFIABLES • *See* Saponification.

WHEAT GERM PROTEIN • The protein derived from wheat germ used in shampoos and emollients.

WHEAT GERMAMIDOPROPYL BETAINE • *See* Quaternary Ammonium Compounds.

WHEAT GERMAMIDOPROPYL DIMETHYLAMINE • *See* Quaternary Ammonium Compounds.

WHEAT GERMAMIDOPROPYL DIMETHYLAMINE HYDROLYZED COLLAGEN • The wheat germ salt of hydrolyzed collagen. *See* Quaternary Ammonium Compounds.

WHEAT GERMAMIDOPROPYL DIMETHYLAMINE HYDROLYZED WHEAT PROTEIN • *See* Quaternary Ammonium Compounds.

WHEAT GERMAMIDOPROPYL DIMETHYLAMINE LACTATE • *See* Quaternary Ammonium Compounds.

WHEAT GERMAMIDOPROPYL ETHYDIMONIUM ETHOSULFATE • *See* Quaternary Ammonium Compounds.

WHEAT GERMAMIDOPROPYLDIMONIUM HYDROXYPROPYL HYDROLYZED WHEAT PROTEIN • Antistatic ingredient in hair products. *See* Quaternary Ammonium Compounds.

WHEAT GLUTEN • Used in powders and creams as a base. A mixture of proteins present in wheat flour and obtained as an extremely sticky, yellowish gray mass by making a dough and then washing out the starch. It consists almost entirely of two proteins, gliadin and glutenin. It contributes to the porous and spongy structure of bread.

WHEAT STARCH • A product of cereal grain. It swells when water is added. Used as a demulcent, emollient, and in dusting and face powders. May cause allergic reactions such as red eyes and stuffy nose.

WHEY PROTEIN • Obtained from the thin, watery part of milk separated from the curds, it is used in emollients.

WHITE • Inorganic pigments are widely used to "color" cosmetics white. The most widely used are zinc oxide and titanium dioxide to whiten face powders. Also used are gloss white (aluminum hydrate), barium sulfate (blanc fixe), and alumina (*see all*).

WHITE CEDAR LEAF OIL • Oil of Arborvitae. Stable, pale yellow volatile oil obtained by steam distillation from the fresh leaves and branch ends of the eastern arborvitae. Has a strong camphoraceous and sagelike scent. Used as a perfume and scent for soaps and room sprays. Also used as a flavoring ingredient. Soluble in most fixed oils. *See* Cedar for toxicity.

WHITE GINGER EXTRACT • The extract of the roots of Hawaiian white ginger, *Hedycium coronarium. See* Ginger.

WHITE LILY EXTRACT • Extract of the bulbs of *Lilium candidum.* Edible bulbs that were made into soup by the Indians, the lily is used in perfumery.

WHITE MUSTARD EXTRACT • The pulverized seeds of *Brassica alba,* native to southern Europe and western Asia and naturalized in the United States. It is used in cosmetics as a counterirritant (*see*). It is irritating to the skin, however, and can cause burns that are slow to heal.

WHITE NETTLE EXTRACT • Obtained from the flowers of *Lamium album. See* Nettles.

WHITE OAK BARK • *Quercus alba.* The extract of *Quercus alba.* Contains tannic acid, quercitol, resin, pectin, and levulin. Used as an astringent.

WHITE SAPONARIA • *Gypsophila paniculata.* A cleansing ingredient. *See* Saponaria Extract.

WHITE TEA • Green tea was all the rage for the last few years; now it is white tea's turn. It's already appeared in skin care products and, of course, tea. Expect this ingredient, which contains antioxidants, to be touted in hair care and skin products.

WHITEHEAD • A noninflammatory closed comedone (*see*) with a white center.

WHOLE DRY MILK • The solid residue produced by the dehydration of cow's milk. *See* Milk.

WILD AGRIMONY EXTRACT • Extract of Wild Pansy. The extract of the herb *Potentilla anserina.* The Indians used to crush the leaves to treat boils and swellings. By the late 1800s, the wild pansy was being ground up and used to treat many skin diseases, including impetigo, skin ulcers, and scabies.

WILD CHERRY • *See* Wild Cherry Bark.

WILD CHERRY BARK • Wild Black Cherry Bark. The dried stem bark of *Prunus serotina,* collected in autumn in North America. Used in lipsticks and cherry flavorings.

WILD GERANIUM • *See* Cranesbill Extract.

WILD GINGER • *Asarum heterotropoides.* Xi Xin. The root is used by Chinese herbalists to treat menstrual problems. Its warm, pungent action relieves spasms. The American wild ginger is not as strong as the Chinese. The Chinese ginger can be mildly toxic. *See* Ginger.

WILD INDIGO ROOT • *Baptisia tinctoria.* Baptisia. Bastard Indigo. A wild uncultivated plant of North America with showy yellow or blue flowers. The root contains alkaloids, glycosides, and resin (*see all*). It is used by herbalists to treat infections of the ear, nose, and throat. Taken both internally and as a mouthwash, it reputedly heals mouth ulcers and sore gums, and helps to control pyorrhea. Used as a coloring.

WILD MARJORAM EXTRACT • Extract of the flowering ends of *Origanum vulgare.* Yellow or greenish-yellow liquid containing about 40 percent terpenes (*see*). Used in perfumery. *See* Marjoram Oil.

WILD MINT EXTRACT • Extract of the leaves and tender twigs of *Mentha arven-sis*. The Cheyenne Indians prepared a decoction of the ground leaves and stems of wild mint and drank the liquid to check nausea. Pulegone and thymol (*see*) are derived from an oil of wild mint. Its odor resembles peppermint.

WILD MINT OIL • *See* Wild Mint Extract.

WILD PANSY • *See* Agrimony Extract.

WILD SARSAPARILLA EXTRACT • The extract of the roots of *Aralia nudicaulis*. *See* Sarsaparilla Extract.

WILD THYME EXTRACT • *Thymus serpillium*. The flowering tops of the plant grown in Eurasia and throughout the United States. The dried leaves are used in emollients and fragrances. Has also been used as a muscle relaxant.

WILD YAM • *Dioscorea villosa*. *See* Yam.

WILD YAM ROOT • *Dioscorea paniculata* or *D. villosa*. Colicroot. Rheumatism Root. Chinese Yam. Japanese researchers in 1936 discovered glycoside saponins of several Mexican yam species from which the steroid saponin (*see*), primarily diosgenin, could be derived. These derivatives were then converted to progesterone, an intermediate in cortisone production. Steroid drugs derived from diosgenin include corticosteroids, oral contraceptives, androgens, and estrogens. American herbalists for more than two centuries used wild yam root to treat painful menstruation, ovarian pain, cramps, and problems of childbirth. One of the most widely prescribed birth control pills in the world, desogen, is made from the wild yam, confirming what the ancient Mexican women knew all along: they used wild yam as a contraceptive. The EU banned progestens in cosmetics.

WILLOW BARK EXTRACT • *Salix alba* or *S. Nigra*. *See* Salicylates and Willow Leaf Extract.

WILLOW LEAF EXTRACT • The extract of the leaves of the willow tree species *Salix*. The willow has been used for its pain-relieving and fever-lowering properties since ancient Greece. The American Indians used willow baths to cool fevers and indeed, the extract of willows contains salicylic acid, a close cousin of aspirin. *See* Salicylates.

WINE EXTRACT • Antioxidant. Promoted to reduce cholesterol and to enhance sexual function in massage creams.

WINTERGREEN EXTRACT • An extract of the leaves of *Gaultheria procumbens*. *See* Wintergreen Oil.

WINTERGREEN OIL • Menthyl Salicylate. *Gaultheria procumbens*. Spiceberry. Teaberry. Checkerberry Extract. Deerberry. Used in toothpaste, tooth powder, and perfumes. Obtained naturally from betula, sweet birch, or teaberry oil. Present in certain leaves and bark, but usually prepared by treating salicylic acid with methanol (*see both*). Also used as a food and beverage flavoring. Wintergreen oil is an old remedy for rheumatism and rheumatic fever, sciatica, edema, diabetes, bladder disorders, and skin diseases. It contains methyl salicylate (*see*). It is still used for eye lotions, gargles, poultices, antiseptic washes, toothpastes, tooth powders, and perfumes, and by herbalists as a diuretic in small amounts. Large doses cause vomiting. Wintergreen is a strong irritant. Ingestion of relatively small amounts may cause severe poisoning and death. Average lethal dose in children is 10 milliliters and in adults 30 milliliters. It is very irritating to the mucous membranes and skin and can be absorbed rapidly through the skin.

WISTERIA • Used in perfumes. The extract from the Asiatic, mostly woody vines of the family that produces showy blue, white, purple, and rose flowers.

WITCH HAZEL • One of the most widely used cosmetic ingredients, it is a skin freshener, local anesthetic, and astringent made from the leaves and/or twigs of *Hamamelis virginiana*. Collected in the autumn. Witch hazel has an ethanol content of 70 to 80 percent and a tannin content of 2 to 9 percent. Witch hazel water, which is what you buy at the store, contains 15 percent ethanol. *See* Ethanol for toxicity.

WITHANIA SOMNIFERA • Aswagandha. Antifungal. An Indian medicinal plant used widely in the treatment of many clinical conditions in India. Its antistressor properties have been investigated for its rejuvenating capacity in adults. It is believed to be able to impart long life, youthful vigor, and intellectual power. Powdered root is considered to be an invigorating and nutritive tonic for healthy people and a restorer of health for children emaciated by famine or disease. Indian practitioners believe that the root can improve the sperm count of men who have low sperm.

WOOD POWDER • Ground wood consisting of mainly cellulose (*see*) and lignin. Used as an abrasive, absorbent, and thickener.

WOODRUFF • *Asperula odorata.* Master of the Woods. Used in perfumes and sachets. Made of the leaves of an herb grown in Europe, Siberia, North America, Africa, and Australia. It is a symbol of spring and has a clean fresh smell.

WOOL FAT • Crude lanolin (*see*).

WOOL WAX ALCOHOLS • Wool Fat. Chemically more like a fat than a wax, it is the deposit sheep make on their wool. Used as emollients. *See* Lanolin Alcohols.

WORMSEED OIL • Chenopodium Oil. Colorless or yellowish oil with a penetrating odor and bitter taste. Distilled from the seeds and leaves of *Chenopodium ambrosioides anthelminticum.* It is used to combat worms. Used in special soaps. A variety of skin outbreaks, including allergic contact dermatitis, photodermatitis, and mechanical injury have been reported. Nothing is known about the nature of the allergens or the phototoxic principles. *See* Quinoa.

WORMWOOD • *Artemisia absinthium.* Absinthe. Flavoring and aromatherapy. A perennial herb native to the Ural Mountains, it was taken to Egypt very early in recorded history and was listed in Ebers Papyrus as useful for headaches and for eliminating pinworms, two uses still prescribed by herbalists. Because it was used to expel tapeworms and other intestinal worms, it was called "wormwood." In Europe and North America, it was believed to counteract poison. It was recommended for insomnia, jaundice, indigestion, sprains, bruises, and inflammations. The aromatic oil of wormwood contains the cineole, thujone, artemisia. Herbalists today recommend an infusion of the leaves and stems to stimulate appetite and soothe stomach pains. Ingestion of the volatile oil or of the liquor, absinthe, distilled from wormwood, may cause gastrointestinal symptoms, abortion, nervousness, stupor, coma, and death. The use of absinthe is banned in many nations.

WRINKLE REMOVERS • Periodically, the cosmetic industry comes up with a magic ingredient that will prevent or cure wrinkles. Among such ingredients in recent years were serum albumen (from bulls) and estrogen. Another wrinkle remover contained some unidentified ingredients that irritated the skin so that it "puffed up" and the wrinkles "filled out." Turtle oil, natural proteins, and polyunsaturates, among many others, were supposed to feed aging skin, but there is no apparent biochemical or physiological activity in any of them. The companies really went wild in the mid-1980s when Christiaan Barnard, M.D., the pioneer South African heart surgeon, lent his name to a Swiss product with "glycel" and mysterious ingredients that reversed the aging process in the skin. Other competitors came out with similar claims. Ironically, around the same time, physicians reported that Retin-A, a vitamin A derivative, actually did have some wrinkle-reducing effects. *See* Retin-A and Tretinoin. It is difficult for the Federal Trade Commission and the FDA to go after promoters of wrinkle creams. By the time the agencies get the manufacturers to court, it has taken several years and a great deal of money and manpower. Then all the manufacturers have to do is open up under different names or change the names of their products and start selling wrinkle creams all over again. The constant advertising that wrinkles are bad also has its deleterious effect on the psyche of women who may have them.

WU WEI ZI • *Schisandra chinensis.* An herb that may have a constricting effect and can be a skin irritant.

X

XANTHAN GUM • A gum produced by a pure culture fermentation of a carbohydrate with *Xanthomonas campestris.* Also called corn sugar gum. Widely used as a thickener, an emulsifier, and a stabilizer.

XANTHENE • Colorants are divided into acid and basic groups. Xanthenes are the second-largest category of certified colors. The acids are derived from fluorescein. The quinoid acid type is represented by FD & C Red No. 3, erythrosine, used frequently in lipsticks. The phenolic formulations, often called "bromo acids," are represented by D & C Red No. 2, used to "stain" lips. The only basic type certified is D & C Red No. 19, also called Rhodamine B. Has been linked to acne.

XANTHINES • Skin conditioners. Occur in animal organs, blood, urine, yeast, potatoes, coffee beans, and tea. First isolated from gallstones. Xanthines are found in chocolate, coffee, tea, and many drugs such as aminophyllin and caffeine (*see*). They stimulate the brain, heart, and muscles. They act as diuretics to reduce body fluid and also dilate the heart's blood vessels.

XANTHIUM STRUMARIUM • Cocklebur. Used by various Native American tribes to relieve constipation, diarrhea, and vomiting. Indigenous Chinese applications as headache remedy, assist with cramping and numbness of the limbs, ulcers, and sinus problems. Antibacterial, antifungal, and styptic (*see*). May be toxic to the liver and should not be ingested by pregnant women since it adversely affects the placenta.

XANTHOPHYLL • Vegetable Lutein. Skin conditioner. A yellow coloring originally isolated from egg yolk, now isolated from petals of flowers. Occurs also in colored feathers of birds. One of the most widespread carotenoid alcohols (a group of red and yellow pigments) in nature. Provisionally listed for use in food. Although carotenoids can usually be turned into vitamin A, xanthophyll has no vitamin A activity. Used in the following product types: mascara, bath oil/salts/soak, after-sun products, facial moisturizers/treatments, and anti-aging products. No toxicity information available.

XANTHOXYLUM AMERICANUM • *See* Zanthoxylum Piperitum Peel Extract.

XERODERMA • Dry skin.

XIMENIA AMERICANA • A widely distributed family of tropical shrubs and trees. An essential oil, it has a scent like sandalwood (*see*) and is used in fragrances.

XI XIN • *See* Ginger.

XIMENIA OIL • Emollient. *See* Plum Extract.

XYLENE • Fragrance ingredient and solvent. Since xylene is an aromatic hydrocarbon, as is chlorine, it warrants further investigation as a cancer-causing ingredient. There has been no definite association, but it is toxic by inhalation or ingestion. Used as a solvent.

XYLENE SULFONIC ACID • A mixture of aromatic acids. *See* Surfactants.

XYLIDINES, THEIR ISOMERS, SALTS AND HALOGENATED AND SULFONATED DERIVATIVES • Used in the manufacture of dyes. Banned in cosmetics by the EU and ASEAN (*see*). On the Canadian Hotlist (*see*). The FDA allows Brown 1 not more than 0.2 percent. Certification required. 6-Xylidine is a chemical intermediate used principally in the production of dyes. It is also a component of tobacco smoke, a degradation product of aniline-based pesticides, and a metabolite of certain drugs, particularly the xylide group of local anesthetics. The National Toxicology Program (NTP) sponsored single-administration, 2-week, and 13-week studies of 2,6-xylidine by gavage in rats. The U.S. Environmental Protection Agency (EPA) sponsored short-term gavage studies and 10-week range-finding feed studies in Charles River CD rats. The compound was found to be carcinogenic. Toxic by ingestion, inhalation, and skin absorption.

XYLITOL • Formerly made from birchwood, but now made from waste products from the pulp industry. Xylitol has been reported to have diuretic effects, but this has not been substantiated. Found in natural sources such as fruits and vegetables, xylitol is a great-tasting bulk sweetener with 40 percent fewer calories than sugar and key health advantages not normally associated with sugar alternatives. It is used in moisturizers and toothpaste. It is used in chewing gum and as an artificial sweetener. It has been reported to sharply reduce cavities in teeth but costs more than sugar.

XYLOBIOSE • Skin conditioner. A sugar made from xylose (*see*) used as a humectant in cosmetics. Has a stimulatory effect on the selective growth of the intestinal bacterium *Bifidobacterium*.

XYLOCAINE • Lidocaine. Used in after-shave lotions. A local anesthetic that interferes with the transmission of nerve impulses, thereby effecting local anesthetic action. Recommended by manufacturers for topical use on mucous membranes only. Can cause allergic reactions. Not permitted in cosmetics in Switzerland. Banned in cosmetics by ASEAN (*see*).

XYLOSE • A flavoring ingredient, humectant, and skin conditioner in cosmetics. A sugar widely distributed in plant material, especially cherry and maple woods. Not found in a free state. Isolated from corn cobs by boiling. Used as a sweetener for diabetics and in tanning and dyeing.

Y

YAM • *Dioscorea paniculata*. Colicroot. Rheumatism Root. Chinese Yam. Japanese researchers in 1936 discovered glycoside saponins of several Mexican yam species from which the steroid saponin (*see*), primarily diosgenin, could be derived. These derivatives were then converted to progesterone, an intermediate in cortisone production. Steroid drugs derived from diosgenin include corticosteroids, oral contraceptives, androgens, and estrogens. American herbalists for more than two centuries used wild yam roots to treat painful menstruation, ovarian pain, and cramps, and problems of childbirth. Wild yam root has also been used to treat gallbladder pain and ease the passage of gallstones. Yam is used in "organic" cosmetics. The EU banned progestogens in cosmetics. *See* Wild Yam.

YARA YARA • Methoxy naphthalene. Leaflets from ether. Used in the manufacture of cosmetics as a solvent. *See* Naphthalene.

YARROW • *Achillea millefolium*. A strong-scented, spicy, wild herb used in astringents and shampoos. Its astringent qualities have caused it to be recommended by herbalists for greasy skins. According to old herbal recipes, it prevents baldness when the hair is washed regularly with it. Used medicinally as an astringent, tonic, and stimulant. May cause a sensitivity to sunlight and artificial light, in which the skin breaks out and swells.

YEAST • A fungus that is a dietary source of folic acid. It produces enzymes that will convert sugar to alcohol and carbon dioxide. Used in skin conditioners.

YEAST BETA-GLUCAN • A carbohydrate fraction obtained from yeast and used as a film former, skin conditioner, and thickener. *See* Yeast.

YEAST EXTRACT • Facial moisturizer. *See* Yeast.

YEAST PALMITATE • A derivative of yeast and palmitic acid (*see both*) used as a hair fixative and skin conditioner.

YELLOW CURLED DOCK • *Rumex crispus.* Curly Dock. Out-Sting. One of the most common wayside plants, the yellow dock flourished on wasteland. The herb has antibacterial properties. English children use it as an antidote for a nettle sting. It was once used as a primary treatment for scurvy and anemia, probably because of its high iron content. It is recommended by herbalists for skin diseases, arthritis, piles, and lung and gallbladder problems. It is used in "organic" cosmetics.

YELLOW DOCK • *See* Yellow Curled Dock.

YELLOW NO. 5 • EU name CI 19140. Japanese name Ki4. U.S. name FD & C Yellow No. 5. All foods containing this coloring, which is the most widely used color additive in food, drugs, and cosmetics, are supposed to identify it on the label. The FDA ordered this so that those allergic to it could avoid it. *See also* Tartrazine and Salicylates.

YELLOW NO. 5 LAKE • EU name CI 19140. Japanese name Ki4. The salt of Yellow No. 5. Used in lipsticks, blushers, nail polish, and face powders.

YELLOW NO. 6 • EU name CI 15985. Japanese name Ki5. Used in colognes, shampoos, hair coloring, hair conditioners, moisturizers, and cleansers. A coal tar color (*see*).

YELLOW NO. 6 LAKE • EU name CI 15985. Japanese name Ki5. Sunset Yellow (uncertified). Used in lipsticks, blushers, and other makeup products as well as suntan gels and creams. *See* FD & C Yellow No. 6 Aluminum Lake.

YELLOW NO. 7 • EU name CI 45350. Japanese name Ki201. U.S. name Acid Yellow 73 (uncertified). A coal tar color (*see*).

YELLOW NO. 7 LAKE • EU name CI 45350. *See* D & C Yellow No. 7.

YELLOW NO. 8 • EU name CI 45350. Japanese name Ki202(1). U.S. name Acid Yellow (uncertified). A coal tar color (*see*) used in permanent wave products.

YELLOW NO. 10 • EU name CI 47005. Japanese name Ki203. Color widely used in shampoos, bath products, hair conditioners, hand and body preparations, deodorants, and dentifrices.

YELLOW NO. 10 LAKE • EU name CI 47005. Japanese name Ki203. Coal tar color (*see*) used in makeup, lipsticks, and hair bleaches and dyes.

YELLOW NO. 11 • EU name CI 47000. Japanese name Ki204. U.S. name Solvent Yellow (uncertified). Coal tar (*see*) coloring used in hair products, nail polishes, moisturizers, suntan gels, fragrances, and body and hand preparations.

YELLOW OCHER • Consists of mainly aluminum silicate and iron oxide and is used as a coloring. Its use is not approved in the United States or European Union.

YERBA SANTA FLUID EXTRACT • Holy Herb. Mountain Balm. Consumptive's Weed. Bear's Weed. Gum Bush. An extract of the leaves of *Eriodictyon californicum.* A fruit flavoring in commercial products derived from evergreen shrubs grown in California, the American Indians smoked or chewed the leaves of this plant as a treatment for asthma. It is still used by herbalists as an expectorant to treat bronchial congestion, urinary tract inflammations, asthma, and hay fever.

YLANG-YLANG OIL • *Cananga odorata.* A light yellow, very fragrant liquid obtained in the Philippines from flowers. Used for perfumes and as a food and beverage flavoring. May cause allergic reactions.

YOGURT • A dairy product produced by the action of bacteria or yeast on milk. Used as a flavoring and hair conditioner. Believed to have emollient properties.

YOGURT FILTRATE • Obtained by removing insoluble matter from fermented skim milk.

YOKUININ • Job's Tears. Yi Yi Ren. Coix. The seed of *Coix lacryma-jobi* from which the outer coat has been removed. In cosmetics, it is used as an abrasive and skin conditioner. In folk medicine, it is used to treat edema, urirnary problems, diarrhea, pustules, carbuncles, abscesses, joint pain, movement muscle spasms, digestive problems, and warts.

YOKUININ EKISU • Extract of yokuinin (*see*).

YOMOGI EKISU • *Artemisia mongolia.* All *artemisia* species produce aromatic oils, and several are culinary herbs or used as flavorings, hallucinogens, vermifuges, and pharmaceuticals. In cosmetics, this one is used as a skin conditioner.

YUCCA ALOIFOLIA • Spanish Bayonet. A stiff yucca with a short trunk found in the southern United States and tropical America; has rigid spine-tipped leaves and clusters of white flowers. Used as a skin conditioner.

YUCCA BREVIFOLIA POWDER • *See* Yucca Extract.

YUCCA EXTRACT • Mohave Extract. Joshua Tree. Adam's Needle. Derived from a southwestern U.S. plant and used as a base for organic cosmetics as a hair fixative and as a root beer flavoring for beverages and ice cream. *Yucca glauca,* often called Mojave yucca or soap weed, was used by the Indians of the Southwest to treat burns and abrasions. Modern scientists have reported it increases cell growth and is an anti-irritant. Used in cleansers.

YUCCA SCHIDIGERA EXTRACT • *See* Yucca Extract.

YUKARI EKISU • Skin conditioner. *See* Eucalyptus Oil.

YUKARI YU • *See* Eucalpytol.

Z

ZANTEDESCHIA AETHIOPICA • Calla Lily Extract. Arum Lily. Many plants in this family are poisonous raw, due to the presence of calcium oxalate crystals. Used in hair care products. Pigs eat the roots, and the leaves are used to heal infected wounds.

ZANTHOXYLUM PIPERITUM PEEL EXTRACT • *Sanshou ekisu.* Sichuan pepper. The leaves have a fresh flavor somewhat in between mint and lime. The peel extract is used as a preservative.

ZEA MAYS • Corn Oil. Abrasive. Bulking ingredient. Antistatic ingredient. May cause acne. *See* Corn Acid.

ZEDOARY • *Curcuma zedoaria.* An Indian plant. The dried rhizomes of this plant are used in perfumes and cosmetics. Has anti-inflammatory and antioxidant properties but can be a skin irritant.

ZEIN • Protein obtained from corn (*see*) used as a film former in hair and skin conditioners.

ZEOLITE • Absorbent and deodorant ingredient. *See* Aluminum Silicate.

ZINC • A white brittle metal insoluble in water and soluble in acids or hot solutions of alkalies. It is a mineral source and added as a nutrient to food. Widely used as an astringent for mouthwashes. Ingestion of the salts can cause nausea and vomiting. It can cause contact dermatitis. GRAS

ZINC ACETATE • Astringent, protectant, and germicide. *See* Acetic Acid and Zinc.

ZINC ASPARTATE • Preservative and skin conditioner. *See* Aspartic Acid and Zinc.

ZINC BORATE • Preservative. *See* Borates and Zinc.

ZINC BOROSILICATE • Thickener. *See* Borates and Zinc.

ZINC CARBONATE • Opacifier and skin protectant. *See* Zinc and Carbonic Acid.

ZINC CHLORIDE • Butter of Zinc. A zinc salt used as an antiseptic and astringent in shaving creams, dentifrices, and mouthwashes. Odorless and water absorbing; also a deodorant and disinfectant. Can cause contact dermatitis and is mildly irritating to the skin. Can be absorbed through the skin.

ZINC CITRATE • *See* Zinc and Citric Acid.

ZINC COCETH SULFATE • Surfactant, cleanser, and emulsifier. *See* Coconut Oil.

ZINC CYSTEINATE • An organic salt that is used as a preservative. *See* Cysteine, L-Form.

ZINC DIBUTYLDITHIOCARBAMATE • Antioxidant and germicide. *See* Zinc and Carbamate.

ZINC DNA • The zinc salt of DNA (*see*). Skin conditioner.

ZINC FORMALDEHYDE SULFOXYLATE • *See* Formaldehyde and Zinc.

ZINC GLUCOHEPTONATE • Skin conditioner. *See* Carboxylic Acid and Heptanoic Acid.

ZINC GLUCONATE • *See* Zinc and Gluconic Acid and Salts.

ZINC GLUTAMATE • Preservative and skin conditioner. The zinc salt of glutamic acid (*see*).

ZINC GLYCYRRHETINATE • Flavoring and skin conditioner. *See* Glycyrrhetinic Acid.

ZINC HYDROLYZED COLLAGEN • The word *animal* was removed from this ingredient's name but not from the ingredient. Hair and skin conditioner. *See* Hydrolyzed Collagen.

ZINC 4-HYDROXYBENZENE SULFONATE • Deodorants, antiperspirants, and astringent lotions. The EU label must read "Avoid contact with eyes." *See* Benzene and Sulfur.

ZINC LACTATE • Zinc salt of lactic acid (*see*). Used as an astringent, a preservative, and a deodorant.

ZINC LAURATE • *See* Zinc and Lauric Acid.

ZINC MYRISTATE • The zinc salt of myristic acid (*see*). Anticaking ingredient and thickener used in makeup and nail polish.

ZINC NEODECANOATE • The zinc salt of neodecanoic acid (*see*). Anticaking ingredient and thickener.

ZINC OLEATE-STEARATE • A white, dry, greasy powder, insoluble in water, soluble in alcohol. An antiseptic and astringent in cosmetic creams. Used medicinally to treat eczema and other skin rashes.

ZINC OXIDE • Flowers of Zinc. Used to impart opacity to face powders, foundation creams, and dusting powders. A creamy white ointment used medicinally as an astringent, antiseptic, and protective in skin diseases. Zinc is believed to encourage healing of skin disorders. It is insoluble in water. In cosmetics, it is also used in baby powder, bleach and freckle creams, depilatories, face packs, antiperspirants, foundation cake makeup, nail whiteners, protective creams, rouge, shaving creams, and white eye shadow. Workers suffer skin eruptions called "zinc pox" under the arm and in the groin when working with zinc. Zinc pox is believed to be caused by the blocking of the hair follicles. Because of its astringent qualities, zinc oxide may be unsuitable for dry skin. Generally harmless, however, when used in cosmetics. Permanently listed as a coloring in 1977. The FDA proposed a ban in 1992 for the use of zinc oxide to treat insect bites and stings because it has not been shown to be safe and effective for stated claims in OTC products, including in astringent (*see*) drug products.

ZINC PALMITATE • Anticaking ingredient and thickener used in blushers. *See* Palmitic Acid.

ZINC PCA • The zinc salt of PCA (*see*). Skin conditioner used in face and neck products.

ZINC PENTADECENE TRICARBOXYLATE • Anticaking ingredient and skin conditioner. *See* Zinc and Carboxylic Acid.

ZINC PEROXIDE • Zinc Superoxide. Disinfectant, antiseptic, deodorant, and astringent applied as a dusting powder alone or with talc or starch. White to yellowish white powder. Liberates hydrogen peroxide, a bleach. It is used in bleach and freckle creams and medicinally as a deodorant for festering wounds and skin diseases.

ZINC PHENOLSULFONATE • A phenol that is used as a topical astringent when mucous membranes are inflamed. Also used in deodorants. Mild redness was observed in twenty-eight-day skin tests. Rats exposed to a spray containing this ingredient for thirteen weeks had depressed brain, liver, testes, and organ/body weight ratios. On the basis of available information, the CIR Expert Panel (*see*) concluded that it is safe as presently used in cosmetic formulations. *See* Phenols.

ZINC PICOLINATE • Oral care ingredient. *See* Pyridine and Zinc.

ZINC PYRIDINETHIONE • Zinc Pyrithione. A bactericide and fungicide used in antidandruff products. Also used as a preservative and hair conditioner. It may be in powders, cleansers such as cold creams, eyeliners, moisturizers, and skin care preparations. A rare sensitizer but may cross-react with ethylene diamine, piperazine, or hydrochloride derivatives (*see all*). Reportedly may be damaging to nerves.

ZINC RESINATE • The zinc salt of rosin (*see*).

ZINC RICINOLEATE • The zinc salt of ricinoleate (*see*). Used as a fungicide, an emulsifier, and a stabilizer.

ZINC ROSINATE • The zinc salt of rosin (*see*).

ZINC SALICYLATE • A zinc salt used as an antiseptic and astringent in dusting powders and antiperspirants. White, odorless needles or crystalline powder. It is omitted from hypoallergenic cosmetics. Causes both skin irritations and allergic reactions.

ZINC SALTS • These salts, if ingested, can produce irritation or corrosion of the gastrointestinal system with pain and vomiting. Used widely in the cosmetic industry in soaps and deodorants, creams, dentifrices, shaving preparations, and astringents. Zinc chloride (*see*) appears to be more corrosive and more toxic than the sulfate. A few grams of the chloride have killed an adult, although recovery has been reported after ingestion of 90 grams. *See* Zinc Sulfate and Zinc Ricinoleate.

ZINC STEARATE • Zinc Soap. A mixture of the zinc salts of stearic and palmitic acids (*see both*). Widely used in cosmetic preparations because it contributes to adhesive properties. Also used as a coloring ingredient. Baby powders of 3 to 5 percent zinc are water repellent and prevent urine irritation. Zinc soap is also used in bath preparations, deodorants, face powders, hair-grooming preparations, hand creams, lotions, and ointments. It is used in tablet manufacture and in pharmaceutical powders and ointments. Inhalation of powder may cause lung problems and produce death in infants from pneumonitis, with lesions resembling those caused by talc but more severe. On the basis of the available information, the CIR Expert Panel (*see*) concluded that it is safe as a cosmetic ingredient.

ZINC SULFATE • White Vitriol. The reaction of sulfuric acid with zinc. Mild crystalline zinc salt used in shaving creams, eye lotions, astringents, styptics, and in gargle spray, skin tonic, and after-shave lotion. Irritating to the skin and mucous membranes. May cause an allergic reaction. Injection under the skin of 2.5 milligrams per kilogram of body weight caused tumors in rabbits.

ZINC SULFIDE • An inorganic zinc salt used as a white pigment and as a fungicide. *See* Zinc Salts.

ZINC SULFOCARBOLATE • *See* Zinc Sulfate.

ZINC THIOSALICYLATE • Antidandruff ingredient and skin conditioner. *See* Zinc Salicylate and Thio-.

ZINC UNDECYLENATE • A zinc salt. Occurs in sweat. Used to combat fungus in cosmetics and on the skin. Made by dissolving zinc oxide (*see*) in diluted undecylenic acid (*see*). Has an odor suggestive of perspiration. *See* Antiperspirant.

ZINC UNDECYLENOYL HYDROLYZED WHEAT PROTEIN • The combination of undecylenic acid and wheat (*see both*) used as an emulsifier and hair and skin conditioner.

ZINC YEAST DERIVATIVE • The derivative of yeast with zinc.

ZINGIBER AROMATICUS EXTRACT • A skin conditioner from the root of ginger (*see*).

ZINGIBER OFFICINALE AND ROOT OIL • Volatile oil obtained from the dried rhizomes of the ginger, Zingiberaceae. It contains L-zingiberene, D-camphene, phellandrene, borneol, eucalyptol (cineol), citral. *See* Ginger.

ZINGIBER ZERUMBET JUICE • Hair conditioner. *See* Ginger.

ZIRCONIUM • Discovered in 1789. Bluish black powder or grayish white flakes used as a bonding ingredient and abrasive; also used in the preparation of dyes. High-quality zirconium is used as a pigment toner and solvent. Zirconium-containing complexes have been used as an ingredient in cosmetics. Mildly acidic, it has been used in body deodorants and antiperspirants. Zirconium hydroxide is used in nail whiteners. Low systemic toxicity, but a disease of the skin has been reported in users of a deodorant containing sodium zirconium lactate. Manufacturers voluntarily removed zirconium from spray antiperspirants in 1976 because the element was found harmful to monkey lungs. The FDA has said that zirconium is safe in formulations other than sprays. Zirconium oxide and zirconium silicate are no longer authorized for use as colorings. Evidence indicates that certain zirconium compounds have caused human skin granulomas and toxic effects in the lungs and other organs of experimental animals. Any aerosol cosmetic product containing zirconium is deemed to be adulterated. On the Canadian Hotlist (*see*). Canada and the United States do not permit it in aerosol dispensers and caution that it should not be applied to irritated or damaged skin. ASEAN has banned it in cosmetics.

ZIRCONIUM CHLOROHYDRATE • *See* Zirconium.

ZIRCONIUM DIOXIDE • An opacifier. *See* Zirconium.

ZIRCONIUM POWDER • Used as an antiperspirant. Not permitted in aerosol cosmetics in Canada. *See* Zirconium.

ZIRCONIUM SILICATE • An abrasive and opacifier. *See* Zirconium and Silicates.

ZIRCONYL CHLORIDE • Zirconium Oxychloride. Used to make other zirconium compounds and to precipitate acid dyes. Acts as a solvent. Mildly acidic. It has been used in deodorants and antiperspirants, but because of skin bumps, particularly under the arm, it has been discontinued. Aluminum zirconyl hydroxychloride is on the Canadian Hotlist (*see*).

ZIRCONYL HYDROXYCHLORIDE • Colorless powder that absorbs moisture. Aluminum zirconyl hydroxychloride is on the Canadian Hotlist (*see*). *See* Zirconium.

ZIZIPHUS • A large genus of American and Asian shrubs. *See* Lotus.

ZOSTERA MARINA • Eel Grass. Skin conditioner. Grasslike flowering plant with dark green, long, narrow, ribbon-shaped leaves. The crisp, sweet rhizomes and leaf bases of eel grass were eaten fresh or dried into cakes for winter food.

ZYMOMONAS FERMENT EXTRACT • A bacterium that ferments xylose (*see*). Used in cosmetics as a skin conditioner and humectant.

APPENDIX

ORGANIZATIONS AND AGENCIES
CONCERNED WITH COSMETIC INGREDIENTS

THE OFFICE OF CONSUMER AFFAIRS, FOOD AND DRUG ADMINISTRATION, HFE-88
Consumer Inquiries: 888-INFO-FDA
5600 Fishers Lane
Rockville, MD 20857
http://www.FDA.gov

Reporting Adverse Events
You can play an important public health role by reporting to the Food and Drug Administration any adverse events or other problems with FDA-regulated products.

Timely reporting allows the agency to take prompt action. Report what happened as soon as possible. Have the following information ready:

- Description of the adverse event
- Name, address, and phone number of the doctor or hospital if emergency treatment was provided
- Name of product and manufacturer
- Any codes or identifying marks on the product label or container
- Name and address of the store where you purchased the product and the date of purchase

To report an emergency that requires immediate action, such as a case of food-borne illness, call the FDA's main emergency number, staffed 24 hours a day: 301-443-1240.

To report a non-emergency adverse event, contact the FDA district office nearest you. Look up the FDA's phone number under the Department of Health and Human Services in the blue U.S. government section of the telephone directory. Or check the phone numbers listed by state at: www.fda.gov/opacom/backgrounders/com-plain.html.

USDA Organic Standards, National Organic Program
202-720-3252
USDA-AMS-TM-NOP, Room 4008 S. Bldg., Ag Stop 0268
1400 Independence Ave SW
Washington, DC 20250
http://www.ams.usda.gov/nop

The FDA's Cosmetics division estimates it may receive only a small percentage of cosmetic complaints reported by consumers. Complaints, the FDA says, are more often filed with poison control centers, state and local agencies, or with the product manufacturer and/or distributor, who are not required to submit their complaint files to the FDA. If you find a website you think is illegally selling cosmetics over the Web, you may report it to the FDA using a form on its website.

UNITED STATES DEPARTMENT OF AGRICULTURE (USDA)

The USDA's Food, Nutrition, and Consumer Services works to harness the Nation's agricultural abundance to end hunger and improve health in the United States. Its agencies administer federal domestic nutrition assistance programs and the Center for Nutrition Policy and Promotion, which links scientific research to the nutrition needs of consumers through science-based dietary guidance, nutrition policy coordination, and nutrition education. It plays a key role in the President's Council on Food Safety and has been instrumental in coordinating a national food safety strategic plan among various partner agencies including the Department of Health and Human Services and the Environmental Protection Agency.

U.S. Department of Agriculture
1400 Independence Ave SW
Washington, DC 20250
http://www.usda.gov

USDA ORGANIC STANDARDS, NATIONAL ORGANIC PROGRAM

Room 4008 S. Bldg., Ag Stop 0268
1400 Independence Ave SW
Washington, DC 20250
202-720-3252
http://www.ams.usda.gov/nop

INTEGRATED RISK INFORMATION SYSTEM (IRIS)

Prepared and maintained by the U.S. Environmental Protection Agency (U.S. EPA)

Health assessment information on a chemical substance is included in IRIS only after a comprehensive review of chronic toxicity data by U.S. EPA health scientists from several Program Offices and the Office of Research and Development. For technical questions about the scientific information content in IRIS contact:

U.S. EPA Risk Information Hotline 1-301-345-2870
FAX: 1-301-345-2876
e-mail: Hotline.IRIS@epamail.epa.gov
http://www.epa.gov/iris/intro.htm

By regular mail:
IRIS
c/o ASRC
6301 Ivy Lane, Suite 300
Greenbelt, MD 20770

NATIONAL TOXICOLOGY PROGRAM

The National Toxicology Program (NTP), within the U.S. Department of Health and Human Services, is an interagency program headquartered at the National Institutes of Health's National Institute of Environmental Health Services (NIEHS) located in Research Triangle Park, NC.

Please send queries, comments, and suggestions to: ntpwm@niehs.nih.gov.

USE YOUR VOTER POWER

If you want regulations strengthened and agencies such as the FDA and USDA well funded so they can more adequately protect our food supply, contact your senators and representatives. The phone number for the House and Senate office buildings is 202-224-3121.

If you want any federal agency, including the White House, the Federal Information Center (FIC) is 800-688-9889. It can be frustrating trying to report something to agencies, especially if they have a "push this number" type of system. Eventually, with persistence, you will be able to not only make yourself feel better; you will be protecting the rest of us from a similar adverse experience.

Other organizations interested in cosmetics:

AMERICAN ACADEMY OF ALLERGY, ASTHMA AND IMMUNOLOGY (AAAAI)

611 East Wells Street
Milwaukee, WI 53202
AAAAI Physician Referral and
Information Line
1-800-822-2762
AAAAI website
www.aaaai.org

ALLERGY AND ASTHMA NETWORK: MOTHERS OF ASTHMATICS

2751 Prosperity Ave, Suite 150
Fairfax, VA 22031
(800) 878-4403
(703) 641-9595
http://www.aanma.org

ASEAN

Association of Southeast Asian Nations. A regional community of ten states with the aim of accelerating economic growth and social progress and promoting peace and security.
http://aseancosmetics.org.

ASTHMA AND ALLERGY FOUNDATION OF AMERICA

1125 15th St. NW, Suite 502
Washington, DC 20036
(800) 7-ASTHMA
(202) 466-7643
http://www.aafa.org

THE BREAST CANCER FUND

In response to the public health crisis of breast cancer, the Breast Cancer Fund identifies—and advocates for elimination of—the environmental and other preventable

causes of the disease. Along with other founding members of the Campaign for Safe Cosmetics, the Breast Cancer Fund helps convince leading salon nail polish manufacturer OPI to remove the most toxic ingredients from its nail polishes and treatments.
1388 Sutter St., Suite 400
San Francisco, CA 94109-5400
(415) 346-8223 or toll-free (866) 760-8223
info@breastcancerfund.org

THE CAMPAIGN FOR SAFE COSMETICS
A national coalition of nonprofit health and environmental organizations. Our collective goal is to protect the health of consumers and workers by requiring the personal care products industry to phase out the use of chemicals linked to cancer, birth defects and other serious health concerns, and replace them with safer alternatives. The Campaign for Safe Cosmetics is working with endorsing organizations, responsible businesses and thousands of citizen activists to shift the cosmetics market toward safer products and to advocate for smarter laws that protect our health from toxic chemicals and encourage innovation of safer alternatives.

Campaign for Safe Cosmetics
(510) 848-5701
info@safecosmetics.org

COSMETIC INGREDIENT REVIEW (CIR)
1101 17th St. NW, Suite 412
Washington, DC 20036-4702
Phone: 202-331-0651 Fax: 202-331-0088
e-mail: cirinfo@cir-safety.org

COSMETICSINFO.ORG
An information website that describes ingredients most commonly used in cosmetics and personal care products in the United States. The Personal Care Products Council and its member companies sponsor the site to provide consumers with easily accessible information.

www.cosmeticsinfo.org

CSPI CENTER FOR SCIENCE IN THE PUBLIC INTEREST
Publishes *Nutrition Action Healthletter*.
Often petitions the FDA about actual and potential problems with food additives.
1875 Connecticut Ave NW, Suite 300
Washington, DC 20009-5728
http://www.cspinet.org/

EUROPEAN UNION
Delegation of the European Commission to the United States
2300 M Street NW, Washington, DC 20037
Phone: (202) 862-9500 Fax: (202) 429-1766
http://www.eurunion.org/legislat/hom.htm

ENVIRONMENTAL WORKING GROUP (EWG)
Its mission is to use the power for public information to protect public health and the environment. Founded in 1993 by Ken Cook and Richard Wiles, the non-profit organization specializes in providing useful resources such as Skin Deep (*see below*) and the Shopper's Guide to Pesticides in Produce to consumers while simultaneously pushing for national policy change.

1436 U St. NW, Suite 100
Washington, DC 2009
202-667-6982
http://www/ewg/prg/

HEALTH CANADA COSMETIC PROGRAM
Consumer Product Safety Bureau
Product Safety Programme
Health Canada
MacDonald Building, 4th Floor,
123 Slater Street
Address Locator: 3504D
Ottawa, Ontario
K1A 0K9
Phone: (613) 957-4467
Fax: (613) 952-3039
http://www.hc-sc.gc.ca/hecs-sesc/cosmetics/index.htmHeadquarters
e-mail: CPS-SPC@hc-sc.gc.ca

THE INTERNATIONAL FRAGRANCE ASSOCIATION (IFRA)
Founded in 1973 in Geneva to represent the fragrance creation houses and the manufacturers of fragrance ingredients. Its main purpose is to promote the safe enjoyment of fragrances worldwide. IFRA represents the fragrance industry regional and national associations worldwide. IFRA is the reflection of the industry's choice to regulate itself, and its activities result in a Code of Practice and Safety Standards, which members must adhere to, in order to achieve the objective of protecting consumers' health and our environment. They emphasize research and development, scientific findings, health and safety concerns as well as environmental protection. Together with the industry's scientific arm the Research Institute for Fragrance Materials (RIFM), IFRA ensures that the establishment of usage Standards for fragrance materials are put into practice according to available scientific recommendations, and that all member companies comply with those Standards. Self-regulation enables the IFRA Standards to be adopted very rapidly by fragrance houses worldwide and by the industry as a whole.

1210 Brussels
Belgium
Phone: +32-2 214 20 60
Fax: +32-2 214 20 69

Chemin de la Parfumerie 5
CH-1214 Vernier, Geneva
Switzerland
Phone: +41-22 431 82 50
Fax: +41-22 431 88 06
http://www.ifraorg.org

PAULA BEGOUN

The author and publisher of seven books on the beauty industry including *Don't Go to the Cosmetics Counter Without Me,* 7th edition. She calls herself the cosmetics cop and now sells her own products on her website.

http://www.cosmeticscop.com

SKIN DEEP

This safety guide to cosmetics and personal care products is the result of efforts by researchers at the Environmental Working Group (*see above*). Skin Deep pairs ingredients in more than forty thousand products against fifty definitive toxicity and regulatory databases, making it one of the largest integrated data resources of its kind.

http://www.skindeep.org

WOMEN'S VOICES FOR THE EARTH CAMPAIGN FOR SAFE COSMETICS

The Campaign for Safe Cosmetics is a coalition working to protect your health by calling for the elimination of chemicals used in the cosmetics industry linked to cancer, birth defects, and other health problems.

Missoula Office—114 W. Pine St., Missoula, MT 59802
Phone: (406) 543-3747 Fax: (406) 543-2557
wve@womenandenvironment.org

WORLD HEALTH ORGANIZATION (WHO)

The directing and coordinating authority for health within the United Nations system.

Avenue Appia 20
1211 Geneva 27
Switzerland
Phone: +41-22 791 21 11
Fax: +41-22 791 31 11

SELECTED REFERENCES

Antczak, Gina and Dr. Steven. *Cosmetics Unmasked.* Hammersmith, London: Thornsons/HarperCollins, 2001.

Castro, Miranda. *The Complete Homeopathy Handbook.* New York: St. Martin's Press, 1990.

CIR (Cosmetic Ingredient Review) Compendium. Washington, DC, 1998, 2001.

Color Additive Status List. Food and Drug Administration, 1992, 2002.

Done, Alan. "Toxic Reactions to Common Household Products." Paper read at the Symposium on Adverse Reactions sponsored by the Drug Service Center for Disease Control, December 1976, San Francisco.

Ellenhorn, Matthew J., and Donald G. Barceloux. *Medical Toxicology: Diagnosis and Treatment of Human Poisoning.* New York: Elsevier Science Publishing Company, 1988.

European Parliament and the Council of European Union, "Directive 2003/15/EC of the European Parliament and of the Council, February 27, 2003, Amending Council Directive 76/768/EEC on the approximation of the laws of the Member States relating to cosmetic products."

FDA's *Cosmetics Handbook.* Washington, DC: U.S. HHS, October 15, 1992.

FDA Cosmetic Labeling, March 26, 2003.

FDA Color Additives, Status List, 2003.

FDA IOM, *Investigations Operations Manual,* 2003.

FDA, Public Meeting on the Challenge of Labeling Food Allergens, August 13, 2001, Washington, DC.

Fisher, Alexander A. *Contact Dermatitis* (3rd ed). Philadelphia: Lea & Febiger, 1986.

GCI. *Global Cosmetic Industry Who's Who, 2002 Annual Directory,* New York.

GCI. *Global Cosmetic Industry, Annual Guide to Personal Care,* July 2002.

Gordon, Lesley. *A Country Herbal.* New York: Mayflower Books, 1980.

Gosselin, Robert, Robert Smith, and Harold Hodge, with Jeannette Braddock. *Clinical Toxicology of Commercial Products.* Baltimore: Williams & Wilkins, 1984.

Greenberg, Leon A., and David Lester. *The Handbook of Cosmetic Materials.* New York: Interscience Publishers, 1954.

Hawley's Condensed Chemical Dictionary (15th ed.), revised by Richard J. Lewis, Sr. New York: Wiley, 2007.

Hoffman, David. *The New Holistic Herbal.* Rockport, MA: Element, Inc., 1991.

"Inspection of Cosmetics." Section 704 of The Food, Drug and Cosmetic Act, February 25, 2003, Washington, DC.

"Intercenter Agreement Between the Center for Drug Evaluation and Research and the Center for Food Safety and Applied Nutrition to Assist FDA in Implementing the Drug and Cosmetic Provision of the Federal Food, Drug and Cosmetic Act for Products that Purport to Be Cosmetics But Meet the Statutory Definition of a Drug," June 2003, Washington, DC.

"International Business Communications Second Annual International Industry Conference: Drug Discovery and Development Approaches to Cosmeceuticals," Short Hills, NJ, February 12–13, 1998.

"Inventory of Ingredients Used in Cosmetic Products." INCI, European Commission, September 8, 2003.

Investigation Operations Manual. Washington, DC: Food and Drug Administration, 1992.

Juo Pei-Shaw, Ph.D. *Concise Dictionary of Biomedicine and Molecular Biology.* Boca Raton, FL: CRC Press, 1995.

Kahn, Julius. "Hypo-Allergenic Cosmetics." *NARD Journal,* February 20, 1967.

Kamm, Minnie Watson. *Old-Time Herbs for Northern Gardens.* Boston: Little, Brown, 1938.

Kibbe, Constance V. *Standard Textbook of Cosmetology* (rev. ed.). Bronx, NY: Milady Publishing, 1981.

Lewis, Richard Sr. *Hazardous Chemicals Desk Reference* (5th ed.). New York: Wiley-Interscience, 2002.

Loprieno, N. *Guidelines for Safety Evaluation of Cosmetics Ingredients Food and Chemical Toxicology.* The Scientific Committee on Cosmetology of the Commission of The European Communities Department of Environmental Sciences. London: Pergamon Press Ltd., 1995.

March, Cyril, and Alexander Fisher. *Cutaneous Reactions to Cosmetics.* Chicago: American Medical Association, 1965.

Martin, Eric W., et al. *Hazards of Medications.* Philadelphia: J. B. Lippincott, 1971.

The Merck Index (8th, 9th, 10th, and 13th eds.). Rahway, NJ: Merck, Sharp and Dohme Research Laboratories, 1968, 1976, 1983, 2001.

The Merck Index (14th ed.). Edited by Maryadele J. O'Neil. Whitehouse Station, NJ: Merck Research Laboratories, 2006.

The Merck Manual (16th ed.). Edited by Robert Berkow. Rahway, NJ: Merck, Sharp and Dohme Research Laboratories, 1992.

Miall, L. Mackenzie, and D. W. A. Sharp. *A New Dictionary of Chemistry* (4th ed.). New York: John Wiley & Sons, 1968.

Microbiology and Cosmetic Section, Cosmetics Programme, Health Canada, Cosmetic Notification System Hot List, November 2003.

Mindell, Earl R. *Earl Mindell's Herb Bible.* New York: Fireside Books, 1992.

Mowrey, Daniel B. *The Scientific Validation of Herbal Medicine.* New Canaan, CT: Keats Publishing, 1986.

Physicians' Desk Reference. Oradell, NJ: Medical Economics, 1988.

PIER (Pacific Island Ecosystem at Risk Project), March 1, 2003. http://www.hear.org/pier.

Principles of Cosmetics for Dermatologists. St. Louis: Mosby, 1982.

"Prospective Study of Cosmetic Reactions, 1977–1980." North American Contact Dermatitis Group. *Journal of the American Academy of Dermatology* 6, no. 5 (May 1982).

Rosen, Meyer (ed.). *Delivery System Handbook for Personal Care and Cosmetic Products.* Norwich, NY: William Andrew, Inc., 2005.

Scheman, Andrew, and David Severson. *Cosmetics Buying Guide.* Yonkers, NY: Consumer Reports Books, 1993.

Steadman's Medical Dictionary (27th ed.). Baltimore: Williams & Wilkins, 1999.

Stehlin, Dori. "Cosmetic Safety More Complex Than at First Blush." *FDA Consumer,* December 1992.

Suspected Carcinogens: A Subfile of the NIOSH Toxic Substance List. Rockville, MD: Tracor Jitco, Inc., U.S. Department of Health, Education and Welfare, 1975.

Suspected Carcinogens: A Subfile of the Registry of Toxic Effects of Chemical Substances. Cincinnati: U.S. Department of Health, Education and Welfare, Public Health Services, Centers for Disease Control, 1976.

Tenth Report on Carcinogens, U.S. Dept. of Health and Human Services, Public Service, National Toxicology Program, Washington, DC, December 2002.

Tierra, Michael. *The Way of Herbs.* New York: Pocket Books, 1990.

Toxicity Testing: Strategies to Determine Needs and Priorities. Washington, DC: National Research Council, National Academy Press, 1984.

Webster's Third New International Dictionary. Chicago: Merriman, 1966.

Weiner, Michael. *Weiner's Herbal 1990 Edition.* Mill Valley, CA: Quantum Books, 1990.

Wenniger, John A., and G. N. McEwen Jr. *CTFA Cosmetic Ingredient Dictionary and Handbook* (7th ed.). Washington, DC: The Cosmetic, Toiletry, and Fragrance Association, 1997.

White, John Henry. *A Reference Book of Chemistry* (3rd ed.). New York: Philosophical Library, 1965.

Winter, Ruth. *Cancer-Causing Ingredients: A Preventive Guide.* New York: Crown, 1979.

———. *A Consumer's Dictionary of Food Additives.* New York: Crown, 2009.

———. *A Consumer's Dictionary of Household, Yard, and Office Chemicals.* New York: Crown, 1992.

———. *A Consumer's Dictionary of Medicines: Prescription, Nonprescription, and Herbal.* New York: Crown, 1994.

———. *A Consumer's Guide to Medicines in Food.* New York: Crown, 1995.

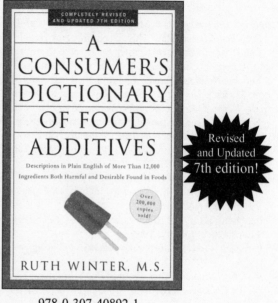